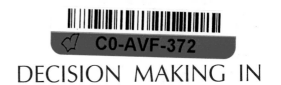

DECISION MAKING IN
Medicine

Harry L. Greene, M.D.

Chief, General Medicine
Associate Chairman of Medicine
Director, Roy P. Drachman Center for Disease
Prevention and Health Promotion
The University of Arizona Health Sciences Center
Tucson, Arizona

William P. Johnson, M.D.

Clinical Assistant Professor of Medicine
The University of Arizona Health Sciences Center
Tucson, Arizona

Michael J. Maricic, M.D.

Clinical Assistant Professor of Medicine
Program Director, Residency Internal Medicine
The University of Arizona Health Sciences Center
Tucson, Arizona

B.C. Decker
An Imprint of Mosby–Year Book, Inc.

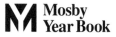 **Mosby Year Book**
Dedicated to Publishing Excellence

Executive Editor: Susan M. Gay
Senior Managing Editor: Lynne Gery
Project Supervisor: Allan S. Kleinberg

Printed in the United States of America

Mosby–Year Book, Inc.
11830 Westline Industrial Drive
St. Louis, Missouri 63146

NOTICE: The authors and publisher have made every effort to ensure that the patient care recommended herein, including choice of drugs and drug dosages, is in accord with the accepted standard and practice at the time of publication. However, since research and regulation constantly change clinical standards, the reader is urged to check the product information sheet included in the package of each drug, which includes recommended doses, warnings, and contraindications. This is particularly important with new or infrequently used drugs.

Library of Congress Cataloging in Publication Data

Decision making in medicine / [edited by] Harry L. Greene, William P.
Johnson, Michael J. Maricic.
        p.   cm. — (Clinical decision making series.)
    Includes bibliographical references and index.
    ISBN 1-55664-226-1
    1. Medicine—Decision making.   I. Greene, Harry L. (Harry
Lemoine), 1942-   . II. Johnson, William P., 1945-   .
III. Maricic, Michael J.   IV. Series
    [DNLM: 1. Decision Making.   2. Diagnosis.   3. Judgment.   WB 141
D294]
R723.5.D42   1993
616—dc20
DNLM/DLC
for Library of Congress   92-49391
                                                              CIP

93 94 95 96 CL/MY 9 8 7 6 5 4 3 2

SECTION EDITORS

CONTRIBUTORS

RODNEY D. ADAM, M.D.
Assistant Professor of Medicine and Microbiology/ Immunology, University of Arizona College of Medicine; and Infectious Disease Physician, The University of Arizona Health Sciences Center, Tucson, Arizona

GEOFFREY L. AHERN, M.D., Ph.D.
Assistant Professor of Neurology and Psychology, The University of Arizona Health Sciences Center; Medical Director, Behavioral Neurology Unit, Department of Neurology, The University of Arizona Health Sciences Center, Tucson, Arizona

FREDERICK R. AHMANN, M.D.
Associate Professor of Medicine, The University of Arizona Health Sciences Center; Chief, Section of Hematology/ Oncology, Veterans Administration Medical Center, Tucson, Arizona

ANWAR AL-HAIDARY, M.B., M.R.C.P., M.Sc.
Clinical Assistant Professor of Medicine, The University of Arizona Health Sciences Center; Staff Physician, Veterans Administration Medical Center, Tucson, Arizona

NEIL M. AMPEL, M.D.
Associate Professor of Medicine, The University of Arizona Health Sciences Center; Staff Physician, Veterans Administration Medical Center, Tucson, Arizona

CATHERINE AZAR, M.D.
Clinical Assistant Professor, Arizona Cancer Center, The University of Arizona Health Sciences Center, Tucson, Arizona

COLIN R. BAMFORD, M.D.
Associate Professor and Associate Head, Department of Neurology, The University of Arizona Health Sciences Center; Director of Clinical Neurophysiology, The University of Arizona Health Sciences Center, Tucson, Arizona

IRIS R. BELL, Ph.D., M.D.
Assistant Professor of Psychiatry, The University of Arizona Health Sciences Center; Director, Program in Geriatric Psychiatry, The University of Arizona Health Sciences Center, Tucson, Arizona

KARIL BELLAH, M.D.
Cardiology Fellow, The University of Arizona Health Sciences Center, Tucson, Arizona

JAMES B. BENJAMIN, M.D.
Associate Professor, Section of Orthopedic Surgery, The University of Arizona Health Sciences Center, Tucson, Arizona

ANDREA BINZER, M.D.
Resident Physician, Department of Medicine, The University of Arizona Health Sciences Center, Tucson, Arizona

JOHN W. BLOOM, M.D.
Associate Professor of Medicine, The University of Arizona Health Sciences Center, Tucson, Arizona

BARBARA BODE, M.D.
Fellow, Section of Rheumatology, The University of Arizona Health Sciences Center, Tucson, Arizona

MARY BORDENAVE, Pharm.D., M.T. (ASCP)
Post Doctoral Fellow, College of Pharmacy, University Medical Center, The University of Arizona Health Sciences Center, Tucson, Arizona

THOMAS W. BOYDEN, M.D.
Associate Professor, University of Arizona College of Medicine; Chief of Endocrinology, Veterans Administration Medical Center, Tucson, Arizona

RIEMKE BRAKEMA, M.D.
Clinical Assistant Professor, The University of Arizona Health Sciences Center, Tucson, Arizona

SAMUEL M. BUTMAN, M.D.
Associate Professor of Medicine, The University of Arizona Health Sciences Center; Director, Cardiac Catheterization Laboratory, University Medical Center, Tucson, Arizona

ANTONIO C. BUZAID, M.D.
Assistant Professor of Medicine, Section of Medical Oncology, Director of Melanoma Unit, and Co-director of Lung Cancer Unit, Yale University School of Medicine, New Haven, Connecticut

JESSICA BYRON, M.D.
Obstetrics and Gynecology, Ironwood Medical Associates, Tucson, Arizona

ANTHONY CAMILLI, M.D.
Clinical Assistant Professor, Division of Respiratory Sciences, The University of Arizona Health Sciences Center, Tucson, Arizona

J. KEVIN CARMICHAEL, M.D., M.S.
Clinical Assistant Professor, Internal Medicine, Section of Infectious Disease and Family and Community Medicine, The University of Arizona Health Sciences Center, Tucson, Arizona

ANTHONY C. CARUSO, M.D.
Assistant Professor of Medicine, The University of Arizona Health Sciences Center; Director, Cardiac Electrophysiology Laboratory, University Medical Center, Tucson, Arizona

ELLEN M. CHASE, B.S.
Assistant Director for Clinical Research, Administration and Outreach, and Director, Clinical Trials Office, Arizona Cancer Center, The University of Arizona Health Sciences Center, Tucson, Arizona

JUNE CLEMENTS, M.D.

Fellow in Transfusion Medicine, Department of Pathology, The University of Arizona Health Sciences Center, Tucson, Arizona

NEIL C. CLEMENTS, Jr., M.D.

Clinical Assistant Professor, Pulmonary Section, Veterans Administration Medical Center, and The University of Arizona Health Sciences Center, Tucson, Arizona

DAVID M. CLIVE, M.D.

Associate Professor of Medicine, Division of Renal Medicine, University of Massachusetts Medical School; Director of Medical Residency Training, University of Massachusetts Medical Center, Worcester, Massachusetts

PONJOLA CONEY, M.D.

Division Director, Reproductive Endocrinology, The University of Arizona Health Sciences Center, Tucson, Arizona

NANCY A. CUROSH, M.D.

Endocrinologist, Providence Medical Center, Portland, Oregon

RICHARD C. DART, M.D., Ph.D.

Director, Rocky Mountain Poison and Drug Center, Denver, Colorado

PAMELA J. DAVIS, M.D.

Clinical Assistant Professor, The University of Arizona Health Sciences Center, Tucson, Arizona

MARK J. DiNUBILE, M.D.

Associate Professor of Medicine, University of Medicine and Dentistry of New Jersey/Robert Wood Johnson Medical School at Camden; Staff, Department of Medicine, Division of Infectious Diseases, Cooper Hospital/University Medical Center, Camden, New Jersey

HILLARY DON, M.D.

Professor of Anesthesiology, University of California, San Francisco, School of Medicine; Staff Anesthesiologist, Veterans Administration Medical Center, San Francisco, California

DEBORAH DOUD, M.D.

Fellow, Section of Rheumatology, The University of Arizona Health Sciences Center, Tucson, Arizona

GEORGE W. DRACH, M.D.

Professor of Surgery and Chief, Division of Urology, The University of Arizona Health Sciences Center, Tucson, Arizona

GREGORY L. EASTWOOD, M.D.

Professor of Medicine and Dean, Medical College of Georgia School of Medicine, Augusta, Georgia

BRIAN L. ERSTAD, Pharm.D.

Assistant Professor, College of Pharmacy, The University of Arizona Health Sciences Center; Clinical Pharmacist, University Medical Center, Tucson, Arizona

GEORGE WILLIAM ESTES, M.D.

Fellow, Infectious Diseases, The University of Arizona Health Sciences Center, Tucson, Arizona

LAURIE L. FAJARDO, M.D.

Assistant Professor of Radiology, The University of Arizona Health Sciences Center; Director, Tucson Breast Center, and Section Head, Mammography and Breast Imaging, The University of Arizona Health Sciences Center, Tucson, Arizona

WILLIAM M. FEINBERG, M.D.

Associate Professor of Neurology, University of Arizona College of Medicine; Neurologist, The University of Arizona Health Sciences Center, Tucson, Arizona

M. BRIAN FENNERTY, M.D., F.A.C.P., F.A.C.G.

Assistant Professor of Medicine, The University of Arizona Health Sciences Center; Director, Gastroenterology Endoscopy Unit, University Medical Center, Tucson, Arizona

PAUL E. FENSTER, M.D.

Associate Professor of Medicine, The University of Arizona Health Sciences Center; Director, Cardiovascular Intensive Care, University Medical Center, Tucson, Arizona

DOUGLAS FISH, M.D.

Clinical Assistant, University of Tennessee Medical Center, Knoxville, Tennessee

DAVID FRAMM, M.D.

Fellow, Section of Cardiology, The University of Arizona Health Sciences Center, Tucson, Arizona

COLLIN FREEMAN, Pharm.D.

Infectious Disease Fellow, Hartford Hospital, Hartford, Connecticut

ERIC P. GALL

Professor and Chief, Section of Rheumatology, Department of Medicine, The University of Arizona Health Sciences Center, Tucson, Arizona

JAMES M. GALLOWAY, M.D.

Fellow, Section of Cardiology, The University of Arizona Health Sciences Center, Tucson, Arizona

LAWRENCE A. GARCIA, M.D.

Junior Assistant Resident, Parkland Memorial Hospital, University of Texas Southwestern Medical Center at Dallas, Dallas, Texas

ALAN J. GELENBERG, M.D.

Professor and Head, Department of Psychiatry, The University of Arizona Health Sciences Center, Tucson, Arizona

DAVID W. GIBSON, M.D.

Resident Physician, Vanderbilt University Medical Center, Nashville, Tennessee

STEPHEN J. GLUCKMAN, M.D.

Professor of Clinical Medicine, Head, Division of General Internal Medicine, and Associate Chief, Department of Medicine, University of Medicine and Dentistry of New Jersey/Robert Wood Johnson Medical School, Camden, New Jersey

MARK C. GOLDBERG, M.D.

Fellow, Section of Cardiology, The University of Arizona Health Sciences Center, Tucson, Arizona

GUILLERMO GONZALEZ-OSETE, M.D.

Clinical Assistant Professor of Medicine, Section of Hematology/Oncology, The University of Arizona Health Sciences Center, Tucson, Arizona

R. SCOTT GORMAN, M.D.

Clinical Associate Professor of Internal Medicine, The University of Arizona Health Sciences Center; Member, Section of General Medicine, The University of Arizona Health Sciences Center, Tucson, Arizona

HARRY L. GREENE, M.D.

Associate Professor and Associate Chairman of Medicine, Chief, General Medicine, The University of Arizona Health Sciences Center, Tucson, Arizona

IRWIN E. HARRIS, M.D.

Assistant Professor of Surgery, The University of Arizona Health Sciences Center; Physician and Orthopedic Surgeon, University Medical Center, Tucson, Arizona

STEVEN T. HARRIS, M.D.

Associate Clinical Professor of Medicine and Radiology, University of California, San Francisco, School of Medicine; Attending Physician, University of California Hospitals and Clinics, San Francisco, California

ALLAN R. HARTSOUGH, M.D.

Clinical Assistant Professor of Obstetrics and Gynecology, The University of Arizona Health Sciences Center, Tucson, Arizona

LEE J. HIXSON, M.D.

Clinical Assistant Professor of Medicine, The University of Arizona Health Sciences Center, Tucson, Arizona

RICHARD F. HOFFMAN, M.D.

Clinical Assistant Professor of Medicine, The University of Arizona Health Sciences Center, Tucson, Arizona

DOUGLAS HUESTIS, M.D.

Professor of Pathology, The University of Arizona Health Sciences Center, Tucson, Arizona

SIMONE A. INCE, M.D.

Resident and House Officer, University of Washington School of Medicine, Seattle, Washington

PHILIP E. JAFFE, M.D.

Clinical Assistant Professor of Medicine, The University of Arizona Health Sciences Center, Tucson, Arizona

WILLIAM P. JOHNSON, M.D.

Clinical Assistant Professor of Medicine, The University of Arizona Health Sciences Center, Tucson, Arizona

MERRILL C. KANTER, M.D.

Assistant Professor and Neurologist, Department of Medicine, University of Texas Health Science Center at San Antonio, San Antonio, Texas

MICHAEL D. KATZ, Pharm.D.

Clinical Associate Professor, College of Pharmacy, The University of Arizona Health Sciences Center; Clinical Pharmacist, University Medical Center, Tucson, Arizona

LISA KAUFMANN, M.D.

Clinical Assistant Professor of Medicine, The University of Arizona Health Sciences Center, Tucson, Arizona

SAMUEL M. KEIM, M.D.

Clinical Assistant Professor of Emergency Medicine, and Residency Director, Emergency Medicine Training Program, The University of Arizona Health Sciences Center, Tucson, Arizona

KARL B. KERN, M.D.

Associate Professor of Medicine, The University of Arizona Health Sciences Center; Associate Director, Cardiac Catheterization Laboratory, University Medical Center, Tucson, Arizona

MYRA M. KERSTITCH, M.D.

Clinical Assistant Professor, The University of Arizona Health Sciences Center, Tucson, Arizona

ROBERT F. KLEIN, M.D.

Associate Professor of Medicine, Division of Endocrinology, Diabetes and Clinical Nutrition, Oregon Health Sciences University School of Medicine; Staff Physician, Veterans Administration Medical Center, Portland, Oregon

STEVEN R. KNOPER, M.D.

Research Assistant Professor, Department of Internal Medicine, Section of Pulmonary and Critical Care Medicine, The University of Arizona Health Sciences Center, Tucson, Arizona

MARCIA KO, M.D.

Clinical Assistant Professor, Department of Internal Medicine, The University of Arizona Health Sciences Center, Tucson, Arizona

WILLIAM H. KREISLE, M.D.

Assistant Clinical Lecturer, The University of Arizona Health Sciences Center, Tucson; Staff, Department of Medicine, Maricopa Medical Center, Phoenix, Arizona

JOHN LACE, M.D., M.S.

Attending Physician, The Everett Clinic, Everett General Hospital, and Providence Hospital, Everett, Washington

NORMAN LEVINE, M.D.

Professor of Medicine and Chief of Dermatology, The University of Arizona Health Sciences Center, Tucson, Arizona

DOUGLAS LINDSEY, M.D., Dr.P.H.

Professor of Surgery Emeritus, The University of Arizona Health Sciences Center; Attending Physician, Emergency Department, University Medical Center, Tucson, Arizona

ROBERT J. LIPSY, Pharm.D.

Adjunct Assistant Professor and Assistant Director, Drug Information, Pharmacy Services, The University of Arizona Health Sciences Center, Tucson, Arizona

FARRELL LLOYD, M.D.

Clinical Assistant, Department of Medicine, The University of Arizona Health Sciences Center, Tucson, Arizona

JOY L. LOGAN, M.D.

Associate Professor of Medicine, The University of Arizona Health Sciences Center; Staff Physician, Veterans Administration Medical Center, Tucson, Arizona

ANA MARÍA LÓPEZ, M.D.

Clinical Assistant, The University of Arizona Health Sciences Center, Tucson, Arizona

CYNTHIA MADDEN, M.D.

Senior Resident, Section of Emergency Medicine, The University of Arizona Health Sciences Center, Tucson, Arizona

RICHARD M. MANDEL, M.D.

Clinical Assistant Professor of Medicine, The University of Arizona Health Sciences Center; Infectious Disease Physician, University Medical Center, Tucson, Arizona

MICHAEL J. MARICIC, M.D.

Clinical Assistant Professor of Medicine, University of Arizona College of Medicine; Program Director, Residency Internal Medicine, The University of Arizona Health Sciences Center, Tucson, Arizona

PATRICIA MAYER, M.D.

Fellow, Section of Rheumatology, The University of Arizona Health Sciences Center, Tucson, Arizona

C. J. McCURDY, M.D.

Clinical Professor, The University of Arizona Health Sciences Center, Tucson, Arizona

ANGELA MURPHY McGHEE, M.D.

Staff Dermatologist, Thomas-Davis Medical Centers, Tucson, Arizona

JAMES L. McGUIRE, M.D.

Associate Professor of Medicine, Stanford University School of Medicine, Stanford; Director, Rheumatology Clinic, and Fellowship Chief, Rheumatology Section, Palo Alto Veterans Affairs Medical Center, Palo Alto, California

KENNETH E. McINTYRE, Jr., M.D.

Associate Professor of Surgery, Section of Vascular Surgery, University of Arizona College of Medicine; Chief, Vascular Surgery Service, Veterans Administration Medical Center, Tucson, Arizona

SUSAN McKENZIE, R.N., M.S.

Cardiac Rehabilitation Staff, The University of Arizona Health Sciences Center, Tucson, Arizona

HUGH S. MILLER, M.D.

Clinical Assistant Professor of Obstetrics and Gynecology, The University of Arizona Health Sciences Center, Tucson, Arizona

JEFFREY I. MILLER, M.D.

Resident in Urology, The University of Arizona Health Sciences Center, Tucson, Arizona

JOHN MISIASZEK, M.D.

Clinical Associate Professor of Psychiatry, The University of Arizona Health Sciences Center; Medical Director, Psychiatry Inpatient Unit, University Medical Center, Tucson, Arizona

MANUEL MODIANO, M.D.

Assistant Professor of Medicine, Hematology/Oncology, and Director, Minority Cancer Control, Arizona Cancer Center, The University of Arizona Health Sciences Center, Tucson, Arizona

ERWIN B. MONTGOMERY, Jr., M.D.

Associate Professor of Neurology, The University of Arizona Health Sciences Center; Attending Staff Neurologist, The University of Arizona Health Sciences Center, Tucson, Arizona

SCOTT W. NOWLIN, M.D.

Clinical Instructor, The University of Arizona Health Sciences Center; General Internist, University Medical Center, Tucson, Arizona

EUGENIE A. M. T. OBBENS, M.D., Ph.D.

Associate Professor of Neurology, The University of Arizona Health Sciences Center, Tucson, Arizona

CYNTHIA A. O'NEIL, M.D.

Clinical Assistant and Chief Resident, Section of Dermatology, Department of Medicine, The University of Arizona Health Sciences Center, Tucson, Arizona

K. J. OOMMEN, M.D.

Associate Clinical Professor, Department of Neurology, The University of Arizona Health Sciences Center; Medical Director, Arizona Comprehensive Epilepsy Program, Tucson, Arizona

PHILIP R. ORLANDER, M.D.

Associate Professor and Acting Director, Division of Endocrinology, University of Texas Medical School at Houston; Acting Chief, Endocrinology, Hermann Hospital, Houston, Texas

STEVEN PALLEY, M.D.

Clinical Assistant Professor of Medicine, The University of Arizona Health Sciences Center, Tucson, Arizona

CAROL S. PORTLOCK, M.D.

Associate Professor, Cornell University Medical College; Acting Chief, Lymphoma Service, Memorial Sloan-Kettering Cancer Center, New York, New York

REBECCA L. POTTER, M.D.

Clinical Associate Professor of Psychiatry, The University of Arizona Health Sciences Center; Staff Psychiatrist and Director of Outpatient Psychiatry Clinic, The University of Arizona Health Sciences Center, Tucson, Arizona

ERIC M. REIMAN, M.D.

Associate Professor of Psychiatry, The University of Arizona Health Sciences Center, Tucson, Arizona

JULIE I. RIFKIN, M.D.

Clinical Assistant Professor of Internal Medicine, University of Colorado School of Medicine; Staff Endocrinologist, Denver General Hospital, Denver, Colorado

ROBERT M. RIFKIN, M.D.

Clinical Assistant Professor of Surgery, Division of Organ Transplantation, University of Colorado School of Medicine; Medical Director, Bone Marrow Transplant Program, Presbyterian Denver Hospital, Denver, Colorado

TERRA A. ROBLES, Pharm.D.

Head, Clinical Pharmacy Services, FHP Healthcare, Tucson, Arizona

STEVEN D. SALAS, M.D.

Medical Resident, The University of Arizona Health Sciences Center, Tucson, Arizona

RICHARD E. SAMPLINER, M.D., F.A.C.P., F.A.C.G.

Professor of Medicine, and Chief, Section of Gastroenterology, The University of Arizona Health Sciences Center, Tucson, Arizona

ROBERT N. SAMUELSON, M.D.

Clinical Assistant Professor of Obstetrics and Gynecology, The University of Arizona Health Sciences Center, Tucson, Arizona

SUSAN FISK SANDER, M.D.

Staff Physician, Veterans Administration Medical Center, Tucson, Arizona

GAIL L. SCHWARTZ, M.D.

Clinical Assistant Professor of Psychiatry, The University of Arizona Health Sciences Center, Tucson, Arizona

MICHAEL E. SCOTT, M.D.

Psychiatry Chief Resident, The University of Arizona Health Sciences Center, Tucson, Arizona

JOSEPH I. SHAPIRO, M.D.

Assistant Professor of Medicine, University of Colorado School of Medicine; Director, Nuclear Magnetic Resonance Spectroscopy, University of Colorado Health Sciences Center, Denver, Colorado

WILLIAM A. SIBLEY, M.D.

Professor of Neurology, The University of Arizona Health Sciences Center, Tucson, Arizona

JEFFREY L. SILBER, M.D.

Assistant Professor of Medicine, University of Medicine and Dentistry of New Jersey/Robert Wood Johnson Medical School at Camden; Staff, Division of Infectious Diseases, Department of Medicine, Cooper Hospital/University Medical Center, Camden, New Jersey

MARK S. SISKIND, M.D.

Clinical Assistant Professor of Medicine, The University of Arizona Health Sciences Center, Tucson, Arizona

GARY H. SMITH, Pharm.D.

Professor of Pharmacy Practice, The University of Arizona Health Sciences Center; Clinical Pharmacist, University Medical Center, Tucson, Arizona

MARTIN SNYDER, D.P.M.

Senior Clinical Lecturer, Department of Medicine, The University of Arizona Health Sciences Center, Tucson, Arizona

JAMES R. STANDEN, M.D., FRCPC

Clinical Professor of Radiology, The University of Arizona Health Sciences Center; Head of Thoracic Radiology, The University of Arizona Health Sciences Center, Tucson, Arizona

LAWRENCE Z. STERN, M.D.

Professor of Internal Medicine, The University of Arizona Health Sciences Center; Director, Mucio F. Delgado Clinic for Neuromuscular Disorders, Tucson, Arizona

JOHN B. SULLIVAN, M.D.

Department of Emergency Medicine, The University of Arizona Health Sciences Center, Tucson, Arizona

RAYMOND TAETLE, M.D.

Professor of Medicine and Pathology, The University of Arizona Health Sciences Center; Chief of Hematology, The University of Arizona Health Sciences Center, Tucson, Arizona

CHARLES W. TAYLOR, M.D.

Assistant Professor of Medicine, The University of Arizona Health Sciences Center; Staff Physician, Arizona Cancer Center, Tucson, Arizona

CATHERINE S. THOMPSON, M.D.

Associate Professor of Medicine, Division of Nephrology, University of Texas Medical School at Houston, Houston, Texas

CYNTHIA THOMSON, M.S., R.D.

Clinical Nutrition Research Specialist, Department of Family and Community Medicine, The University of Arizona Health Sciences Center, Tucson, Arizona

LYNN M. TOLANDER, M.D.

Clinical Neurologist, Iowa Physicians Clinic, Des Moines, Iowa

M. ANGELO TRUJILLO, M.D.

Fellow in Gastroenterology, Department of Medicine, The University of Arizona Health Sciences Center, Tucson, Arizona

DAVID B. VAN WYCK, M.D.

Associate Professor of Medicine, The University of Arizona Health Sciences Center; Associate Head of Medicine, University Medical Center and Chief, Medical Service, Veterans Administration Medical Center, Tucson, Arizona

ALBERTA L. WARNER, M.D.

Clinical Assistant Professor, Section of Cardiology, The University of Arizona Health Sciences Center; Cardiologist, The University of Arizona Health Sciences Center, Tucson, Arizona

BRUCE WEINSTEIN, M.D.

Professor and Chairman, Department of Obstetrics and Gynecology, Medical College of Ohio, Toledo, Ohio

SETH WEISSMAN, M.D.

Clinical Assistant Professor of Medicine, Stanford University School of Medicine; Staff Physician, Stanford Medical Group, Stanford, California

JEANETTE K. WENDT, M.D.

Clinical Assistant Professor of Neurology, The University of Arizona Health Sciences Center, Tucson, Arizona

CAROL A. WOLFE, M.D.

Clinical Assistant Professor, The University of Arizona Health Sciences Center, Tucson, Arizona

PREFACE

Decision Making in Medicine is a book for the practitioner, resident physician, medical student, nurse practitioner, or physician assistant seeking guidelines for diagnosis and therapy. It endeavors to bridge the gap between the didactics of a larger textbook and the practice of seasoned clinicians.

The topics are organized by sign, symptom, problem, or laboratory abnormality. One then follows a decision-tree approach to arrive at the proper diagnosis or family of diagnoses to consider. In other cases the algorithm leads to the appropriate therapy or course of action.

A book of this type assumes that there can be an orderliness to medicine and to the work-up of common complaints. Such an approach offers uniformity, a means to control costs and order tests in an appropriate manner, and the possibility of a consistent quality approach to the same presenting complaints.

Medicine cannot be taught by cookbooks. Much of the flavor of medicine comes from the interplay of individual physician style and patient preference; we cannot put that in a book. The approaches presented here reflect the expertise and preferences of the individual authors, but there is much latitude for the reader's art of medicine.

I want to thank the contributing authors and editors who have successfully put their daily practice into a systematic approach and given us solid paths to follow. My co-editors, William P. Johnson, M.D., and Michael J. Maricic, M.D., have done an excellent job with their tireless review and revision of the manuscripts. I also want to thank Mosby–Year Book for the outstanding assistance they have provided throughout this process. Special thanks go to Lynne Gery, Allan Kleinberg, Wendy Buckwalter, and Dana Dreibelbis who were supportive and set high standards of quality every step of the way. Finally, this book would not have been possible without the administrative and technical support of my friends Luz Palomarez; Christine Lucas; Mary Ann Bell, R.N., M.Ed., G.N.P.; and Cindy Sierra, and others who reviewed and sharpened the manuscripts from typing to copy editing to final review.

Harry L. Greene, M.D.

This book is dedicated to our students, past, present, and future, and to the important people in our lives who gave us the time and inspiration to write

CONTENTS

GENERAL MEDICINE

Fatigue 2
R. Scott Gorman

Eating Disorders 4
Carol A. Wolfe

Involuntary Weight Loss 6
Bruce Weinstein

Obesity 10
Scott W. Nowlin

Sexual Dysfunction 12
C. J. McCurdy

Edema 14
David W. Gibson
Harry L. Greene

Chronic Pain 18
Andrea Binzer
William P. Johnson

Persistent Excessive Sweating 20
Lisa Kaufmann

Acute Red Eye 22
Lisa Kaufmann

Chronic Red Eye 26
Lisa Kaufmann

Rhinitis 28
Seth Weissman

Tinnitus 30
Susan Fisk Sander

Hearing Loss 32
Susan Fisk Sander

Perioperative Evaluation 34
William P. Johnson
Farrell Lloyd

INTERNAL MEDICINE

Cardiology

Bradycardia 42
David Framm
Paul E. Fenster
Karl B. Kern

Narrow QRS Complex Tachycardia 44
Anthony C. Caruso
Karl B. Kern

Wide QRS Complex Tachycardia 46
Anthony C. Caruso

Stable Angina 48
Karil Bellah
Samuel M. Butman

Unstable Angina 50
Karil Bellah
Samuel M. Butman

Systolic Murmur 52
Alberta L. Warner

Diastolic Murmur 54
Alberta L. Warner

Hypertension 56
Pamela J. Davis

Hypotension 60
Mark C. Goldberg

Palpitations 62
Karl B. Kern
Paul E. Fenster

Syncope 64
Anthony C. Caruso

Large Cardiac Silhouette 66
James R. Standen

Congestive Heart Failure 68
Karil Bellah

Acute Pulmonary Edema 70
James M. Galloway
Paul E. Fenster

Cor Pulmonale 72
Mark C. Goldberg
Karl B. Kern

Right Ventricular Failure 74
Mark C. Goldberg
Karl B. Kern

Cardiac Arrest 76
James M. Galloway
Karl B. Kern

Cardiac Dyspnea 78
David Framm
Paul E. Fenster
Karl B. Kern

Acute Myocardial Infarction .80
Paul E. Fenster
James M. Galloway

Counseling After Myocardial Infarction 82
Susan McKenzie
Karl B. Kern

Dermatology

Pigmented Lesions 84
Norman Levine

Leg Ulcer. 86
Cynthia A. O'Neil

Urticaria 88
Norman Levine

Generalized Pruritus. 90
Norman Levine

Palpable Purpura 92
Norman Levine

Livedo Reticularis. 94
Angela Murphy McGhee

Endocrinology

Hyperlipidemia. 96
Nancy A. Curosh
Thomas W. Boyden

Hypoglycemia. 100
Nancy A. Curosh

Hyperglycemia 102
Philip R. Orlander
Thomas W. Boyden

Hypocalcemia. 104
Philip R. Orlander

Hypercalcemia 106
Philip R. Orlander
Thomas W. Boyden

Tests of Thyroid Function 108
Julie I. Rifkin
Thomas W. Boyden

Hypothyroidism 109
Julie I. Rifkin
Thomas W. Boyden

Hyperthyroidism. 110
Julie I. Rifkin
Thomas W. Boyden

Goiter 112
Julie I. Rifkin
Thomas W. Boyden

Thyroid Nodule 114
Julie I. Rifkin
Thomas W. Boyden

Painful Thyroid. 116
Nancy A. Curosh

Thyroid Function Tests in Nonthyroidal Illness 118
Julie I. Rifkin

Adrenal Mass 120
Nancy A. Curosh

Cushing's Syndrome. 122
Nancy A. Curosh

Pituitary Tumor. 124
Philip R. Orlander

Secondary Amenorrhea 126
Nancy A. Curosh

Hirsutism. 128
Nancy A. Curosh

Gynecomastia 130
Nancy A. Curosh
Thomas W. Boyden

Gastroenterology

Acute Abdominal Pain 132
Steven Palley

Chronic Abdominal Pain 134
Lee J. Hixson

Nausea and Vomiting 136
Steven Palley

Anorexia 138
M. Angelo Trujillo

Dysphagia 140
Philip E. Jaffe

Heartburn 142
Richard E. Sampliner

Noncardiac Chest Pain 144
M. Brian Fennerty

Belching 146
Gregory L. Eastwood

Dyspepsia 148
Lee J. Hixson

Jaundice 150
Richard E. Sampliner

Ascites 152
Richard E. Sampliner

Biliary Colic 154
Philip E. Jaffe

Gastrointestinal Bleeding 156
Gregory L. Eastwood

Rectal Bleeding 160
Steven Palley

Acute Diarrhea 162
M. Brian Fennerty

Chronic Diarrhea 164
Lee J. Hixson

Constipation 166
Philip E. Jaffe

Anorectal Pain 168
M. Angelo Trujillo

Guaiac-Positive Stools 170
M. Brian Fennerty

Flatulence 172
Gregory L. Eastwood

Fecal Incontinence 174
Philip E. Jaffe

Asymptomatic Increased Transaminases 176
Steven Palley

Elevated Serum Iron 178
M. Brian Fennerty

Elevated Serum Amylase 180
M. Angelo Trujillo

Hematology/Oncology

Anemia 182
Raymond Taetle

Polycythemia 184
Raymond Taetle

Leukocytosis 186
Robert M. Rifkin

Leukopenia 188
William H. Kreisle
Manuel Modiano

Disseminated Intravascular Coagulation 190
Raymond Taetle

Deep Venous Thrombosis 192
Guillermo Gonzalez-Osete
Manuel Modiano

Coagulation Abnormalities 194
Manuel Modiano

Transfusion Therapy: Platelets 198
June Clements
Douglas Huestis

Transfusion Therapy: Red Blood Cells 200
June Clements
Douglas Huestis

Transfusion Therapy: Granulocytes. 202
June Clements
Douglas Huestis

Transfusion Reactions and Complications 204
June Clements
Douglas Huestis

Hodgkin's Disease 206
Carol S. Portlock

Chronic Myelogenous Leukemia. 208
Robert M. Rifkin

Abnormal Serum Protein Electrophoresis 210
Antonio C. Buzaid

Breast Mass. 212
Laurie L. Fajardo

Lymphadenopathy 214
Guillermo Gonzalez-Osete
Manuel Modiano

Adjuvant Therapy Choices in Breast Cancer 216
Ellen M. Chase
Manuel Modiano

Carcinoma of Unknown Primary Site. 218
Antonio C. Buzaid

Neutropenia and Fever 220
Antonio C. Buzaid

Pathologic Fractures. 222
Irwin E. Harris

Clinical Consideration for Bone Marrow Transplant
Candidates 226
Catherine Azar
Mary Bordenave

Secondary Malignancies in Patients Previously
Treated for Cancer 228
Charles W. Taylor

Superior Vena Caval Syndrome. 230
Frederick R. Ahmann

Spinal Cord Compression 232
Guillermo Gonzalez-Osete
Manuel Modiano

Infectious Disease

Foreign Travel: Immunizations and Infections 234
Rodney D. Adam

Acute and Subacute Meningitis. 236
Steven D. Salas
Richard M. Mandel

Chronic Meningitis. 240
Jeffrey L. Silber
Mark J. DiNubile

Aseptic Meningitis Syndrome 242
Douglas Fish
Richard M. Mandel

Sexually Transmitted Disease 244
George William Estes
Richard M. Mandel

Approach to the Newly Diagnosed HIV-Positive
Patient. 248
J. Kevin Carmichael

The Acutely Ill HIV-Positive Patient 250
Douglas Fish
Richard M. Mandel

Pulmonary Infections in the HIV-Infected Patient 252
Neil M. Ampel

Central Nervous System Infections in the
HIV-Infected Patient. 254
Neil M. Ampel

Sepsis. 256
Neil M. Ampel

Toxic Shock Syndrome 258
Simone A. Ince
Richard M. Mandel

Staphylococcus aureus Bacteremia. 260
Jeffrey L. Silber
Mark J. DiNubile

Hepatitis Exposure 262
Stephen J. Gluckman
Mark J. DiNubile

Fever of Unknown Origin 264
Seth Weissman
Richard M. Mandel

Nephrology

Chronic Renal Failure 266
Anwar Al-Haidary
Joy L. Logan

Acute Renal Failure 268
Anwar Al-Haidary
David B. Van Wyck

Proteinuria. 270
Anwar Al-Haidary
David B. Van Wyck

Hematuria. 272
Anwar Al-Haidary
David B. Van Wyck

Kidney Stones 274
James L. McGuire
David B. Van Wyck

Renal Cysts and Masses 276
David B. Van Wyck

Metabolic Acidosis. 278
Hillary Don

Metabolic Alkalosis 280
Hillary Don

Hyponatremia. 282
Anwar Al-Haidary

Hypernatremia 284
Anwar Al-Haidary

Hypokalemia. 286
Catherine S. Thompson
David M. Clive

Hyperkalemia 288
Catherine S. Thompson
David M. Clive

Hypomagnesemia. 290
Anwar Al-Haidary
David B. Van Wyck

Hypophosphatemia 292
Mark S. Siskind
Robert F. Klein
Steven T. Harris

Choosing a Chronic Dialysis Modality 294
Joseph I. Shapiro

Selection of Patients for Transplantation. 296
Joseph I. Shapiro

Fever in a Transplant Patient. 298
Joseph I. Shapiro

Neurology

Acute Headache. 300
Jeanette K. Wendt

Chronic Headache 302
Jeanette K. Wendt

Transient Ischemic Attacks .304
Merrill C. Kanter

Transient Monocular Visual Loss 306
Merrill C. Kanter

Completed Stroke. 308
Merrill C. Kanter

Progressing Stroke 310
Merrill C. Kanter

Memory Loss 312
Geoffrey L. Ahern

Dizziness. 316
William A. Sibley

Seizures. 318
K. J. Oommen

Status Epilepticus 320
K. J. Oommen

Weakness 322
Lynn M. Tolander

Gait Disturbances...........................326
William A. Sibley

Tremor.....................................328
Erwin B. Montgomery, Jr.

Parkinson's Disease 330
Erwin B. Montgomery, Jr.

Peripheral Neuropathy.......................332
Lynn M. Tolander

Hyperkinesias 336
Erwin B. Montgomery, Jr.

Muscle Cramps and Aches 340
Lawrence Z. Stern

Acute Behavior Change.......................342
Geoffrey L. Ahern

Chronic Behavior Change 344
Geoffrey L. Ahern

Disturbances of Smell and Taste.................348
Eugenie A. M. T. Obbens

Sleep Disturbance 350
Colin R. Bamford

Coma......................................354
Geoffrey L. Ahern

Brain Death.................................356
William M. Feinberg

Pulmonary Disease

Hemoptysis.................................358
Anthony Camilli

Stridor 360
Neil C. Clements, Jr.

Wheezing 362
Neil C. Clements, Jr.

Cough 364
Steven R. Knoper

Pulmonary Dyspnea.........................366
Anthony Camilli

Pleural Effusion.............................368
Steven R. Knoper

Mediastinal Adenopathy 370
Anthony Camilli

Solitary Pulmonary Nodule 372
John Lace

Multiple Pulmonary Nodules..................374
John Lace

Diffuse Interstitial Lung Disease 376
Anthony Camilli

Pulmonary Infiltrates in Patients with AIDS 378
John W. Bloom

Positive Tuberculin Skin Test...................380
Anthony Camilli

Respiratory Symptoms and Occupational Exposure to
Asbestos 382
Anthony Camilli

Rheumatology

Monoarticular Arthritis.......................384
Deborah Doud

Polyarticular Arthritis 386
Deborah Doud

Seronegative Arthritis 388
Michael J. Maricic

Soft Tissue Pain 390
Michael J. Maricic

Neck Pain 392
Michael J. Maricic

Shoulder Pain 394
James B. Benjamin

Low Back Pain 396
Barbara Bode

Hip Pain 398
James B. Benjamin

Hand and Wrist Pain 400
Michael J. Maricic

Knee Pain 402
Michael J. Maricic

Foot Pain. 404
Martin Snyder

Scleroderma 406
Barbara Bode

Keratoconjunctivitis Sicca (Sjögren's Syndrome) 408
Marcia Ko

Raynaud's Phenomenon. .410
Patricia Mayer

Osteopenia 412
Michael J. Maricic

Hyperuricemia and Gout. 414
Eric P. Gall

Diffuse Muscle Pain and Stiffness: Polymyalgia
Rheumatica and Giant Cell Arteritis 416
Michael J. Maricic

Joint Hypermobility 418
Patricia Mayer

Temporomandibular Pain 422
Michael J. Maricic

Positive Antinuclear Antibody Test 424
Marcia Ko

Elevated Alkaline Phosphatase Level 426
Michael J. Maricic

Elevated Creatine Kinase Level 428
Patricia Mayer

EMERGENCY MEDICINE, GYNECOLOGY, UROLOGY, BEHAVIORAL MEDICINE, AND PHARMACOLOGY

Emergency Medicine

Acute Pulseless Extremity. 432
Kenneth E. McIntyre, Jr.

Foreign Body Ingestion 434
Riemke Brakema

Caustic Ingestion and Exposure. 438
Cynthia Madden
Richard C. Dart

Human and Animal Bites. 440
Douglas Lindsey

Snake Venom Poisoning .442
Richard C. Dart

Hypothermia. 444
Cynthia Madden
John B. Sullivan

Drowning and Near-Drowning 446
Samuel M. Keim

Gynecology

Vaginal Discharge 450
Robert N. Samuelson

Cervicitis. 452
Hugh S. Miller

Abnormal Vaginal Bleeding. 454
Hugh S. Miller

Vaginal Bleeding in Pregnancy 456
Allan R. Hartsough

Acute Abdominal Pain in Women 458
Robert N. Samuelson

Urinary Tract Infection in Women 460
Michael D. Katz

Nipple Discharge 462
Allan R. Hartsough

Abnormal Pap Smear. 464
Hugh S. Miller

Premenstrual Syndrome 466
Jessica Byron

Contraceptive Choices. 468
Ana María López

Use of Oral Contraceptives 472
Terra A. Robles

Infertility 476
PonJola Coney

Urology

Acute Dysuria or Pyuria in Men 478
Richard F. Hoffman

Scrotal Mass 480
William P. Johnson

Prostate Nodule or Enlargement 482
Jeffrey I. Miller
George W. Drach

Prostatitis. 484
Jeffrey I. Miller
George W. Drach

Urinary Incontinence 486
William P. Johnson

Male Infertility 488
PonJola Coney

Behavioral Medicine

Alcoholism 490
Michael E. Scott
Myra M. Kerstitch

Anxiety 492
Eric M. Reiman

Depression 494
Iris R. Bell

Emotional Disorders with Somatic Expression 496
John Misiaszek

Grief 498
Gail L. Schwartz

Psychosis. 500
Alan J. Gelenberg

Smoking Cessation 502
Harry L. Greene
Lawrence A. Garcia

Suicidal Patient. 506
Rebecca L. Potter

Pharmacology

Acute Anticoagulation 508
Michael D. Katz
Robert J. Lipsy

Long-Term Anticoagulation 512
Michael D. Katz

Anaphylaxis 514
Michael D. Katz

Adverse Drug Reactions. 518
Robert J. Lipsy

Nonsurgical Antimicrobial Prophylaxis. 520
Brian L. Erstad
Collin Freeman

Antimicrobial Prophylaxis in Surgical Patients. 522
Brian L. Erstad

Choosing Appropriate Antimicrobial Therapy 524
Michael D. Katz

History of Hypersensitivity to Beta-Lactam
Antibiotics. 526
Michael D. Katz

Use and Monitoring of Aminoglycoside
Antibiotics. 528
Brian L. Erstad

Use and Evaluation of Serum Drug Levels. 530
Collin Freeman
Brian L. Erstad

Evaluation of a Drug Study 532
Gary H. Smith

Evaluation of a Drug for Clinical Use or Inclusion
in a Formulary 534
Terra A. Robles

Inpatient Parenteral Nutrition 536
Michael D. Katz

Inpatient Enteral Nutrition 542
Michael D. Katz
Cynthia Thomson

DECISION MAKING IN
Medicine

GENERAL MEDICINE

FATIGUE

R. Scott Gorman, M.D.

A. Fatigue is one of the most common presenting complaints in a physician's office. It may be described as weakness, lethargy, lassitude, tiredness, or just a sense of not being well. Although studies have shown that no organic cause can be found for most cases of fatigue, the physician's role is to search for an organic cause rather than just dismissing the condition as psychologic. The history and physical examination are essential tools in helping identify the cause of fatigue.

B. Abnormal physical findings may help distinguish between fatigue (a symptom) and actual weakness (a sign). Weakness may indicate a neurologic disease (e.g., amyotrophic lateral sclerosis) or a muscular disease (e.g., polymyalgia rheumatica). Other physical findings may suggest other causes of fatigue such as the tremor of hyperthyroidism, the elevated jugular venous pressure of congestive heart failure, the wheezing of chronic obstructive pulmonary disease, or the lymphadenopathy of HIV disease. Specific diagnostic tests may then confirm the diagnosis and assess the extent of impairment. These disease-specific tests may include assessment of thyroid function, monitoring of ESR, or spirometric tests, among others.

C. Even when the physical examination is unrevealing, the history may suggest an underlying disease as the cause. For example, a history of fevers and night sweats suggests an infectious cause. The evaluation of such a patient differs from that of one who presents with a history of heavy snoring, morning headaches, and daytime somnolence. The duration of the fatigue may also be important. Fatigue of more than 6 months' duration may be considered chronic. Some patients with chronic fatigue may suffer from the poorly understood "chronic fatigue syndrome." The symptoms associated with this syndrome suggest that an infectious agent may be the cause, although none has yet been clearly identified. As with abnormal physical findings, the history may lead to the ordering of specific diagnostic tests that may confirm the diagnosis and assess the extent of impairment.

D. A wide variety of commonly used drugs, both prescribed and nonprescribed, can cause fatigue; e.g., beta blockers, antihistamines, and anticholinergics. Alcohol can cause fatigue, not only by its direct effect, but also through its ability to cause a sleep disturbance. Changing prescription drugs and eliminating nonprescribed drugs may alleviate the problem. A trial of discontinuance of alcohol may resolve the fatigue for others. An inability to stop certain drugs and alcohol may signal the need for substance abuse intervention.

E. Anxiety and depression, and the stress associated with these conditions, are the most common identifiable nonorganic causes of fatigue. Some patients may be aware of their anxiety or depression and accompanying stress, and they may even identify these conditions as a cause of their fatigue. In others, determining the presence of anxiety or depression may not be so easy. A good history must include questions about home and work situations as well as an assessment of sleeping, sexual, eating, and bowel patterns.

F. The history and physical examination frequently do not reveal the cause of fatigue. Many fatigue-causing conditions may be discovered by screening laboratory studies.

G. Screening laboratory studies are useful in three circumstances: (1) the patient with an unrevealing history and physical examination whose fatigue may have an occult organic cause, (2) the anxious or depressed patient who may have a metabolic or other abnormality that is causing the anxiety or depression, and (3) the patient who uses drugs or alcohol but who fails to have a change in fatigue after the drugs or alcohol are changed or discontinued. A wide variety of disease processes may subtly present as fatigue. Anemia, diabetes mellitus, adrenal insufficiency, azotemia, hyperthyroidism and hypothyroidism, chronic hepatitis, occult malignancy, and occult infections are frequently detected with screening laboratory studies. Further diagnostic tests may be needed after the screening studies to confirm or better evaluate detected abnormalities.

H. If no organic cause of fatigue is detected, further evaluation is indicated. A formal psychologic evaluation may be useful to assess the possibility of occult anxiety or depression. Specific pharmacologic intervention or counseling may then be required. In other cases of chronic fatigue, no psychologic abnormality is found. A trial of antidepressant medications may be considered for these individuals.

References

Gilroy FJ. Fatigue. In: Greene HL, ed. Introduction to clinical medicine. Philadelphia: BC Decker, 1991:155.

Hayden S. A practical approach to chronic fatigue syndrome. Cleveland Clin J Med 1991; 58:116.

Holmes GP, Kaplan JE, Gentz NM, et al. Chronic fatigue syndrome: a working case definition. Ann Intern Med 1988; 108:387.

Jarrett WA. Lethargy in general practice. Practitioner 1981; 225:731.

Manu P, Lane TJ, Matthews DA. The frequency of the chronic fatigue syndrome in patients with symptoms of persistent fatigue. Ann Intern Med 1988; 109:554.

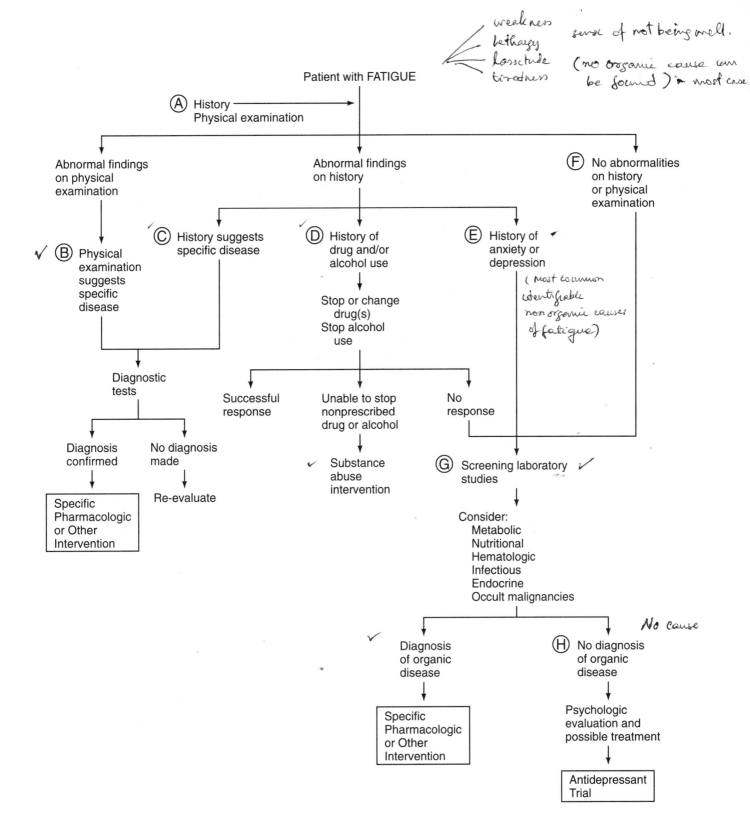

Patient with FATIGUE

weakness
lethargy
lassitude
tiredness

sense of not being well.
(no organic cause can be found) in most case

(A) History
Physical examination

Abnormal findings on physical examination

Abnormal findings on history

(F) No abnormalities on history or physical examination

(B) Physical examination suggests specific disease

(C) History suggests specific disease

(D) History of drug and/or alcohol use

(E) History of anxiety or depression

(Most common identifiable non organic causes of fatigue)

Stop or change drug(s)
Stop alcohol use

Diagnostic tests

Successful response

Unable to stop nonprescribed drug or alcohol

No response

Diagnosis confirmed

No diagnosis made

Specific Pharmacologic or Other Intervention

Re-evaluate

Substance abuse intervention

(G) Screening laboratory studies

Consider:
Metabolic
Nutritional
Hematologic
Infectious
Endocrine
Occult malignancies

No cause

Diagnosis of organic disease

(H) No diagnosis of organic disease

Specific Pharmacologic or Other Intervention

Psychologic evaluation and possible treatment

Antidepressant Trial

EATING DISORDERS

Carol A. Wolfe, M.D.

A. The primary care physician's role in detecting eating disorders during routine medical examinations is extremely important. The patient with an eating disorder is typically an adolescent or young adult white female of middle to upper-middle socioeconomic class. Males also have eating disorders but much less commonly.

B. Bulimia tends to start at a later age than anorexia, and these patients present much later in the course of the disease. They are aware of their abnormal eating problems and attempt to hide them because of embarrassment. The two most common complaints on review of systems are swelling of the hands and feet and abdominal bloating. These are vague and indirect indications, and therefore clues on physical examination are often important to an early diagnosis. Ulceration or calluses on the dorsum of the hand or on the proximal interphalangeal joints can be caused by the teeth during manual triggering of the gag reflex to induce vomiting. This is more often seen early in the disease, because most patients are soon able to vomit spontaneously. Dental erosions or a dull gray discoloration of teeth caused by recurrent exposure to gastric acid is often present. Salivary gland hypertrophy is a common physical finding in bulimics. Unexplained muscle weakness due to hypokalemia should trigger suspicion of ipecac abuse. When emetine, the active ingredient in ipecac, is absorbed in large enough doses it can cause a primary myositis. Male bulimics are often found among wrestlers and jockeys who purge to lose weight quickly.

C. Bulimic patients should be evaluated for life-threatening medical problems. The most common of these are fluid and electrolyte abnormalities, dehydration, hypotension, hypokalemia, and alkalosis. Other rare medical emergencies include esophageal rupture, pneumomediastinum, cardiac myositis from emetine overdose, and pancreatitis.

D. Anorexia nervosa is easiest to detect during physical examination. Weight continually 15% below that expected for height is required for diagnosis. These patients rarely come to ask for help, however, and are unaware of their malnutrition because denial is a large part of the disease. Usually there is a history of an attempt at weight loss starting in the teenage years, and abnormal eating habits develop from that time with severe restriction of food. Food rituals, such as storing food in a certain place in the refrigerator, can occur. There is an intense fear of gaining weight and an abnormal self-image. Despite being very thin, these patients perceive themselves as fat. They often present with a history of amenorrhea. Anorexics engage in excess physical activity, and this often predates the onset of overt anorexia nervosa. They often participate in purging activities, including self-induced vomiting, excessive diuretic use, and cathartic use.

E. Anorexics are often hospitalized because of severe malnutrition or for fluid and electrolyte disorders seen with the bulimic variant. These patients often need tube feeding to regain a minimal weight and be stabilized. There may be multiple physical problems, mostly relating to malnutrition, and sudden death due to cardiac arrest associated with prolongation of the QT interval may occur. Amenorrhea, osteoporosis, euthyroid sick syndrome, hypercarotenemia, abnormal temperature regulation, decreased gastric emptying, constipation, elevated liver enzymes, anemia, and hypoalbuminemia are other physical problems. Most are treated by providing adequate nutrition.

F. There are many atypical presentations of eating disorders. Many women in our culture are distressed with their body shape and do not necessarily have an eating disorder, but if they are abnormally thin a psychiatric evaluation should be considered. Many women set abnormally low weight goals for themselves to compete in professions such as ballet, sports, or modeling. Unlike the typical anorexia nervosa patients, these patients know they are thin, but if they are unwilling to achieve a healthy minimal weight, they should be referred for psychiatric evaluation. There is a subclinical group of patients with eating disorders who intermittently, under periods of stress, have binge-purge episodes. Binge eating is not uncommon in many women during times of stress, but any history of purging suggests a self-destructive behavior, and psychiatric evaluation should be considered.

G. After hospitalization or if hospitalization is not necessary, psychiatric evaluation and help from an experienced nutritionist are begun. Often there is an associated depression that requires antidepressant medication. Some patients may have problems with alcohol or other substance abuse. Goals should be agreed on by the treatment group. If relapse occurs, goals and types of therapy should be re-evaluated. If there are recurrent medical emergencies, contracts with patients to limit high-risk behavior and mandatory hospitalization for failure to comply can be helpful, along with frequent monitoring.

References

Herzog DB, Copeland PM. Eating disorders. N Engl J Med 1985; 313:295.
Isner JM, et al. Anorexia nervosa and sudden death. Ann Intern Med 1985; 102:49.
McKenna MS. Eating disorders. Psychiatr Ann 1989; 19:464.
Mitchell JE, et al. Medical complications and medical management of bulimia review. Ann Intern Med 1987; 107:71.

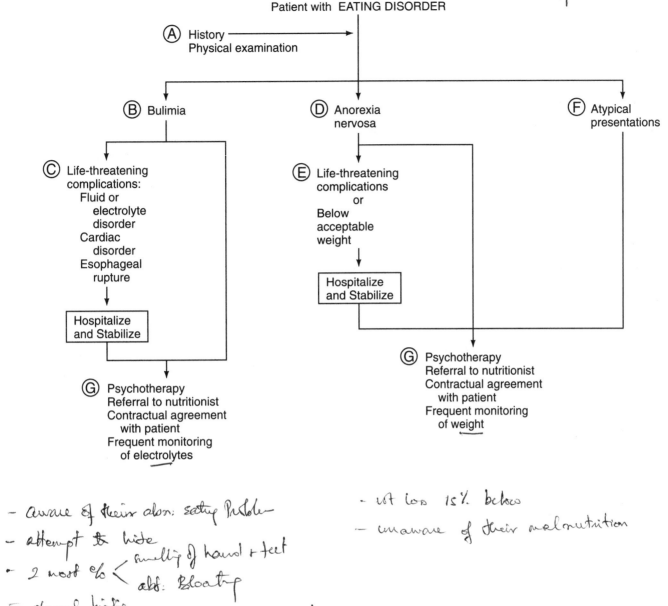

Patient with EATING DISORDER

white ♀, adolescent or young adult
middle to upper middle socioeconomic
class

(A) History
Physical examination

(B) Bulimia

(C) Life-threatening
complications:
Fluid or
electrolyte
disorder
Cardiac
disorder
Esophageal
rupture

Hospitalize
and Stabilize

(G) Psychotherapy
Referral to nutritionist
Contractual agreement
with patient
Frequent monitoring
of electrolytes

(D) Anorexia
nervosa

(E) Life-threatening
complications
or
Below
acceptable
weight

Hospitalize
and Stabilize

(F) Atypical
presentations

(G) Psychotherapy
Referral to nutritionist
Contractual agreement
with patient
Frequent monitoring
of weight

- aware of their abn: eating Problem
- attempt to hide
- 2 most c/o < swelling of hand + feet
              abd: Bloating
- physical finding

- wt loss 15% below
- unaware of their malnutrition

5

INVOLUNTARY WEIGHT LOSS

Bruce Weinstein, M.D.

Involuntary weight loss (IWL) can be associated with serious organic disease or no physical illness at all (Table 1). Clinical studies attempting to establish causes of IWL have shown differing results. In studies focusing primarily on hospitalized patients, organic illnesses have predominated, while ambulatory studies have shown a substantial prevalence of nonphysical causes, particularly psychiatric ones. All studies, however, found a significant number of patients whose IWL remained unexplained. The nonspecificity of weight loss and its association with malignant diseases can lead to extensive and expensive diagnostic testing. However, there is no evidence to support exhaustive testing performed in an unfocused manner. A strategy emphasizing the history and physical examination (H&P), a few basic screening laboratory tests, and directed diagnostic testing is recommended.

A. Many patients who claim to have lost weight have not done so. Before evaluating a person for IWL, document the weight loss. If this cannot be done through the medical record, IWL can be presumed if two of the following criteria are met: the patient (1) can numerically quantify the amount of weight loss, (2) exhibits physical evidence of weight loss (such as appearing cachectic or demonstrating a recent change in clothing or belt size), or (3) can produce a friend or relative who can verify the weight loss. Although what constitutes "significant" weight loss is unknown, several studies have arbitrarily defined it as a 5% or greater loss in body weight within a 6-month period.

B. When the medical history includes an illness that is known to cause IWL (e.g., diabetes mellitus, breast cancer), it is prudent to first evaluate, through the H&P

and appropriate laboratory studies, for exacerbation or recurrence of the illness.

C. Carefully direct the H&P toward specific organic and nonphysical conditions that can cause IWL. Specific abnormalities can then be pursued with appropriate laboratory or diagnostic testing. In addition, all patients with IWL should receive five basic screening tests at the initial evaluation: (1) CBC, (2) 12-panel chemistry profile (SMA-12), (3) urinalysis, (4) chest film, and (5) stool guaiac. The use of thyroid function tests to detect apathetic hyperthyroidism in geriatric patients without overt symptoms of hyperthyroidism is supported by the results of one study but not by another.

D. Patients who on the initial H&P show abnormalities suggestive of an organic cause of IWL and who show an abnormality on any of the five basic screening tests are likely to have an organic cause for IWL. Conversely, patients whose H&P do not suggest a physical cause of IWL and whose basic screening test results are completely normal are likely to have a nonphysical cause of IWL. In other words, an organic cause is usually apparent early in the evaluation. The basic initial evaluation is a useful guide in pursuing a more focused investigation. Although it is a possible cause, "occult" cancer has never been shown to be a common cause of IWL. Accordingly, when a nonphysical illness is suspected, it may be helpful to pursue more detailed psychosocial questioning to help elucidate the cause of IWL. Watchful waiting should not be undervalued as a diagnostic tool when the cause of IWL is not readily apparent.

(Continued on page 8)

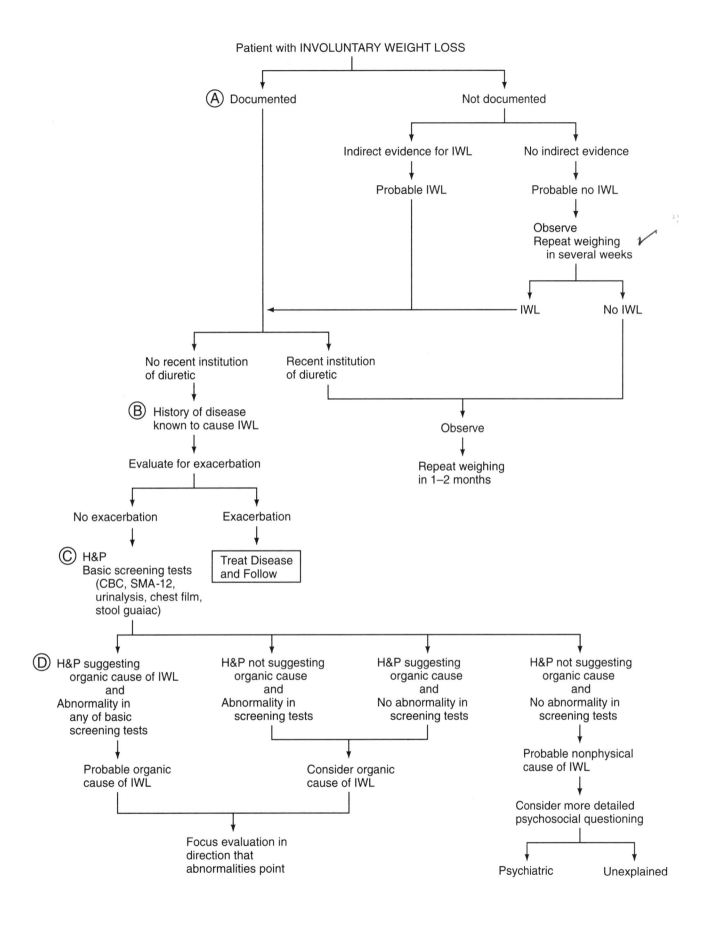

Patient with INVOLUNTARY WEIGHT LOSS

Ⓐ Documented

Not documented

Indirect evidence for IWL

No indirect evidence

Probable IWL

Probable no IWL

Observe
Repeat weighing
in several weeks

IWL

No IWL

No recent institution
of diuretic

Recent institution
of diuretic

Ⓑ History of disease
known to cause IWL

Evaluate for exacerbation

Observe

Repeat weighing
in 1–2 months

No exacerbation

Exacerbation

Ⓒ H&P
Basic screening tests
(CBC, SMA-12,
urinalysis, chest film,
stool guaiac)

Treat Disease
and Follow

Ⓓ H&P suggesting
organic cause of IWL
and
Abnormality in
any of basic
screening tests

H&P not suggesting
organic cause
and
Abnormality in
screening tests

H&P suggesting
organic cause
and
No abnormality in
screening tests

H&P not suggesting
organic cause
and
No abnormality in
screening tests

Probable organic
cause of IWL

Consider organic
cause of IWL

Probable nonphysical
cause of IWL

Consider more detailed
psychosocial questioning

Focus evaluation in
direction that
abnormalities point

Psychiatric

Unexplained

TABLE 1 Causes of Weight Loss

Study population:	Mixed Outpatient (30%)/ Inpatient (70%) V.A. Hospital	Inpatient Medical Service	Primary Care Outpatients		Geriatric Outpatients
Study design:	Prospective	Retrospective	Retrospective	Prospective	Retrospective
Number of patients:	91	154	107	117	45
Causes of Weight Loss:					
Physical Cause Found	65%	66%	40%	35%	56%
Neoplastic disease	19%	36%	—	7%	16%
Gastrointestinal	14%	17%	—	9%	11%
Cardiovascular	9%				
Nutritional/alcohol related	8%			5%	2%
Hyperthyroidism	1%	2%	—	2%	9%
Medication effect	2%			4%	9%
Other physical cause	12%	11%	—	8%	9%
Psychiatric cause found	9%	10%	22%	56%	20%
No apparent cause	26%	23%	36%	9%	24%
References:	A	B	C	D	E

A. Modified from Marton et al.
B. Modified from Rubinovitz et al.
C. Modified from Levine.
D. Modified from Weinstein et al. and additional unpublished data of the authors.
E. Modified from Thompson and Morris.

References

Levine MA. Unintentional weight loss in the ambulatory setting: etiologies and outcomes (Abstract). In: Abstracts submitted to the Society of General Internal Medicine, Seattle, Wash., May 1−4, 1991. Program supplement 1191:5.

Marton KI, Sox HC, Krupp J. Involuntary weight loss: diagnostic and prognostic significance. Ann Intern Med 1981; 95:568.

Robbins LJ. Evaluation of weight loss in the elderly. Geriatrics 1989; 44:31.

Rubinovitz M, Pitlik SD, Leifer M, et al. Unintentional weight loss: a retrospective analysis of 154 cases. Arch Intern Med 1986; 146:186.

Thompson MP, Morris LK. Unexplained weight loss in the ambulatory elderly. J Am Geriatr Soc 1991; 39:497.

Weinstein BR, Stephenson WP, Ellison RC, Greene HL. Involuntary weight loss in the primary care setting (Abstract). In: Abstracts submitted to the Society for Research and Education in Primary Care Internal Medicine, Washington, D.C., May 1, 2, 1986. Clin Res 1986; 34:844A.

OBESITY

Scott W. Nowlin, M.D.

In the United States, obesity affects about 34 million adults between the ages of 20 and 74. Morbidity and mortality rates are high. Effective treatment is difficult.

A. "Overweight" can be defined as an increase in body weight above some arbitrary standard defined in relation to height. Up to 20% above the upper limits of "ideal" is considered overweight. Obesity means an abnormally high proportion of body fat (Table 1). Anthropometric measurements such as height, weight, and skinfold thickness are useful for determining the degree of overweight or obesity in a patient. A person who is >20% above the upper limits of "ideal" body weight can be considered obese. The Metropolitan Life Insurance Company's Tables of Heights and Weights are commonly used to determine "ideal" body weight, the ideal weight for height being that weight at which longevity is the greatest.

B. On initial evaluation of the obese patient, one must consider a variety of possible causes. Unfortunately, <1% of obese patients have an identifiable endocrine dysfunction. In most cases, obesity results from an imbalance of energy intake versus energy expenditure. Multiple twin and adoption studies have indicated that human fatness is under strong genetic control. Rare genetic diseases such as the Laurence-Moon-Biedl syndrome are associated with obesity through unknown mechanisms.

C. Medications such as the phenothiazines and the tricyclic antidepressants can lead to obesity by increasing appetite. Corticosteroids also increase appetite and are associated with central or truncal obesity.

D. Obesity predisposes individuals to many other diseases. Diabetes mellitus, hypertension, and cardiovascular disease are more common in obese individuals. About 85% of patients in the US with type II diabetes mellitus are obese. Obesity is an independent risk factor for the development of coronary artery disease. Other associated disorders include cholesterol, gallstones, hyperlipidemia, venous circulatory disease, osteoarthritis, gout, and cancer. Women have an increased incidence of cancer of the breast, endometrium, ovary, and biliary system. Men have an increased incidence of cancer of the colon, rectum, and prostate.

E. Before beginning a treatment program for obesity, assess the patient's motivation and commitment. Educate the patient about the benefits of weight loss and the health benefits attained. Long-term success depends on a combination approach using diet, exercise, and behavior modification. Social and psychological support are also important.

F. Exercise should (1) promote increased energy expenditure, (2) promote fat loss and the maintenance of lean body mass, (3) be safe for the participating individual, and (4) promote increases in activity levels within the individual's lifestyle.

G. Low calorie diets should be nutritionally balanced and provide macronutrients in the following distribution: carbohydrates (≥50% of total energy intake), fat (<30%), and protein (15–20%). The usual energy intake for such diets is 1000–1200 kcal/day. When energy intake is <1000 kcal/day, vitamin and mineral supplements are usually necessary.

H. Very low calorie diets (VLCDs) provide 400–800 kcal/day. They supply protein of high biologic value and are prescribed for severely or morbidly obese patients (BMI >35). Medical supervision and supplementation with vitamins and minerals are necessary. The VLCD allows rapid weight loss while preserving lean body mass by providing dietary protein; it usually lasts 12–16 weeks. Behavior modifications and close follow-up are also necessary.

I. Behavior changes in eating patterns to affect weight loss are the crux of behavior modification. Behavioral assessment of obese persons involves attention to three points: (1) the antecedents of eating that promote excessive intake, (2) slowing the act of eating, and (3) selectively emphasizing the consequences of certain behaviors (e.g., rewarding appropriate eating behaviors).

J. Gastric surgery should be considered only in morbidly obese patients who have been unsuccessful with conventional means of weight loss. The other approaches to weight loss, including dietary management and exercise, are still important in those who undergo surgery.

TABLE 1   Parameters of Obesity

	Men	Women
Triceps plus subscapular skinfold (mm)	>43	>58
Body fat (% body weight)	>25	>30
Body mass index (BMI) $\dfrac{\text{(weight in kg)}}{\text{(height in m)}^2}$	>30	>30

Adapted from Bray GA. Obesity: an endocrine perspective. In: DeGroot LJ, ed. Endocrinology. 2nd ed. Philadelphia: WB Saunders, 1989:2303.

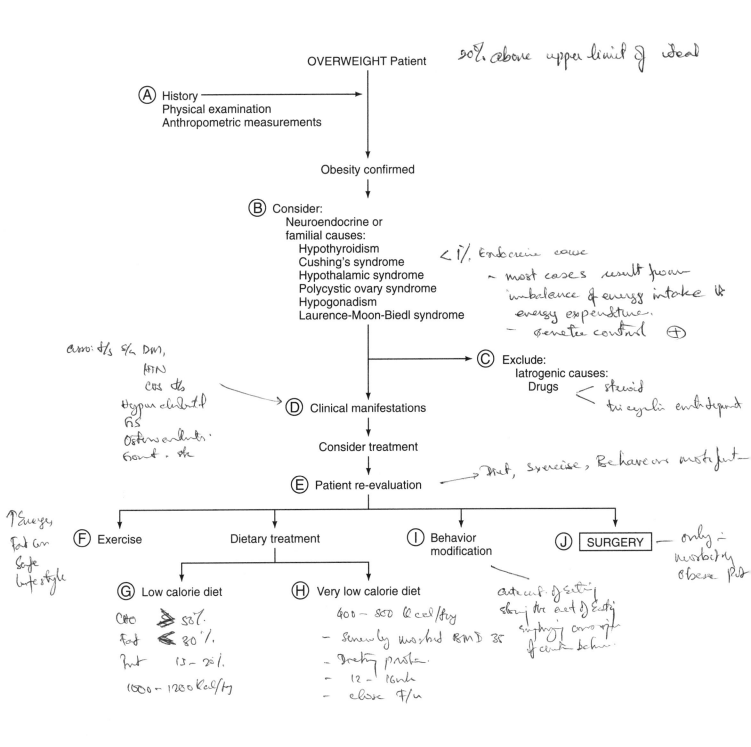

OVERWEIGHT Patient

20% above upper limit of ideal

(A) History
Physical examination
Anthropometric measurements

Obesity confirmed

(B) Consider:
Neuroendocrine or
familial causes:
Hypothyroidism
Cushing's syndrome
Hypothalamic syndrome
Polycystic ovary syndrome
Hypogonadism
Laurence-Moon-Biedl syndrome

< 1% Endocrine cause
– most cases result from
imbalance of energy intake &
energy expenditure.
– genetic control ⊕

(C) Exclude:
Iatrogenic causes:
Drugs *< steroid, tricyclic antidepres.*

assoc: t/s s/a DM,
HTN
CVS dis
Hyperlipidt.
GS
Osteoarthts.
Gout. etc

(D) Clinical manifestations

Consider treatment

(E) Patient re-evaluation *→ Diet, exercise, Behaviour modifict—*

(F) Exercise   Dietary treatment   (I) Behavior modification   (J) [SURGERY] *— only in morbidly obese Pts*

↑Energy
Fat loss
Safe
lifestyle

(G) Low calorie diet   (H) Very low calorie diet

CHO ≥ 55%
Fat ≤ 30%
Prot 15 – 20%
1000 – 1200 Kcal/hy

400 – 800 Kcal/day
– Severely morbid BMI 35
– Dietary protein.
– 12 – 16wk
– close F/u

acute of Eating
during the act of Eating
emptying content
of gastric before.

References

Bray GA. Obesity: an endocrine perspective. In: DeGroot LJ, ed. Endocrinology. 2nd ed. Philadelphia: WB Saunders, 1989:2303.
Council on Scientific Affairs. Treatment of obesity in adults. JAMA 1988; 260:2547.
Pi-Sunyer FX. Obesity. In: Wyngaarden JB, Smith LH, eds. Cecil textbook of medicine. 18th ed. Philadelphia: WB Saunders, 1989:1219.

The Surgeon General's report on nutrition and health. Washington, DC: US Dept. of Health and Human Services, Public Health Service, 1988:275.
Wadden TA, Van Itallie TB, Blackburn GL. Responsible and irresponsible use of very-low calorie diets in the treatment of obesity. JAMA 1990; 263:83.

SEXUAL DYSFUNCTION

C. J. McCurdy, M.D.

A. An essential part of a complete medical evaluation is sexual history. Only 3% of patients spontaneously offer sexual complaints, while 16–50% of patients acknowledge sexual problems when a sexual history is obtained. Make the inquiry in a nonthreatening, nonjudgmental fashion and include sexual activity, relationship(s), self-satisfaction, partner satisfaction, and perceived dysfunction.

B. Premature ejaculation is usually associated with situational factors, sexual anxiety, or unrealistic sexual expectations. Counseling and supportive therapy should include sexual education, increased coital frequency, and instruction on the squeeze technique.

C. Neurologic, endocrine, vascular, and penile disorders can all result in impotence in male patients. Thorough physical examination and laboratory screening are useful in determining the cause of impotence. To differentiate between psychologic and organic causes, test for nocturnal erections by using a strain gauge or stamp test. The absence of nocturnal erections indicates an organic cause.

D. The complaint of decreased sexual desire can be associated with acute and chronic medical illnesses, acute and chronic psychologic or emotional illness, substance abuse, and medication affect. Situational factors commonly associated with decreased libido can usually be determined by a careful history: marital discord, job stress, fatigue. Decreased or absent emission requires an evaluation for retrograde ejaculation, hypogonadism, or pituitary disease. A near-normal level of testosterone is required to stimulate the prostate and seminal vesicles. Therefore, if the semen volume is normal, the cause of decreased libido is unlikely to be an endocrine disorder.

E. Female patients with orgasmic dysfunction can often benefit from education about female anatomy and female sexual response. Instruction on self-manipulation and relaxation techniques and marital counseling may be helpful. A history of sexual abuse or rape warrants psychotherapy.

F. Complaints of painful intercourse can be divided into two distinct categories: pain with vaginal penetration, and deep-thrust dyspareunia. Pain with penetration may be secondary to lower genitourinary tract pathology, including vaginitis, cystitis, scarring, and vaginismus. The cause of deep-thrust dyspareunia usually involves the upper genital tract and includes endometriosis, leiomyomas, pelvic inflammatory disease, pelvic adhesive disease, and ovarian pathology.

References

Bachmann GA, Leiblum SR, Grill J. Brief sexual inquiry in gynecologic practice. Obstet Gynecol 1989; 73:425.

Klingman EW. Office evaluation of sexual function and complaints. Clin Geriatr. Med 1991; 7:15.

Reamy K. Sexual counseling for the nontherapist. Clin Obstet Gynecol 1984; 27:781.

Sanderson MO, Maddock JW. Guidelines for assessment and treatment of sexual dysfunction. Obstet Gynecol 1989; 73:130.

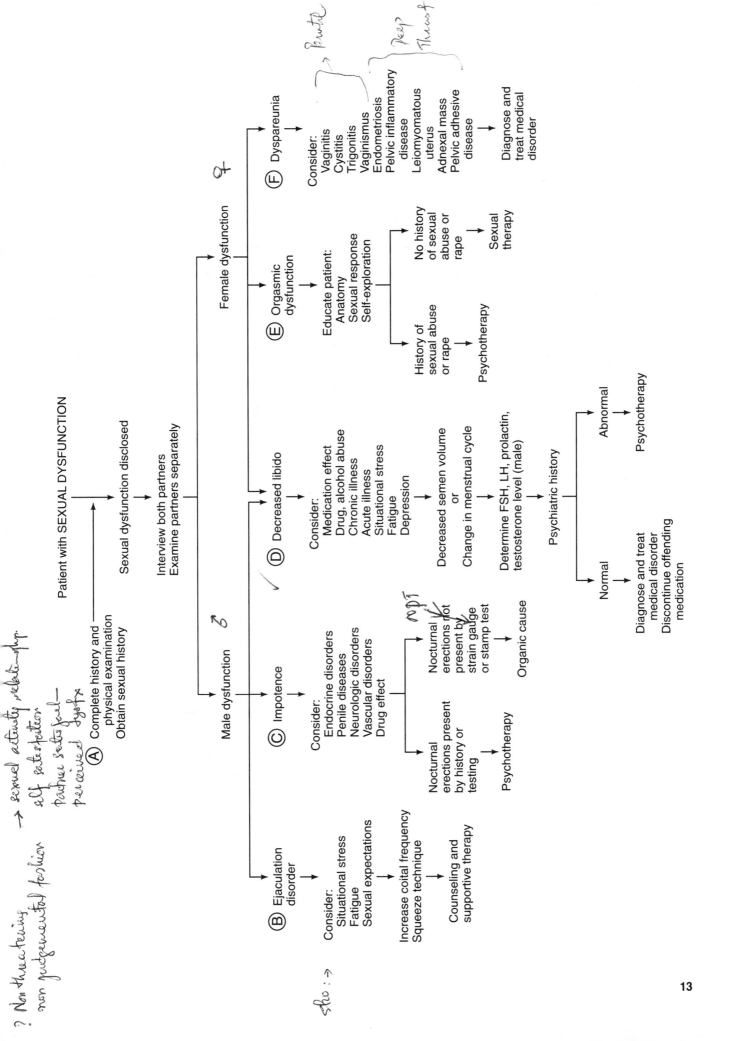

Patient with SEXUAL DYSFUNCTION

Ⓐ Complete history and physical examination
Obtain sexual history

Sexual dysfunction disclosed

Interview both partners
Examine partners separately

Male dysfunction ♂

Female dysfunction ♀

Ⓑ Ejaculation disorder

Consider:
Situational stress
Fatigue
Sexual expectations

Increase coital frequency
Squeeze technique

Counseling and supportive therapy

Ⓒ Impotence

Consider:
Endocrine disorders
Penile diseases
Neurologic disorders
Vascular disorders
Drug effect

Nocturnal erections present by history or testing

Psychotherapy

Nocturnal erections not present by strain gauge or stamp test

Organic cause

Ⓓ Decreased libido

Consider:
Medication effect
Drug, alcohol abuse
Chronic illness
Acute illness
Situational stress
Fatigue
Depression

Decreased semen volume
or
Change in menstrual cycle

Determine FSH, LH, prolactin, testosterone level (male)

Psychiatric history

Normal

Diagnose and treat medical disorder
Discontinue offending medication

Abnormal

Psychotherapy

Ⓔ Orgasmic dysfunction

Educate patient:
Anatomy
Sexual response
Self-exploration

History of sexual abuse or rape

Psychotherapy

No history of sexual abuse or rape

Sexual therapy

Ⓕ Dyspareunia

Consider:
Vaginitis
Cystitis
Trigonitis
Vaginismus
Endometriosis
Pelvic inflammatory disease
Leiomyomatous uterus
Adnexal mass
Pelvic adhesive disease

Diagnose and treat medical disorder

13

EDEMA

David W. Gibson, M.D.
Harry L. Greene, M.D.

Edema is an abnormal collection of fluid in the interstitial space that may be localized or generalized. Fluid movement between the intravascular and extravascular space is related to the interacting forces of hydrostatic pressure, colloid oncotic pressure, and capillary permeability, as well as to the effects of lymphatic drainage. Normally there exists an equilibrium among these forces, and no net fluid accumulation takes place. Edema occurs when there is a decrease in plasma oncotic pressure, an increase in hydrostatic pressure, an increase in capillary permeability, or a combination of these factors. Edema can also be present when lymphatic flow is obstructed.

A. The history and physical examination focus on the causes of edema and seek to ascertain whether it is generalized or localized.

B. Generalized edema can be documented by weight gain and is often associated with increased capillary hydrostatic pressure as seen in congestive heart failure (CHF), in renal failure with increased sodium and water load, after expansion of the intravascular volume from IV fluids, or in conditions of sodium retention. Edema may occur after corticosteroid therapy or with estrogens or other medications. Edema involving the whole body (e.g., anasarca) may extend to involve the peritoneal cavity (e.g., ascites) or the pleural space (e.g., hydrothorax). In patients with generalized edema the first step is to estimate central venous pressure by determining jugular venous pressure (JVP). The distance from the manubrium sterni to the fluid meniscus in the jugular vein should be 2 cm or less at 45° or 5 cm from the left atrium.

C. In patients with generalized edema and normal JVP, serum albumin and urinary protein should be determined.

D. If serum albumin is normal, perform urinalysis, looking for abnormal urinary sediment, and check BUN and creatinine to evaluate the possibility of renal pathology. If urinalysis findings are normal, order thyroid function tests (TFTs) to look for myxedema.

Remaining patients should be considered as possibly having idiopathic edema or drug-induced edema.

E. If serum albumin is decreased, perform urinalysis to check for proteinuria. More than 3.5 g protein suggests nephrotic syndrome; <3.5 g in a normal urinalysis suggests another cause, such as hepatitis or hepatic infiltration disease. Liver function tests (LFTs) should be checked and, if abnormal, evaluation for liver pathology performed. If LFT results are normal, check prealbumin and cholesterol to evaluate for malnutrition. If the prealbumin is <20 mg/dl and the cholesterol is low, malnutrition is suggested. If the prealbumin is >20 mg/dl, a capillary leak, abnormal protein synthesis, or protein-losing enteropathy are all possibilities.

F. In patients with an elevated JVP and generalized edema, order chest radiography to look for cardiomegaly.

G. If cardiomegaly is found, order echocardiography to look for pericardial effusion; pericardial thickening, as in acute or chronic pericarditis; abnormal contractility of the heart, as might be seen in CHF; or signs of infiltrative cardiac problems, such as hypertrophic obstructive cardiomyopathy, amyloid, or neoplasm.

H. If cardiac size is normal on the chest film, evaluate the lung fields for pulmonary hypertension. Such a finding should lead to evaluation for cor pulmonale. Clear lung fields should prompt echocardiography, to seek pericardial constriction.

I. Regional edema or localized edema is often due to increased capillary pressure. Some causes include chronic venous insufficiency; incompetent venous valves; vascular obstructions, either extrinsic owing to neoplasm, lymph nodes, surgery, fibrosis, or radiation, or intrinsic owing to deep venous thrombosis, surgery, infection, immobility, trauma, or a hypercoagulable state (e.g., protein C deficiency, protein S deficiency, antithrombin III deficiency, or in the presence of neoplasms).

(Continued on page 16)

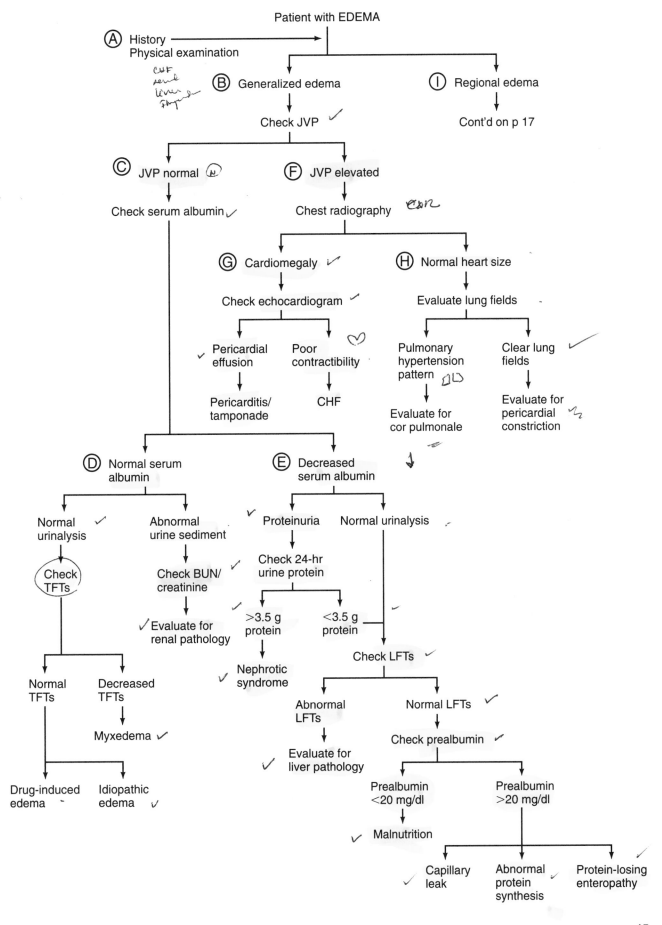

Patient with EDEMA

(A) History
Physical examination

(B) Generalized edema → Check JVP

(I) Regional edema → Cont'd on p 17

(C) JVP normal → Check serum albumin

(F) JVP elevated → Chest radiography

(G) Cardiomegaly → Check echocardiogram

Pericardial effusion → Pericarditis/tamponade

Poor contractibility → CHF

(H) Normal heart size → Evaluate lung fields

Pulmonary hypertension pattern → Evaluate for cor pulmonale

Clear lung fields → Evaluate for pericardial constriction

(D) Normal serum albumin

Normal urinalysis → Check TFTs

Normal TFTs

Decreased TFTs → Myxedema

Drug-induced edema

Idiopathic edema

Abnormal urine sediment → Check BUN/creatinine → Evaluate for renal pathology

(E) Decreased serum albumin

Proteinuria → Check 24-hr urine protein

>3.5 g protein → Nephrotic syndrome

<3.5 g protein

Normal urinalysis

Check LFTs

Abnormal LFTs → Evaluate for liver pathology

Normal LFTs → Check prealbumin

Prealbumin <20 mg/dl → Malnutrition

Prealbumin >20 mg/dl

Capillary leak

Abnormal protein synthesis

Protein-losing enteropathy

J. When regional edema is present, its location should be noted. If it is in one or both upper extremities, JVP should be determined.

K. Patients with upper extremity edema and normal JVP should undergo a Doppler study, impedance plethysmography (IPG), or venography to look for venous obstruction from either intrinsic or extrinsic causes with a negative study for lymphatic obstruction.

L. Patients with upper extremity edema and elevated JVP should be evaluated for superior vena cava syndrome with a chest x-ray and CT scan.

M. If the regional edema is confined to the lower extremities, note whether it is unilateral or bilateral. Historical features specifically directed towards trauma, a hypercoagulable state, history of neoplasm, or conditions that might cause lymphatic or venous obstruction should be sought.

N. If the history is negative, order a Doppler study or IPG. If this study is positive, venography may be indicated to evaluate venous thrombosis versus extrinsic compression. If the Doppler study is negative, rhabdomyolysis, musculoskeletal edema, or localized vascular defects may be present.

O. Patients with a positive history of lower extremity edema should undergo IPG, Doppler study, or venography of the lower extremity. Again, a positive study may suggest venous thrombosis, with treatment for this. A negative study may suggest lymphatic obstruction. This can be evaluated with lymphangiography.

References

Braunwald E. Edema. In: Braunwald E, et al., eds. Harrison's principles of internal medicine. 11th ed. New York: McGraw-Hill, 1988:149.

Greene HL, Kahn KL. Edema. In: Greene HL, Glassock RJ, Kelly MA, eds. Introduction to clinical medicine. Philadelphia: BC Decker, 1991.

Healey PM, Jacobson EJ. Edema. In: Healey PM, Jacobson EJ, eds. Common medical diagnoses: an algorithmic approach. Philadelphia: WB Saunders, 1990:28.

Spittell JA, Schirger A. Peripheral edema. In: Taylor RB, ed. Difficult diagnosis. Philadelphia: WB Saunders, 1985:130.

Regional edema
(Cont'd from p 15)

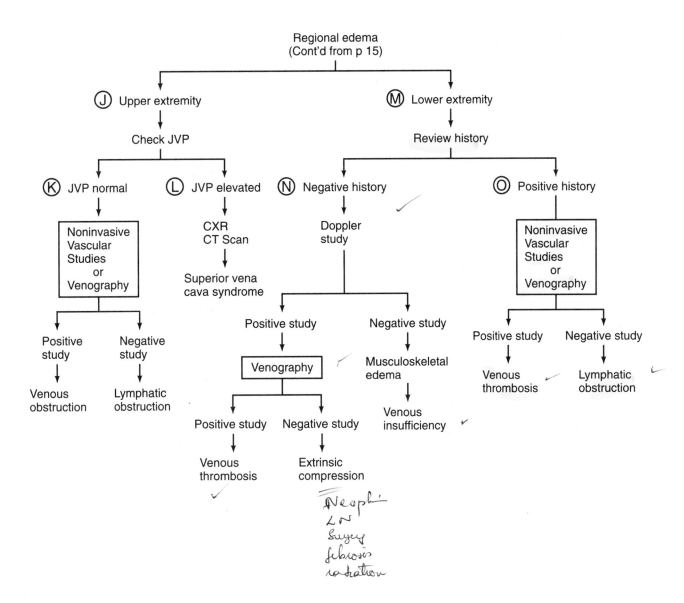

Ⓙ Upper extremity

Check JVP

Ⓚ JVP normal

Noninvasive
Vascular
Studies
or
Venography

Positive
study

Venous
obstruction

Negative
study

Lymphatic
obstruction

Ⓛ JVP elevated

CXR
CT Scan

Superior vena
cava syndrome

Ⓜ Lower extremity

Review history

Ⓝ Negative history

Doppler
study

Positive study

Venography

Positive study

Venous
thrombosis

Negative study

Extrinsic
compression

Negative study

Musculoskeletal
edema

Venous
insufficiency

Ⓞ Positive history

Noninvasive
Vascular
Studies
or
Venography

Positive study

Venous
thrombosis

Negative study

Lymphatic
obstruction

[handwritten] Neopl̄
LN
Surgery
fibrosis
radiation

CHRONIC PAIN

Andrea Binzer, M.D.
William P. Johnson, M.D.

A. The information needed to evaluate the patient includes a detailed history of the pain complaint(s), an understanding of pain characteristics (Table 1), response to past treatments, a thorough understanding of the patient's history (i.e., a review of the often voluminous medical records and psychosocial history), and the temporal relationship of all these factors to the onset and exacerbation of pain.

B. Acute pain is often associated with an increase in circulation, ventilation, and metabolism and a decrease in urinary and GI function. Patients are in obvious pain, and often there are associated findings of pallor, diaphoresis, and nausea.

C. Chronic pain is defined as any pain continuing beyond the usual course of an acute injury process. It can be dangerous to place an arbitrary time limit, such as 6 months, on this definition. For example, the pain of a broken wrist should last, at most, 2 weeks. Any continuing pain may indicate a reflex sympathetic dystrophy. This is a cause of chronic pain in which early recognition and treatment lead to complete recovery. Waiting 6 months to consider this pain chronic could leave the patient with a permanent disability. Patients with constant pain develop vegetative signs: disturbances in sleep and appetite, constipation, increased irritability, decreased libido, psychomotor retardation, and lowered pain tolerance. Patients with intermittent chronic pain (e.g., those with recurrent bouts of neuralgia, headaches, or angina) may have responses similar to those with acute pain.

D. A multidisciplinary pain team may include an internist, psychiatrist, physiatrist, pharmacist, anesthesiologist, neurosurgeon, nurse, dentist, psychologist, physical therapist, and occupational therapist.

E. Chronic benign pain is a diagnostic and management challenge. If possible, it is sometimes useful to localize the pain to the target organ most affected.

F. Some patients do not fit nicely into any of the usual chronic benign pain subcategories. The approach to this group of patients needs to be individualized.

G. All chronic pain patients go through proven psychologic changes while coping with their pain. Psychological and environmental factors play a great role in chronic pain, with 30% of patients becoming clinically depressed. However, psychogenic pain occurs when the pain is a result of psychological mechanisms. The fact that a physician cannot find a specific organic cause for the pain is insufficient, by itself, to warrant a psychiatric diagnosis. Positive evidence for a psychiatric diagnosis must be found. (DSM-3-R criteria should be applied.)

H. A multidisciplinary pain center (MPC) should have on its staff a variety of health care providers capable of assessing and treating physical, psychosocial, medical, vocational, and social aspects of chronic pain. At least three medical specialties should be represented on the staff of an MPC. If one of the physicians is not a psychiatrist, physicians from two specialties and a clinical psychologist are the minimum required. The MPC may take place in either an inpatient or outpatient setting. A MPC should establish protocols for patient management and assess their efficiency periodically. With benign pain the emphasis should be on pain management and rehabilitation, with little or no use of controlled medications.

I. Malignant pain is managed like benign pain; however, narcotic analgesia is less of an issue. A multidisciplinary team can also help with the management of malignant pain, for which therapies other than narcotics can be very useful.

TABLE 1 Pain terminology

Nociceptors	Nerve endings in skin, tissue, and viscera activated by potentially damaging stimuli
Central (neuropathic)	Results from injury, or changes in, somatosensory pathways; may persist without demonstrable nociceptive stimuli.
Allodynia	Perception of non-nociceptive stimuli (e.g., light touch) as painful
Causalgia	Continuous burning pain, usually after nerve injury; may be associated with allodynia, sympathetic dysfunction, and glossy skin
Deafferentation	Central pain that follows direct injury to the peripheral or central nervous system; associated sensations include causalgia, dysesthesia, formications, and/or allodynia
Dysesthesia	An unpleasant sensation (e.g., pins and needles)
Hyperesthesia	Excessive sensitivity to touch, pain, and other sensations
Hyperalgesia	Exaggerated sensitivity to painful stimuli
Hyperpathia	Increased sensitivity to stimuli
Hypoesthesia	Decreased sensitivity to touch, pain, and other sensations
Hypoalgesia	Decreased sensitivity to painful stimuli
Neuralgia	Pain in distribution of a single nerve; usually the result of trauma or irritation

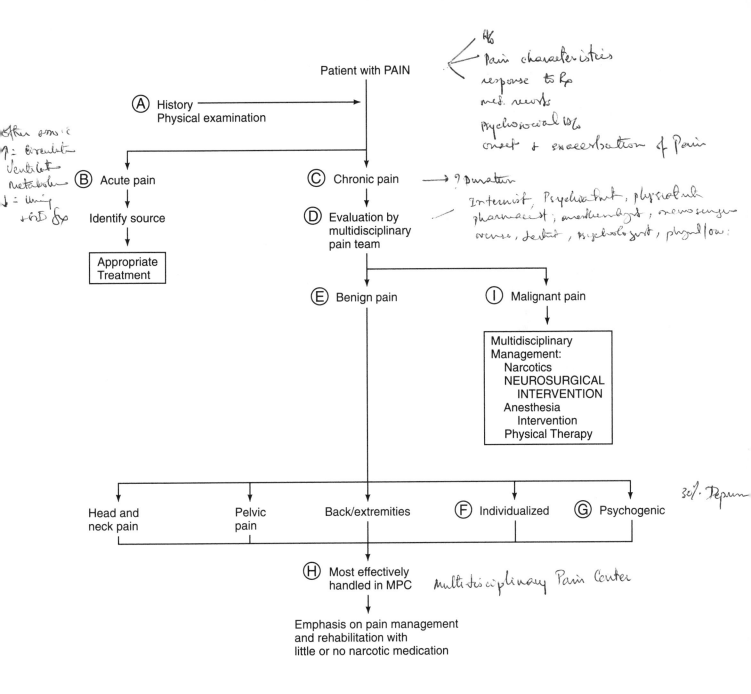

Patient with PAIN

(A) History
Physical examination

(B) Acute pain

Identify source

Appropriate Treatment

(C) Chronic pain

(D) Evaluation by multidisciplinary pain team

(E) Benign pain

(I) Malignant pain

Multidisciplinary Management:
Narcotics
NEUROSURGICAL INTERVENTION
Anesthesia
Intervention
Physical Therapy

Head and neck pain

Pelvic pain

Back/extremities

(F) Individualized

(G) Psychogenic

(H) Most effectively handled in MPC

Emphasis on pain management and rehabilitation with little or no narcotic medication

References

Bonica JJ, ed. The management of pain. 2nd ed. Philadelphia: Lea & Febiger, 1990.

Reuler JB, Girard DE, Nardone DA. The chronic pain syndrome: misconceptions and management. Ann Intern Med 1980; 93:588.

Vasudevan SV, Lynch NT. Pain centers: organization and outcome. In: Rehabilitation medicine—adding life to years (Special Issue). West J Med 1991; 154:532.

Wise MG, Rundell JR. Consultation psychiatry. Washington, D.C.: American Psychiatric Press, 1988.

PERSISTENT EXCESSIVE SWEATING

Lisa Kaufmann, M.D.

A. Several dermatologic conditions are associated with localized hyperhidrosis. There is increased sweating in areas of vitiligo, granulosis rubra nasi, dyshidrotic eczema, pachydermoperiostosis, epidermolysis bullosa, pachyonychia congenita, nail-patella syndrome, palmoplantar keratodermas, and others. These conditions should be detectable on physical examination.

B. Although anxiety or stimulants may increase sweating, some people have severe hyperhidrosis without obvious psychiatric disorder. Such patients often have a family history of hyperhidrosis. Severe hyperhidrosis may cause difficulty with hand work, infection due to the moist environment (especially in the feet), and considerable social distress. Topical treatments have varying success. Removal of the axillary sweat glands or sympathectomy have been reported to give good results in severe cases (see references).

C. A structural lesion in the sympathetic nervous system may cause abnormalities in sweating. Cerebrocortical tumors, stroke, or infection may cause contralateral hyperhidrosis through release of inhibition. When injured sympathetic nerves regrow, connections may develop between the parasympathetic and sympathetic nerves. This can result in sweating of the innervated skin, as seen with gustatory sweating. Spinal cord disease (including syringomyelia, spinal cord injury, tabes dorsalis) may cause segmental areas of hyperhidrosis. Thoracic sympathetic nerve trunk injury may also cause localized hyperhidrosis. A large area of anhidrosis, as in severe diabetic autonomic neuropathy or after a sympathectomy involving more than one limb, may result in compensatory hyperhidrosis of other areas.

D. Many chemicals may cause sweating, either during withdrawal states (as from alcohol or opiates) or with use (e.g., alcohol, some tricyclic antidepressants, cholinergic and adrenergic agents, and acetylcholinesterase inhibitors). Chronic ingestion of mercury or arsenic can cause excessive sweating.

E. Malaria, tuberculosis, brucellosis, abdominal abscesses, rheumatic fever, and endocarditis may commonly present with fevers and sweats as the predominant symptoms, but any infection producing a fever may cause sweating through the hypothalamic temperature regulatory centers as the fever falls. Even after a severe febrile illness resolves, patients may continue to have sweats for days to months.

F. Certain malignant conditions, including lymphoma, monocytic leukemia, and renal carcinoma, classically cause fevers, but fever with associated sweats may also be found in other malignancies. Carcinoid syndrome may cause excessive sweating. Rheumatologic diseases associated with excessive sweating include rheumatoid arthritis and Raynaud's.

G. Other endocrine causes of hyperhidrosis include menopause, pregnancy, diabetes mellitus, gout, obesity, porphyria, rickets, and hyperpituitarism. In some cases of hypoglycemia, CNS dysfunction and sweats may occur in the absence of other adrenergic symptoms.

References

Champion RH. Disorders of the sweat glands. In: Rook A, Wilkinson DS, Ebling FTG, et al., eds. Textbook of dermatology. London: Blackwell Scientific Publications, 1986:1881.

Hurley HJ. The eccrine sweat glands. In: Moscella SC, Hurley HJ, eds. Dermatology. Philadelphia: WB Saunders, 1985:1341.

Patient with PERSISTENT EXCESSIVE SWEATING

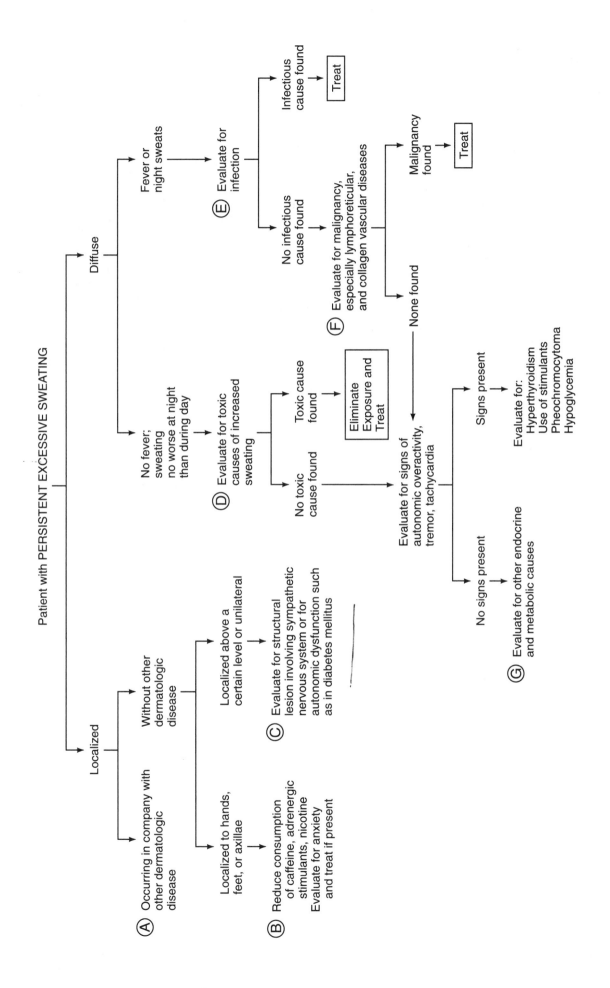

A Occurring in company with other dermatologic disease

Localized

Without other dermatologic disease

Localized to hands, feet, or axillae

B Reduce consumption of caffeine, adrenergic stimulants, nicotine Evaluate for anxiety and treat if present

Localized above a certain level or unilateral

C Evaluate for structural lesion involving sympathetic nervous system or for autonomic dysfunction such as in diabetes mellitus

Diffuse

No fever; sweating no worse at night than during day

D Evaluate for toxic causes of increased sweating

Toxic cause found

Eliminate Exposure and Treat

No toxic cause found

Evaluate for signs of autonomic overactivity, tremor, tachycardia

Signs present

Evaluate for:
Hyperthyroidism
Use of stimulants
Pheochromocytoma
Hypoglycemia

No signs present

G Evaluate for other endocrine and metabolic causes

Fever or night sweats

E Evaluate for infection

Infectious cause found

Treat

No infectious cause found

F Evaluate for malignancy, especially lymphoreticular, and collagen vascular diseases

Malignancy found

Treat

None found

ACUTE RED EYE

Lisa Kaufmann, M.D.

Although most cases of red eye can be successfully treated by the primary care physician, some uncommon causes of red eye require ophthalmologic intervention. In some conditions, such as acute glaucoma or penetrating ocular trauma, emergent ophthalmologic intervention can save sight. General points in evaluation of a red eye that should trigger serious concern about possible urgent eye disease include visual loss, corneal haziness, opacities in the eye, new pupillary irregularities, ciliary flush, noticeable alterations in pressure of a red eye by finger examination of the lid, previous serious eye disease such as iritis, glaucoma, or ocular pain not due to a superficial corneal abrasion. Even if these are *absent* and the initial diagnosis is of a less serious cause of red eye, failure to respond to appropriate therapy in 2–3 days should trigger re-evaluation. Ocular topical steroids should generally be avoided unless an opthalmologist has prescribed them.

A. Blurred vision is a common complaint in conjunctivitis due to tears and mucus, but it should clear with blinking. Any blurred vision that does not clear with blinking, or any sudden decrease in visual acuity, should receive urgent ophthalmologic evaluation. Recurrence of a red eye in a patient with a history of uveitis or glaucoma may indicate a flare-up of disease even if no visual symptoms are present.

B. Laceration of the globe or a history of metal or rock fragments entering the eye (as may occur when machining or metal working without adequate protective eye wear) should prompt an urgent ophthalmology examination, since foreign bodies in the globe may lead rapidly to serious infections or foreign body reactions. Blood visible in the vitreous may be due to an underlying retinal detachment, and blood in the anterior chamber may lead to scarring. Both conditions should be urgently referred to ophthalmology.

C. Patients with a history of chemical burns of the eye should receive copious irrigation with sterile saline for at least 5 minutes and should be seen as soon as possible by an ophthalmologist.

D. Corneal ulcers may be traumatic, bacterial (including *Pseudomonas,* which may produce a bluish green exudate; gonococcal, which can rapidly appear if the hyperacute purulent conjunctivitis of initial gonococcal infection is not treated and which may perforate; or viral, especially herpes, which may cause a classic dendritic appearance or may look like a scratch. Amebae may cause corneal ulcers, especially in contact lens wearers who cold sterilize their lenses. Fungi can cause ulcers even in normal hosts. Because of the wide variety of organisms that may cause corneal ulcers, these patients need microscopic examination of smears and cultures to guide therapy. In most cases this requires urgent ophthalmologic evaluation.

(Continued on page 24)

Possible Urgent eye dx. → Visual loss
corneal haziness
opacities of eye
unequal pupil
ciliary flush
alteration of pressure by finger exam
previous eye dx
- glaucoma
- iritis

failure to respond therapy in 2 - 3 d

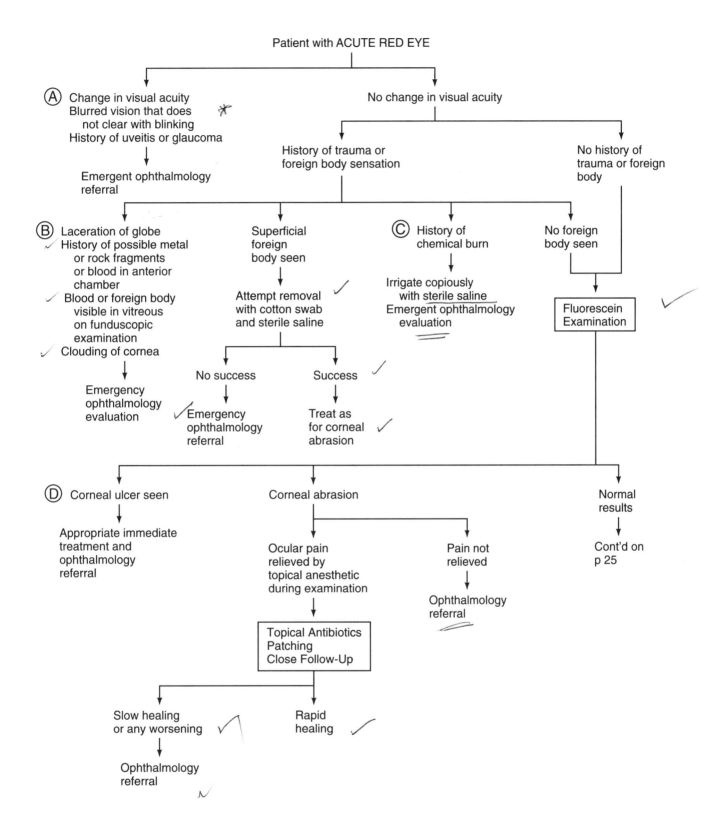

Patient with ACUTE RED EYE

A Change in visual acuity
Blurred vision that does
not clear with blinking
History of uveitis or glaucoma

No change in visual acuity

Emergent ophthalmology
referral

History of trauma or
foreign body sensation

No history of
trauma or foreign
body

B Laceration of globe
History of possible metal
or rock fragments
or blood in anterior
chamber
Blood or foreign body
visible in vitreous
on funduscopic
examination
Clouding of cornea

Superficial
foreign
body seen

C History of
chemical burn

No foreign
body seen

Attempt removal
with cotton swab
and sterile saline

Irrigate copiously
with sterile saline
Emergent ophthalmology
evaluation

Fluorescein
Examination

Emergency
ophthalmology
evaluation

No success

Success

Emergency
ophthalmology
referral

Treat as
for corneal
abrasion

D Corneal ulcer seen

Corneal abrasion

Normal
results

Appropriate immediate
treatment and
ophthalmology
referral

Ocular pain
relieved by
topical anesthetic
during examination

Pain not
relieved

Cont'd on
p 25

Ophthalmology
referral

Topical Antibiotics
Patching
Close Follow-Up

Slow healing
or any worsening

Rapid
healing

Ophthalmology
referral

E. A localized area of painless, wedge-shaped hemorrhage over an otherwise normal sclera, with an otherwise normal eye examination, usually represents a subconjunctival hematoma that will resolve spontaneously. If it recurs, evaluate for disorders of hemostasis.

F. Episcleritis causes a localized area of erythema over the sclera, usually pie shaped, with an otherwise normal ocular examination. It usually responds well to short-term topical vasoconstrictor therapy. If it recurs, obtain ophthalmologic consultation.

G. Sexually transmitted diseases (STDs) such as chlamydia and syphilis may cause conjunctivitis. Trachoma and other ocular infections may be acquired abroad. Complete evaluation may require ophthalmologic or infectious disease consultation and is beyond the scope of this chapter.

H. Erythema or increased vascularity that is more intense around the edge of the iris than over the remainder of the sclera usually indicates serious eye disease. It can be seen with iritis and acute glaucoma, and with other causes of intraocular inflammation. Absence of a ciliary flush does not rule out serious eye disease.

References

Coles WH. Ophthalmology: a diagnostic text. Baltimore: Williams & Wilkins, 1984, chapters 1, 2, 6, 9.

Havener W. Diagnosis and management of the red eye. In: Synopsis of ophthalmology. St. Louis: Mosby–Year Book, 1984:255.

Trobe J. The emergent eye. Emerg Med, 1978; 10:25.

Normal results of fluorescein examination
(Cont'd from p 23)

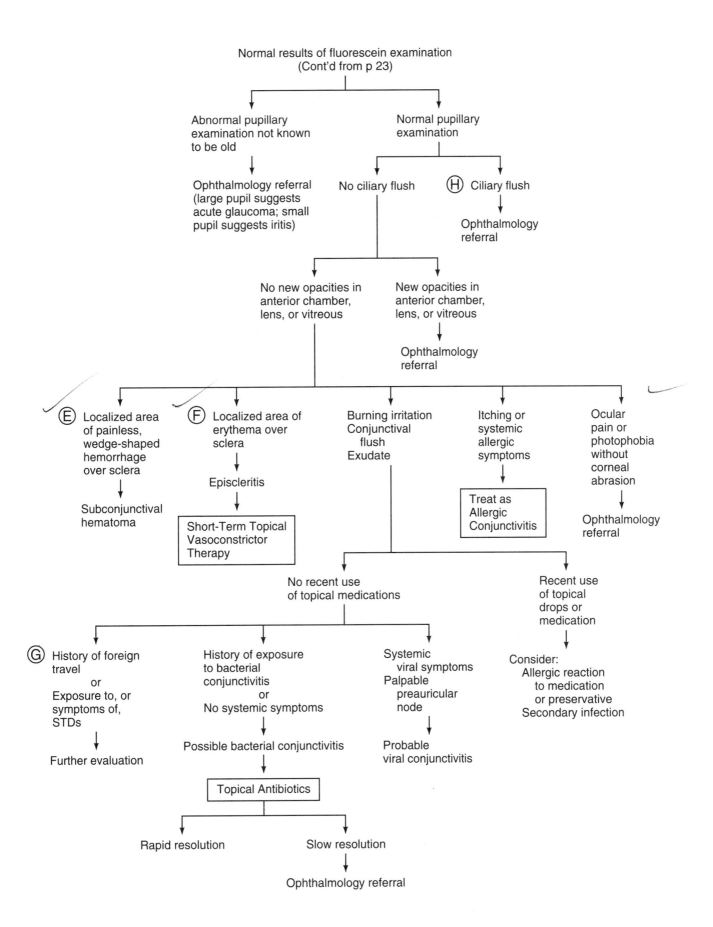

Abnormal pupillary examination not known to be old

Ophthalmology referral (large pupil suggests acute glaucoma; small pupil suggests iritis)

Normal pupillary examination

No ciliary flush

(H) Ciliary flush

Ophthalmology referral

No new opacities in anterior chamber, lens, or vitreous

New opacities in anterior chamber, lens, or vitreous

Ophthalmology referral

(E) Localized area of painless, wedge-shaped hemorrhage over sclera

Subconjunctival hematoma

(F) Localized area of erythema over sclera

Episcleritis

Short-Term Topical Vasoconstrictor Therapy

Burning irritation Conjunctival flush Exudate

Itching or systemic allergic symptoms

Treat as Allergic Conjunctivitis

Ocular pain or photophobia without corneal abrasion

Ophthalmology referral

No recent use of topical medications

Recent use of topical drops or medication

Consider: Allergic reaction to medication or preservative Secondary infection

(G) History of foreign travel
or
Exposure to, or symptoms of, STDs

Further evaluation

History of exposure to bacterial conjunctivitis
or
No systemic symptoms

Possible bacterial conjunctivitis

Topical Antibiotics

Systemic viral symptoms Palpable preauricular node

Probable viral conjunctivitis

Rapid resolution

Slow resolution

Ophthalmology referral

CHRONIC RED EYE

Lisa Kaufmann, M.D.

A. Any of these findings suggest intraocular or retro-ocular diseases, which require ophthalmologic referral. These include tumors (e.g., an intraocular melanoma may present as a localized area of increased vascularity on the sclera), uveitis, and glaucoma.

B. Patients may become sensitized to nonprescription drops, which usually may simply be discontinued. Sensitization to chronic prescription drops, either the active ingredient or the preservative, should generate a referral back to the prescribing ophthalmologist. Ill-fitting or improperly cleaned contact lenses may also cause chronic red eye in contact lens users; the lenses should be evaluated in such cases.

C. Many systemic diseases may manifest as red eye: infectious diseases such as tuberculosis, nutritional deficiencies such as vitamin A deficiency, mucous membrane immune-mediated diseases such as Stevens-Johnson syndrome, alcoholism, and many others. A careful history and physical examination will reveal associated findings for most of these disorders.

D. The tear film normally contains mucous, aqueous, and oil layers. A defect in mucus or oil production may produce irritation even if aqueous production remains intact. Autoimmune diseases involving the lacrimal gland, such as Sjögren's syndrome, may produce dry eyes. Defective blinking (due to weakness as in Bell's palsy or to lid deformity) may cause serious dry eyes. There may be decreased tear production with advancing age, especially noticeable when humidity is low. A careful drug history is important because anticholinergics (including tricyclic antidepressants), diuretics, and some other medications may cause dry eyes.

E. Blepharitis is inflammation of the lid margins. This may be irritant (related to eye makeup or seborrheic dermatitis), related to infection (usually staphylococcal), or both.

F. Chronic conjunctivitis may be due to Chlamydia (including trachoma), syphilis, chronic viral infection, or multiple other causes.

References

Coles WH. Ophthalmology: a diagnostic text. Baltimore: Williams & Wilkins, 1984: Chapters 1, 2, 6, 9.

Havener W. Diagnosis and management of the red eye. In: Synopsis of ophthalmology. St. Louis: Mosby–Year Book, 1984: 255.

Trobe J. The emergent eye. Emerg Med 1978:25.

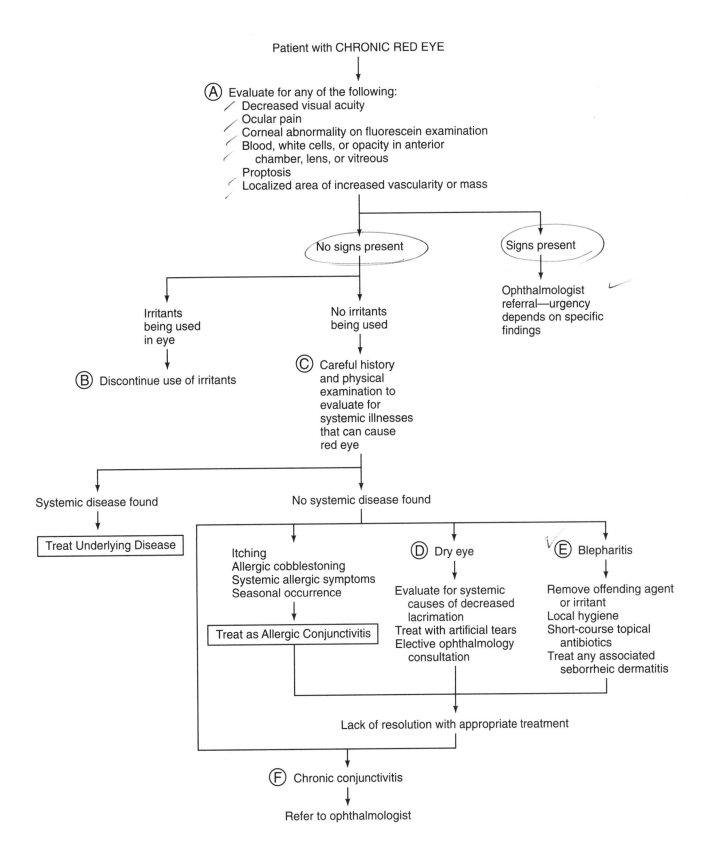

Patient with CHRONIC RED EYE

A Evaluate for any of the following:
  Decreased visual acuity
  Ocular pain
  Corneal abnormality on fluorescein examination
  Blood, white cells, or opacity in anterior
    chamber, lens, or vitreous
  Proptosis
  Localized area of increased vascularity or mass

No signs present   Signs present

Ophthalmologist referral—urgency depends on specific findings

Irritants being used in eye   No irritants being used

B Discontinue use of irritants

C Careful history and physical examination to evaluate for systemic illnesses that can cause red eye

Systemic disease found   No systemic disease found

Treat Underlying Disease

Itching
Allergic cobblestoning
Systemic allergic symptoms
Seasonal occurrence

D Dry eye

E Blepharitis

Treat as Allergic Conjunctivitis

Evaluate for systemic causes of decreased lacrimation
Treat with artificial tears
Elective ophthalmology consultation

Remove offending agent or irritant
Local hygiene
Short-course topical antibiotics
Treat any associated seborrheic dermatitis

Lack of resolution with appropriate treatment

F Chronic conjunctivitis

Refer to ophthalmologist

RHINITIS

Seth Weissman, M.D.

A. Because many of these clinical entities have similar presentations, it is important to perform a careful examination of conjunctivae, nares, tympanic membranes, teeth, and pharynx in addition to transillumination.

B. In a patient with previously normal sinuses, complete opacity provides strong evidence of infection. Dullness may signify infection in about one third of patients. Normal transillumination usually indicates absence of infection. False positives occur with chronic sinusitis, solid tumors, and bony abnormalities.

C. Clues to viral rhinitis include clear mucoid nasal secretions with abundant neutrophils, exposure to persons with similar symptoms, and occurrence in fall or spring. Sore or scratchy throat is seen in 50% of patients; cough in 30%.

D. Symptomatic treatment includes rest, hydration, early continuous use of nasal decongestants, and analgesics. Aspirin should be avoided because of epidemiologic evidence linking Reye's syndrome to its use in children and adolescents with influenza or varicella infections.

E. Clues to acute sinusitis include purulent nasal discharge, facial pain, pain with mastication, toothache, and recent upper respiratory infection. Fever is noted in <50% of patients. Radiographs are very sensitive but expensive. They may be necessary to confirm the diagnosis in patients with equivocal results on transillumination, with an unusual presentation, or where empiric therapy has failed.

F. In a recent series, 50% of isolates from adult patients with community-acquired maxillary sinusitis showed either *Streptococcus pneumoniae* or unencapsulated *Haemophilus influenzae*. In acute disease, anaerobes can be found in 10% of cases and are usually associated with dental disease. Reasonable empiric antibiotic therapy could be a 10-day course of amoxicillin or trimethoprim-sulfamethoxazole. Topical decongestants are a helpful adjunct. Antihistamine use may result in increased thickness of secretions and probably is not indicated.

G. Potential complications of acute sinusitis include osteomyelitis, dacrocystitis, epidural or subdural abscess, meningitis, dural sinus thrombosis, and brain abscess. Nosocomial sinusitis (due to nasotracheal intubation or nasal packing) usually occurs in the second week of hospitalization and is often caused by gram-negative organisms. Fungal sinusitis (invasive aspergillosis, mucormycosis) is seen in severely immunocompromised patients and those with diabetes mellitus or chronic renal failure. It can be aggressive and lethal if not treated promptly with surgical debridement and antifungal agents. Noninvasive aspergillus may cause sinusitis uncommonly in immunocompetent patients. CT scan and antral puncture should be considered earlier in immunocompromised patients, those with nosocomial or post-traumatic infections, or those who show evidence of craniofacial complications. Nasal swabs or irrigation do not give useful information in determining the microbes responsible for causing sinusitis. The role of sinoscopy is evolving, and it may be useful in complicated cases.

H. Prolonged, repeated episodes of sinusitis may lead to irreversible changes in the mucosal lining of the sinuses and subsequent chronic sinusitis. This may be associated with polyposis and adenoid hyperplasia. Anaerobes are cultured in up to 50% of cases, but antibiotic therapy is seldom successful. The clinician can treat any coexisting allergic or obstructive components that may be contributing to the symptoms, and needs to eliminate dental infection as an underlying cause, but many of these patients ultimately require surgical intervention.

I. Allergic rhinitis is commonly associated with sneezing, tearing, and itching of nose, eyes, conjunctivae, and pharynx. Examination may reveal boggy turbinates, nasal obstruction, conjunctival injection, and periorbital swelling. Allergies may be seasonal (pollens in spring/summer or ragweed in summer/fall) or perennial (mold). Treatment consists of avoidance of identified allergens, pharmocologic therapy, and immunotherapy if other forms of treatment fail and symptoms persist for more than 6 weeks per year.

J. Negative skin test responses with common inhalant antigens indicate that the rhinitis is nonallergic. IgE is elevated in 30–40% of patients with allergic rhinitis, and eosinophils in the nasal smear and an increased blood eosinophil count may be seen.

K. Vasomotor rhinitis is perennial and has no correlation with specific antigens. It is often worsened by changes in temperature and humidity, exposure to noxious odors, spicy foods, or ethanol, and emotional upset or sexual arousal. The nasal smear is unremarkable.

L. Rhinitis medicamentosa may be due to a rebound effect from use of nasal sprays as well as to estrogens (including oral contraceptives), reserpine, hydralazine, or alpha-methyldopa.

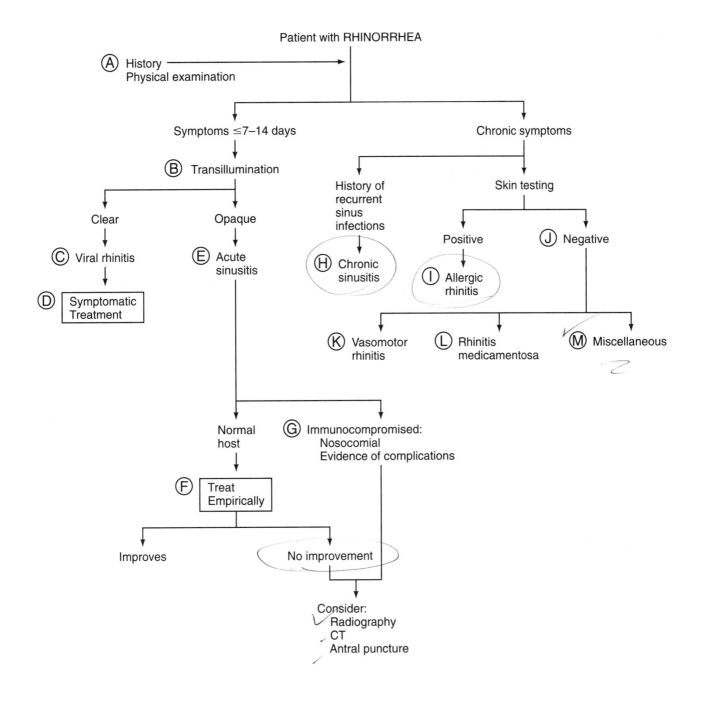

Patient with RHINORRHEA

Ⓐ History
Physical examination

Symptoms ≤7–14 days

Ⓑ Transillumination

Clear

Ⓒ Viral rhinitis

Ⓓ Symptomatic Treatment

Opaque

Ⓔ Acute sinusitis

Normal host

Ⓕ Treat Empirically

Improves

No improvement

Ⓖ Immunocompromised:
Nosocomial
Evidence of complications

Consider:
Radiography
CT
Antral puncture

Chronic symptoms

History of recurrent sinus infections

Ⓗ Chronic sinusitis

Skin testing

Positive

Ⓘ Allergic rhinitis

Ⓙ Negative

Ⓚ Vasomotor rhinitis

Ⓛ Rhinitis medicamentosa

Ⓜ Miscellaneous

M. Miscellaneous causes of rhinitis include structural abnormalities, congenital and post-traumatic changes, tumor, pregnancy, hypothyroidism, mucociliary defects, and opioid withdrawal.

References

Daley CL, Sande M. The runny nose: infection of the paranasal sinuses. Infect Dis Clin North Am 1988; 2:131.

Gwaltney JM. Rhinovirus. In: Mandel GL, ed. Principles and practice of infectious diseases. 3rd ed. New York: Churchill Livingstone, 1990:1399.

Gwaltney JM. Sinusitis. In: Mandel GL, ed. Principles and practice of infectious diseases. 3rd ed. New York: Churchill Livingstone, 1990:510.

Kapikian AZ. The common cold. In: Wyngaarden JB, ed. Cecil textbook of medicine. 18th ed. Philadelphia: WB Saunders, 1988:1753.

Salvaggio JE. Allergic rhinitis. In: Wyngaarden JB, Smith LH, eds. Cecil textbook of medicine. 18th ed. Philadelphia: WB Saunders, 1988:1951.

TINNITUS

Susan Fisk Sander, M.D.

A. Tinnitus is a perceived sound that cannot be related to an external source. Particular attention should be paid to any history of noise exposure, previous ear surgery, drug exposure, trauma, diabetes mellitus, hyper- or hypothyroidism, cerebrovascular accidents (CVAs), or multiple sclerosis. Associated symptoms such as hearing loss, vertigo, and otalgia should be noted. Hearing loss is the most common associated symptom, and increasing intensity of tinnitus correlates with worsening hearing loss. Tinnitus may be divided into subjective (observed only by the patient) and objective (observed by patient and examiner) forms. Objective tinnitus is uncommon and its cause is usually found. Subjective tinnitus is common and its cause is more difficult to determine.

B. Tinnitus cerebre is defined as a perceived sound that is not localized to either ear and is diffuse. Encephalitis of the temporal lobe and psychiatric illnesses must be considered. Auditory hallucinations are noted primarily in patients with psychosis.

C. Tinnitus aurium is a perceived sound that does not come from an external source and is localized to one or both ears. It is divided into vibratory (perceived by both examiner and patient) and nonvibratory (totally subjective) forms.

D. Nonvibratory tinnitus lesions may be attributed to defects in the cochlea (75%), CNS (18%), and middle ear (4%). In patients with hearing loss that is not treatable by a surgical procedure, a hearing device may improve tinnitus. Hearing aids and masking devices may be used together for patients who do not respond to hearing aids alone. Recent literature supports the use of auditory brain response in evaluating the site of the lesion; it objectivizes tinnitus and helps determine the type and frequency of the masking device.

E. Eustachian tube patency may be noted with weight loss, in high-estrogen states as associated with birth control pills, and post partum. This may result in patients experiencing autophony, or hearing of their own voice.

References

Deweese DD, Saunders WH, Schuller DE, Schleuning AJ III. Otolaryngology—Head and neck surgery. 7th ed. St. Louis: Mosby—Year Book, 1988.

Meyerhoff WL, Cooper JC. Tinnitus. In: Paparella MM, ed. Otolaryngology. 2nd ed. Philadelphia: WB Saunders, 1980:1861.

Shulman A. Diagnosis of tinnitus. In: Kitahara M, ed. Tinnitus: pathophysiology and management. New York: Igaku-Shoin, 1988:53.

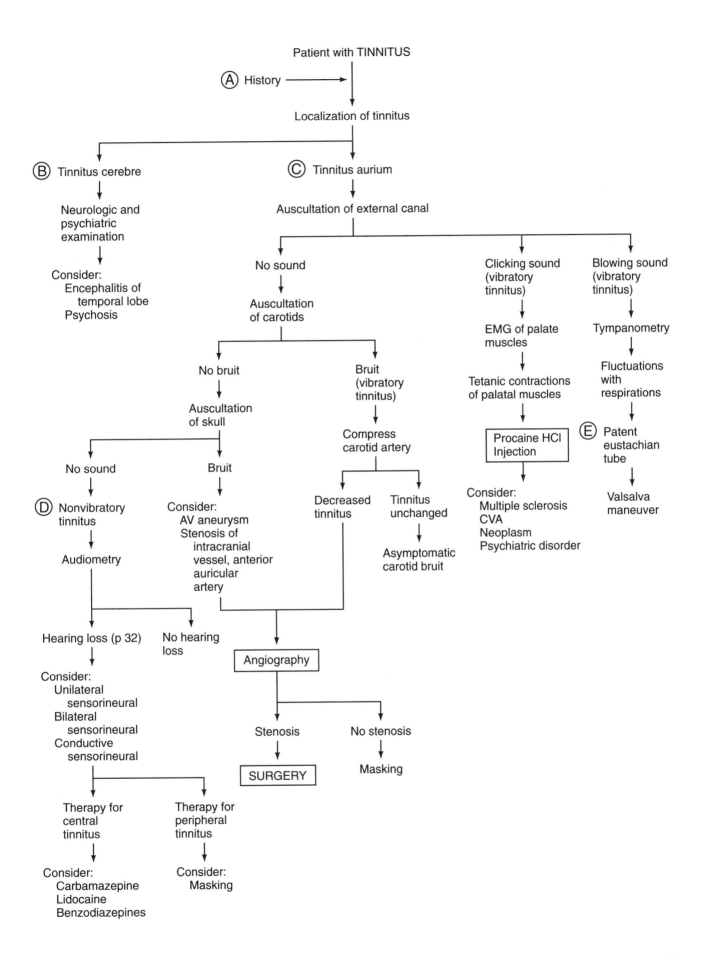

Patient with TINNITUS

Ⓐ History →

Localization of tinnitus

Ⓑ Tinnitus cerebre

Neurologic and
psychiatric
examination

Consider:
 Encephalitis of
  temporal lobe
 Psychosis

Ⓒ Tinnitus aurium

Auscultation of external canal

No sound

Auscultation
of carotids

No bruit

Auscultation
of skull

No sound

Ⓓ Nonvibratory
tinnitus

Audiometry

Hearing loss (p 32)   No hearing
                        loss

Consider:
 Unilateral
  sensorineural
 Bilateral
  sensorineural
 Conductive
  sensorineural

Therapy for   Therapy for
central   peripheral
tinnitus   tinnitus

Consider: Consider:
 Carbamazepine   Masking
 Lidocaine
 Benzodiazepines

Bruit

Consider:
 AV aneurysm
 Stenosis of
  intracranial
  vessel, anterior
  auricular
  artery

Bruit
(vibratory
tinnitus)

Compress
carotid artery

Decreased   Tinnitus
tinnitus   unchanged

                Asymptomatic
                carotid bruit

Angiography

Stenosis   No stenosis

SURGERY   Masking

Clicking sound
(vibratory
tinnitus)

EMG of palate
muscles

Tetanic contractions
of palatal muscles

Procaine HCl
Injection

Consider:
 Multiple sclerosis
 CVA
 Neoplasm
 Psychiatric disorder

Blowing sound
(vibratory
tinnitus)

Tympanometry

Fluctuations
with
respirations

Ⓔ Patent
 eustachian
 tube

Valsalva
maneuver

HEARING LOSS

Susan Fisk Sander, M.D.

A. Approximately 50% of the 16 million hearing-impaired Americans are >65 years old. Particular attention should be paid to any history of acoustic or physical trauma or barotrauma; deafness; exposure to ototoxins; recent upper respiratory infection; or associated symptoms such as otalgia, tinnitus, or vertigo.

B. Physical examination of the ear should include otoscopy and evaluation of the external auditory canal, tympanic membrane, and ossicles. Rule out otitis externa, foreign body in the external canal, ceruminal impaction, canal cholesteatoma, exostosis, tympanic membrane perforation, effusions (hemorrhagic, purulent, or serous), and ossicular discontinuity. Weber's and Rinne's tests are performed in all patients with hearing loss to further define sensorineural or conductive hearing loss. Weber's test is performed by placing a tuning fork on the central forehead. Lateralization of the sound to one ear is consistent with either a conductive defect to the affected ear or a sensorineural defect to the opposite ear. No lateralization indicates either a normal result or bilaterally symmetric sensorineural or conductive defects. This test, in conjunction with Rinne's test, supports either a sensorineural or a conductive disorder.

C. Audiography includes pure tone testing of air and bone thresholds, speech reception, speech discrimination, and acoustic impedance. Sensorineural losses reveal a pattern in which both air and bone thresholds are depressed as compared with normal. In conductive hearing loss the bone conduction threshold is greater than air conduction thresholds. In mixed deficits the air conduction is less than bone conduction, both being depressed.

D. Sensorineural hearing loss is defined as a lesion in the organ of Corti or in the central pathways, including the eighth nerve and auditory cortex. Metabolic examination of bilateral progressive sensorineural deficits include evaluation for diabetes mellitus, hyper- and hypothyroidism, anemia, hypo- and hypertension, and renal disease. Infection evaluation includes an FTA-Abs for neurosyphilis. Syphilis may present with a waxing and waning, usually bilateral sensorineural hearing loss. Many medications have been noted to affect hearing. The aminoglycoside antibiotics and diuretics are the most common drugs causing hearing loss; others include quinine, chloroquine, and antineoplastics such as cis-platinum. Therapy is aimed at the underlying cause: removal of the offending drug, treatment of the autoimmune disease, and antibiotics for syphilis. For acoustic trauma and presbycusis, a hearing aid evaluation is warranted.

E. Congenital hearing deficits include maternal viral infections during pregnancy (e.g., cytomegalovirus, rubella, and mumps). Other possibilities include Rh incompatibility, anoxia at birth, and exposure to fetal ototoxins.

F. Hereditary disorders of hearing loss are numerous and include Waardenburg's syndrome, Crouzon's disease, Paget's disease, Alport's disease, and Pendred's disease.

G. Temporal bone fractures occur longitudinally or transversely. The longitudinal fracture usually results in middle ear damage and is associated with a conductive hearing loss. The transverse fracture may damage the facial nerve and the labyrinth and result in a sensorineural deficit. Both require referral to an otolaryngologist.

H. Conductive hearing loss is defined as a lesion involving the outer and middle ear to the level of the oval window. Physical examination has assessed external and middle ear sources: atresias of the external canal, ceruminal impaction, exostosis, foreign bodies, canal cholesteatoma, external otitis, tympanic membrane perforation or sclerosis, effusions, and ossicular damage. Tuberculous infection of the inner ear must be included in the differential diagnosis; it has the classic presentation of multiple perforations of the typanic membrane. Therapy should address the underlying problem: removal of the foreign body or cerumen, antituberculous drugs, and removal of excessive cartilage in exostosis.

References

Cody DT, Kern EB, Pearson BW. Diseases of the ears, nose and throat. Chicago: Year–Book, 1981.

Deweese DD, Saunders WH, Schuller DE, Schleuning AJ III. Otolaryngology–Head and neck surgery. 7th ed. St. Louis: Mosby–Year Book, 1988.

Levine S. Diseases of the inner ear. In: Adams GL, ed. Boie's fundamentals of otolaryngology, 6th ed. Philadelphia: WB Saunders, 1989:123.

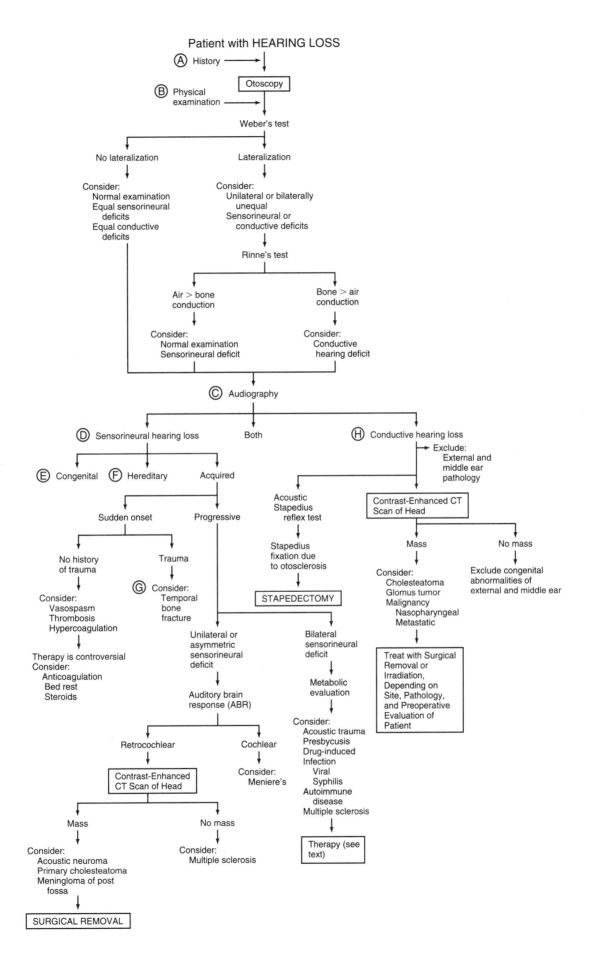

Patient with HEARING LOSS

Ⓐ History

Otoscopy

Ⓑ Physical examination

Weber's test

No lateralization

Consider:
Normal examination
Equal sensorineural deficits
Equal conductive deficits

Lateralization

Consider:
Unilateral or bilaterally unequal
Sensorineural or conductive deficits

Rinne's test

Air > bone conduction

Consider:
Normal examination
Sensorineural deficit

Bone > air conduction

Consider:
Conductive hearing deficit

Ⓒ Audiography

Ⓓ Sensorineural hearing loss

Both

Ⓗ Conductive hearing loss

→ Exclude:
External and middle ear pathology

Ⓔ Congenital   Ⓕ Hereditary   Acquired

Acoustic Stapedius reflex test

Contrast-Enhanced CT Scan of Head

Sudden onset   Progressive

Stapedius fixation due to otosclerosis

Mass

No mass

No history of trauma   Trauma

STAPEDECTOMY

Consider:
Cholesteatoma
Glomus tumor
Malignancy
Nasopharyngeal
Metastatic

Exclude congenital abnormalities of external and middle ear

Consider:
Vasospasm
Thrombosis
Hypercoagulation

Ⓖ Consider:
Temporal bone fracture

Therapy is controversial
Consider:
Anticoagulation
Bed rest
Steroids

Unilateral or asymmetric sensorineural deficit

Bilateral sensorineural deficit

Treat with Surgical Removal or Irradiation, Depending on Site, Pathology, and Preoperative Evaluation of Patient

Auditory brain response (ABR)

Metabolic evaluation

Consider:
Acoustic trauma
Presbycusis
Drug-induced
Infection
  Viral
  Syphilis
Autoimmune disease
Multiple sclerosis

Retrocochlear   Cochlear

Contrast-Enhanced CT Scan of Head

Consider:
Meniere's

Therapy (see text)

Mass   No mass

Consider:
Acoustic neuroma
Primary cholesteatoma
Meningioma of post fossa

Consider:
Multiple sclerosis

SURGICAL REMOVAL

PERIOPERATIVE EVALUATION

William P. Johnson, M.D.
Farrell Lloyd, M.D.

General internists are frequently asked to perform a medical consultation for surgical patients. The duties of the consultant may be divided into perioperative evaluation and postoperative care. In fulfilling this task, the consultant identifies patient factors that could increase the risk of the operation and provides recommendations on how to minimize the surgical risk. Preoperative risks may be patient related, procedure related, provider related, and anesthetic related. The focus of this chapter is patient-related risk.

A. Advances in anesthetic and surgical techniques have made operative death uncommon, the usual risk of mortality being 0–0.01%, but with a range of 0.01% (low) to >20% (high). When asked to evaluate a patient for surgery, the internist estimates the risk on the basis of as much objective data as possible. The initial assessment involves determining the status of the patient's health and the urgency of the surgery. If there is evidence of major organ system impairment, how severe is the impairment, and does it affect or increase the operative risk? If there is no reason to delay the surgery, what perioperative management is appropriate for the individual patient? An acceptable description of risk may be the following: low risk (0–0.01% mortality), low but increased (0.01 –0.09% mortality), significant risk (1–5% mortality), moderate risk (5–10% mortality), high risk (>10%– <20%), and very high risk (>20%). Note that risk assessment is based on a calculated mortality rate, but morbidity is also an important component in the final recommendations.

B. Various authors have reviewed the cardiac risk of noncardiac surgery. An important step toward objective classification of cardiac risk was the development by Goldman and co-workers of a Multifactorial Cardiac Risk Index (MCRI) (Table 1). The MCRI is useful when used as adjunctive data, especially if the patient has multiple risk factors. Since the development of the MCRI, other authors have modified the index, but there is no convincing evidence that any one is better than the others. The outcomes predicted by the MCRI are death and life-threatening complications; a patient may still develop a lesser cardiac event that the MCRI was not designed to predict. Of note, 31 of the 53 possible risk points are in concern areas that might be corrected preoperatively.

C. Although pulmonary disease presents less risk of death with surgery than cardiac disease does, respiratory complications are common and potentially serious. Chronic obstructive pulmonary disease (COPD) is the primary risk, in part because adequate flow rates are necessary to generate an effective cough. Factors that increase the chance of postoperative pulmonary complications in a patient with COPD include a smoking history, obesity, age >60 years, duration of anesthesia >3 hours, and type of surgery. Pulmonary function tests alone cannot always identify a patient at risk of serious respiratory complication, but they are probably the most reliable objective indicator of operative risk. When the operative site is the thoracic cavity, there may be a need for more sophisticated pulmonary function assessment.

TABLE 1 Multifactorial Cardiac Risk Index

Variable	Points
S3 gallop or increased jugular venous distension (JVD)	11
MI in past 6 mo	10
Rhythm other than sinus	7
Age >70 years	5
Emergency surgery	4
Intraperitoneal, intrathoracic, or aortic operation	3
Suspected critical aortic stenosis	3
Poor general medical condition (K^+ <3.0, Po_2 <60 mm Hg or Pco_2 >50 mm Hg, BUN $\geq$50, creatinine 3 mg/dl, chronic liver disease or patient bedridden)	3

Operative risks may be classed as:		
	I (low)	0–5 points
	II	6–12 points
	III	13–25 points
	IV (high)	>25 points

From Goldman L. Cardiac risks and complications of noncardiac surgery. Ann Intern Med 1983; 98:504.

(Continued on page 36)

Patient for PREOPERATIVE ASSESSMENT

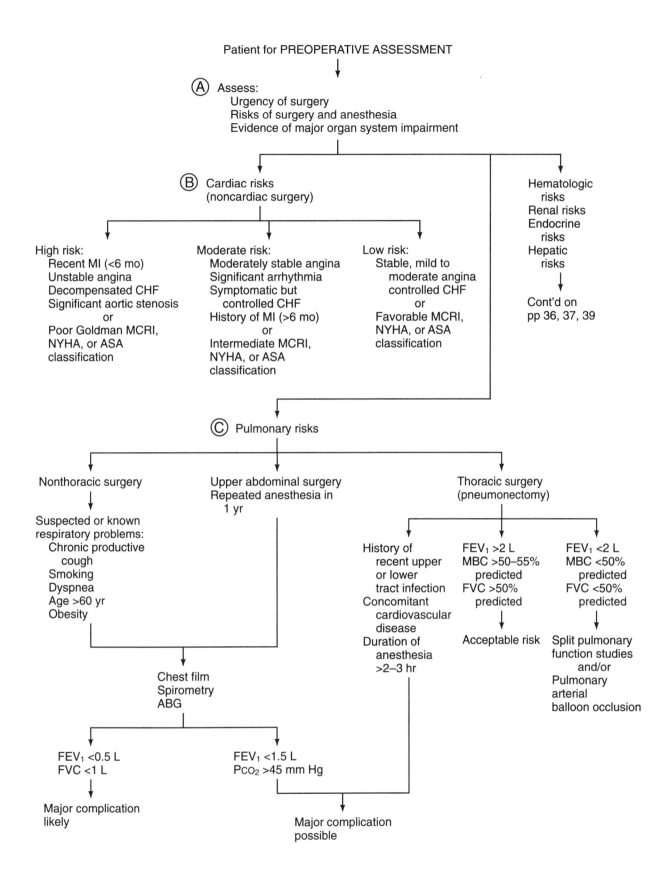

(A) Assess:
  Urgency of surgery
  Risks of surgery and anesthesia
  Evidence of major organ system impairment

(B) Cardiac risks
  (noncardiac surgery)

High risk:
  Recent MI (<6 mo)
  Unstable angina
  Decompensated CHF
  Significant aortic stenosis
  or
  Poor Goldman MCRI,
  NYHA, or ASA
  classification

Moderate risk:
  Moderately stable angina
  Significant arrhythmia
  Symptomatic but
    controlled CHF
  History of MI (>6 mo)
  or
  Intermediate MCRI,
  NYHA, or ASA
  classification

Low risk:
  Stable, mild to
    moderate angina
    controlled CHF
  or
  Favorable MCRI,
  NYHA, or ASA
  classification

Hematologic
  risks
Renal risks
Endocrine
  risks
Hepatic
  risks

Cont'd on
pp 36, 37, 39

(C) Pulmonary risks

Nonthoracic surgery

Suspected or known
respiratory problems:
  Chronic productive
    cough
  Smoking
  Dyspnea
  Age >60 yr
  Obesity

Upper abdominal surgery
Repeated anesthesia in
  1 yr

Thoracic surgery
(pneumonectomy)

History of
  recent upper
  or lower
  tract infection
Concomitant
  cardiovascular
  disease
Duration of
  anesthesia
  >2–3 hr

FEV_1 >2 L
MBC >50–55%
  predicted
FVC >50%
  predicted

Acceptable risk

FEV_1 <2 L
MBC <50%
  predicted
FVC <50%
  predicted

Split pulmonary
function studies
and/or
Pulmonary
arterial
balloon occlusion

Chest film
Spirometry
ABG

FEV_1 <0.5 L
FVC <1 L

Major complication
likely

FEV_1 <1.5 L
PCO_2 >45 mm Hg

Major complication
possible

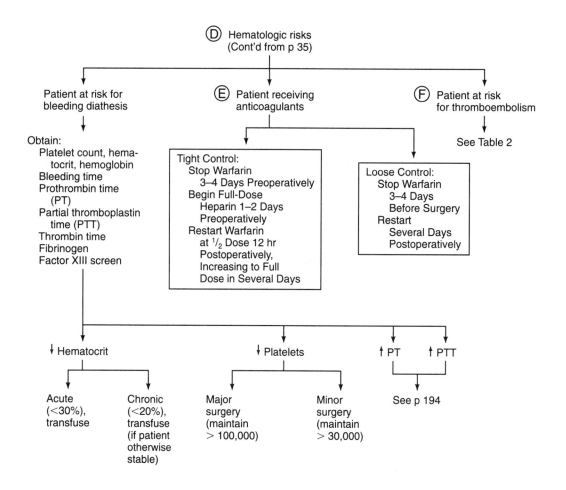

D. Four elements of blood are usually considered preoperatively: RBCs, WBCs, platelets, and clotting factors. Other issues related to hematologic risk include patients taking chronic anticoagulants and those at risk for thromboembolism (Table 2).

E. Perioperative management of patients requiring chronic anticoagulant therapy can be "tight" or "loose," depending on the indication for chronic therapy. Tight control can be considered for mechan-

ical prosthetic heart valves in the mitral position, dialysis patients whose shunts have previously clotted, and persons who have demonstrated a tendency toward embolization.

F. Prophylaxis of thromboembolism can benefit certain subsets of surgical patients. These recommendations are summarized in Table 2. Note that studies to date have not included vascular operations.

TABLE 2   Prophylaxis of Thromboembolism in Surgical Procedures

Type of Surgery	Prophylaxis	Regimen*
General	Low-dose heparin	5000 U SC bid
Urology†	Low-dose heparin	5000 U SC bid
Gynecology†	Low-dose heparin	5000 U SC bid
Neurosurgery		
Extracranial	Low-dose heparin	5000 U SC bid
Intracranial	Pneumatic compression	
Orthopedic (hip and knee)	Two-step warfarin	10 days preoperatively, begin keeping PT 2–3 sec prolonged; give twice dose postoperatively to increase PT to 1.5 times control
	Adjusted-dose heparin	Begin 2 days preoperatively at 3500 U tid; check PTT 6 hr after AM dose and adjust dose to keep in 30- to 40-sec range
	Pneumatic compression	

*Duration of prophylaxis: 5–7 days, or until ambulatory.
†For open prostatectomies and gynecologic cancer operations, consider stronger prophylaxis, such as one of the orthopedic regimens.
PT, Prothrombin time; PTT, partial thromboplastin time.

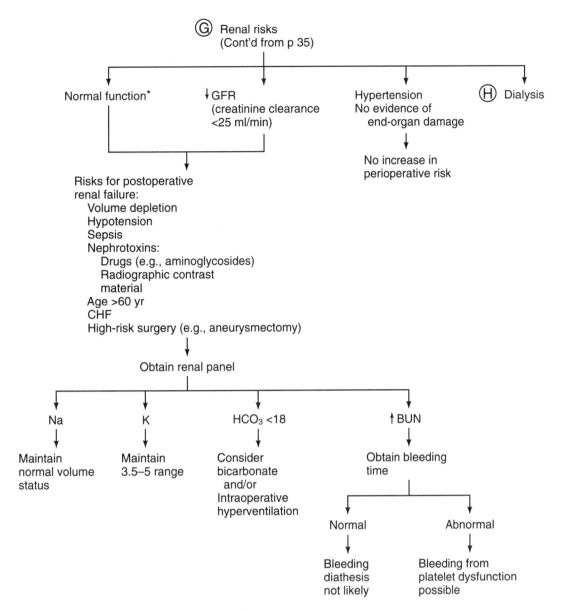

G Renal risks
(Cont'd from p 35)

Normal function*

↓GFR
(creatinine clearance
<25 ml/min)

Hypertension
No evidence of
end-organ damage

H Dialysis

No increase in
perioperative risk

Risks for postoperative
renal failure:
  Volume depletion
  Hypotension
  Sepsis
  Nephrotoxins:
    Drugs (e.g., aminoglycosides)
    Radiographic contrast
    material
  Age >60 yr
  CHF
  High-risk surgery (e.g., aneurysmectomy)

Obtain renal panel

Na

K

HCO_3 <18

↑BUN

Maintain
normal volume
status

Maintain
3.5–5 range

Consider
bicarbonate
 and/or
Intraoperative
hyperventilation

Obtain bleeding
time

Normal

Abnormal

Bleeding
diathesis
not likely

Bleeding from
platelet dysfunction
possible

*If patient has abnormal renal function, the risks have even greater significance.

G. Acute renal failure (ARF) after surgery or trauma is very difficult to manage and carries a high mortality rate. The recognition and treatment of factors predisposing to ARF is important. Surgery can generally be performed in patients with chronic renal disease if precautions are taken to prevent ARF. The surgical complications of renal disease depend primarily on the severity rather than the type of disease. As the glomerular filtration rate (GFR) approaches 25 ml/min, the complication rate rises. Generally, patients with uncomplicated urinary tract infections can be treated before surgery without significantly increasing the operative risk.

H. Dialysis is best avoided in the 4 hours before surgery. However, to avoid hyperkalemia, it is recommended that patients on maintenance hemodialysis be dialyzed within 24 hours of their operation. Any patient with a vascular access requires antimicrobial prophylaxis to prevent endarteritis.

(Continued on page 38)

I. Diabetes mellitus is the most prevalent endocrine disorder in surgical patients. Other than hyperglycemia, the most common postoperative complications in diabetic patients are infection and cardiovascular events. How tightly blood sugar should be controlled in surgical patients is an unsettled issue. There are few data to support tight rather than moderate control in this setting.

J. Management of patients on adrenal-suppressing doses of corticosteroids is an important element of perioperative assessment and is discussed elsewhere (p 122).

K. In most clinical situations patients with hyper- or hypothyroidism may undergo necessary nonelective procedures before correction to the euthyroid state without a significant increase in perioperative mortality. Surgery is generally delayed in elective cases until the patient is euthyroid. An important exception is coronary artery bypass grafting (CABG) in hypothyroid patients, since correction to the euthyroid state may increase perioperative cardiac events.

L. The greatest operative risk relating to the liver occurs in patients with chronic liver dysfunction, particularly those with progressive hepatic failure. Although Childs' classification was designed for patients undergoing portosystemic shunting, a modification of it is also prognostically useful in nonshunt operations (Table 3). Preoperatively, the medical consultant should concentrate on correcting clotting and electrolyte abnormalities, reducing ascites, alleviating encephalopathy, and improving nutritional status. Postoperative complications include pulmonary conditions (atelectasis, pneumonia), renal difficulties (hepatorenal syndrome, acute tubular necrosis), bleeding, encephalopathy, and impairment of wound healing. The patient's volume status should be closely monitored. All anesthetic agents reduce blood flow to the liver and enhance the surgical risks in patients with liver disease.

TABLE 3 Modified Childs' Index for Grading Severity of Liver Disease

Clinical or Laboratory Feature	Points Scored for Increasing Abnormality*		
	1	2	3
Encephalopathy	None	Mild–moderate	Severe
Ascites	None	Slight	Moderate
Bilirubin	<2 mg/dl	2–3 mg/dl	>3 mg/dl
Albumin	>3.5 g/L	2.8–3.4 g/L	<2.8 g/L
Prothrombin time	<4 sec	4–6 sec	>6 sec

*5–6 points, good risk; 7–9 points, moderate risk; 10–15 points, poor risk.
Adapted from Pugh RNH, et al. Transection of the oesophagus for bleeding oesophageal varices. Br J Surg 1973; 60:646, by permission of the publishers Butterworth-Heinemann Ltd.

References

Detsky A. Predicting cardiac complications in patients undergoing non-cardiac surgery. J Gen Intern Med 1986; 1:211.

Goldman L. Cardiac risks and complications of noncardiac surgery. Ann Intern Med 1983; 98:504.

Hou S. Hospital-acquired renal insufficiency: a prospective study. Am J Med 1983; 74:243.

Kroenke K. Preoperative evaluation: the assessment and management of surgical risk. J Gen Intern Med 1987; 2:257.

Luce JM. Preoperative evaluation and preoperative management of patients with pulmonary disease. Postgrad Med 1980; 67:201.

Mohr D. Preoperative evaluation of pulmonary risk factors. J Gen Intern Med 1988; 3:277.

Pasulka PS, et al. The risks of surgery in obese patients. Ann Intern Med 1986; 104:540.

Plumpton FS, et al. Corticosteroid treatment and surgery. Anaesthesia 1969; 24:3.

Pugh RNH, et al. Transection of the oesophagus for bleeding oesphageal varices. Br J Surg 1973; 60:646.

Shusternan N. Risk factors and outcome of hospital-acquired acute renal failure. Am J Med 1987; 83:65.

Weinberg AD, et al. Outcome of anesthesia and surgery in hypothyroid patients. Arch Intern Med 1983; 143:893.

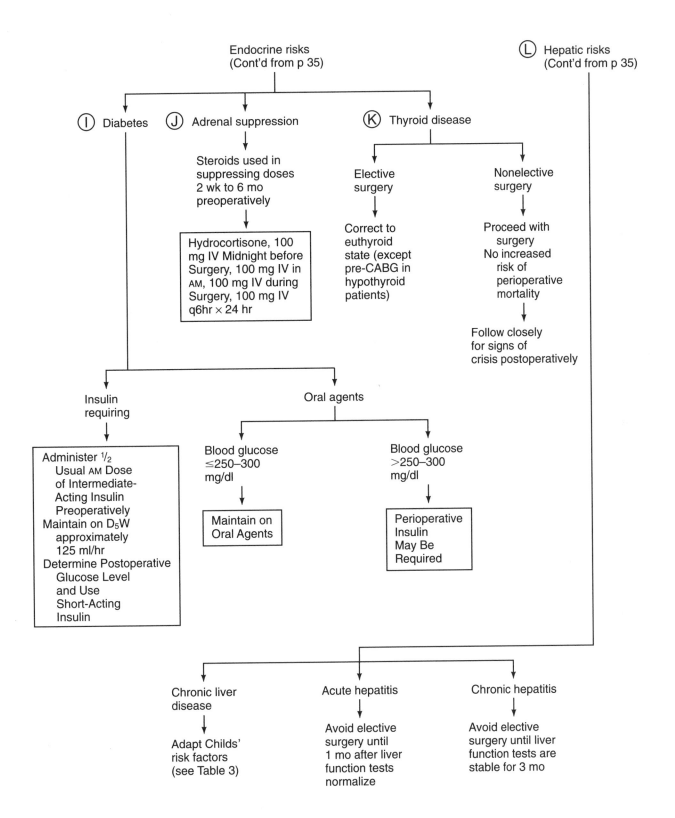

Endocrine risks
(Cont'd from p 35)

Ⓛ Hepatic risks
(Cont'd from p 35)

Ⓘ Diabetes   Ⓙ Adrenal suppression   Ⓚ Thyroid disease

Adrenal suppression: Steroids used in suppressing doses 2 wk to 6 mo preoperatively

Hydrocortisone, 100 mg IV Midnight before Surgery, 100 mg IV in AM, 100 mg IV during Surgery, 100 mg IV q6hr × 24 hr

Thyroid disease:
Elective surgery → Correct to euthyroid state (except pre-CABG in hypothyroid patients)

Nonelective surgery → Proceed with surgery No increased risk of perioperative mortality → Follow closely for signs of crisis postoperatively

Diabetes:
Insulin requiring

Administer ½ Usual AM Dose of Intermediate-Acting Insulin Preoperatively Maintain on D5W approximately 125 ml/hr Determine Postoperative Glucose Level and Use Short-Acting Insulin

Oral agents

Blood glucose ≤250–300 mg/dl → Maintain on Oral Agents

Blood glucose >250–300 mg/dl → Perioperative Insulin May Be Required

Chronic liver disease → Adapt Childs' risk factors (see Table 3)

Acute hepatitis → Avoid elective surgery until 1 mo after liver function tests normalize

Chronic hepatitis → Avoid elective surgery until liver function tests are stable for 3 mo

INTERNAL MEDICINE

CARDIOLOGY

BRADYCARDIA

David Framm, M.D.
Paul E. Fenster, M.D.
Karl B. Kern, M.D.

Bradycardia is a common clinical problem, particularly in the elderly. It is most important in the selection of therapy to be certain that the described symptoms are the result of a slow heart rate (HR). No definitive rate requirement can be established, since some athletes may do well with rates at 30–40/min, while some patients with underlying cardiac or CNS disease may be truly symptomatic when the rate falls below 60/min.

A. History is crucial in establishing a relationship between the observed rate and symptoms. Subtle symptoms, often mental or personality changes, can often best be observed and documented by family members. Medication use is critical in the consideration of reversible causes for bradycardia. A history of underlying heart disease, ischemic or valvular, is also helpful.

B. If reversible causes for the bradycardia are found, they should be eliminated and the resolution of the slow arrhythmia documented. If the bradycardia persists, further work-up is indicated.

C. If no precipitating or reversible cause for the bradycardia can be identified, a rhythm strip or ECG should be examined to distinguish patients with sinus node disease or Mobitz I AV block from those with higher-degree atrioventricular (AV) block (Mobitz II and complete heart block).

D. Patients with sinus node disease or Mobitz I AV block should be carefully evaluated for symptoms. If they are asymptomatic, an exercise test (treadmill) can be helpful to document appropriate increases in HR with exercise. If no increase is seen, careful periodic monitoring to ascertain any worsening of rhythm disturbance is warranted.

E. Symptomatic patients with sinus node disease or low-grade AV block (Mobitz I) should undergo Holter monitoring. If evidence for tachy-brady syndrome is found, a pacemaker will probably be needed to allow adequate therapy for both the rapid rhythm (using drugs) and the slow rhythm (using a permanent pacemaker). If only bradycardia is evident, a pacemaker may be indicated, depending on the symptoms and their correlation with the bradycardia.

F. High-grade AV block (Mobitz II or greater) has a poor long-term prognosis, often proceeding to complete heart block. A permanent pacer is indicated for such patients.

G. Any hemodynamic instability secondary to a slow HR should be immediately treated.

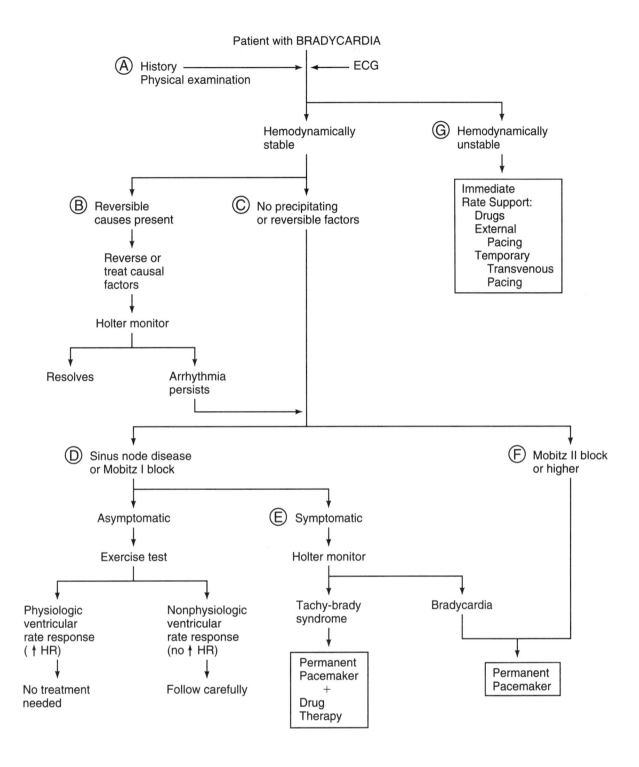

Patient with BRADYCARDIA

A) History ——————— ECG
Physical examination

Hemodynamically
stable

G) Hemodynamically
unstable

Immediate
Rate Support:
  Drugs
  External
    Pacing
  Temporary
    Transvenous
    Pacing

B) Reversible
causes present

C) No precipitating
or reversible factors

Reverse or
treat causal
factors

Holter monitor

Resolves   Arrhythmia
                  persists

D) Sinus node disease
or Mobitz I block

F) Mobitz II block
or higher

Asymptomatic

E) Symptomatic

Exercise test

Holter monitor

Physiologic
ventricular
rate response
(↑ HR)

Nonphysiologic
ventricular
rate response
(no ↑ HR)

Tachy-brady
syndrome

Bradycardia

No treatment
needed

Follow carefully

Permanent
Pacemaker
+
Drug
Therapy

Permanent
Pacemaker

NARROW QRS COMPLEX TACHYCARDIA

Anthony C. Caruso, M.D.
Karl B. Kern, M.D.

Evaluation of patients with narrow complex tachycardia poses a challenge to the physician, for clearly there are many different tachyarrhythmias that on superficial examination appear to be identical. Supraventricular tachycardia is a broad term for a variety of rhythm disturbances that originate at or above the atrioventricular (AV) node. This includes atrial fibrillation and atrial flutter, which are usually rather distinct in presentation, as well as sinus tachycardia, sinus node re-entry tachycardia (SNRT), ectopic atrial tachycardia, accelerated junctional rhythm, multifocal atrial tachycardia, AV node re-entrant tachycardia (AVNRT), and sometimes new accessory pathway-mediated tachycardias such as the orthodromic atrioventricular re-entrant tachycardia (AVRT) found in Wolff-Parkinson-White (WPW) syndrome.

A. The foremost consideration in evaluating narrow complex tachycardia is hemodynamic stability. If the patient is unstable, immediate cardioversion is warranted, regardless of the QRS morphology or exact diagnosis.

B. Stable patients can be more carefully evaluated with a 12-lead ECG. The major initial decision is whether or not P waves are visible.

C. If P waves are present and identical to the sinus P scan previous to the tachycardia, sinus tachycardia is likely. The hallmark of SNRT is an abrupt onset and offset of narrow complex tachycardia in which the P wave has the same axis configuration as the P wave during sinus rhythm.

D. The appearance of P waves distinctly different from the sinus P wave is helpful. Ectopic atrial tachycardia is characterized by a single P wave morphology distinct from that of the sinus P wave. This tachycardia is often initiated by a premature atrial beat late in diastole. An inverted P wave (retrograde P) (often best seen in leads II, III, or AVF) is indicative of paroxysmal supraventricular tachycardia (PSVT). PSVT in the elderly population is most commonly AVNRT in which the P wave is usually seen buried within the ST segment. This tachycardia, along with orthodromic AVRT of WPW, responds well to vagal maneuvers, with 50% of patients returning to sinus rhythm. A delta wave on a resting ECG alerts the clinician to an accessory pathway, but in patients with a concealed accessory pathway there is no antegrade conduction and consequently no delta wave. Atrial flutter is recognized by the typical sawtooth pattern of atrial waves at a rate of 280–300 beats per minute. Atrial flutter P waves are best seen in leads II, III, AVF, or V.

E. If multiple distinct forms of P waves are evident, the likely diagnosis is multifocal atrial tachycardia (MAT).

F. If distinct P waves are absent, carefully consider the baseline between QRS complexes and the regularity of the R-R interval. If a chaotic baseline and irregularly irregular R-R intervals are found, the diagnosis is most likely atrial fibrillation.

G. If the baseline is R-R and the interval remains regular, the diagnosis is almost certainly an accelerated junctional tachycardia.

References

Bär FW, Brugada P, Dossen WRM, Wellens HJJ. Differential diagnosis of tachycardia with narrow QRS complex. Am J Cardiol 1984; 54:555.

Brugada P, Smeets JLRM, Wellens HJJ. Spectrum of supraventricular tachycardias. Am J Cardiol 1989; 62:4L.

Levine JH, Michael JR, Guarnieri T. Treatment of multifocal atrial tachycardia with verapamil. N Engl J Med 1985; 312:21.

Mehta D, Ward DE, Wafa S, Camm AJ. Relative efficacy of various physical maneuvers in the termination of junctional tachycardia. Lancet 1988; 1:1187.

Rankin AC, McGovern BA. Adenosine or verapamil for the acute treatment of supraventricular tachycardia? Ann Intern Med 1991; 114:513.

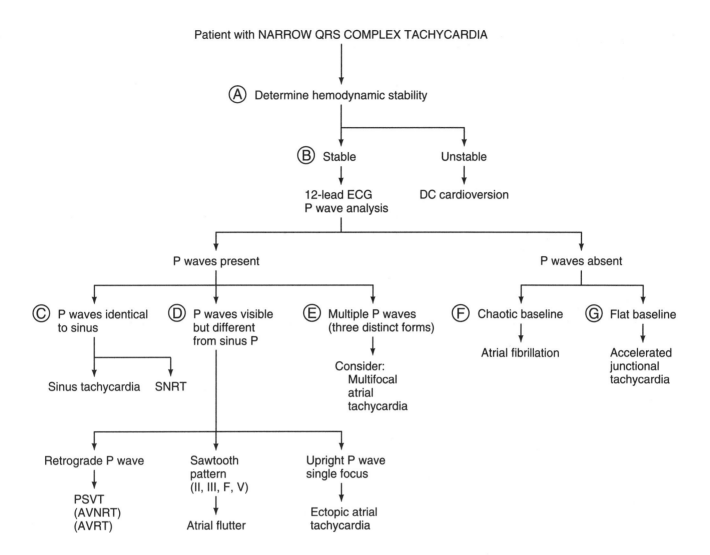

Patient with NARROW QRS COMPLEX TACHYCARDIA

(A) Determine hemodynamic stability

(B) Stable | Unstable

12-lead ECG
P wave analysis | DC cardioversion

P waves present | P waves absent

(C) P waves identical to sinus | (D) P waves visible but different from sinus P | (E) Multiple P waves (three distinct forms) | (F) Chaotic baseline | (G) Flat baseline

Sinus tachycardia   SNRT | Consider: Multifocal atrial tachycardia | Atrial fibrillation | Accelerated junctional tachycardia

Retrograde P wave | Sawtooth pattern (II, III, F, V) | Upright P wave single focus

PSVT (AVNRT) (AVRT) | Atrial flutter | Ectopic atrial tachycardia

WIDE QRS COMPLEX TACHYCARDIA

Anthony C. Caruso, M.D.

Wide QRS tachycardia poses a complex set of problems, because the treatment of supraventricular tachycardias with aberrant conduction is clearly different from that of acute ventricular tachycardia. Inability to distinguish one from the other may lead to catastrophic consequences.

A. The first step in the management of all tachycardias is an assessment of hemodynamic stability. In patients found to have a wide QRS complex tachycardia who are hemodynamically unstable, immediate cardioversion with 200 joules is the appropriate response; pharmacologic interventions at this point would only delay a safe and effective therapy. In patients found to be hemodynamically stable, a 12-lead ECG provides valuable information in distinguishing a supraventricular from a ventricular cause of wide QRS complex tachycardia.

B. Patients who have an irregular R-R interval must be distinguished from those with a regular R-R interval.

C. In those with an irregular RR interval who have a history of either congenital or an acquired long QT and are found to have atrioventricular (AV) dissociation, the diagnosis is one of probable polymorphic ventricular tachycardia (VT), and the appropriate therapy is administration of 2 g magnesium sulfate IV. Should this fail to convert the patient to sinus rhythm, isoproterenol infusion to shorten QT intervals is effective. In patients with recent myocardial infarction or unstable angina, this therapy may be hazardous. An equally effective approach is the use of transient cardiac pacing to maintain adequate QT reduction. Of course, correction of electrolyte abnormalities is essential.

D. In patients found to have an irregular R-R rate with classic bundle branch block (BBB) morphology in which no AV dissociation is obvious, the most likely cause is atrial fibrillation with aberrancy, and esmolol, digitalis, or verapamil may be initiated to control ventricular response. This should be performed only if there is no evidence of a delta wave. In patients with rapid ventricular response across an accessory pathway, cardiac collapse has been known to occur with the administration of verapamil.

E. In patients found to have a regular R-R interval, an attempt should be made to identify P waves on a 12-lead ECG, and in patients with clear AV dissociation the diagnosis is one of probable VT. Treatment at this point would be lidocaine with an initial bolus of 1.5 mg/kg followed by 0.8 mg/kg at 8-, 16-, and 24-min intervals. A maintenance infusion of 30 μg/kg/min is then initiated with appropriate titration via plasma levels of lidocaine. If this is unsuccessful, it is recommended to proceed with procainamide: a 15 mg/kg loading dose administered at 35 mg/min followed by a maintenance dose of 4 mg/min. This regimen will achieve adequate steady state levels quickly with dose adjustment via drug level determination. If lidocaine or procainamide fails to control VT, bretylium may be administered at a 5 mg/kg loading dose administered over 30 minutes followed by 1–2 mg/min constant infusion.

F. In patients who have wide complex tachycardia with a regular R-R interval and AV synchrony, supraventricular tachycardia (SVT) may be suspected. However, in all cases of wide complex tachycardia one should always be wary of VT. Consequently, in patients with suspected SVT with aberrant conduction, it is recommended that adenosine rather than verapamil be used for the management of this disorder. While AV dissociation virtually establishes a diagnosis of VT, the presence of AV association does not exclude VT. In patients in whom an assessment of AV synchrony cannot be made, procainamide should be administered. This will successfully treat most cases of paroxsymal supraventricular tachycardia (PSVT) and provide reasonable management of VT.

References

McGovern B, Garan H, Ruskin JN. Precipitation of cardiac arrest by verapamil in patients with Wolff-Parkinson-White syndrome. Ann Intern Med 1986; 104:791.

Rankin AC, Goldroyd K, Chong E, et al. Value and limitations of adenosine in the diagnosis and treatment of narrow and broad complex tachycardias. Br Heart J 1989; 62:195.

Tzivoni D, Banai S, Schuger C, et al. Treatment of torsades de pointes with magnesium sulfate. Circulation 1988; 77:392.

Wellens HJJ, Bar FW, Vanagt EJ, et al. The differentiation between ventricular tachycardia and supraventricular tachycardia with aberrant conduction: the value of the electrocardiogram. In: Wellens HJJ, Kulbertus HE, eds. What's new in electrocardiography. Boston: Martinus Nijhoff, 1981.

Woosley RL and Shand DG. Pharmacokinetics of antiarrhythmic drugs. Am J Cardiol 1978; 41:986.

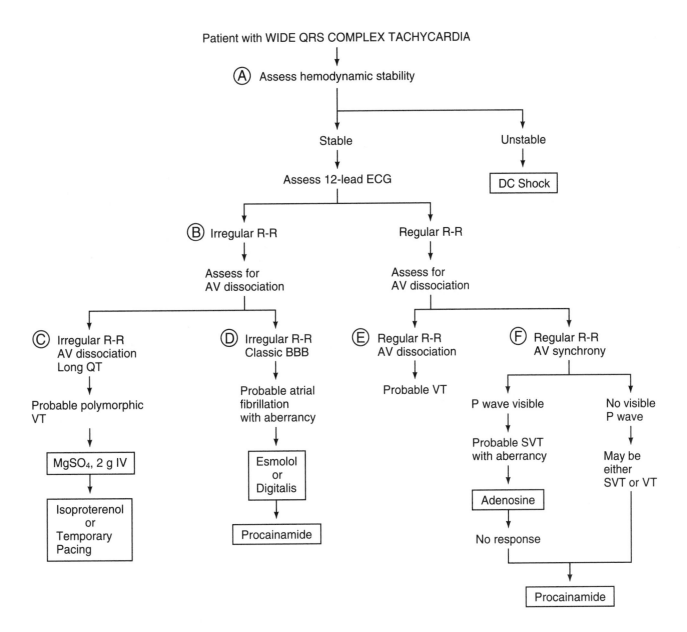

Patient with WIDE QRS COMPLEX TACHYCARDIA

Ⓐ Assess hemodynamic stability

Stable — Unstable

Assess 12-lead ECG — DC Shock

Ⓑ Irregular R-R — Regular R-R

Assess for AV dissociation — Assess for AV dissociation

Ⓒ Irregular R-R AV dissociation Long QT

Ⓓ Irregular R-R Classic BBB

Ⓔ Regular R-R AV dissociation

Ⓕ Regular R-R AV synchrony

Probable polymorphic VT

Probable atrial fibrillation with aberrancy

Probable VT

P wave visible — No visible P wave

MgSO₄, 2 g IV

Esmolol or Digitalis

Probable SVT with aberrancy

May be either SVT or VT

Isoproterenol or Temporary Pacing

Procainamide

Adenosine

No response

Procainamide

STABLE ANGINA

Karil Bellah, M.D.
Samuel M. Butman, M.D.

A. The evaluation of chronic stable angina should provide the clinician with documentation of coronary disease as the cause of chest pain, determine the efficacy of therapy, and select patients at high risk for infarction or death so that revascularization can be performed early and safely. When the diagnosis of chronic stable angina is made, evaluation and modification of risk factors should begin with cholesterol reduction, control of hypertension, weight loss, and smoking cessation.

B. The choice of stress testing is determined by the patient's resting ECG and ability to exercise, and the clinician's familiarity with the study.

C. The most common stress test is the exercise treadmill test (ETT) in which the grade and rate of the treadmill are increased incrementally to achieve an increase in heart rate that correlates with an increase in oxygen consumption. The sensitivity of this test is about 65% (35% false-negative) and the specificity 90% (10% false-positive) when at least 85% of the predicted maximal heart rate is achieved. False-positive results are particularly common in patients on digitalis and diuretics or with hypertensive disease, hypertrophy, hypokalemia, Wolff-Parkinson-White syndrome, interventricular conduction defects, and left bundle branch block.

D. When a false-positive result is likely, the study can be performed with thallium imaging (Th-ETT), radionuclide angiography, or stress echocardiography.

E. Patients with a good chance of completing an exercise test proceed with Th-ETT, but if exercise tolerance or ability is questionable an alternative is dipyridamole-thallium testing.

F. A nondiagnostic study is one in which an adequate heart rate is not achieved owing to poor conditioning, other medical factors, or cardiac medications (beta blockers and calcium channel blockers). A nondiagnostic study should be followed by a dipyridamole-thallium study. Patients with claudication, lung disease, arthritis, or other debilitating diseases should be spared a probable nondiagnostic study, and a dipyridamole-thallium study should be performed.

G. A positive stress test provides information to enable the clinician to stratify patients into high- and low-risk groups.

H. The criteria for high-risk patients with ETT include early onset of ST depression, >2 mm ST depression, ST changes at a low heart rate and level of exercise, or a drop in systolic blood pressure. Studies have shown that the degree of ST depression correlates with a higher incidence of left main and multivessel disease. Patients in the high-risk group are more likely to have a cardiac event and poorer survival than those in the low-risk group. Likewise, with thallium studies the increasing number of segments with reperfusion defects correlates with increasing severity of coronary disease (i.e., more myocardium at risk), and the same has been shown with wall motion abnormalities with stress echocardiography. Using radionuclide angiography, an exercise ejection fraction (EF) $\geq$50% is associated with a very good prognosis (regardless of resting EF), but one $\leq$35% is substantially worse (50% risk of cardiac event in 3 years). Irrespective of the method of stress testing chosen, all patients who fall into the high-risk group should undergo cardiac catheterization and appropriate revascularization with percutaneous coronary angioplasty (PTCA) or coronary artery bypass grafting (CABG), if needed.

I. The decision of which patients should have surgical therapy or medical therapy for coronary artery disease has been evaluated by three large, ongoing studies. Clearly, patients with refractory angina on maximally tolerated medical therapy should receive PTCA or CABG for relief of symptoms. Patients with left main disease have prolonged survival with surgical therapy, as do those with three-vessel disease and two-vessel disease with proximal LAD stenosis and who have decreased EF and evidence of ischemia. At present, there are no studies directly comparing CABG with PTCA in this group of patients. PTCA is considered an important means of revascularization for many patients with the appropriate anatomic lesion.

References

Bonow RO. Prognostic implications of exercise radionuclide angiography in patients with coronary artery disease. Mayo Clin Proc 1988; 63:630.

Brown KA. Prognostic value of thallium 201 myocardial perfusion imaging: a diagnostic tool comes of age. Circulation 1991; 83:363.

Helfant RH. Stable angina pectoris: Risk stratification and therapeutic options. Circulation 1990; 82 (Suppl II):66.

Kirklin JW, Akins CW, Blackstone EH, et al. Guidelines and indications for coronary artery bypass graft surgery. J Am Coll Cardiol 1991; 17:543.

Schlant RC, Blomquist CG, Brandenberg RO, et al. Guidelines for exercise testing. J Am Coll Cardiol 1986; 8:725.

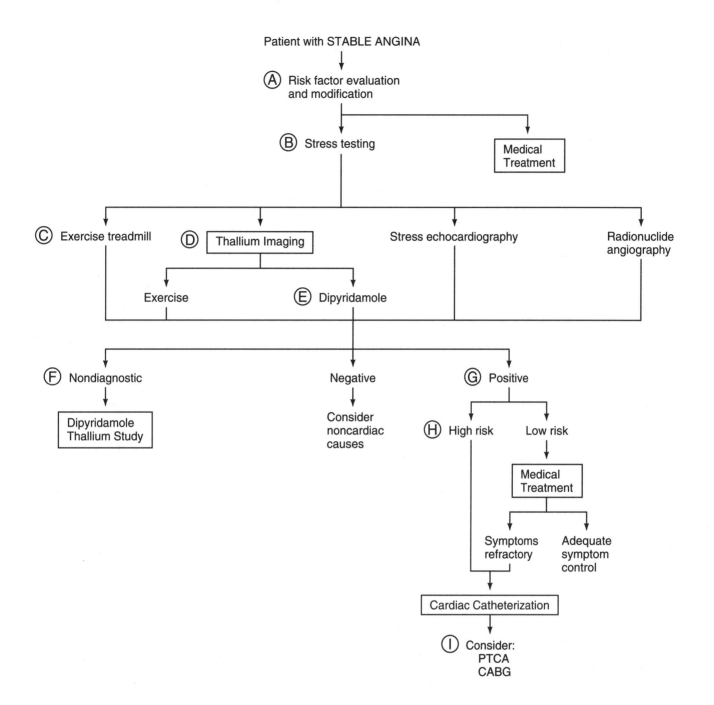

Patient with STABLE ANGINA

(A) Risk factor evaluation and modification

(B) Stress testing

Medical Treatment

(C) Exercise treadmill

(D) Thallium Imaging

Exercise

(E) Dipyridamole

Stress echocardiography

Radionuclide angiography

(F) Nondiagnostic

Dipyridamole Thallium Study

Negative

Consider noncardiac causes

(G) Positive

(H) High risk

Low risk

Medical Treatment

Symptoms refractory

Adequate symptom control

Cardiac Catheterization

(I) Consider:
PTCA
CABG

UNSTABLE ANGINA

Karil Bellah, M.D.
Samuel M. Butman, M.D.

Unstable angina is a clinical syndrome defined by one of the following entities: (1) new-onset angina or ischemia, (2) intensification (quality, duration, or inciting factors) of pre-existing angina, or (3) angina that occurs at rest. The natural history of unstable angina has been studied. Approximately 10–15% of patients with unstable angina suffer acute myocardial infarction (MI) during that hospitalization, and 10–40% experience an MI within the next year. The incidence of death is 1–5% in the hospital and 5–25% over the next year. Approximately one third of patients with unstable angina undergo coronary artery bypass grafting (CABG) within 1 year. In addition, 40–60% of patients with acute infarctions experience antecedent unstable angina. The goal of therapy for unstable angina should be to decrease the risk of infarction and death.

A. Persons presenting with new-onset angina have a better prognosis than those who experience a change in symptoms or develop angina at rest. New-onset angina probably represents progressive luminal narrowing that has advanced to a critical obstruction of coronary blood flow. Persons with new-onset angina have less severe coronary disease, higher left ventricular ejection fractions, and lower mortality rates.

B. The most frequent ECG changes with unstable angina are T wave changes (present 62% of the time) including T wave inversion, flattening, or pseudonormalization (upright T waves with angina that are inverted at baseline). ST segment depression is present in 20–30% of patients with unstable angina chest pain. The absence of ECG changes does not rule out significant coronary disease.

C. When symptoms are easily controlled with medical treatment, a less invasive work-up is justified. Exercise treadmill testing is a reasonable approach in patients with new-onset but easily controlled angina. A positive exercise stress test in patients with new-onset angina should be followed by cardiac catheterization, even if symptoms are adequately controlled by medical therapy.

D. In patients with new-onset angina who have positive ECG changes or refractory symptoms, cardiac catheterization is indicated. Likewise, any patient with an impressive change in anginal pattern or rest pain should undergo catheterization.

E. The incidence of left main artery stenosis is 10–15% in patients with unstable angina. Fifty percent of patients have three-vessel disease, while 5–10% have no significant coronary artery disease. The remaining 20–35% have one- or two-vessel disease at the time of catheterization. Therefore, cardiac catheterization plays a decisive role in selection of the appropriate therapy, as patients with left main and three-vessel disease have improved survival with CABG and should be referred for cardiothoracic surgery. Cardiac catheterization should be performed only in patients in whom revascularization is a viable option. Those who are not candidates for revascularization should not be subjected to the minimal, but significant risks of the procedure.

References

Ambrose JA, et al. Angiographic evolution of coronary artery morphology in unstable angina. J Am Coll Cardiol 1986; 7:472.

Butman SM, Olson HG, Butman LK. Early exercise testing after stabilization of unstable angina: correlation with coronary angiographic findings and subsequent cardiac events. Am Heart J 1986; 111:11.

Myler RK, Shaw RE, Stertzer SH, et al. Unstable angina and coronary angioplasty. Circulation 1990; 82 (Suppl II):11-88.

Parisi AF, Khari S, Deupree RH, et al. Medical compared with surgical management of unstable angina: 5-year mortality and morbidity in the Veterans Administration study. Circulation 1989; 80:1176.

Théroux P, Duimet H, McCans J, et al. Aspirin, heparin, or both to treat acute unstable angina. N Engl J Med 1988; 319:1105.

Patient with UNSTABLE ANGINA

History ──────────→
Physical examination

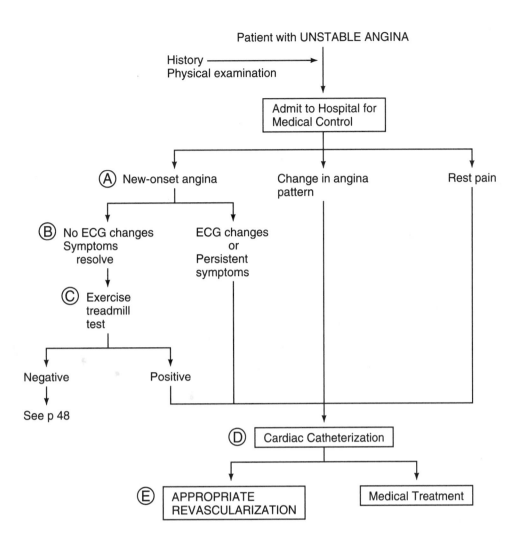

Admit to Hospital for
Medical Control

Ⓐ New-onset angina

Change in angina
pattern

Rest pain

Ⓑ No ECG changes
Symptoms
resolve

ECG changes
or
Persistent
symptoms

Ⓒ Exercise
treadmill
test

Negative

Positive

See p 48

Ⓓ Cardiac Catheterization

Ⓔ APPROPRIATE
REVASCULARIZATION

Medical Treatment

SYSTOLIC MURMUR

Alberta L. Warner, M.D.

A. After it has been determined whether a murmur occurs during systole or diastole, the next step is to listen carefully during respiration. Systolic murmurs of right-side origin usually increase during inspiration, whereas left-sided systolic murmurs increase during expiration.

B. It may be difficult to identify a murmur as regurgitant or ejection. If the patient has occasional ectopy or an irregular rhythm, listen for change in intensity after a pause. An ejection or outflow murmur increases in intensity after a pause, whereas a regurgitant murmur remains unchanged. One must also identify the relationship of the murmur to the first and second heart sounds. An ejection murmur cannot begin until the aortic or pulmonic valve opens, after the isovolumetric contraction period, and thus well after S_1. In contrast, a regurgitant murmur usually begins as soon as the pressure in the ventricle rises above that in the atrium, and thus with S_1. Further, regurgitant murmurs usually do not end until after the aortic component of S_2 into the isovolumetric relaxation period. Although the classic regurgitant murmur is holosystolic, regurgitant murmurs may be early systolic (as in acute mitral regurgitation [MR]) or late systolic (as in mitral valve prolapse [MVP]). Hence, a systolic murmur that begins with S_1 or continues into S_2 is usually regurgitant.

C. The presence of other heart sounds gives clues to the origin of a systolic murmur. An ejection sound, which is high pitched and occurs shortly after S_1, may be present with pulmonic stenosis (PS) or aortic stenosis (AS). Abnormal splitting of S_2, such as the wide fixed split S_2 of an atrial septal defect, or the paradoxically split S_2 of severe AS, aids in diagnosis. The clicks of MVP are distinguished by their movement away from S_1 with squatting and toward S_1 with standing.

D. An "innocent" murmur is one caused by normal turbulence across the pulmonic or aortic valve in a patient with a normal cardiovascular system. Murmurs that occur in high-output states such as anemia or sepsis are due to turbulent flow, but are not necessarily innocent by definition. Innocent murmurs are ejection murmurs that decrease or even disappear with maneuvers that decrease venous return (Valsalva, standing) and increase with maneuvers that increase venous return (squatting). As discussed, the presence of an ejection sound or abnormal splitting of S_2 identifies AS or PS. Innocent flow murmurs can be identified by their soft quality, short duration, occurrence only in early systole, and localization along the left sternal border. The key is the absence of apparent cardiac pathology on history taking or thorough examination. ECG and chest films are normal, whereas left ventricular hypertrophy is evident with AS. Echo-Doppler evaluation is a reliable diagnostic tool for clarification or confirmation of a diagnosis and a means to quantitate more accurately the severity of a valvular lesion.

E. To further characterize a systolic murmur, dynamic auscultation should be used during Valsalva, squatting, and standing maneuvers. The murmur of hypertrophic cardiomyopathy (HCM) can be especially distinguished with these maneuvers. Maneuvers that decrease venous return, such as Valsalva or standing from a squatting position, increase the intensity of the murmur of HCM. The murmur of AS may decrease in intensity, whereas that of MR or ventricular septal defect (VSD) may remain unchanged. Conversely, maneuvers that increase venous return, such as squatting, decrease the murmur of HCM, whereas other systolic murmurs increase or remain unchanged. An exception to this is the murmur of MVP, which may begin earlier in systole with the Valsalva maneuver, and later in systole with the squatting maneuver. This is distinguished from the murmur of HCM, which varies in intensity rather than in timing with these maneuvers.

F. The murmurs of MR and VSD demonstrate similar changes in response to maneuvers. MR is distinguished by its localization at the apex, whereas the murmur of VSD is localized at the lower left sternal border. Furthermore, the presence of right ventricular hypertrophy on ECG or chest film supports the diagnosis of VSD, as opposed to that of MR in which left ventricular and left atrial enlargement predominate.

References

Ewy GE. Bedside evaluation of the cardiac patient. Hosp Med 1980; 16:11.

Grewe K, Crawford MH, O'Rourke RA. Differentiation of cardiac murmurs by dynamic auscultation. Curr Probl Cardiol 1988; 10:671.

Lembo NJ, Dell'Italia LJ, Crawford JH, et al. Bedside diagnosis of systolic murmurs. N Engl J Med 1988; 318:1572.

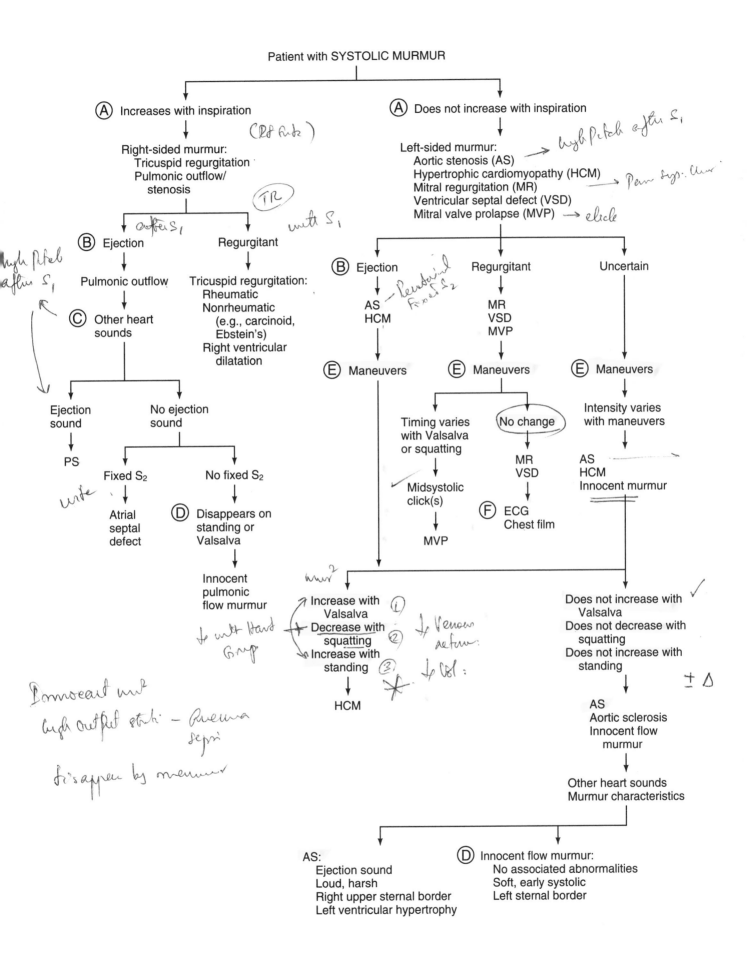

Patient with SYSTOLIC MURMUR

(A) Increases with inspiration *(Rt ratr)*

Right-sided murmur:
 Tricuspid regurgitation
 Pulmonic outflow/
  stenosis

(TR)

(A) Does not increase with inspiration → *high Pitch after S₁*

Left-sided murmur:
 Aortic stenosis (AS) → *high Pitch after S₁*
 Hypertrophic cardiomyopathy (HCM) → *Pan Sys. Chur*
 Mitral regurgitation (MR)
 Ventricular septal defect (VSD)
 Mitral valve prolapse (MVP) → *click*

(B) Ejection *after S₁*   Regurgitant *with S₁*

Pulmonic outflow

Tricuspid regurgitation:
 Rheumatic
 Nonrheumatic
  (e.g., carcinoid,
  Ebstein's)
 Right ventricular
  dilatation

high Pitch after S₁

(C) Other heart
 sounds

Ejection
sound

No ejection
sound

PS

write

Fixed S₂

Atrial
septal
defect

No fixed S₂

(D) Disappears on
 standing or
 Valsalva

Innocent
pulmonic
flow murmur

*Innocent mur
high output stati - Anemia
                    Sepsi
disappear by maneuver*

(B) Ejection → *Peristernal Fixed S₂*

AS
HCM

(E) Maneuvers

Regurgitant

MR
VSD
MVP

(E) Maneuvers

Uncertain

(E) Maneuvers

Timing varies
with Valsalva
or squatting

Midsystolic
click(s)

MVP

(No change)

MR
VSD

(F) ECG
 Chest film

Intensity varies
with maneuvers

AS
HCM
Innocent murmur

mur?

*↑ with Hand
Grip*

↗ Increase with
 Valsalva ①
→ Decrease with
 squatting ②
↘ Increase with
 standing ③

*↓ Venous
return:*

↓ Vol:

HCM

Does not increase with ✓
 Valsalva
Does not decrease with
 squatting
Does not increase with
 standing

± Δ

AS
Aortic sclerosis
Innocent flow
 murmur

Other heart sounds
Murmur characteristics

AS:
 Ejection sound
 Loud, harsh
 Right upper sternal border
 Left ventricular hypertrophy

(D) Innocent flow murmur:
 No associated abnormalities
 Soft, early systolic
 Left sternal border

53

DIASTOLIC MURMUR

Alberta L. Warner, M.D.

A. The presence of a diastolic murmur usually indicates cardiovascular pathology. As with systolic murmurs, careful auscultation during respiration should be performed. Augmentation of a diastolic murmur during inspiration suggests a right-sided murmur, either tricuspid stenosis or pulmonic regurgitation. Left-sided diastolic murmurs, as mitral stenosis or aortic regurgitation (AR), soften with inspiration and increase during expiration.

B. Tricuspid stenosis and pulmonic regurgitation may be distinguished by their differences in location and pitch. Tricuspid stenosis is heard as a low-pitched diastolic rumble along the lower left sternal border, whereas pulmonic regurgitation presents with a higher-pitched murmur at the upper left sternal border. Tricuspid stenosis, which is relatively rare, is almost always rheumatic in origin and is usually associated with rheumatic mitral valve disease. The presence of prominent A waves in the jugular venous pulse and of ascites supports a diagnosis of significant tricuspid stenosis, which may be masked by concomitant mitral stenosis on auscultation.

C. Pulmonic regurgitation often occurs secondary to pulmonary hypertension and is referred to as a Graham Steell murmur. A right ventricular lift along the left sternal border, an increased pulmonic component of the second heart sound, and associated tricuspid regurgitation suggest pulmonic regurgitation due to pulmonary hypertension.

D. As with right-sided murmurs, the murmurs of mitral stenosis and aortic regurgitation can usually be distinguished by their quality and localization. AR is heard best along the left sternal border, with the patient upright or leaning forward, and has a high-pitched blowing quality. AR due to aortic root dilatation rather than leaflet incompetence is frequently heard best at the right upper sternal border. In contrast, mitral stenosis is low-pitched, requiring the bell of the stethoscope to hear the characteristic "rumble," and is heard best at the apex with the patient in a left lateral decubitus position.

E. An Austin Flint murmur is a low-pitched diastolic murmur that occurs in severe AR owing to impaired opening of the anterior leaflet of the mitral valve against the regurgitant aortic jet. The absence of an opening snap or the presence of left ventricular (LV) enlargement support the diagnosis of an Austin Flint murmur due to AR, rather than that of mitral stenosis. Amyl nitrate, which lowers systemic vascular resistance, increases the murmur of mitral stenosis but decreases diastolic murmurs due to AR.

F. Acute AR due to aortic dissection, infective endocarditis, or trauma presents clinically quite differently from chronic AR and must be identified. Owing to the increase in LV load, congestive heart failure may occur early and suddenly. The pulse pressure usually is not increased in acute AR; hence peripheral findings of chronic AR such as Duroziez' sign or Quincke's sign are not present. On auscultation, S_1 may be soft owing to early closure of the mitral valve, and an S_3 sound is often present. The murmur of acute AR is shorter and lower-pitched than that of chronic AR because of the rapid rise in LV pressure. Indeed, a shortening or diminishing AR murmur may herald acute worsening of AR.

References

Braunwald E. Valvular heart disease. In: Braunwald E, ed. Heart disease: a textbook of cardiovascular medicine. Philadelphia: WB Saunders, 1988:1023.

Fuster V, Shub C, Giuliani E, McGoon D. Acquired valvular heart disease. In: Brandenburg RO, ed. Cardiology: Fundamentals and practice. Chicago: Year–Book, 1987:1271.

Grewe K, Crawford MH, O'Rourke RA. Differentiation of cardiac murmurs by dynamic auscultation. Curr Probl Cardiol 1988; 10:671.

Patient with DIASTOLIC MURMUR

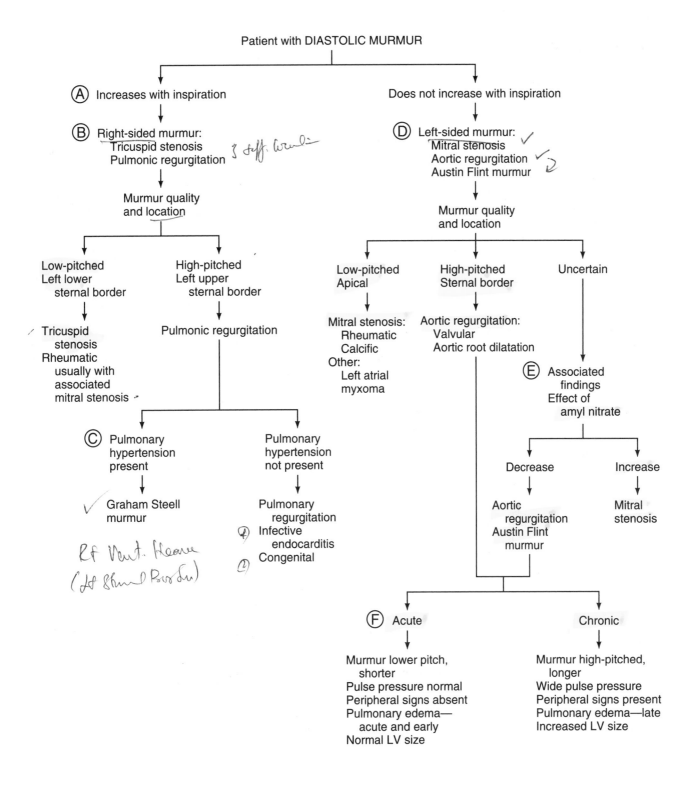

(A) Increases with inspiration

(B) Right-sided murmur:
    Tricuspid stenosis
    Pulmonic regurgitation   *3 stiff. Coronli*

Murmur quality
and location

Low-pitched
Left lower
sternal border

High-pitched
Left upper
sternal border

Tricuspid
stenosis
Rheumatic
usually with
associated
mitral stenosis

Pulmonic regurgitation

(C) Pulmonary
hypertension
present

Pulmonary
hypertension
not present

Graham Steell
murmur

*Rf Vent. Heave
(Lt Strnd Border)*

Pulmonary
regurgitation
① Infective
endocarditis
② Congenital

(D) Left-sided murmur:
    Mitral stenosis
    Aortic regurgitation
    Austin Flint murmur

Does not increase with inspiration

Murmur quality
and location

Low-pitched
Apical

Mitral stenosis:
    Rheumatic
    Calcific
Other:
    Left atrial
    myxoma

High-pitched
Sternal border

Aortic regurgitation:
    Valvular
    Aortic root dilatation

Uncertain

(E) Associated
findings
Effect of
amyl nitrate

Decrease

Increase

Aortic
regurgitation
Austin Flint
murmur

Mitral
stenosis

(F) Acute

Chronic

Murmur lower pitch,
    shorter
Pulse pressure normal
Peripheral signs absent
Pulmonary edema—
    acute and early
Normal LV size

Murmur high-pitched,
    longer
Wide pulse pressure
Peripheral signs present
Pulmonary edema—late
Increased LV size

HYPERTENSION

Pamela J. Davis, M.D.

Hypertension (HTN) is the most common reason for a patient to see an internist in the United States today and the most common indication for the use of prescription medication. Approximately 58 million Americans have HTN, defined as elevated blood pressure (BP): systolic blood pressure (SBP) ≥140 mm Hg and/or diastolic blood pressure (DBP) ≥90 mm Hg. The prevalence of HTN increases with age and is greater in blacks than in whites. Risks of cardiovascular (CV) complications increase with increasing levels of BP. HTN with no definable cause is termed primary, idiopathic, or essential HTN. HTN due to a specific organ or metabolic defect is termed secondary HTN.

A. HTN should not be diagnosed on the basis of a single measurement. Individuals commonly experience a transient, moderate elevation in BP when under stress (e.g., in an emergency room or a doctor's office or while in pain). Elevated BP readings in this setting may be spurious and should be repeated. The following measurement techniques are recommended: (1) the patient should be seated, with arm bared, supported, and positioned at heart level, and should rest quietly for 5 minutes before measurement; (2) there should be no tobacco or caffeine intake within 30 minutes before measurement; (3) an appropriate cuff size should be used to ensure an accurate measurement (the bladder should encircle four fifths of arm circumference and two thirds of its length); and (4) SBP and DBP should be recorded at least twice and averaged, using the disappearance of sound (phase V) for the DBP reading.

B. There are three reasons for evaluating a patient with HTN: (1) to determine the type of HTN, specifically looking for secondary causes; (2) to assess the impact of HTN on target organs; and (3) to estimate the patient's risk profile for development of CV disease. The history should emphasize the onset of HTN; any family history of CV disease; any personal history of diabetes mellitus, renal disease, hyperlipidemia, medications, and weight gain or loss; lifestyle factors such as alcohol, tobacco, and illicit drug use; sodium intake; and pertinent psychosocial and environmental factors such as stress and food preferences. In the review of systems, secondary HTN symptoms may be elicited. Headache, sweating, weight loss, palpitations (pheochromocytoma), muscle cramps, weakness, polyuria (hyperaldosteronism), leg claudication (coarctation), menstrual irregularities, easy bruising, or personality changes (Cushing's syndrome) are a few symptoms that may be revealed.

C. Observe the patient's overall appearance, noting any stigmata of disease. Focus on weight measurements, funduscopic examination, thyroid evaluation, careful cardiopulmonary review, and evaluation of peripheral vasculature. Most patients with established HTN of several years' duration exhibit varying degrees of retinopathy. Narrowing of the arteriolar wall (grade I) and obscuring of veins as they cross behind arteries (grade II) are seen in the early stages of end-organ damage. More serious disease is indicated by hemorrhages and exudate (grade III), which may progress to papilledema (grade IV). Examine the neck for carotid bruits and increased jugular venous pressure; the heart for increased rate and size, clicks, murmurs, and S_3 and S_4 heart sounds; the abdomen for bruits and masses; and the lungs for bibasilar rales. Measure arm and leg BP and perform simultaneous radio-femoral pulse palpation. Finally, a simple neurologic examination may uncover evidence of a previous stroke or other neurologic deficit. On the basis of the history and physical examination, most secondary causes of HTN can be excluded and overall CV status largely determined.

D. The diagnostic tests ordered may depend on the patient's presentation, but these tests are essential in the routine evaluation of HTN: CBC; urinalysis; determinations of serum potassium, creatinine, BUN, calcium, fasting blood glucose, cholesterol, and high-density lipoproteins; and ECG. These tests usually provide sufficient information about the presence of end-organ damage from HTN and the likelihood that complications will develop from the BP elevation. When the history, physical examination, or laboratory evaluation suggests a secondary cause of HTN, obtain additional specific studies as indicated.

(Continued on page 58)

Patient with ELEVATED BLOOD PRESSURE (≥140/90)

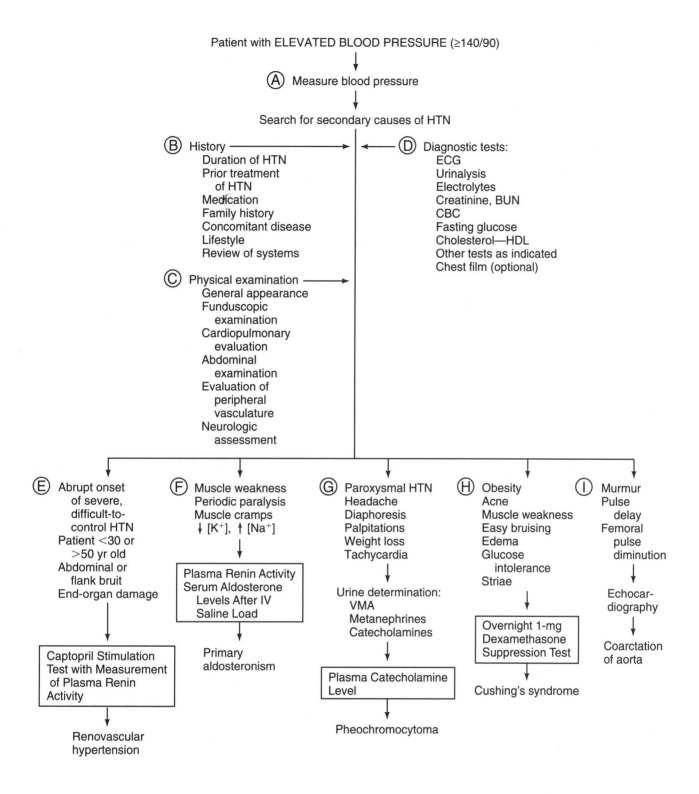

Ⓐ Measure blood pressure

Search for secondary causes of HTN

Ⓑ History
    Duration of HTN
    Prior treatment
        of HTN
    Medication
    Family history
    Concomitant disease
    Lifestyle
    Review of systems

Ⓓ Diagnostic tests:
    ECG
    Urinalysis
    Electrolytes
    Creatinine, BUN
    CBC
    Fasting glucose
    Cholesterol—HDL
    Other tests as indicated
    Chest film (optional)

Ⓒ Physical examination
    General appearance
    Funduscopic
        examination
    Cardiopulmonary
        evaluation
    Abdominal
        examination
    Evaluation of
        peripheral
        vasculature
    Neurologic
        assessment

Ⓔ Abrupt onset
    of severe,
    difficult-to-
    control HTN
    Patient <30 or
    >50 yr old
    Abdominal or
    flank bruit
    End-organ damage

Captopril Stimulation
Test with Measurement
of Plasma Renin
Activity

Renovascular
hypertension

Ⓕ Muscle weakness
    Periodic paralysis
    Muscle cramps
    ↓ [K⁺], ↑ [Na⁺]

Plasma Renin Activity
Serum Aldosterone
Levels After IV
Saline Load

Primary
aldosteronism

Ⓖ Paroxysmal HTN
    Headache
    Diaphoresis
    Palpitations
    Weight loss
    Tachycardia

Urine determination:
    VMA
    Metanephrines
    Catecholamines

Plasma Catecholamine
Level

Pheochromocytoma

Ⓗ Obesity
    Acne
    Muscle weakness
    Easy bruising
    Edema
    Glucose
        intolerance
    Striae

Overnight 1-mg
Dexamethasone
Suppression Test

Cushing's syndrome

Ⓘ Murmur
    Pulse
        delay
    Femoral
        pulse
        diminution

Echocar-
diography

Coarctation
of aorta

E. Renovascular disease, one of the more common causes of secondary HTN (1–5% of HTN patients), results in renal hypoperfusion and renovascular hypertension (RVH). Suspect RVH when there is an abrupt onset of severe, difficult-to-control HTN in a female <30 or >50 years of age, abdominal or flank bruits, azotemia induced by angiotensin-converting enzyme inhibitors, and evidence of end-organ damage. The two major causes of RVH are atherosclerosis and fibromuscular dysplasia of the renal artery. The former is found in the older population and the latter in a younger age group. The diagnosis is suggested by the captopril stimulation test. All antihypertensive drugs, including diuretics, are discontinued for 1 week. The patient is seated for 30 minutes before and throughout the test. Plasma renin angiotensin (PRA) levels are drawn initially and 60 minutes after oral administration of a 50-mg captopril tablet. An increase in PRA at 60 minutes is the hallmark of RVH. Sampling of renal vein renin usually corroborates RVH.

F. Primary aldosteronism is the syndrome resulting from the secretion of excessive amounts of aldosterone. Most cases involve a unilateral adrenal adenoma occurring with equal frequency on either side. The disease, known as Conn's syndrome, is seen in patients 30 to 50 years old, and in women more than in men. Many patients have clinical and biochemical features characteristic of primary aldosteronism, but a solitary adenoma is not found at surgery. Instead, these patients have bilateral adreno-cortical hyperplasia. Clinical features include HTN, hypokalemia, hypernatremia, excessive urinary potassium, weakness, headache, muscle cramping, and polydipsia.

The ECG reveals signs of left ventricular enlargement and prominent U waves, denoting potassium depletion. Edema is usually absent. The diagnosis is made by measurement of plasma renin activity that fails to increase during volume depletion and hypersecretion of aldosterone that fails to suppress appropriately during volume expansion (salt loading).

G. Pheochromocytoma occurs in ≤1% of HTN patients, generally in the fourth to sixth decades of life. It is a catecholamine-producing tumor arising from the adrenal medulla (only a small percentage originate from extra-adrenal sites). The distinctive clinical features of pheochromocytoma are related to excessive production of catecholamines. Clinical features are extremely variable, with paroxysmal HTN occurring in 50% of cases. Typical paroxysms consist of marked BP elevation, headache, sweating, palpitations, pallor, nausea, and abdominal discomfort. Attacks may be spontaneous or precipitated by emotion, smoking, exercise, or postural change. On rare occasions it is associated with neurofibromatosis, Von Hippel-Lindau syndrome, and medullary carcinoma of the thyroid. The diagnosis is based on elevated levels of catecholamines and their metabolites in urine. Assays of urinary catecholamines and metanephrines are usually sufficient to diagnose pheochromocytoma in most patients, but when results are equivocal and "pheo" is suggested clinically, plasma catecholamines should be measured. After diagnosis the tumor is located by CT scan of the abdomen. About 90% of pheochromocytomas are in an adrenal gland, with a 2:1 preference for the right over the left side.

H. Cushing's syndrome is caused by cortisol excess. The syndrome carries an excessive mortality rate because of its association with CV disease. HTN, present in >80% of patients with Cushing's syndrome, is the major risk factor for the development of premature CV disease. Bruising, myopathy, HTN, edema, hirsutism, striae, and various neuropsychiatric disturbances ranging from a mild decrease in energy to severe depression are found in the syndrome. The extent of the work-up of patients with suspected Cushing's syndrome varies with the clinical situation. An overnight 1-mg dexamethasone suppression test is adequate for most patients with only minimal suggestive features. The plasma cortisol is measured at 8 AM the next morning.

I. Coarctation of the aorta is a constriction of the lumen of the aorta, just below the origin of the left subclavian artery. The lesion occurs in 7% of patients with congenital heart disease and is twice as common in males as in females. Symptoms may include headache, cold extremities, fatigue, and claudication of lower extremities. HTN in the upper extremities and marked delay or diminution of femoral pulses are detected on physical examination. The ECG may reveal left ventricular hypertrophy of varying degree. Chest radiography may reveal cardiomegaly, rib notching, and the "3" sign from dilation of the aorta above and below the constriction. Two-dimensional echocardiography is used to identify the site of the coarctation.

References

Littenberg B, Garber AM, Sox HC Jr. Screening for hypertension. Ann Intern Med 1990; 112:192.

Marks P. Endocrine hypertension. Intern Med Specialist. 1987; 8:155.

1988 Report of the Joint National Commission (JNC) on Detection, Evaluation and Treatment of High Blood Pressure. US Department of Health and Human Services. NIH Pub 88-1088. High Blood Pressure.

Postma CT, Van der Steen PHM. Horsnagels WHL, et al. The captopril test in the detection of renal vascular disease in hypertensive patients. Arch Intern Med 1988; 150:625.

HYPOTENSION

Mark C. Goldberg, M.D.

The systolic pressure at which a patient can be considered hypotensive is variable. When systolic blood pressure drops below 80 mm Hg, symptoms and signs of a generalized inadequacy in tissue perfusion are often noted. Chronically hypertensive patients may manifest these symptoms and signs long before their systolic pressure reaches 80 mm Hg.

A. If the cause of hypotension does not declare itself immediately on presentation, the symptoms and signs of inadequate tissue perfusion will alert the examiner to the rapid need for investigation. An altered sensorium; diaphoresis; tachycardia; a drop in urine output; tachypnea; and cool, clammy skin are typically present. A history and physical examination in conjunction with basic laboratory studies (including chest films and ECG) usually provide a diagnosis.

B. ECG monitoring begins on presentation of the hypotensive patient. The prevalence of coronary artery disease makes acute myocardial infarction (MI) a likely cause of hypotension in the middle-aged and elderly population. In the setting of acute MI, malignant arrhythmias may be effectively treated with DC cardioversion if they need to be treated immediately. In situations unrelated to an ischemic event, supraventricular and ventricular arrhythmias may cause hypotension by reducing the ventricular filling period. Pharmacologic therapy is occasionally indicated, but cardioversion is most often preferred in hypotensive patients.

C. In patients with acute MI and hypotension, Swan-Ganz catheterization is used to direct therapy. A moderately elevated left-sided filling pressure suggests substantial loss of left ventricular (LV) muscle, which may result in progression to cardiogenic shock. Conversely, a normal-to-low pulmonary capillary wedge pressure (PCWP) with an elevated right ventricular (RV) pressure is found in RV infarction. This usually arises when an inferior infarction involves the right ventricle. If the PCWP tracing shows large V waves, acute papillary muscle rupture must be suspected. Oxygen saturations may be performed on blood withdrawn from ports located at various positions on the catheter. If RV saturation exceeds right atrial (RA) saturation, a ventricular septal defect may be diagnosed.

D. The chest film in cardiac tamponade often shows an enlarged cardiac silhouette. Patients in congestive heart failure have Kerley B lines, interstitial edema, and pulmonary effusions in addition to an enlarged cardiac silhouette.

E. A crude gauge of volume status may be obtained from the BUN/creatinine ratio. The hemoglobin may be followed in a bleeding patient, although it is not useful in acute situations.

F. Cardiac tamponade may be considered a state of relative volume depletion in that ventricular filling is compromised although the patient is euvolemic. Both echocardiography and Swan-Ganz catheterization may be used to confirm the diagnosis. On echocardiography, evidence of RA or RV collapse in addition to specific Doppler flow patterns are diagnostic. The Swan-Ganz catheter shows an equalization of pressures throughout the heart brought about by external compression of the heart.

G. Pneumothorax may be diagnosed on chest film by a shift in mediastinal location and loss of pulmonary markings in the periphery of the affected hemithorax.

References

Forrester JS, Diamond MD, Chatterjee K. Medial therapy of acute myocardial infarction by application of hemodynamic subsets. N Engl J Med 1976; 295:1356.

Fox AC, Glassman E. Surgical remediable complications of myocardial infarction. Prog Cardiovasc Dis 1979; 21:461.

Yakaitis RW, Ewy GA, Otto CW, et al. Influence of time and therapy on ventricular defibrillation in dogs. Crit Care Med 1986; 8:157.

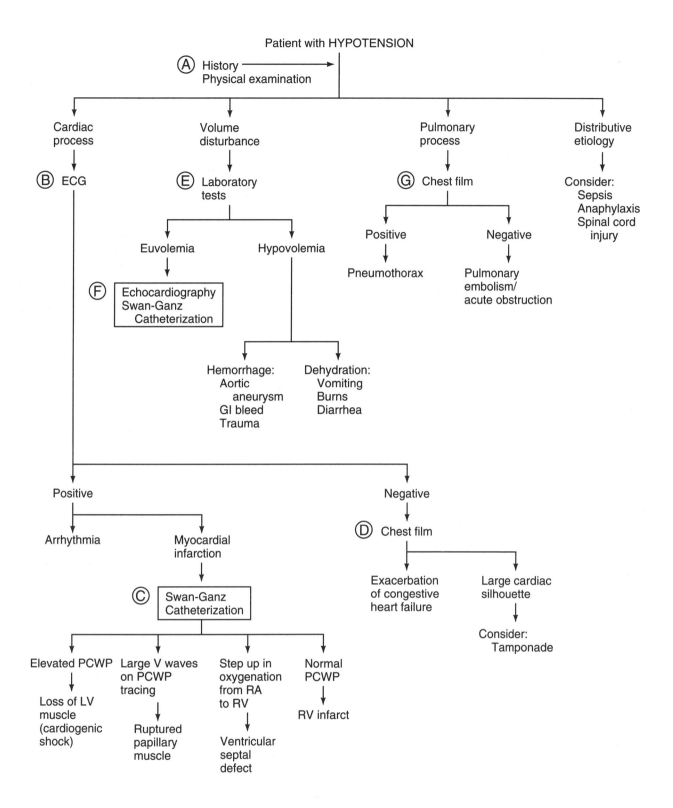

PALPITATIONS

Karl B. Kern, M.D.
Paul E. Fenster, M.D.

Palpitations are a common problem. Recent evidence suggests a more cautious approach to antiarrhythmic therapy in dealing with such problems.

A. The history and physical examination should be targeted towards revealing any reversible cause for the palpitations. Most important is the patient's current use of medications. Stimulants, including caffeine and smoking, should also be carefully reviewed. Metabolic, pulmonary, and neurologic/psychiatric causes should then be considered.

B. Important in the work-up of palpitations is the relative frequency at which they occur. If they are infrequent but bothersome, an event monitor may be a real help. Such a device can be worn for up to 1 week and has the ability to continuously monitor the patient's rhythm, but to record the rhythm only when specific buttons are activated. Some devices can even "go back in time" and record up to 15–30 seconds before the moment when the recording button is activated.

C. Results from the monitoring period may be varied. Some patients may experience their symptoms and yet show no correlation on the monitor to a rhythm disturbance. No cardiac treatment is then necessary.

D. Supraventricular arrhythmias may cause palpitations. If atrial fibrillation is discovered, an assessment of underlying organic heart disease is helpful, since thromboembolism is common in patients with heart disease and atrial fibrillation.

E. Discovery of atrial premature contractions (APCs) or even supraventricular tachycardia (SVT) may first be dealt with as benign and with reassurance. If symptoms are troublesome, therapy may be indicated. (See pp 44 and 46.)

F. If ventricular ectopy is the cause of palpitations, the underlying status of myocardial disease is an impor-

tant factor in considering treatment. If there is no evidence of coronary artery disease (CAD) or left ventricular dysfunction, reassurance, even for nonsustained ventricular tachycardia, appears to be the best therapeutic choice.

G. If there is left ventricular dysfunction, treatment of the underlying condition is most helpful.

H. The presence of CAD should lead to Holter or EPS (electrophysiologic study)-guided treatment for any serious form of ventricular ectopy. Alternatives are empiric amiodarone therapy or an implantable device (automatic implantable cardioverter-defibrillator [AICD]) if documented, serious ventricular ectopy is found.

I. Bradycardia can also be a cause of palpitations. Most commonly, medications are involved. If bradycardia is not due to a reversible cause, such as drugs, and the degree of block is advanced (Mobitz II or worse), pacemaker therapy is worth considering.

References

Burkart F, Pfisterer M, Kiowski W, et al. Effect of antiarrhythmic therapy on mortality in survivors of myocardial infarction with symptomatic complex ventricular arrhythmias: Basel Antiarrhythmic Study of Infarct Survival (BASIS). J Am Coll Cardiol 1990; 16:1711.

Cardiac Arrhythmia Suppression Trial. Preliminary report: effect of encainide and flecainide on mortality in a randomized trial of arrhythmia suppression after myocardial infarction. N Engl J Med 1989; 321:406.

Report of the stroke prevention in preliminary atrial fibrillation study. N Engl J Med 1990; 322:863.

Stanton MS, Prystowsky EN, Fineberg NS, et al. Arrhythmogenic effects of antiarrhythmic drugs: a study of 506 patients treated for ventricular tachycardia or fibrillation. J Am Coll Cardiol 1989; 14:209.

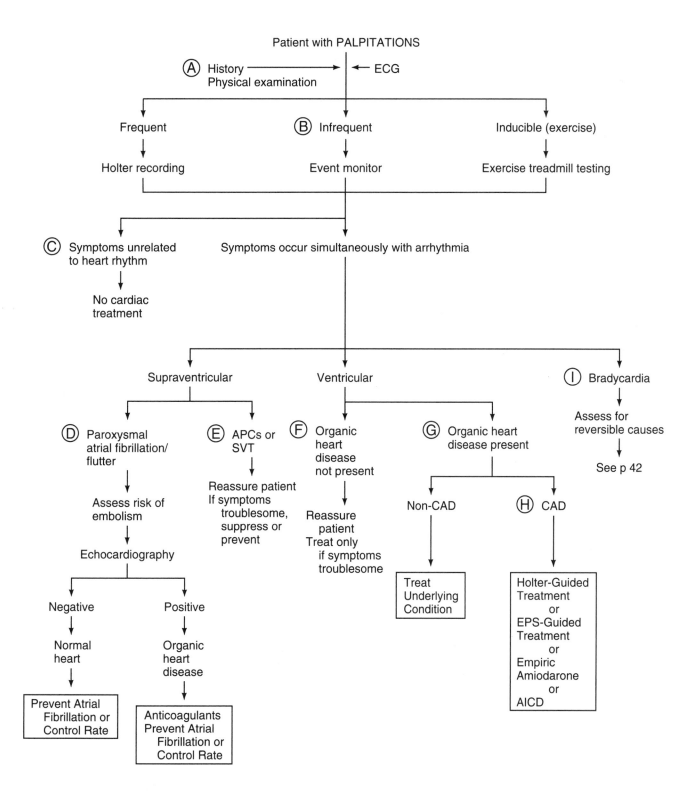

Patient with PALPITATIONS

(A) History ——————→ ← ECG
Physical examination

Frequent   (B) Infrequent   Inducible (exercise)

Holter recording   Event monitor   Exercise treadmill testing

(C) Symptoms unrelated to heart rhythm   Symptoms occur simultaneously with arrhythmia

No cardiac treatment

Supraventricular   Ventricular   (I) Bradycardia

Assess for reversible causes

See p 42

(D) Paroxysmal atrial fibrillation/ flutter

(E) APCs or SVT

(F) Organic heart disease not present

(G) Organic heart disease present

Reassure patient If symptoms troublesome, suppress or prevent

Assess risk of embolism

Reassure patient Treat only if symptoms troublesome

Non-CAD

(H) CAD

Echocardiography

Treat Underlying Condition

Holter-Guided Treatment or EPS-Guided Treatment or Empiric Amiodarone or AICD

Negative   Positive

Normal heart

Organic heart disease

Prevent Atrial Fibrillation or Control Rate

Anticoagulants Prevent Atrial Fibrillation or Control Rate

SYNCOPE

Anthony C. Caruso, M.D.

Syncope is defined as a temporary loss of consciousness and postural tone with spontaneous resolution. Although syncope is a common problem, accounting for up to 6% of medical admissions and 3% of all ER visits, the causes are myriad, the work-up seemingly unending, and the results often inconclusive. A reassuring point is that the patient who has a diagnosis of syncope of undetermined origin following an extensive work-up as described in this chapter is at low risk for suffering a fatal event, although the morbidity of frequent episodes of syncope should not be minimized.

A. A detailed history is important. The events leading up to syncope (e.g., micturition, postural changes, exercise), prodromal symptoms or auras, and the presence of witnesses and their impressions are extremely valuable. A history of other medical problems such as hypoglycemia and neurologic disease and a complete knowledge of current medications is essential. Physical examination should include orthostatic blood pressure determinations, cardiovascular examination, and thorough neurologic assessment. Although carotid hypersensitivity is an uncommon cause of syncope, carotid sinus massage may be performed at this time if there are no contraindications. Blood chemistry studies, including glucose and electrolytes, and a 12-lead ECG conclude the initial evaluation.

B. In patients with a history of seizure disorder, focal neurologic findings, a recent history of head trauma or other factors suggesting a neurologic etiology, CT of the head, and EEG are beneficial.

C. In patients with a strong cardiac history or who show evidence of obstructive coronary disease, valvular heart disease, or dysrhythmia, a careful cardiac work-up should be pursued before a neurologic work-up. A simple 12-lead ECG may reveal evidence of heart block or sinus node dysfunction but rarely leads to a diagnosis of tachydysrhythmias as the cause of syncope. Since 26% of all episodes of syncope are due to cardiac causes and there is an increased risk of sudden death (up to 30% mortality) if syncope has a cardiac cause, it is prudent to screen carefully for a cardiac etiology if the history and physical examination do not suggest a neurologic basis.

D. Echocardiography is helpful for evaluation of structural cardiac defects associated with syncope, including aortic stenosis, hypertrophic cardiomyopathy (HCM), atrial myxomas, and mitral stenosis. If a cardiac etiology seems possible and no history of cardiac disease is known, echocardiography can help determine the presence of normal or abnormal left ventricular (LV) function. In patients with preserved LV function, the head-up tilt test may be helpful but lacks

specificity. This method of assessing neurocardiac syncope has undergone a resurgence of interest in recent years, although the mechanism for neurocardiac syncope remains unclear. We recommend that the head-up tilt should be to at least 60° after a baseline supine assessment of at least 20 min (the initial tilt should be for up to 45 min if catecholamines are not to be used) or until the patient becomes symptomatic. After baseline assessment the patient is returned to the supine position for 5 min, then returned to a 60° tilt with the administration of a 2-μg isoproterenol IV bolus. This should be repeated with incremental doses of isoproterenol at 4, 6, and 8 μg after rest periods of 5 min in the supine position, or until symptomatic. The patient should remain in the upright tilt position for up to 10 min after each administration of isoproterenol or until symptoms develop.

E. The ambulatory Holter monitor is helpful when the patient has frequent episodes of syncope or presyncope, but in patients whose episodes are infrequent, a cardiac event monitor is often necessary. In patients with depressed LV function (LVEF < 40%) and a history of myocardial infarction who are found to have nonsustained ventricular tachycardia, a signal-averaged ECG is often useful.

F. A negative signal-averaged ECG has excellent negative predictive accuracy and gives reassurance that the patient is at low risk for cardiac sudden death. Up to 50% of patients with a positive signal-averaged ECG will be found to have inducible ventricular tachycardia on electrophysiologic studies (EPS).

G. The use of invasive EPS in the work-up of syncope remains controversial. Clearly there are problems with the sensitivity and specificity of invasive testing of sinoatrial and atrioventricular nodal function. We recommend that EPS be reserved for patients with a high pretest probability of a tachyarrhythmia as the cause of syncope, because the sensitivity and specificity of inducible ventricular tachycardia in patients with no structural heart disease are only 40 and 60%, respectively. It is strongly urged that patients with a positive signal-averaged ECG or a history of myocardial infarction, depressed LV function, and nonsustained ventricular tachycardia undergo EPS, because the incidence of ventricular tachycardia in this population is increased and the consequence of missing this diagnosis may be catastrophic.

H. Exercise treadmill testing (ETT) is often helpful in a patient with a history of exercise-induced syncope, but is otherwise of little value, since myocardial ischemia is a rare cause of syncope.

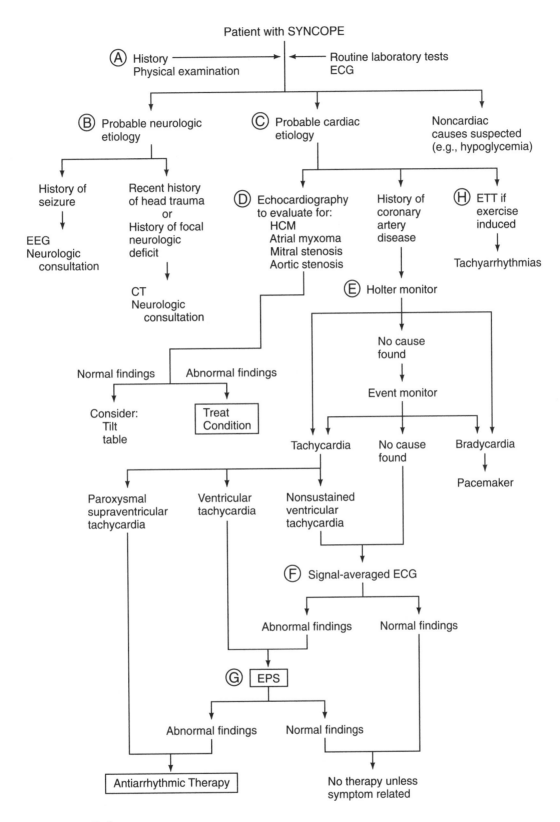

Patient with SYNCOPE

(A) History ——— Physical examination ←—— Routine laboratory tests / ECG

(B) Probable neurologic etiology

(C) Probable cardiac etiology

Noncardiac causes suspected (e.g., hypoglycemia)

History of seizure → EEG Neurologic consultation

Recent history of head trauma or History of focal neurologic deficit → CT Neurologic consultation

(D) Echocardiography to evaluate for:
HCM
Atrial myxoma
Mitral stenosis
Aortic stenosis

History of coronary artery disease

(H) ETT if exercise induced → Tachyarrhythmias

(E) Holter monitor

Normal findings → Consider: Tilt table

Abnormal findings → Treat Condition

No cause found → Event monitor

Tachycardia

No cause found

Bradycardia → Pacemaker

Paroxysmal supraventricular tachycardia

Ventricular tachycardia

Nonsustained ventricular tachycardia

(F) Signal-averaged ECG

Abnormal findings

Normal findings

(G) EPS

Abnormal findings

Normal findings

Antiarrhythmic Therapy

No therapy unless symptom related

References

Dimarco JP. Electrophysiologic studies in patients with unexplained syncope. Circulation 1987; 75:140.

Kapoor WN, Cha R, Petersen JR, et al. Prolonged electrocardiographic monitoring in patients with syncope. Am J Med 1987; 82:20.

Kapoor WN, Karpf M, Wieand S, et al. A prospective evaluation and follow-up of patients with syncope. N Engl J Med 1983; 309:197.

Strasberg B, Rechavie E, Sagie A, et al. The head-up tilt table test in patients with syncope of unknown origin. Am Heart J 1989; 118:923.

LARGE CARDIAC SILHOUETTE

James R. Standen, M.D.

Cardiomegaly on chest films is a common finding in many heart diseases. In some conditions there is generalized enlargement of the cardiac silhouette; in others there is a dilatation of some cardiac chambers and sparing of the rest. Chamber dilatation may be due to volume overload (e.g., aortic regurgitation) or decomposition from pressure overload (e.g., aortic stenosis). Identification of the pattern of enlargement and specifically of which individual chambers and great vessels are involved often provides a specific diagnosis.

A. The pulmonary vascular pattern gives useful insights into cardiac function. Decreased pulmonary vascularity is seen in severe forms of constrictive pericarditis, cardiac tamponade, and obstructive lesions of the right side of the heart (e.g., pulmonary stenosis and tetralogy of Fallot). Increased pulmonary vascularity, with normal upper and lower lobe distribution, is usually seen in left-to-right shunt lesions when the shunt ratio is >2:1 (e.g., atrial septal defect). Pulmonary venous hypertension with redistribution of flow to the upper lungs (with or without pulmonary edema) results from impaired diastolic function of the left ventricle and/or emptying of the left atrium. Vascular redistribution begins when the pulmonary venous pressure (wedge pressure) exceeds 15–20 mm Hg. In the acute situation, pulmonary edema results when the pressure exceeds the oncotic pressure of plasma at 25–30 mm Hg. In chronic states (e.g., mitral stenosis) compensatory mechanisms such as increased lymphatic drainage may prevent pulmonary edema even though the pulmonary venous pressure considerably exceeds that of the plasma proteins. Pulmonary arterial hypertension may be due to postcapillary pulmonary venous hypertension (e.g., mitral stenosis), obliteration of the capillary bed (e.g., cor pulmonale in emphysema), or precapillary obstruction (e.g., primary pulmonary hypertension). When persistent, it causes dilatation of the central pulmonary arteries, with oligemia or "pruning" of the smaller peripheral branches. Recognition of specific heart chamber, pulmonary vascular, and great vessel abnormalities on chest films can help direct which further investigations are appropriate (e.g., echocardiography, nuclear studies, cardiac catheterization) and what particular information is required from them. Localized enlargements of specific cardiac chambers may lead to distinct diagnoses.

B. Left ventricular (LV) enlargement alone results from decompensated aortic stenosis or systemic hypertension. In some cases of aortic stenosis, a prominent ascending aorta is seen from post-stenotic dilatation.

C. LV and aortic enlargement results commonly from aortic regurgitation.

D. LV and left atrial (LA) enlargement indicates mitral regurgitation.

E. LA and pulmonary artery (PA) enlargement with vascular redistribution to the upper lobes results from mitral stenosis. A "double density" sign for left atrial enlargement is often seen.

F. Increased pulmonary vascularity (i.e., shunt vascularity) may result from several lesions, with consequent increased left-to-right pulmonary flow. Right ventricular (RV) and sometimes right atrial (RA) enlargement with shunt vascularity is seen with atrial septal defect. LV and LA enlargement with shunt vascularity indicates ventricular septal defect. LV, LA, and aortic enlargement with shunt vascularity indicates patent ductus arteriosus.

G. RV and central PA enlargement with "pruning" of the pulmonary vascular pattern peripherally is seen with primary pulmonary hypertension, cor pulmonale, or multiple pulmonary emboli.

References

Daves ML. Cardiac roentgenology. Chicago: Year–Book, 1981.

Fraser RG, Pare JAP. Diagnosis of diseases of the chest. 3rd ed. Philadelphia: WB Saunders, 1990.

Taveras JM, Ferrucci JT. Radiology: diagnosis–imaging–intervention. Philadelphia: JB Lippincott, 1990.

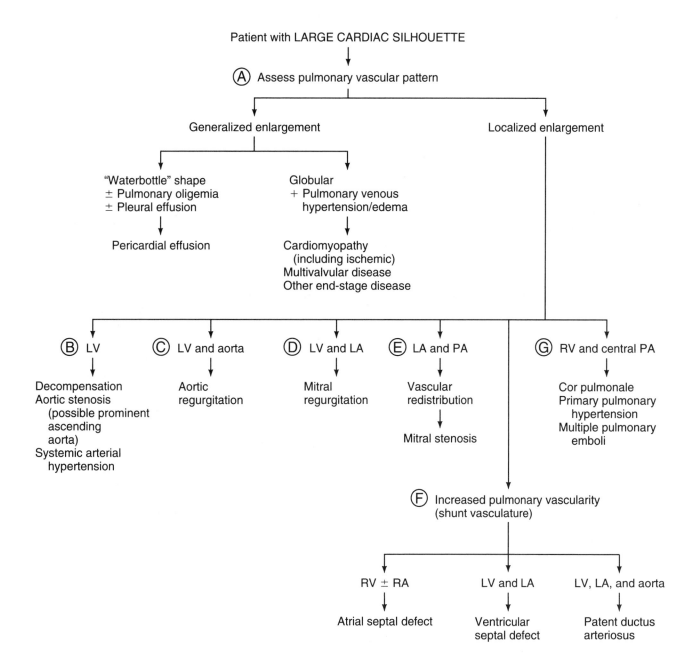

Patient with LARGE CARDIAC SILHOUETTE

Ⓐ Assess pulmonary vascular pattern

Generalized enlargement   Localized enlargement

"Waterbottle" shape   Globular
± Pulmonary oligemia   + Pulmonary venous
± Pleural effusion   hypertension/edema

Pericardial effusion   Cardiomyopathy
                             (including ischemic)
                             Multivalvular disease
                             Other end-stage disease

Ⓑ LV   Ⓒ LV and aorta   Ⓓ LV and LA   Ⓔ LA and PA   Ⓖ RV and central PA

Decompensation   Aortic   Mitral   Vascular   Cor pulmonale
Aortic stenosis   regurgitation   regurgitation   redistribution   Primary pulmonary
  (possible prominent   hypertension
  ascending   Mitral stenosis   Multiple pulmonary
  aorta)   emboli
Systemic arterial
  hypertension

Ⓕ Increased pulmonary vascularity
   (shunt vasculature)

RV ± RA   LV and LA   LV, LA, and aorta

Atrial septal defect   Ventricular   Patent ductus
                       septal defect   arteriosus

CONGESTIVE HEART FAILURE

Karil Bellah, M.D.

Heart failure is a common disease affecting approximately 2 million Americans. The prevalence of this disease in persons 50–59 years of age is 1%. This number doubles every decade, so that 10% of the US population > 80 years old is affected. Heart failure has a very grave prognosis, with a 5-year mortality rate of 62% in men and 42% in women. Heart failure is not a single disease entity with one cause; rather, there are many causes. An improved clinical outcome can be achieved with many forms of heart failure, so that it is important to determine the cause of heart failure and treat it appropriately.

A. Valvular heart disease accounts for 5–10% of cases of heart failure and includes lesions caused by rheumatic heart disease, myxomatous valves, and degenerative (usually calcified) valves. Both stenotic and regurgitant lesions can lead to heart failure by creating either pressure (stenotic) or volume (regurgitant) overload on the heart.

B. Approximately 40–60% of patients with heart failure have coronary artery disease (CAD). In patients with known or suspected CAD, an echocardiographic (ECHO) or radionuclide ventriculography (RVG) study is indicated to assess the ejection fraction (EF). Many patients with CAD have systolic failure with a low EF due to replacement of functioning myocardium with scar tissue created by myocardial infarction(s). Patients with systolic heart failure benefit from afterload reduction, diuretics, and digitalis therapy.

C. Many patients with documented heart failure have a normal EF. The cause of heart failure in these patients is diastolic dysfunction resulting from impaired relaxation and filling of the left ventricle. Diastolic dysfunction can be caused by acute ischemia, which may be silent and thus not detected on a resting ECHO study.

D. If there is no evidence of systolic or diastolic dysfunction, a cardiac stress test (treadmill, thallium, stress ECHO, or RVG) should be performed to rule out CAD. Right and left heart catheterization may also be indicated if the diagnosis of CAD and cause of heart failure are still in question.

E. Hypertensive heart disease is very prevalent, especially in the elderly, and may be found in up to 75% of heart failure patients. The initial problem is decreased ventricular compliance causing impaired relaxation and ventricular filling. This may be severe and is usually associated with ventricular hypertrophy. With appropriate antihypertensive therapy (angiotensin-converting enzyme inhibitors, calcium channel blockers, and, to a lesser extent, beta-adrenergic blockers), the hypertrophy regresses and an improvement in diastolic function may also occur. As the disease progresses, systolic failure may result, but this is much less common.

F. Even though a patient has hypertensive disease, CAD may also be contributing to the heart failure if wall motion abnormalities are demonstrated on ECHO. A combination of hypertension and CAD are often the cause of heart failure, and each should be appropriately treated.

G. When the history and physical examination do not assist in determining the cause of the heart failure, an ECHO can provide very useful information. Evidence of restrictive, constrictive, and hypertrophic heart disease may be seen, and if so should be followed up with cardiac catheterization. One should consider obtaining a cardiac biopsy at the time of catheterization if an infiltrative disease process (such as amyloid) is suspected but not confirmed by ECHO.

H. Many diseases can cause a dilated cardiomyopathy, but the most common ones are postviral and idiopathic, accounting for 10–30% of patients with heart failure. The role of biopsy in this group of patients has been examined; when acute viral myocarditis is suspected, there is a moderate yield from the biopsy (20–65%). However, when the biopsy is performed to obtain a diagnosis of unexplained heart failure, the yield is low and does not warrant the risk of the procedure. Other causes of heart failure in this group are rare and include alcohol, metal intoxication, cardiotoxic medications, and other systemic diseases. When these rare causes are suspected, a prudent and exhaustive evaluation is warranted.

I. When the ECHO is normal in a patient with symptoms of heart failure, a right and left heart catheterization may provide useful information and uncover unsuspected coronary or pulmonary vascular disease. When this is not the case, chronic lung disease, anemia, obesity, physical deconditioning, depression, or an endocrine abnormality should be considered as the cause of the symptoms.

References

Applegate RJ, Little WC. Systolic and diastolic dysfunction in CHF. Cardiology 1991; 57.

Chesebro JH, Burnett JC. Cardiac failure: characteristics and clinical manifestations. In: Brandenburg RO, Fuster V, Giuliani ER, McGoon DC, eds. Cardiology: fundamentals and practice. Chicago: Year–Book Medical Publishers, 1989.

Chow LC, Dittrich HC, Shabetai R. Endomyocardial biopsy in patients with unexplained heart failure. Ann Intern Med 1988; 109:535.

Kannel WB, Belanger AJ. Epidemiology of heart failure. Am Heart J 1991; 121:951.

Patient with CONGESTIVE HEART FAILURE

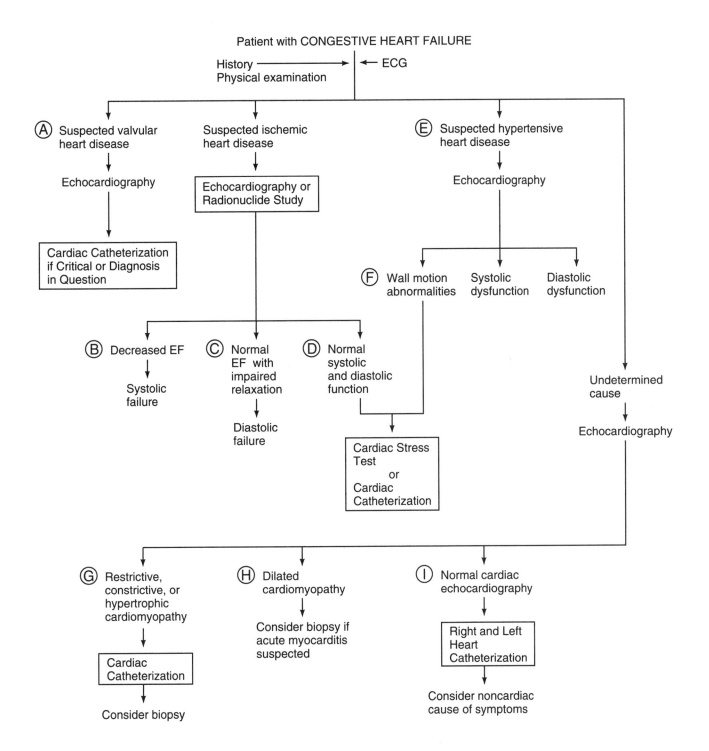

ACUTE PULMONARY EDEMA

James M. Galloway, M.D.
Paul E. Fenster, M.D.

A. Significant historical data include any history of heart disease (including ischemic, valvular, or congestive heart failure), pulmonary disease, recent acute illness, fevers, chills, sweats, sputum production, chronic renal failure, or other chronic illness. Also, determine current medication and drug usage.

B. Direct particular attention in the physical examination to BP, pulse rate, the presence or absence of a pulsus paradoxus, jugular venous pressure, pulmonary status, heart murmurs, the presence or absence of an S_3, and peripheral edema.

C. Initial laboratory evaluation should include arterial blood gases, CBC with differential, electrolytes, BUN, creatinine, ECG, and chest film. A pulse oximeter to determine peripheral oxygenation status may be helpful and provide a rapid assessment of the severity of the hypoxia.

D. A number of priorities can be addressed simultaneously. In urgent cases therapeutic interventions should be initiated immediately upon patient arrival, even while the history and physical examination are being performed. In most patients the assumption of a sitting position, IV administration of a potent diuretic, and high-flow O_2 and IV morphine and/or sublingual nitroglycerin results in significant clinical improvement. Diuretics commonly used include furosemide, 20–40 mg, or bumetanide, 0.5–1.0 mg. IV furosemide acutely exerts a direct venodilating effect that produces venous pooling and reduces central venous pressure (CVP) before the onset of diuresis. IV morphine is effective in reducing CVP and afterload as well as reducing anxiety. Sublingual nitroglycerin, 0.4–0.8 mg, also reduces CVP. Morphine or nitroglycerin may worsen hypotension. High concentrations of O_2 (50–100%) should be initiated at once. O_2 therapy should not be withheld in hypoxic patients with acute dyspnea despite a history of chronic obstructive pulmonary disease and concern about CO_2 retention, although initial low-concentration or low-flow rates may be prudent. If higher levels of O_2 are required, assess the need for intubation frequently.

E. Clinically, an adequate response to therapy is indicated by improvement in pulse rate, respiratory rate and depth, skin color, pulmonary status, and overall appearance. A reasonable goal for adequate oxygenation is to maintain PaO_2 of 90–100 mm Hg.

F. In patients believed to be in initially unresponsive cardiogenic pulmonary edema with adequate BP, the use of afterload reduction to improve cardiac output and reduce pulmonary congestion may be of significant benefit. A continuous infusion of IV nitroprusside or nitroglycerin can be given. IV nitroglycerin has the added advantage of antianginal properties. The IV use of positive inotropes can also be considered in this group of patients (as well as those with low BP) to increase cardiac output. Continuous infusions of dobutamine or dopamine may be given and titrated to optimal response. The placement of a pulmonary artery (PA) catheter is generally recommended to guide therapy while these agents are used.

G. Although the differential diagnosis of acute pulmonary edema is extensive, most patients who present with this condition have a history of heart disease and have had progression of underlying disease (e.g., worsening valvular disease, recurrent ischemia), dietary indiscretion, a recent change in medications (through noncompliance, the addition of a cardiodepressant medication, or a recent decrease in needed cardiac medications), an increase in metabolic demands (including infection, anemia, pregnancy, atrioventricular (AV) shunt, hyperthyroidism), or (particularly in hospitalized patients) volume overload.

H. Myocardial etiologies include systolic and diastolic dysfunction due to primary or secondary myocardial disease. These conditions include dilated cardiomyopathies with many possible causes (hypertensive, ischemic, infectious, toxic, idiopathic), restrictive cardiomyopathies (amyloidosis, sarcoidosis, hemochromatosis), and hypertrophic cardiomyopathy.

I. Acute pulmonary edema with no easily discernible cause may have cardiac or noncardiac causes. Cardiogenic etiologies include transient ischemic or arrhythmic events, occult valvular disease (e.g., infectious endocarditis), pericardial disease (e.g., tamponade and constriction), metabolic causes (e.g., hyperthyroidism and hypothyroidism), initial late presentations of congenital heart disease, and heart disease related to connective tissue disorders. Noncardiac causes include diffuse pulmonary infections, aspiration, toxic pulmonary insults (e.g., smoke, chlorine gas), narcotic overdose, gram-negative septicemia, hemorrhagic pancreatitis, lymphatic blockage due to carcinomatosis, fibrosis or inflammatory disease, neurogenic disorders, and high-altitude pulmonary edema. Echocardiography can differentiate cardiogenic from noncardiogenic etiologies and thus determine further therapeutic interventions. If echocardiography is nondiagnostic, further evaluate noncardiogenic or transient cardiogenic etiologies.

J. Initial evaluation for transient arrhythmias (besides the initial ECG) should generally consist of a Holter monitor and/or a signal-averaged ECG. If these suggest significant ventricular arrhythmias, electrophysiologic evaluation may be in order to best define the arrhythmia and its ideal therapy. Provocative testing for transient ischemia generally consists of a treadmill

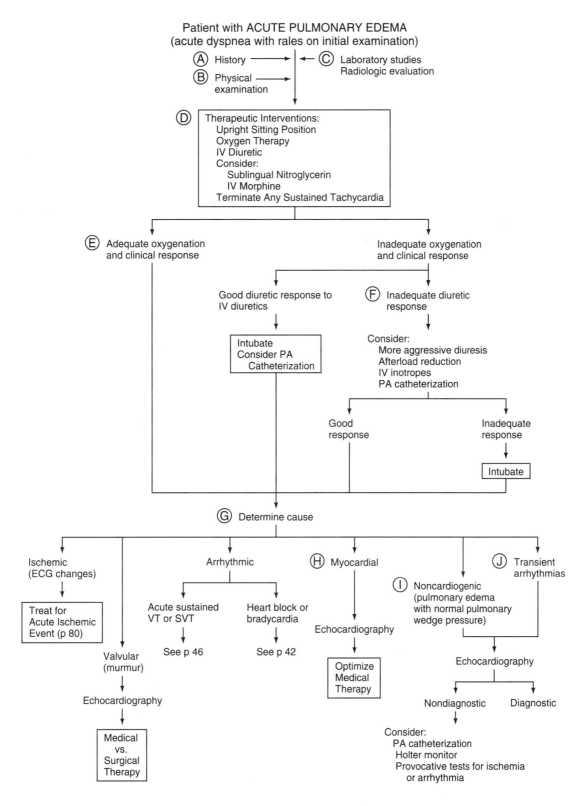

Patient with ACUTE PULMONARY EDEMA
(acute dyspnea with rales on initial examination)

(A) History → ← (C) Laboratory studies
                     Radiologic evaluation
(B) Physical →
    examination

(D) Therapeutic Interventions:
    Upright Sitting Position
    Oxygen Therapy
    IV Diuretic
    Consider:
        Sublingual Nitroglycerin
        IV Morphine
        Terminate Any Sustained Tachycardia

(E) Adequate oxygenation   Inadequate oxygenation
    and clinical response   and clinical response

Good diuretic response to   (F) Inadequate diuretic
IV diuretics   response

Intubate   Consider:
Consider PA   More aggressive diuresis
Catheterization   Afterload reduction
                                 IV inotropes
                                 PA catheterization

                    Good   Inadequate
                    response   response

                                            Intubate

(G) Determine cause

Ischemic   Arrhythmic   (H) Myocardial   (I) Noncardiogenic   (J) Transient
(ECG changes)   (pulmonary edema   arrhythmias
                                                          with normal pulmonary
                                                          wedge pressure)
Treat for   Acute sustained   Heart block or
Acute Ischemic VT or SVT   bradycardia
Event (p 80)   Echocardiography
                See p 46   See p 42
Valvular   Optimize   Echocardiography
(murmur)   Medical
                                  Therapy   Nondiagnostic   Diagnostic
Echocardiography

Medical   Consider:
vs.   PA catheterization
Surgical   Holter monitor
Therapy   Provocative tests for ischemia
                                                           or arrhythmia

exercise test, with or without the use of thallium or echocardiographic imaging.

References

Chesebro JG, Burnett JL. Cardiac failure: characteristics and clinical manifestations. In: Giuliani ER, Fuster V, Gersh BJ, et al, eds. Cardiology: fundamentals and practice. 2nd ed. St Louis: Mosby-Year Book, 1991.

Ingram RH, Braunwald F. Dyspnea and pulmonary edema. In: Braunwald E, Isselbacher KJ, Petersdorf RJ, et al, eds. Harrison's principles of internal medicine. 11th ed. New York: McGraw-Hill, 1987.

Ruggie N. Congestive heart failure. Med Clin North Am 1986; 70:829.

COR PULMONALE

Mark C. Goldberg, M.D.
Karl B. Kern, M.D.

Cor pulmonale can be defined as cardiac dysfunction that occurs as a result of some process affecting respiratory structure or function, or both. The process responsible for right ventricular (RV) hypertrophy and ultimately dilatation must be intrinsic to the lung. The most frequently implicated causes of cor pulmonale are (1) diseases of the pulmonary parenchyma such as emphysema, chronic bronchitis, asthma, or interstitial lung disease; (2) diseases of the pulmonary vasculature such as primary pulmonary hypertension (HTN) or recurrent thromboembolic events; (3) disorders in the mechanism or mechanics of respiration, e.g., sleep apnea or kyphoscoliosis; and (4) chronic exposure to low Po_2. Disorders that cause RV failure but are not intrinsic to the lung, e.g., mitral stenosis or congenital cardiac defects, must be excluded before the diagnosis of cor pulmonale can be made.

A. The history and physical findings in chronic cor pulmonale vary widely, frequently overshadowed by those of the underlying disease. A 59-year-old man with emphysema may give a history of tobacco abuse and complain of dyspnea, cough, and sputum production; a 23-year-old woman with primary pulmonary HTN may give a history of dyspnea and exertional syncope. Likewise, the physical findings in cor pulmonale vary according to the cause. An accentuated pulmonary closure sound and the ability to feel the pulmonary valve close in the second intercostal space on the left are two of the earliest findings in pulmonary HTN. RV heave, an indication of RV hypertrophy, and the murmurs of tricuspid and pulmonic insufficiency tend to occur later in the course and indicate more severe disease. Other physical findings in cor pulmonale include tachypnea; cyanosis; increased jugular venous pressure with prominent A wave reflecting noncompliance of hypertrophied RV; RV heave; RV S_3, S_4; murmurs of tricuspid and pulmonic insufficiency; hepatomegaly; ascites; and peripheral edema.

B. The chest film is an integral part of the work-up. Cor pulmonale secondary to thoracic deformities such as kyphoscoliosis may be dramatically illustrated. The chest film may specifically suggest the diagnosis of chronic diffuse interstitial fibrosis, bronchiectasis, tuberculosis, or sarcoidosis. Often the chest film is normal, especially in cases of primary pulmonary HTN or chronic pulmonary embolism. Findings on chest films most often reflect the underlying disease process. However, if the pulmonary HTN is of long standing, the main pulmonary artery may have dilated. In the lateral chest film the hypertrophied RV may be seen occupying what was previously the retrosternal air space. Occasionally the "pruned tree" appearance of branching pulmonary arteries is observed. Pulmonary function testing may be useful in distinguishing between obstructive and restrictive disorders. Obstruction due to emphysema and chronic bronchitis may be noted, as well as that due to scarring or tumor in the tracheobronchial tree. Restrictive lung disease due to thoracic cage, respiratory muscle, parenchymal, or pleural abnormalities can be diagnosed.

C. This diagnosis should most often be suspected in persons living at a high altitude. In many patients with mild or moderate disease the resting Po_2 is normal if the arterial blood gas (ABG) testing is performed at a lower altitude. With exercise, desaturation will occur. This reflects the hyperactivity of the pulmonary vasculature in a group of patients who seem predisposed to pulmonary HTN when exposed to a low Po_2.

D. The ECG in cor pulmonale should indicate RV hypertrophy. Criteria most frequently used include right axis deviation; delayed intrinsicoid deflection in V_1; R/S ratio in V_1 >1, or <1 in V_5, V_6; QR pattern in V_1; and R wave V_1 + S wave V_5 and V_6 >10.5. These findings are further supported when ST depression and T wave inversion are noted in the precordium and when P pulmonale is seen in the right atrium.

E. Echocardiography reveals the anatomic changes in RV function that have occurred as a result of pulmonary HTN. The RV may be hypertrophied or dilated. Color echocardiography may show tricuspid or pulmonic insufficiency. Pulmonary artery pressures may be quantitated on Doppler study.

F. If doubt remains that a congenital shunt may be the underlying cause of pulmonary HTN or RV failure, cardiac catheterization or a nuclear medicine shunt study will be necessary.

References

Alpert JS, Kwin RS, Dalen JE. Pulmonary hypertension. Curr Prob Cardiol 1981; 5:1.

Brent BN, et al. Physiologic correlates of right ventricular ejection fraction chronic obstructive pulmonary disease: a combined radionuclide and hemodynamic. Am J Cardiol 1982; 50:255.

Dexter L. Pulmonary vascular disease in acquired and congenital heart disease. Arch Intern Med 1979; 139:922.

Fernandez-Bonetti P, et al. Peripheral airways obstruction in idiopathic pulmonary artery hypertension (primary). Chest 1983; 83:732.

Patient with COR PULMONALE

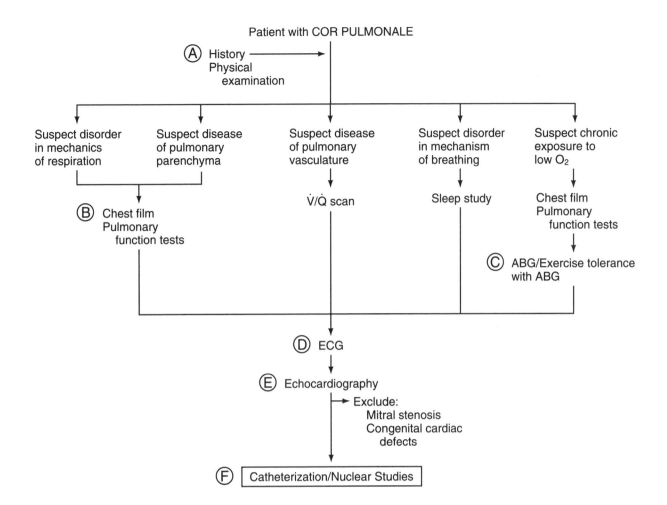

RIGHT VENTRICULAR FAILURE

Mark C. Goldberg, M.D.
Karl B. Kern, M.D.

Right ventricular (RV) failure describes failure of the right ventricle as a pump. In this state, pressure builds up in the venous system behind the right ventricle, hydrostatic forces exceed osmotic forces, and the net result is a transudation of fluid. The symptoms of RV failure reflect the underlying increase in venous pressures. The causes, however, are myriad. Almost any type of cardiac disease may lead to RV failure. Pulmonary processes may also lead to RV failure; when this occurs, the term cor pulmonale is applied. Regardless of the cause, approach to the diagnosis of RV failure begins with a complete history and physical examination, ECG, and chest film. Analysis of preliminary data leads to hypotheses concerning the cause of RV dysfunction, which can be more specifically targeted for investigation.

A. The distinction between right and left ventricular failure may become difficult late in the course of the disease when both ventricles have become dysfunctional. Early symptoms include fatigue and peripheral edema. Physical examination may reveal elevated jugular venous pressure, an enlarged and perhaps pulsatile liver, tricuspid regurgitation, and an RV S_3. An occasional patient may present with ascites and jaundice.

B. The chest film in RV failure may be helpful. When the disease process involves a state in which pulmonary pressures are chronically elevated, the pulmonary artery may be dilated. Often the lateral chest film shows the right ventricle occupying what was previously the retrosternal air space. In cor pulmonale, the chest film may specifically suggest an underlying cause, e.g., chronic diffuse interstitial fibrosis or bronchiectasis.

C. When RV failure is secondary to cor pulmonale, valvular heart disease, or a shunt, the ECG should show RV hypertrophy. If RV failure is secondary to ischemic heart disease, a concurrent inferior myocardial infarction is most often seen on ECG. If infarction is acute, a V4 R lead may show ST elevation consistent with RV infarction.

D. If history and physical are compatible with sleep apnea, a sleep study is in order.

E. If cor pulmonale is a likely cause of RV failure, pulmonary function testing may be useful in distinguishing between obstructive and restrictive disorders. Obstruction due to emphysema and bronchitis, as well as tumor in the tracheobronchial tree, may be diagnosed. Restrictive lung disease due to thoracic cage, respiratory muscle, parenchymal, or pleural abnormalities can also be diagnosed.

F. Pulmonary embolism is initially investigated with a ventilation-perfusion ($\dot{V}/\dot{Q}$) scan. Pulmonary angiography may be required in follow-up.

G. Echocardiography may show a hypertrophied or dilated right ventricle. Color echocardiography may show tricuspid and pulmonic insufficiency as well as mitral and pulmonic stenosis. Pulmonary artery pressures may be quantitated using Doppler. If doubt remains that a congenital shunt may be the underlying cause of pulmonary hypertension or RV failure, cardiac catheterization will be necessary. Catheterization is always performed before shunt or valve repair.

References

Cintron GB, Hernandez E, Linares E, et al. Bedside recognition, incidence and clinical course of right ventricular infarction. Am J Cardiol 1981; 47:224.

Fishman AP. Chronic cor pulmonale. Am Rev Respir Dis 1976; 114:775.

Guilleminault C, Tilkian A, Dement WC. The sleep apnea syndromes. Annu Rev Med 1976; 27:465.

McDonald IG, Hirsh J, Hale GS, et al. Major pulmonary embolism, a correlation of clinical findings, haemodynamics, pulmonary angiography, and pathological physiology. Br Heart J 1972; 34:356.

Shah PK, Maddahi J, Berman DS, et al. Scintigraphically detected predominate right ventricular dysfunction in acute myocardial infarction: clinical, hemodynamic correlates and implications for therapy and prognosis. J Am Coll Cardiol 1985; 6:1264.

Patient with RIGHT VENTRICULAR FAILURE

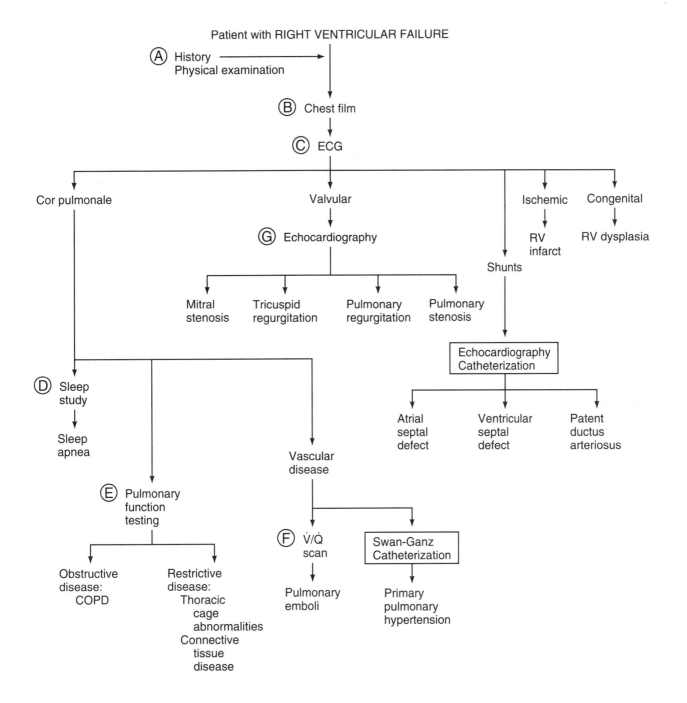

CARDIAC ARREST

James M. Galloway, M.D.
Karl B. Kern, M.D.

The following guidelines, as suggested by the American Heart Association's Advanced Cardiac Life Support Task Force, were written to provide useful help for most patients. However, they were not written to preclude other measures that may be indicated in a particular patient.

A. If the cardiac arrest is a witnessed arrest but a monitor-defibrillator is not immediately available and the patient is pulseless, a solitary precordial thump may be attempted in an effort to convert the patient. Although this is rarely successful, it may be of benefit and costs little time.

B. Cardiac arrest is a common final pathway of several arrhythmias amenable to defibrillation. In one report of cardiac arrest occurring in ambulatory patients during ECG monitoring, 62% had ventricular tachycardia as the initial rhythm that rapidly evolved into ventricular fibrillation, 8% had primary ventricular fibrillation, and 13% had torsades de pointes.

C. Because the probability of survival after a cardiac arrest declines rapidly as the time to defibrillation increases, early defibrillation is essential for a successful outcome. Therefore, as soon as a monitor-defibrillator is available, the patient's rhythm must be identified. If the rhythm is ventricular tachycardia or ventricular fibrillation and the pulse is absent, the patient should be defibrillated immediately. This step should precede CPR if a monitor-defibrillator is immediately available.

D. The importance of properly performed CPR cannot be overemphasized. Effective CPR is essential in the patient in whom early defibrillation either is not immediately available or is initially unsuccessful. External CPR is the most widely used technique to support the circulation and ventilation of a cardiac arrest patient. However, in a hospital setting, with individuals trained and experienced in the performance of thoracotomy, open chest or internal cardiac compression may be used. Standard closed-chest CPR is now recommended to be 80–100 compressions/min with 2-inch compression depth and an accompanying ventilator breath after every fifth compression. If resuscitative efforts are not immediately successful, a central line should be placed to ensure optimal delivery of medications in the central circulation.

E. The current recommended dosage of epinephrine is given in the decision tree. However, the ideal dosage of epinephrine is unknown at this time. Recent animal studies have revealed that higher dosages improved cerebral and myocardial blood flow. Anecdotal human reports have been published suggesting benefit.

Several randomized studies are under way to answer this question.

F. Adequate ventilation can be accomplished in the early stages of cardiac arrest treatment with alternative measures, e.g., mouth to mouth, bag to mouth. However, if initial attempts to restore circulation fail, intubation should be performed. An additional benefit of intubation is the ability to then measure end-tidal carbon dioxide levels; these have proved the best available measure of CPR effectiveness in individual patients. Such information can be used to tailor CPR effects to the needs of each cardiac arrest victim.

G. Electromechanical dissociation (EMD) is determined to be present when there is evidence of an organized cardiac rhythm without the generation of a pulse. This rhythm carries a grave prognosis, and a careful search must be made for reversible causes. The most common causes include hypovolemia, hypoxia, tension pneumothorax, pericardial tamponade, massive myocardial infarction, and massive pulmonary embolus.

H. Fine ventricular fibrillation can mimic asystole and is more amenable to therapy. Therefore, it is important to check at least two different ECG leads to define this rhythm. If there is a suspicion of fine ventricular fibrillation, an attempt at defibrillation is reasonable.

I. In a pulseless patient, regardless of whether the arrest was witnessed or not, blind defibrillation (without documentation of the rhythm first) can be performed. In the unusual situation when a defibrillator is available but a monitor is not, blind defibrillation should be initiated at 200 J and subsequently, if no pulse returns, with 200–300 J, followed if necessary by 360 J.

References

Brown CG, Herman HA, Davis EA, et al. The effect of graded doses of epinephrine on regional myocardial blood flow during cardiopulmonary resuscitation in survival. Circulation 1987; 75:491.
De Luna AB, Coumel P, Leclercq JF. Ambulatory sudden cardiac death: mechanism of production of fatal arrhythmia on the basis of data from 157 cases. Am Heart J 1989; 117:151.
Kern KB, Ewy GA. Future directions in cardiopulmonary resuscitation. American College of Cardiology: Learning Center Highlights, Winter, 1990:11.
1985 National Conference on Standards and Guidelines for Cardiopulmonary Resuscitation and Emergency Cardiac Care. JAMA 1986; 255:2905.
Textbook of advanced cardiac life support. American Heart Association, 1987.

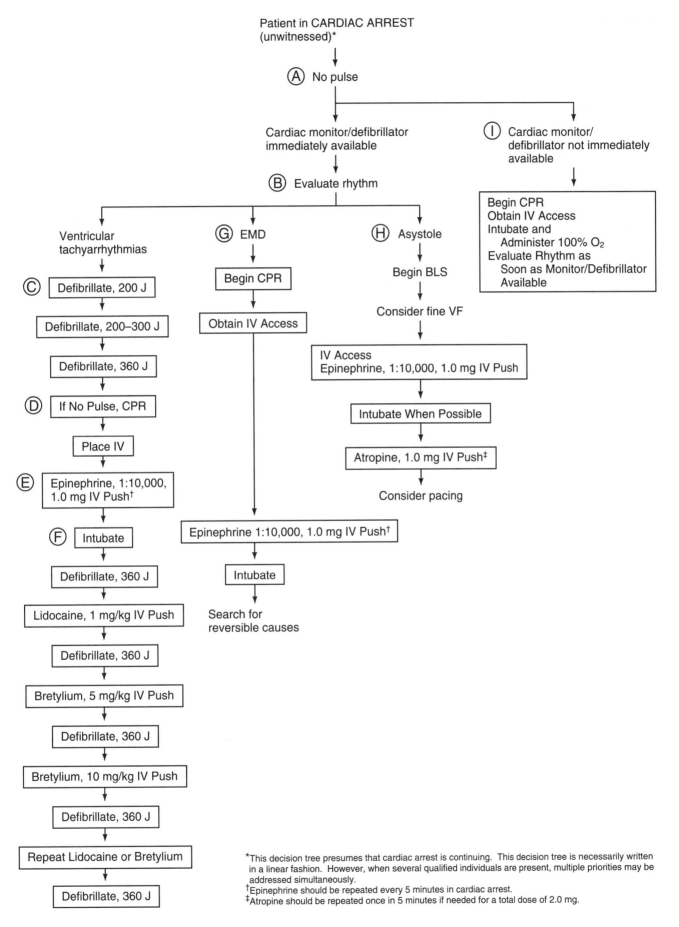

Patient in CARDIAC ARREST
(unwitnessed)*

Ⓐ No pulse

Cardiac monitor/defibrillator
immediately available

Ⓘ Cardiac monitor/
defibrillator not immediately
available

Ⓑ Evaluate rhythm

Begin CPR
Obtain IV Access
Intubate and
    Administer 100% O₂
Evaluate Rhythm as
    Soon as Monitor/Defibrillator
    Available

Ventricular
tachyarrhythmias

Ⓖ EMD

Ⓗ Asystole

Ⓒ Defibrillate, 200 J

Begin CPR

Begin BLS

Defibrillate, 200–300 J

Obtain IV Access

Consider fine VF

Defibrillate, 360 J

IV Access
Epinephrine, 1:10,000, 1.0 mg IV Push

Ⓓ If No Pulse, CPR

Intubate When Possible

Place IV

Atropine, 1.0 mg IV Push‡

Ⓔ Epinephrine, 1:10,000,
1.0 mg IV Push†

Consider pacing

Ⓕ Intubate

Epinephrine 1:10,000, 1.0 mg IV Push†

Defibrillate, 360 J

Intubate

Lidocaine, 1 mg/kg IV Push

Search for
reversible causes

Defibrillate, 360 J

Bretylium, 5 mg/kg IV Push

Defibrillate, 360 J

Bretylium, 10 mg/kg IV Push

Defibrillate, 360 J

Repeat Lidocaine or Bretylium

Defibrillate, 360 J

*This decision tree presumes that cardiac arrest is continuing. This decision tree is necessarily written
  in a linear fashion. However, when several qualified individuals are present, multiple priorities may be
  addressed simultaneously.
†Epinephrine should be repeated every 5 minutes in cardiac arrest.
‡Atropine should be repeated once in 5 minutes if needed for a total dose of 2.0 mg.

CARDIAC DYSPNEA

David Framm, M.D.
Paul E. Fenster, M.D.
Karl B. Kern, M.D.

A. The history and physical examination of a patient with dyspnea can be very helpful. Any known cardiac or pulmonary disease should be carefully explored. Metabolic, hematologic, renal, or neuromuscular diseases should also be considered. Physical examination may reveal such overt causes as congestive heart failure or pneumonia, thus directing the diagnostic work-up and therapeutic plan.

B. If the diagnosis remains uncertain, it is important to determine the severity of the symptoms. If these are mild or episodic, an exercise treadmill can provide a useful objective assessment of functional capacity.

C. If symptoms are severe and functional capacity is limited, a chest film is an important first step. Three distinct patterns may be identified, depending on the presence of pulmonary disease and the size of the cardiac silhouette.

D. A chest film showing evidence of pulmonary disease and a normal-sized heart can be followed up by specific tests as needed. Pulmonary function tests (PFTs) can help differentiate obstructive and restrictive disease as well as the location of the obstructive process.

E. If no evidence of overt pulmonary disease is seen on the chest film and the cardiac silhouette is likewise normal, PFTs, including arterial blood gases (ABGs), are needed. When these are abnormal, a ventilation-perfusion ($\dot{V}/\dot{Q}$) scan or pulmonary angiography can define possible pulmonary emboli as the source of dyspnea.

F. When the chest film reveals an enlarged heart or vascular redistribution, an echocardiographic Doppler study can differentiate between several potential causes of dyspnea. Pericardial disease, represented by either pericardial fluid (and potential tamponade) or pericardial constriction (from scarring), can be identified by echocardiography. Valvular disease and its severity can be assessed by echocardiographic and Doppler studies. If left ventricular (LV) dysfunction is seen on echocardiography, Doppler studies can determine whether systolic dysfunction or both systolic and diastolic dysfunction are present. When systolic contraction is preserved, a Doppler study can demonstrate diastolic dysfunction: a potential cause of dyspnea that is often overlooked. Segmental wall motion abnormalities detected on echocardiography may be the result of ischemic disease and should be further evaluated with an exercise test or catheterization.

References

Lukas DS. Dyspnea. In: MacBryde CM, Blacklow RS, eds. Signs and symptoms: applied pathologic physiology and clinical interpretation. Philadelphia: JB Lippincott, 1970:341.

Neil JVL. Dyspnea. In: Horwitz LD, Groves BM, eds. Signs and symptoms in cardiology. Philadelphia: JB Lippincott, 1985:28.

Swan HJC, Ganz W, Forrester JS. Catheterization of the heart in man with the use of a flow-directed balloon-tipped catheter. N Engl J Med 1970; 283:447.

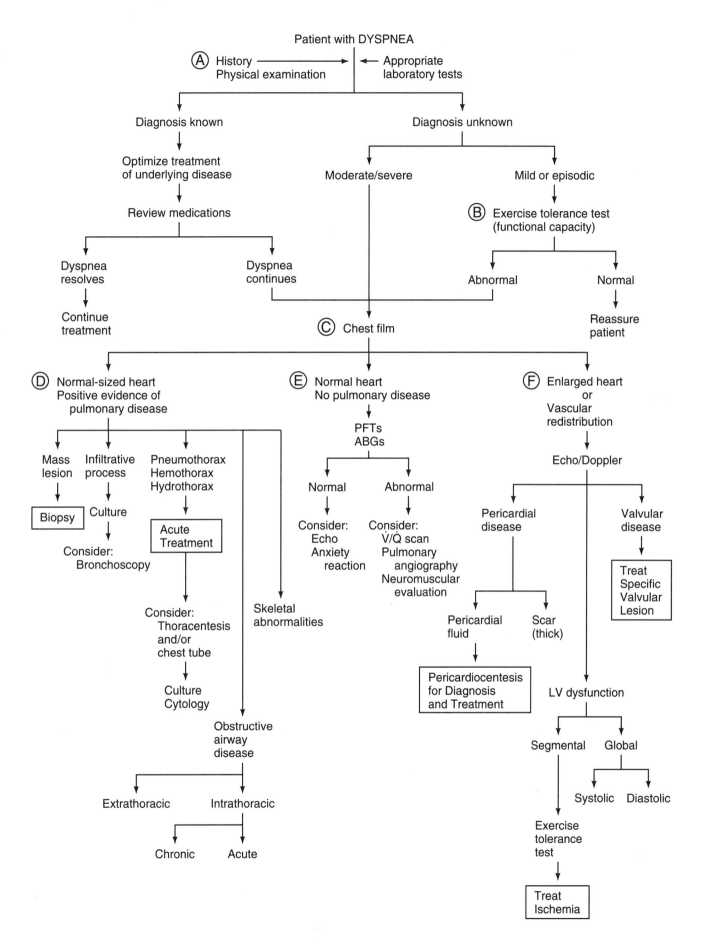

Patient with DYSPNEA

(A) History → ← Appropriate
Physical examination   laboratory tests

Diagnosis known   Diagnosis unknown

Optimize treatment   Moderate/severe   Mild or episodic
of underlying disease

Review medications   (B) Exercise tolerance test
                                                                 (functional capacity)

Dyspnea   Dyspnea   Abnormal   Normal
resolves   continues

Continue   (C) Chest film   Reassure
treatment   patient

(D) Normal-sized heart   (E) Normal heart   (F) Enlarged heart
Positive evidence of   No pulmonary disease   or
pulmonary disease   Vascular
                                    PFTs   redistribution
                                    ABGs
                                                             Echo/Doppler
Mass   Infiltrative Pneumothorax
lesion process   Hemothorax   Normal   Abnormal
                      Hydrothorax   Pericardial   Valvular
                                       Consider: Consider: disease   disease
Biopsy   Culture   Echo   V̇/Q̇ scan
                       Acute   Anxiety   Pulmonary
                       Treatment   reaction   angiography   Treat
Consider: Neuromuscular   Specific
Bronchoscopy   evaluation   Pericardial Scar Valvular
                                                               fluid   (thick) Lesion
                       Consider:
                       Thoracentesis   Pericardiocentesis
                       and/or   for Diagnosis
            Skeletal chest tube   and Treatment LV dysfunction
            abnormalities
                       Culture
                       Cytology   Segmental Global

                       Obstructive
                       airway   Systolic Diastolic
                       disease

Extrathoracic   Intrathoracic   Exercise
                                                              tolerance
                                                              test
            Chronic   Acute
                                                              Treat
                                                              Ischemia

79

ACUTE MYOCARDIAL INFARCTION

Paul E. Fenster, M.D.
James M. Galloway, M.D.

A. Important initial measures in the treatment of patients with suspected acute myocardial infarction (AMI) are cardiac monitoring, O_2 therapy, pain and anxiety relief with IV morphine, bed rest, and adequate sedation. Supplemental O_2 should be provided at least for the initial hours for all patients suspected of having acute ischemic pain. Lower flow rates may be prudent in patients with chronic obstructive pulmonary disease. Pain after the initial hours may indicate continuing ischemia of jeopardized myocardium. Thus efforts to limit myocardial O_2 demand (including adequate sedation, pain control, and anti-ischemic medication) are important.

B. Sublingual nitroglycerin or nifedipine is effective in the treatment of coronary artery spasm, another cause of ST segment elevation. If these medications cause resolution of the chest discomfort and ECG changes, admit the patient and evaluate for evidence of AMI. If infarction is ruled out, a stress test should be performed. If this is negative for ischemia, treat the patient for coronary artery spasm with calcium channel blockers and/or nitrates.

C. Thrombolytic therapy significantly reduces mortality in patients with AMI and ST segment elevation who are treated within 1 hour of the onset of symptoms. As time passes, however, its efficacy is dramatically reduced. The GISSI study found no benefit to patients treated after 6 hours of chest pain, although the ISIS-2 trial suggested benefit when streptokinase (STK) was administered up to 24 hours after onset of pain. The most widely studied thrombolytic drugs are STK and tissue plasminogen activator (tPA). Although tPA has a higher early recanalization rate, the late patency of the infarct vessel is comparable for the two drugs. Clinical trials comparing the drugs document similar reductions in mortality rates and improvements in ventricular function.

D. Aspirin (ASA) is recommended whether or not thrombolytic therapy is employed. The addition of subcutaneous heparin to STK and ASA has been associated with no additional reduction in mortality but with a significantly increased risk of hemorrhagic stroke.

E. Maintenance of a patent infarct artery after thrombolytic therapy is important. In the Heparin-Aspirin Reperfusion Trial, early IV heparin significantly improved the early infarct artery patency rate in tPA-treated patients. However, in ISIS-3, 12-hour delayed subcutaneous heparin did not improve the clinical outcome with tPA. Therefore, when tPA is administered, IV heparin is probably beneficial during the first 24 hours; thereafter, ASA may be as beneficial.

F. Acute IV beta blocker therapy followed by oral therapy reduces acute mortality and the rate of reinfarction and cardiac arrest in patients who are not receiving concomitant thrombolytic therapy. Combining a beta blocker with thrombolytic therapy has resulted in a reduction in reinfarction and mortality rates. Chronic oral beta blocker therapy begun in the first few days after AMI also improves survival rates and decreases the incidence of reinfarction.

G. The prophylactic use of lidocaine is controversial. In some studies, routine lidocaine administration was associated with a mortality rate higher than that in placebo-treated controls. Its use is currently recommended in patients with acute (or suspected) AMI with ventricular tachyarrhythmias or ventricular premature beats that are frequent, multiform, or closely coupled. Lidocaine may not be needed if a beta blocker is administered.

H. Ventricular arrhythmias are a major cause of death in the year after AMI. Electrophysiologic study (EPS) helps determine the risk of arrhythmic death, but is invasive, so patients must be carefully selected. Noninvasive tests can indicate low-risk patients and can be combined to better define the high-risk patient, who may then undergo EPS. A reasonable approach is to sequentially perform a signal-averaged ECG, a Holter monitor to look for ventricular tachycardia, and then an echocardiographic or nuclear study to determine if EF < 40%. If all three tests are abnormal, EPS is indicated. If any one test is normal, the arrhythmic risk is low and further arrhythmia evaluation unnecessary.

I. Although there are no uniform recommendations for an ideal time for stress testing after AMI, its importance in risk stratification cannot be overemphasized. Patients who have received thrombolytic therapy should undergo a submaximal stress test early, possibly before hospital discharge. Such patients may require a second (symptom-limited) stress test 4–8 weeks after AMI to determine safe activity levels or exercise prescription. However, for most patients a single symptom-limited stress test at 3 weeks is safe and cost effective, with few deaths or reinfarctions occurring between hospital discharge and stress testing. Another alternative is submaximal testing 7–10 days after AMI (which can be performed on an outpatient basis) with a follow-up symptom-limited test at 4–6 weeks.

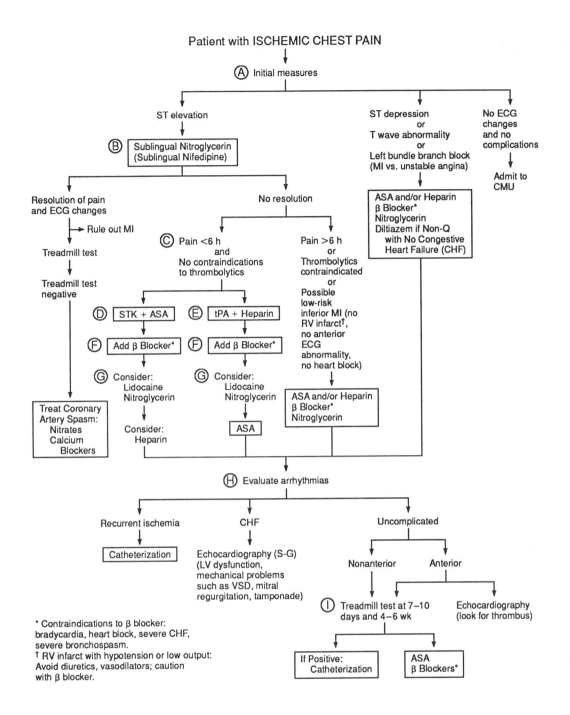

Patient with ISCHEMIC CHEST PAIN

Ⓐ Initial measures

ST elevation

ST depression
or
T wave abnormality
or
Left bundle branch block
(MI vs. unstable angina)

No ECG
changes
and no
complications

Admit to
CMU

Ⓑ Sublingual Nitroglycerin
(Sublingual Nifedipine)

Resolution of pain
and ECG changes

No resolution

ASA and/or Heparin
β Blocker*
Nitroglycerin
Diltiazem if Non-Q
with No Congestive
Heart Failure (CHF)

Rule out MI

Treadmill test

Treadmill test
negative

Ⓒ Pain <6 h
and
No contraindications
to thrombolytics

Pain >6 h
or
Thrombolytics
contraindicated
or
Possible
low-risk
inferior MI (no
RV infarct†,
no anterior
ECG
abnormality,
no heart block)

Ⓓ STK + ASA   Ⓔ tPA + Heparin

Ⓕ Add β Blocker*   Ⓕ Add β Blocker*

Ⓖ Consider:
Lidocaine
Nitroglycerin

Ⓖ Consider:
Lidocaine
Nitroglycerin

ASA and/or Heparin
β Blocker*
Nitroglycerin

Treat Coronary
Artery Spasm:
Nitrates
Calcium
Blockers

Consider:
Heparin

ASA

Ⓗ Evaluate arrhythmias

Recurrent ischemia

Catheterization

CHF

Echocardiography (S-G)
(LV dysfunction,
mechanical problems
such as VSD, mitral
regurgitation, tamponade)

Uncomplicated

Nonanterior   Anterior

Ⓘ Treadmill test at 7–10
days and 4–6 wk

Echocardiography
(look for thrombus)

* Contraindications to β blocker:
bradycardia, heart block, severe CHF,
severe bronchospasm.
† RV infarct with hypotension or low output:
Avoid diuretics, vasodilators; caution
with β blocker.

If Positive:
Catheterization

ASA
β Blockers*

References

Fenster PE. Thrombolytic therapy: controversies in the management of acute myocardial infarction. Hosp Formul 1990; 25:622.

Gruppo Italiano per lo studio della streptochinasi nell'infarto Miocardico (GISSI). Effectiveness of intravenous thrombolytic treatment in acute myocardial infarction. Lancet 1986; 1:397.

Guidelines for the Early Management of Patients with Acute Myocardial Infarction. A Report of the American College of Cardiology/American Heart Association Task Force on Assessment of Diagnostic and Therapeutic Cardiovascular Procedures (Subcommittee to Develop Guidelines for the Early Management of Patients with Acute Myocardial Infarction). J Am Coll Cardiol 1990; 16:249.

Hsia J, Hamilton WP, Kleiman N, et al. A comparison between heparin and low dose aspirin as adjunctive therapy with tissue plasminogen activator for acute myocardial infarction. N Engl J Med 1990; 323:1433.

ISIS-2 Collaborative Group. Randomized trial of intravenous streptokinase, oral aspirin, both or neither among 17,187 cases of suspected acute myocardial infarction: ISIS-2. Lancet 1988; 2:349.

Lopez LM, Mehta JL. Anticoagulation in coronary artery disease: heparin and warfarin trials. Cardiovasc Clin 1987; 18:215.

COUNSELING AFTER MYOCARDIAL INFARCTION

Susan McKenzie, R.N., M.S.
Karl B. Kern, M.D.

Counseling is an important aspect of care after a myocardial infarction (MI). Necessary components include education of the patient and determination of proper or optimal activity level.

A. Secondary prevention of coronary heart disease (CHD) through risk factor modification is an important beneficial strategy that complements both medical and surgical interventions in attempting to reduce the risk of further CHD events. The three most important controllable risk factors for CHD are hypertension, elevated serum cholesterol, and smoking. Successful control of hypertension and serum cholesterol is achieved through diet modification and pharmacologic management. Smoking cessation has been identified as the single most important lifestyle change to reduce morbidity and mortality after an MI. Other controllable risk factors are diabetes, obesity, and stress. Management of these factors by means of support groups and behavior modification also reduce the incidence of subsequent cardiac events. Education about risk factor modification should begin in inpatient cardiac rehabilitation and continue through all phases of outpatient rehabilitation. Patients should progress in activity from bed exercises with active and passive range of motion to sitting in a chair and performing activities of daily living and to walking in the halls of the hospital ward. Specific objectives of a cardiac rehabilitation program include: (1) restoring individuals with cardiovascular disease to their optimal physiologic, psychosocial, and vocational status; (2) prevention of progression or reversal of the underlying atherosclerosis process in patients who have or are at high risk for CHD; and (3) reduction of risk of sudden death and reinfarction and alleviation of angina pectoris in CHD patients.

B. During phase I (inpatient) cardiac rehabilitation or before phase II (outpatient) cardiac rehabilitation, risk stratification of MI patients is carried out on the basis of their prognosis for future CHD events and survival. The type and duration of supervision and frequency of monitoring in the rehabilitation setting is guided by the level of risk (low, moderate, or high). The patient's medical history, clinical course, physiologic variables, and test results assist the risk stratification process.

C. Low-risk individuals (approximately 50% of all MI patients) include those with an uncomplicated hospital course, no evidence of myocardial ischemia after MI, functional capacity ≥7 METS, normal left ventricular function (LVEF >50%), and absence of significant ventricular ectopy.

D. Intermediate- or moderate-risk patients include those with ST segment depression <2 mm, reversible thallium defects, moderate to good LVEF (35–49%), and stable angina pectoris.

E. High-risk patients include those with previous MI or infarct involving ≥35% of the left ventricle, LVEF <35% at rest, fall in exercise systolic blood pressure on exercise tolerance test, persistent or recurrent ischemic pain 24 hours or more after hospital admission, functional capacity <5 METS with hypotensive blood pressure response or positive ST depression at low levels of exercise, congestive heart failure in the hospital, >2 mm ST segment depression at peak heart rate ≤135 beats/min, or high-grade ventricular ectopy.

F. Symptom-limited exercise testing is performed 3–6 weeks after MI helps determine functional capacity (resumption of physical activity including occupational work). If, on the exercise tolerance test, patients achieve a 9-MET level without symptoms, they can safely participate in home activity programs and return to work. If they experience cardiac abnormalities during the symptom-limited exercise test, continued attendance in a supervised rehabilitation program with intermittent monitoring is suggested. All post-MI patients should have eventual exercise goals of 30–45 minutes of exercise per day, 3–4 days per week at moderate intensities (3–7 METS), with an annual review by a cardiologist, including an exercise tolerance test.

References

American Association of Cardiovascular and Pulmonary Rehabilitation. Guidelines for cardiac rehabilitation programs. Human Kinetics, 1991.

DeBusk RF. Evaluation of patients after recent acute myocardial infarction. Ann Intern Med 1989; 110:485.

Leon AS, et al. Scientific evidence of the value of cardiac rehabilitation services with emphasis on patients following myocardial infarction—section I: exercise conditioning component. J Cardiopulm Rehabil 1990; 10:79.

Miller NH, et al. The efficacy of risk factor intervention and psychosocial aspects of cardiac rehabilitation. J Cardiopulm Rehabil 1990; 10:198.

Patient Ready for POST–MYOCARDIAL INFARCTION REHABILITATION

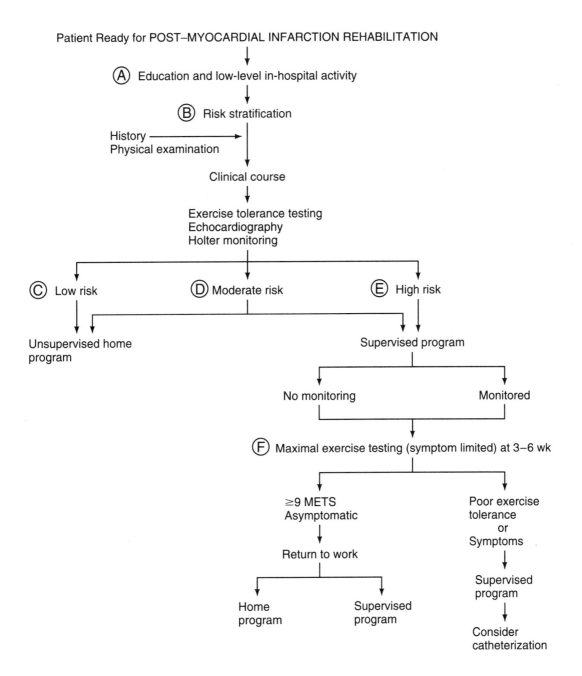

Ⓐ Education and low-level in-hospital activity

Ⓑ Risk stratification

History ——————→
Physical examination

Clinical course

Exercise tolerance testing
Echocardiography
Holter monitoring

Ⓒ Low risk   Ⓓ Moderate risk   Ⓔ High risk

Unsupervised home
program

Supervised program

No monitoring   Monitored

Ⓕ Maximal exercise testing (symptom limited) at 3–6 wk

≥9 METS   Poor exercise
Asymptomatic   tolerance
                              or
                            Symptoms

Return to work   Supervised
                            program

Home   Supervised   Consider
program   program   catheterization

DERMATOLOGY

PIGMENTED LESIONS

Norman Levine, M.D.

Skin color is determined mainly by the amount and distribution of melanin, a pigmented polymer produced by melanocytes. Hyperpigmentation is almost always the result of either production of too much melanin or abnormal distribution of pigment, although foreign materials such as heavy metals or drug metabolites (e.g., amiodarone) can produce a color change in the skin.

A. Nevus of Ota is present at birth in about 60% of cases. There usually is patchy blue-brown pigmentation in the distribution of the fifth cranial nerve, including the eye. A mongolian spot is a blue macule present at or near birth that occurs in 95% of black and 10% of white newborns. Of the lesions, 75% are over the sacrum and they may be as large as 10 cm in diameter. They disappear by age 5 years.

B. Café au lait spots present at birth as well-marginated tan macules. Six or more lesions >1.5 cm in diameter are diagnostic of neurofibromatosis. Congenital nevi range in size from 2 mm to >20 cm in diameter. Giant lesions regress to melanoma in up to 5% of cases. Although small Nevus of Ota and medium-sized lesions are associated with melanoma, the incidence of malignant transformation is far less than in the large congenital nevi. These nevi present as deeply pigmented, verrucous papules, often with coarse hair.

C. Freckles arise at age 2–4 years and can be differentiated from a nevus or a lentigo by the fact that they darken with sun exposure in the summer and fade in the winter. Melasma occurs commonly in pregnant women or in those on oral contraceptives, but men may also develop this condition. Mottled, tan-brown macules coalesce into irregular patches on the face. Minocycline can produce gray-brown discoloration in old acne scars or in a pattern of more diffuse hyperpigmentation over the anterior legs or trunk. Phenothiazines may cause a blue-gray color, particularly in sun-exposed skin. Hydroxychloroquine may produce irregular gray plaques on the legs. Patients taking amiodarone may develop slate-gray hyperpigmentation on the face, particularly after chronic sun exposure. Systemic disorders such as Addison's disease, uremia, and hemochromatosis produce a uniform generalized pattern of hyperpigmentation.

D. A nevus (mole) is a localized benign proliferation of melanocytes. The average individual has 40 nevi, which appear during the first three decades of life and regress after age 65. These are uniformly pigmented macules or papules <5 mm in diameter, with sharp margination. Seborrheic keratoses usually occur after age 35 years and are well-defined, verrucous, hyperpigmented papules and plaques without surrounding inflammation or pigment incontinence. Dermatofibromas often occur after minor trauma such as an insect bite or a razor cut. They are firm, smooth, brown papules that often pucker in the center when compressed from the edges ("button sign"). Becker's nevus usually appears during teenage years as a solitary, thickened, uniformly brown plaque on the trunk. Over time, the lesion acquires coarse, dark hairs. A lentigo ("liver spot") is a discrete tan-brown macule <5 mm in diameter that may occur on any part of the skin, but particularly on the dorsal hands and the face. Sunlight does not increase its color and it does not fade over time.

E. After cutaneous trauma or inflammatory dermatoses, an irregular pattern of macular hyperpigmentation may ensue and may be permanent. The diagnosis of melanoma depends on recognition of irregularity of surface, margin, and color along with incontinence of pigment beyond the main body of the lesion. The surface may be flat at one pole, ulcerated in the center, and raised at the edge. The margins may be notched or feathered. Red, white, or blue hues may be interspersed throughout the tumor. If melanoma is in the differential diagnosis, an excisional biopsy is indicated.

References

Fulk CS. Primary disorders of hyperpigmentation. J Am Acad Dermatol 1984; 10:1.

Rhodes AR. Pigmented birthmarks and precursor melanocytic lesions of cutaneous melanoma identifiable in childhood. Pediatr Clin North Am 1983; 30:435.

Sober AJ, Fitzpatrick TB, Mihm MC Jr. Primary melanoma of the skin: recognition and management. J Am Acad Dermatol 1980; 3:179.

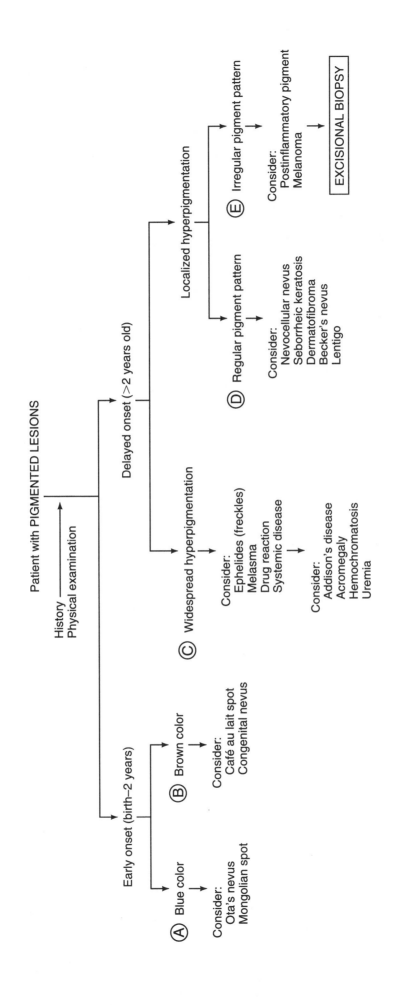

Patient with PIGMENTED LESIONS

History ⟶ Physical examination

Early onset (birth–2 years)

Ⓐ Blue color

Consider:
Ota's nevus
Mongolian spot

Ⓑ Brown color

Consider:
Café au lait spot
Congenital nevus

Delayed onset (>2 years old)

Ⓒ Widespread hyperpigmentation

Consider:
Ephelides (freckles)
Melasma
Drug reaction
Systemic disease

Consider:
Addison's disease
Acromegaly
Hemochromatosis
Uremia

Localized hyperpigmentation

Ⓓ Regular pigment pattern

Consider:
Nevocellular nevus
Seborrheic keratosis
Dermatofibroma
Becker's nevus
Lentigo

Ⓔ Irregular pigment pattern

Consider:
Postinflammatory pigment
Melanoma

⟶ EXCISIONAL BIOPSY

LEG ULCER

Cynthia A. O'Neil, M.D.

A. The cause of a leg ulcer can usually be determined by history and physical examination alone. It is therefore important to ask the patient about trauma and any history of diseases such as coronary artery disease, deep venous thrombosis, and diabetes mellitus. One should inquire about symptoms of vasculitis, chronic inflammatory disorders, and neoplasms. The physical examination should focus on evidence of edema, varicosities, arterial insufficiency, neuropathy, and infection.

B. Arterial ulcers account for 5% of all leg ulcers. They result from impairment of blood flow and have multiple causes, including emboli/thrombi, arteriosclerosis, Buerger's disease, hypertension, vasospasm, vasculitis, and hematologic disorders. Patients complain of pain at rest that is exacerbated with leg elevation and relieved with dependency. The ulcers are characterized by a pale or eschar-covered base with minimal granulation tissue, usually occurring on the distal foot. Other important signs of arterial involvement are coolness of the extremities, decreased pulses and capillary refill, and decreased hair on the distal legs.

C. Chronic venous insufficiency accounts for about 90% of all leg ulcers. Venous stasis results from a dysfunction of venous outflow, most commonly caused by defective valves (usually secondary to deep venous thromboses or a congenital defect). Patients present with edema and, in contrast to those with arterial disease, have relatively little pain. On physical examination an ulcer with exudate and granulation tissue is often seen over the medial malleolus. Varicosities, brown hemosiderin pigment, and dermatitis support the diagnosis.

D. Neurotrophic ulcers are caused by the repeated trauma or pressure on weight-bearing areas where there is impaired cutaneous sensation. Diabetes mellitus accounts for most of these ulcers, but other causes include other forms of vascular disease (polyarteritis nodosa), lead/arsenic polyneuropathies, alcoholic polyneuropathy, sarcoidosis, leprosy, and syphilis.

E. Infection is another etiologic factor in leg ulcers. It occurs most commonly after primary inoculation of a pathogen, although dissemination from a primary focus elsewhere is also possible. Lesions are inflamed and purulent and may have draining sinuses. A biopsy at the ulcer margin should be performed and the tissue sent to be cultured for bacterial, fungal, mycobacterial, and viral pathogens.

F. Lack of response of an ulcer to therapy or rapid growth of a lesion that was previously stable should lead one to suspect neoplasm. An elevated ulcer edge with central crust or granulation tissue is characteristic of many tumors, and a biopsy of the ulcer margin should be performed.

G. Traumatic ulcers are diagnosed by history. Some patients with self-induced disease may not be willing to divulge the cause and may, in fact, be inappropriately unconcerned. These ulcers are characterized by bizarre shapes that have minimal surrounding erythema.

References

Krull EA. Chronic cutaneous ulcerations and impaired healing in human skin. J Am Acad Dermatol 1985; 12:394.

Spittle JA. Diagnosis and management of leg ulcers. Geriatrics 1983; 38:57.

Tofgren EP. Chronic venous insufficiency. Cardiovasc Clin 1983; 13:133.

Young JR. Differential diagnosis of leg ulcers. Cardiovasc Clin 1983; 13:171.

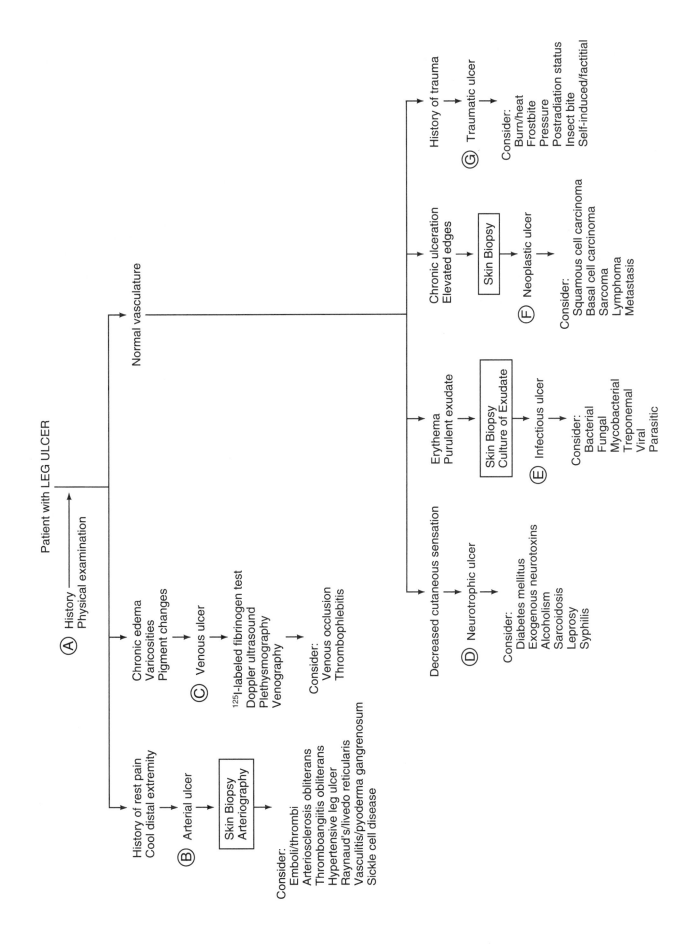

Patient with LEG ULCER

Ⓐ History
Physical examination

History of rest pain
Cool distal extremity

Ⓑ Arterial ulcer

Skin Biopsy
Arteriography

Consider:
Emboli/thrombi
Arteriosclerosis obliterans
Thromboangiitis obliterans
Hypertensive leg ulcer
Raynaud's/livedo reticularis
Vasculitis/pyoderma gangrenosum
Sickle cell disease

Normal vasculature

Chronic edema
Varicosities
Pigment changes

Ⓒ Venous ulcer

¹²⁵I-labeled fibrinogen test
Doppler ultrasound
Plethysmography
Venography

Consider:
Venous occlusion
Thrombophlebitis

Decreased cutaneous sensation

Ⓓ Neurotrophic ulcer

Consider:
Diabetes mellitus
Exogenous neurotoxins
Alcoholism
Sarcoidosis
Leprosy
Syphilis

Erythema
Purulent exudate

Skin Biopsy
Culture of Exudate

Ⓔ Infectious ulcer

Consider:
Bacterial
Fungal
Mycobacterial
Treponemal
Viral
Parasitic

Chronic ulceration
Elevated edges

Skin Biopsy

Ⓕ Neoplastic ulcer

Consider:
Squamous cell carcinoma
Basal cell carcinoma
Sarcoma
Lymphoma
Metastasis

History of trauma

Ⓖ Traumatic ulcer

Consider:
Burn/heat
Frostbite
Pressure
Postradiation status
Insect bite
Self-induced/factitial

URTICARIA

Norman Levine, M.D.

Urticaria is a vascular reaction of the skin characterized by evanescent edematous plaques (wheals, hives). Angioedema differs only in that the edema extends into the deep dermis and subcutaneous tissue. About 15% of the population develop this problem at some time in life. In about 60% of cases the lesions resolve in <6 weeks (acute urticaria); in the remaining patients the disease persists longer, usually in the form of recurrent episodes.

A. In approximately 25% of cases a definite cause can be uncovered, and in the vast majority of these patients the history and physical examination alone are sufficient to determine the cause.

B. The most common cause of acute urticaria is a drug reaction. The agents often implicated are sulfonamides, penicillin derivatives, barbiturates, diuretics, and anti-inflammatory agents. Medications taken within 14 days of the onset of the urticaria are the most likely offenders. Certain foods such as nuts, shellfish, and eggs may produce urticaria in susceptible individuals. Focal infections such as sinusitis or genitourinary infections, and systemic infections such as viral hepatitis or infectious mononucleosis, occasionally produce urticaria. In rare instances, patients may develop localized wheals after direct contact with an offending agent (contact urticaria).

C. Certain chronic skin diseases have lesions that appear urticarial and must be differentiated from urticaria. Urticaria pigmentosa (mastocytosis) presents with stable brown papules that urticate when rubbed. The lesions of urticarial vasculitis are wheals that persist for several days and often have a violaceous color. These diagnoses can be confirmed by a skin biopsy.

D. Many cases of chronic urticaria are secondary to physical stimuli that produce hives in susceptible patients. Dermographism occurs in 5% of the population and consists of wheals that develop 1–3 minutes after skin stroking. Stimuli as innocuous as toweling after bathing or rubbing one's eyes can produce hives. Less commonly, patients develop wheals after cold, heat, water, or sun exposure. Patients with cholinergic urticaria develop 2- to 4-mm wheals within 2–20 minutes after general overheating of the body, such as occurs after vigorous exercise.

E. In patients with chronic urticaria that are not secondary to physical stimuli, a routine noninvasive laboratory screen is indicated. However, abnormal laboratory test results rarely uncover an occult cause of urticaria in the face of a normal history and physical examination.

F. In many patients an identifiable cause of chronic urticaria is never uncovered. In some of these, there may be psychogenic influences that exacerbate the urticarial episodes. Others may have a genetic tendency that makes them more prone to hives from a variety of stimuli.

References

Hirschmann JV, Lawlor F, English JSC, et al. Cholinergic urticaria: a clinical and histologic study. Arch Dermatol 1987; 123:462.

Jacobson KW, Branch CB, Nelson HS. Laboratory tests in chronic urticaria, JAMA 1980; 243:1644.

Sorensen HT, Christensen B, Kaerulff E. A two-year follow-up of children with urticaria in general practice. Scand J Prim Health Care 1987; 5:24.

Wong RC, Fairley JA, Ellis CN. Dermographism: a review. J Am Acad Dermatol 1984; 11:643.

Patient with URTICARIA

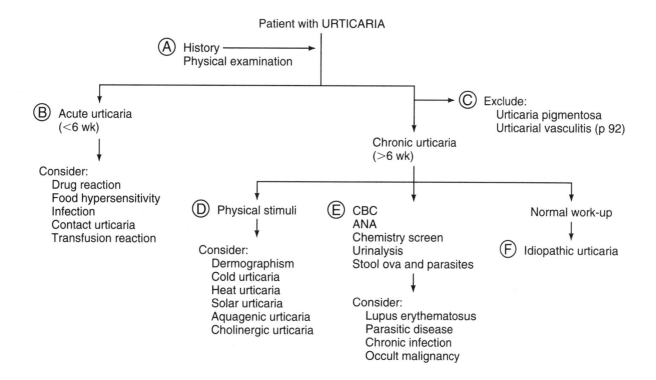

Ⓐ History
Physical examination

Ⓑ Acute urticaria
(<6 wk)

Consider:
 Drug reaction
 Food hypersensitivity
 Infection
 Contact urticaria
 Transfusion reaction

Ⓒ Exclude:
 Urticaria pigmentosa
 Urticarial vasculitis (p 92)

Chronic urticaria
(>6 wk)

Ⓓ Physical stimuli

Consider:
 Dermographism
 Cold urticaria
 Heat urticaria
 Solar urticaria
 Aquagenic urticaria
 Cholinergic urticaria

Ⓔ CBC
ANA
Chemistry screen
Urinalysis
Stool ova and parasites

Consider:
 Lupus erythematosus
 Parasitic disease
 Chronic infection
 Occult malignancy

Normal work-up

Ⓕ Idiopathic urticaria

GENERALIZED PRURITUS

Norman Levine, M.D.

Pruritus is defined as an unpleasant sensation that provokes the desire to scratch. Regardless of the underlying cause, most patients have maximal itching at bedtime. There are many pruritic dermatoses, but relatively few of these cause generalized itching. Generalized pruritus can be divided into those conditions in which there is an associated dermatosis and those in which pruritus is a symptom of a noncutaneous disease.

A. Physical examination alone is sufficient to diagnose most primary cutaneous pruritic diseases. In the absence of an obvious primary lesion, a medical history may uncover occult dermatoses. For example, xerotic (dry) skin often itches just after bathing. Scabies may affect multiple household members and can be a venereally transmitted condition. Atopic dermatitis often appears in successive generations and is associated with asthma and allergic rhinitis.

B. The two most common causes of generalized pruritus are xerosis and atopic dermatitis. Xerosis is most prominent on the anterior legs and lateral arms. The plaques have fine fissures that look like a cracked pot ("erythema craquele"). The lesions of atopic dermatitis are thickened (lichenified) and excoriated.

C. Diagnosis can often be confirmed by a skin biopsy. If scabies is suspected, examine the superficial contents of a burrow.

D. In the absence of an obvious cutaneous cause of generalized pruritus, empirically treat for xerosis with moisturizers. If the pruritus persists, a laboratory work-up is indicated and should include a hemogram, serum chemistries, glucose tolerance test, thyroid function studies, urinalysis, and chest radiography.

E. Pruritus rarely predates the diagnosis of systemic malignancy except in Hodgkin's disease, where 6% of cases present with pruritus alone.

F. Polycythemia vera is associated with pruritus after quick temperature change (e.g., bathing). Itching occurs commonly in leukemia and rarely in iron deficiency states, even in the absence of other signs and symptoms.

G. Pruritus is often the first symptom of biliary cirrhosis and extrahepatic biliary obstruction. An elevated serum alkaline phosphatase level is characteristic.

H. The pruritus of diabetes mellitus occurs in <5% of patients and is not correlated with disease severity.

I. Hyperthyroidism may produce generalized pruritus that improves when the patient becomes euthyroid. Most cases of pruritus with hypothyroidism are secondary to xerosis.

J. Chronic renal failure commonly produces generalized pruritus in patients with BUN >50 mg/dl. Dialysis may produce paroxysms of intense itching.

K. Consider psychogenic pruritus only after all other causes have been ruled out, although this is a common cause of itching. If after a routine work-up there are no localizing signs of carcinoma, further evaluation is usually not indicated.

References

Denman ST. A review of pruritus. J Am Acad Dermatol 1986; 14:375.

Kantor GR, Lookingbill DP. Generalized pruritus and systemic disease. J Am Acad Dermatol 1983; 9:375.

Martin J. Pruritus. Int J Dermatol 1985; 24:634.

Paul R, Paul R, Jansen CT. Itch and malignancy prognosis in generalized pruritus: a 6-year follow-up of 125 patients. J Am Acad Dermatol 1987; 16:1179.

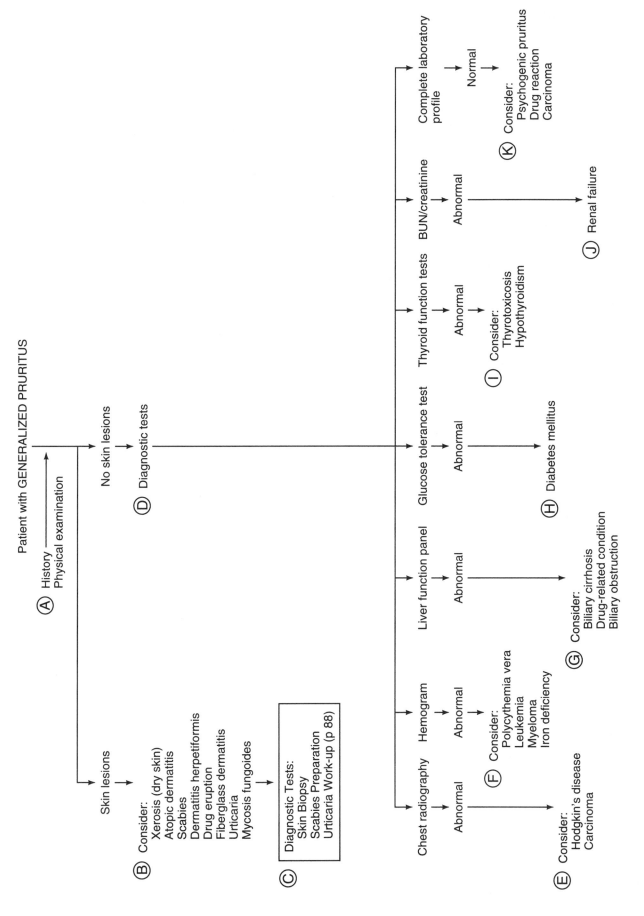

Patient with GENERALIZED PRURITUS

(A) History
Physical examination

Skin lesions

(B) Consider:
Xerosis (dry skin)
Atopic dermatitis
Scabies
Dermatitis herpetiformis
Drug eruption
Fiberglass dermatitis
Urticaria
Mycosis fungoides

(C) Diagnostic Tests:
Skin Biopsy
Scabies Preparation
Urticaria Work-up (p 88)

No skin lesions

(D) Diagnostic tests

Chest radiography

Abnormal

(E) Consider:
Hodgkin's disease
Carcinoma

Hemogram

Abnormal

(F) Consider:
Polycythemia vera
Leukemia
Myeloma
Iron deficiency

Liver function panel

Abnormal

(G) Consider:
Biliary cirrhosis
Drug-related condition
Biliary obstruction

Glucose tolerance test

Abnormal

(H) Diabetes mellitus

Thyroid function tests

Abnormal

(I) Consider:
Thyrotoxicosis
Hypothyroidism

BUN/creatinine

Abnormal

(J) Renal failure

Complete laboratory profile

Normal

(K) Consider:
Psychogenic pruritus
Drug reaction
Carcinoma

PALPABLE PURPURA

Norman Levine, M.D.

Palpable purpura is defined as a skin lesion that is purpuric and has substance. It can be a papule, vesicle, or pustule. These lesions are highly indicative of inflammatory destruction of cutaneous blood vessel walls (vasculitis). Immune-mediated mechanisms of damage are often operative. Many clinically distinct disorders fall under the general heading of vasculitis, but the pathologic processes are similar in most of them.

A. The presence of palpable purpura is considered septic vasculitis until proved otherwise. Underlying causes of sepsis should therefore be ruled out before any other work-up. Signs and symptoms of sepsis include fever, chills, mental status changes, tachycardia, tachypnea, and hypotension. In this clinical setting, several blood cultures and a skin biopsy of a purpuric lesion for light microscopy, bacterial smear, and culture are indicated.

B. Although there are few distinguishing clinical features of the skin lesions in septic vasculitis that would lead to the diagnosis of a specific infection, there occasionally are clues. In staphylococcal sepsis, showers of purpuric pustules appear. Gram stain reveals the offending organism. In gonococcemia, there are relatively few acral purpuric papules and vesicles that subsequently develop into pustules. Patients with meningococcemia have an explosive onset of hundreds of hemorrhagic papules over the whole body. In Rocky Mountain spotted fever, palpable purpuric lesions occur after several days of illness, and only after the lesions have progressed from pink macules to red papules to purpuric papules.

C. In many cases, palpable purpura of the skin mirrors systemic vasculitides, most of which are immune mediated. Although laboratory abnormalities are common in systemic vasculitis, there are few abnormalities pathognomonic for given diseases. Thus, the work-up includes measurements of organ function and immune status along with the history and physical examination.

D. Henoch-Schönlein purpura is a small vessel vasculitis, usually occurring in children, that involves the skin (palpable purpura), joints, kidneys, and gastrointestinal tract. In 90% of cases this follows an upper respiratory infection and lasts for 7–14 days. There may be recurrences. Several chronic disorders are characterized by granuloma formation involving blood vessels that can produce palpable purpuric lesions. Wegener's granulomatosis is a disease involving the skin, kidneys, and upper respiratory tract.

Allergic granulomatosis (Churg-Strauss syndrome) occurs in asthmatics who develop palpable purpura, hypertension, chronic pneumonitis, and a neuropathy. Polyarteritis nodosa is a vasculitis of small and medium-sized arteries with involvement of the skin, kidneys, pulmonary system, nervous system, and joints. The skin lesions may be purpuric papules, subcutaneous nodules, and/or cutaneous ulcerations along with livedo reticularis (p 94). Urticarial vasculitis is a multisystem disorder with recurrent crops of purpuric wheals lasting several days. Some of these patients have associated hypocomplementemia. This is differentiated from other forms of vasculitis by the relatively evanescent nature of the lesions and by the fact that the lesions appear more urticarial.

E. In many cases, palpable purpura (vasculitis) occurs in an otherwise clinically healthy patient. A limited laboratory work-up, including skin biopsy, is indicated to rule out occult immune complex diseases such as essential mixed cryoglobulinemia and hyperglobulinemic purpura, and purely cutaneous vasculitides such as erythema elevatum diutinum.

F. Hypersensitivity vasculitis does not have pathognomonic criteria but depends on a constellation of signs and symptoms. Most patients are >16 years of age and may have a history of intake of a medication that could be causative. They present with palpable purpura and blanching red papules and macules, usually on the lower extremities.

References

Calabrese LH, Michel BA, Bloch DA, et al. The American College of Rheumatology 1990 criteria for the classification of hypersensitivity vasculitis. Arthritis Rheum 1990; 33:1108.

Eckstein E, Callen JP. Cutaneous leukocytoclastic vasculitis: clinical and laboratory features of 82 patients seen in private practice. Arch Dermatol 1984; 120:484.

Jorizzo JL, Solomon AR, Zanolli MD. Neutrophilic vascular reactions. J Am Acad Dermatol 1988; 19:983.

Lightfoot RW, Michel BA, Block DA, et al. The American College of Rheumatology 1990 criteria for the classification of polyarteritis nodosa. Arthritis Rheum 1990; 33:1088.

Mills JA, Michel BA, Bloch DA, et al. The American College of Rheumatology 1990 criteria for the classification of Henoch-Schönlein in purpura. Arthritis Rheum 1990; 33:1114.

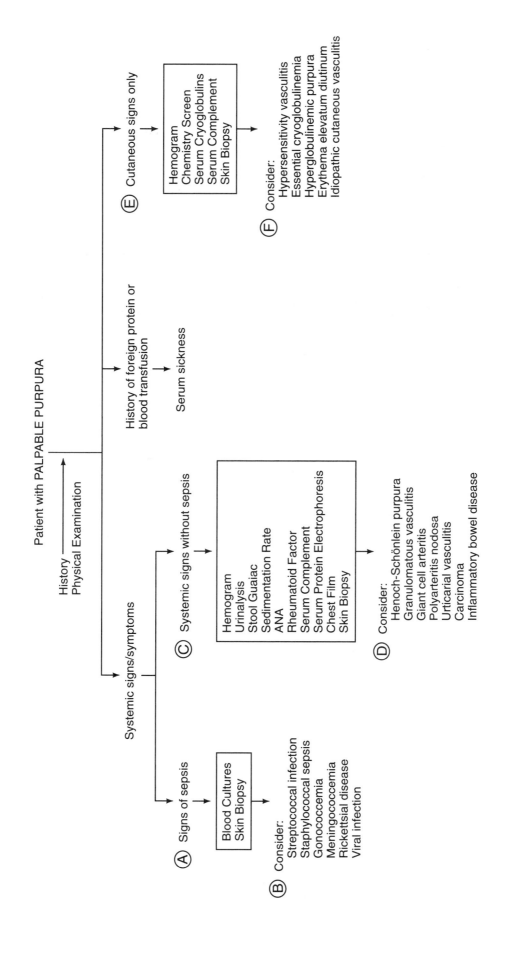

Patient with PALPABLE PURPURA

History —— Physical Examination

Systemic signs/symptoms

Ⓐ Signs of sepsis

Blood Cultures
Skin Biopsy

Ⓑ Consider:
Streptococcal infection
Staphylococcal sepsis
Gonococcemia
Meningococcemia
Rickettsial disease
Viral infection

Ⓒ Systemic signs without sepsis

Hemogram
Urinalysis
Stool Guaiac
Sedimentation Rate
ANA
Rheumatoid Factor
Serum Complement
Serum Protein Electrophoresis
Chest Film
Skin Biopsy

Ⓓ Consider:
Henoch-Schönlein purpura
Granulomatous vasculitis
Giant cell arteritis
Polyarteritis nodosa
Urticarial vasculitis
Carcinoma
Inflammatory bowel disease

History of foreign protein or blood transfusion

Serum sickness

Ⓔ Cutaneous signs only

Hemogram
Chemistry Screen
Serum Cryoglobulins
Serum Complement
Skin Biopsy

Ⓕ Consider:
Hypersensitivity vasculitis
Essential cryoglobulinemia
Hyperglobulinemic purpura
Erythema elevatum diutinum
Idiopathic cutaneous vasculitis

LIVEDO RETICULARIS

Angela Murphy McGhee, M.D.

Livedo reticularis is a netlike (reticulate) mottling of the skin encountered with some frequency in medical practice, in both pediatrics and adult medicine. It may represent a normal variant or may be a sign of a serious systemic disorder.

A. The age of the patient is important in evaluating the cause of livedo reticularis. If the livedo pattern is first observed in the adult, it is associated more often with underlying diseases than when seen in the child.

B. When the skin appears mottled upon exposure to cold but returns to normal when the body is warmed over a period of minutes to hours, physiologic factors are operative.

C. In adults the pattern (symmetry versus asymmetry) and location (extremities, trunk, generalized) can help determine the cause of a livedo reticularis pattern. In general, symmetric involvement, especially of the extremities, is usually physiologic, whereas asymmetric, patchy, or truncal involvement often indicates pathologic change.

D. Long-standing livedo reticularis without ulcerations and no other signs or symptoms is the idiopathic variant, but this can be diagnosed only after other causes are excluded. However, in patients with abrupt-onset livedo without ulcerations, the rheumatologic diseases should be considered.

E. Fixed livedo accompanied by leg ulcerations represents a variant that usually occurs in women <40 years of age. It is the result of long-standing microvascular stasis. Although fixed, the livedo pattern is accentuated by the cold. Rarely, there is an associated arterial disease elsewhere, such as endarteritis obliterans or arteriosclerosis. The livedo pattern in these instances is widespread and the disease progressive. Rheumatic diseases with accompanying vasculitis should also be considered here. The work-up should include CBC, ESR, ANA, renal panel, and skin biopsy.

F. The clinical picture of fixed livedo in a discontinuous pattern, especially that of recent onset, suggests an underlying pathologic condition such as systemic lupus erythematosus (SLE), systemic vasculitis, malignancies, hypo- or hyperparathyroidism, infections (tuberculosis, syphilis), emboli, pancreatitis, reactions to drugs (e.g., amantadine), and hematologic disorders (e.g., thrombocythemia).

References

Champion RH. Cutaneous reactions to cold. In: Rook R, et al, eds. Textbook of dermatology. 4th ed. Palo Alto: Blackwell, 1986:627.

Edwards EA, Coffman JD. Cutaneous changes in peripheral vascular disease. In: Fitzpatrick TB, et al, eds. Dermatology in general medicine. 3rd ed. San Francisco: McGraw-Hill, 1987:2007.

From L, Assaad, D. Vascular neoplasms, pseudoneoplasms, and hyperplasias. In: Fitzpatrick TB, et al, eds. Dermatology in general medicine. 3rd ed. San Francisco: McGraw-Hill, 1987:1070.

Jacobs AH. Vascular malformations. In: Schachner LA, Hansen RC, eds. Pediatric dermatology. New York: Churchill Livingstone, 1988:1037.

Picascia DD, Pellegrini JR. Livedo reticularis. Cutis 1987; 39:429.

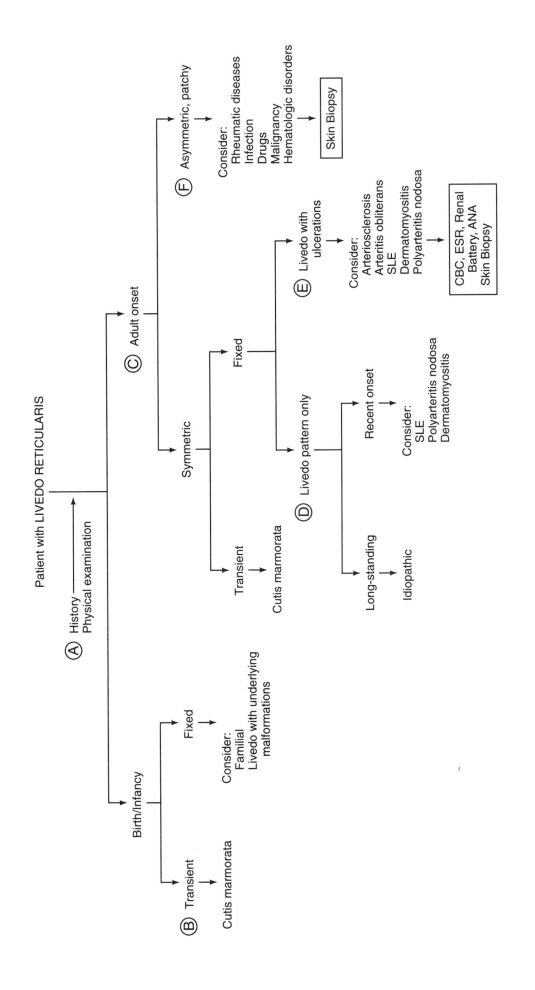

Patient with LIVEDO RETICULARIS

Ⓐ History — Physical examination

Birth/Infancy

Ⓑ Transient

Cutis marmorata

Fixed

Consider:
Familial
Livedo with underlying malformations

Ⓒ Adult onset

Symmetric

Transient

Cutis marmorata

Fixed

Ⓓ Livedo pattern only

Long-standing

Idiopathic

Recent onset

Consider:
SLE
Polyarteritis nodosa
Dermatomyositis

Ⓔ Livedo with ulcerations

Consider:
Arteriosclerosis
Arteritis obliterans
SLE
Dermatomyositis
Polyarteritis nodosa

CBC, ESR, Renal
Battery, ANA
Skin Biopsy

Ⓕ Asymmetric, patchy

Consider:
Rheumatic diseases
Infection
Drugs
Malignancy
Hematologic disorders

Skin Biopsy

ENDOCRINOLOGY

HYPERLIPIDEMIA

Nancy A. Curosh, M.D.
Thomas W. Boyden, M.D.

Hyperlipidemia can be due to hypercholesterolemia, hypertriglyceridemia, or both. Hypertriglyceridemia is a risk factor for pancreatitis. Hypercholesterolemia is an important risk factor for atherosclerosis. Since coronary artery disease (CAD) is a leading cause of death in the United States and is usually asymptomatic in the early stages, it is important to identify people at high risk as early as possible. The other major risk factors for CAD are male gender, family history of coronary heart disease before 55 years of age, cigarette smoking, hypertension, diabetes mellitus, cerebrovascular or peripheral vascular disease, obesity, and a high-density lipoprotein cholesterol (HDL-C) level <35 mg/dl. If a patient has a cholesterol level >240 mg/dl, or 200–240 mg/dl with two or more risk factors, further investigation is needed.

A. Before diagnosing and treating disorders of lipid metabolism, consider secondary causes of hyperlipidemia. Significant hypercholesterolemia can be caused by hypothyroidism, liver disease, nephrosis, porphyria, dysproteinemias, progestins, and anabolic steroids. Secondary causes of hypertriglyceridemia include poorly controlled diabetes mellitus, systemic lupus erythematosus, renal failure, excessive alcohol consumption, glycogen storage diseases, and various medications, including thiazide diuretics, beta blockers, estrogens, and corticosteroids. These can usually be discovered by a careful history and physical examination and confirmed by appropriate laboratory tests. Eliminate offending agents and treat underlying medical conditions as completely as possible. If hyperlipidemia remains after these corrections, further investigation is warranted.

B. The NIH developed a classification of lipid disorders based on the lipoprotein class that is elevated (Table 1). This classification system can serve as a framework for the diagnosis of hyperlipidemic conditions. Initial classification begins with the measurement of plasma or serum cholesterol, triglyceride, and HDL-C in a sample obtained after an overnight fast. If the fasting triglyceride is <400 mg/dl, VLDL-C can be approximated by triglyceride divided by five. LDL-C is calculated by the formula, LDL-C = total cholesterol − (VLDL-C + HDL-C). In most cases, measuring and comparing HDL-C, triglyceride, and cholesterol elevations permits sufficient categorization to determine the proper course of treatment.

C. HDL-C is considered a good cholesterol. A low level (<35 mg/dl) of HDL-C is an independent risk factor for CAD. HDL-C levels can be increased by weight reduction, cessation of cigarette smoking, and regular vigorous exercise. In patients at very high risk of CAD but unable to elevate their HDL-C, it may be prudent to consider drug therapy, although no long-term studies have been done to prove benefit.

D. Patients with type IIA or IIB hypercholesterolemia due to the autosomal dominant disorder familial hypercholesterolemia often have xanthomas that aid the diagnosis. Heterozygotes may develop corneal arcus and tendinous xanthomas. Homozygotes may also develop planar and tuberous xanthomas of the extensor surfaces of the hands, elbows, buttocks, and knees. These patients are at substantial risk of premature CAD (homozygotes frequently die in their teens). Early identification is important so that aggressive therapy can be instituted.

E. Overweight patients with hypercholesterolemia should be encouraged to lose weight, since this can decrease VLDL-C and LDL-C and increase HDL-C. All patients with hypercholesterolemia should follow a diet low in saturated fat and cholesterol. Usually a 6-month trial of intensive dietary therapy is recommended before drug therapy is started. However, diet therapy can be expected to decrease total cholesterol by only 10–20% even in the most compliant patients.

F. In patients whose cholesterol and triglyceride are elevated to nearly equal levels, consider type III hyperlipidemia, a rare hereditary disorder causing premature atherosclerosis and peripheral vascular disease. Many patients have pathognomonic palmar xanthomas. Tuberoeruptive xanthoma may also be seen. Definitive diagnosis can be made by lipoprotein electrophoresis or ultracentrifugal subfractionation.

TABLE 1   NIH Classification of Lipid Disorders

Type	Elevated Lipoprotein
I	Chylomicrons
IIA	LDL-C
IIB	LDL-C and VLDL-C
III	IDL-C
IV	VLDL-C
V	VLDL-C and chylomicrons

LDL-C, Low-density lipoprotein cholesterol; VLDL-C, very-low-density lipoprotein cholesterol; IDL-C, intermediate-density lipoprotein cholesterol.

(Continued on page 98)

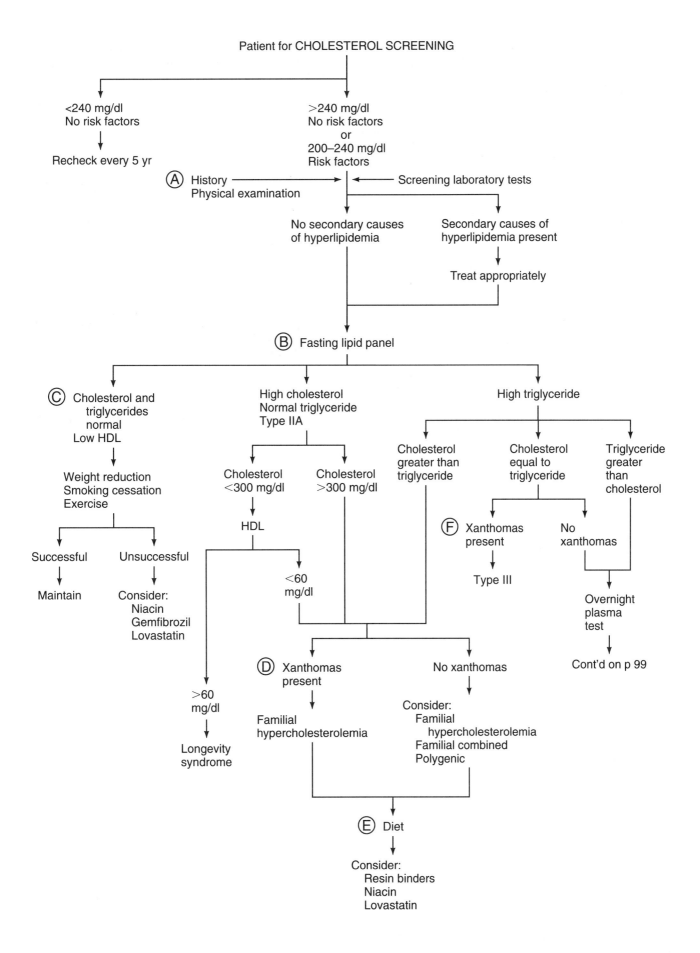

Patient for CHOLESTEROL SCREENING

<240 mg/dl
No risk factors

Recheck every 5 yr

>240 mg/dl
No risk factors
or
200–240 mg/dl
Risk factors

Ⓐ History
Physical examination → ← Screening laboratory tests

No secondary causes
of hyperlipidemia

Secondary causes of
hyperlipidemia present

Treat appropriately

Ⓑ Fasting lipid panel

Ⓒ Cholesterol and
triglycerides
normal
Low HDL

Weight reduction
Smoking cessation
Exercise

Successful

Maintain

Unsuccessful

Consider:
Niacin
Gemfibrozil
Lovastatin

High cholesterol
Normal triglyceride
Type IIA

Cholesterol
<300 mg/dl

HDL

>60
mg/dl

Longevity
syndrome

<60
mg/dl

Cholesterol
>300 mg/dl

Ⓓ Xanthomas
present

Familial
hypercholesterolemia

No xanthomas

Consider:
Familial
hypercholesterolemia
Familial combined
Polygenic

Ⓔ Diet

Consider:
Resin binders
Niacin
Lovastatin

High triglyceride

Cholesterol
greater than
triglyceride

Cholesterol
equal to
triglyceride

Triglyceride
greater
than
cholesterol

Ⓕ Xanthomas
present

Type III

No
xanthomas

Overnight
plasma
test

Cont'd on p 99

G. Triglycerides are elevated in types I, IV, and V hyperlipidemias. Type I is a rare disorder caused by a deficiency of lipoprotein lipase that results in markedly elevated chylomicrons. This disease begins in childhood or early adulthood with bouts of abdominal pain and recurrent pancreatitis. There is no increased risk of CAD. Treatment consists of severe dietary restriction of fats. If plasma from type I patients is allowed to stand overnight at 4° C, the chylomicrons form a creamy layer that floats to the top; the remainder of the plasma is clear. In type IV the entire plasma is turbid, indicating excess VLDL-C. Type V patients have both a turbid plasma and a creamy supernatant. Type V patients frequently have eruptive xanthomas, lipemia retinalis, hepatosplenomegaly, and associated conditions such as obesity, hyperglycemia, and hyperuricemia. With some treatment they may revert to the less severe type IV pattern.

H. If triglyceride levels are >1000 mg/dl, the patient has an increased risk of pancreatitis, so treatment should be instituted to lower triglycerides. Treatment benefits are less clear at lower triglyceride levels. Patients with autosomal dominant familial hypertriglyceridemia may have only a slight increase in risk for CAD, but patients with familial combined hyperlipidemia have a substantial risk of CAD. This disease can be differentiated from other forms of hyperlipidemia only by family screening studies. Approximately one-third of affected family members have a type IIA pattern, one-third a type IIB pattern, and one-third a type IV pattern. If the patient has known risk factors for CAD or pancreatitis, treatment should be instituted. It is unclear, however, if treatment is beneficial for patients with no obvious risk factors. Watchful waiting may be all that is necessary.

I. Dietary treatment for hypertriglyceridemia primarily consists of calorie restriction and weight loss. If excessive, dietary fat should be decreased and regular alcohol use eliminated. In addition, these patients often respond very well to diets high in fish. Oily fish such as salmon, sardines, and mackerel are preferred, since these are rich in beneficial omega-3 fatty acids.

References

Garber AM, Sox HC, Littenberg B. Screening asymptomatic adults for cardiac risk factors: the serum cholesterol level. Ann Intern Med 1989; 110:622.

Lavie CJ, Gau GT, Squires RW, Kottke BA. Management of lipids in primary and secondary prevention of cardiovascular diseases. Mayo Clin Proc 1988; 63:605.

Schaefer EJ. Hyperlipoproteinemias and other lipoprotein disorders. In: Becker KL, ed. Principles and practice of endocrinology and metabolism. Philadelphia: JB Lippincott, 1990:1229.

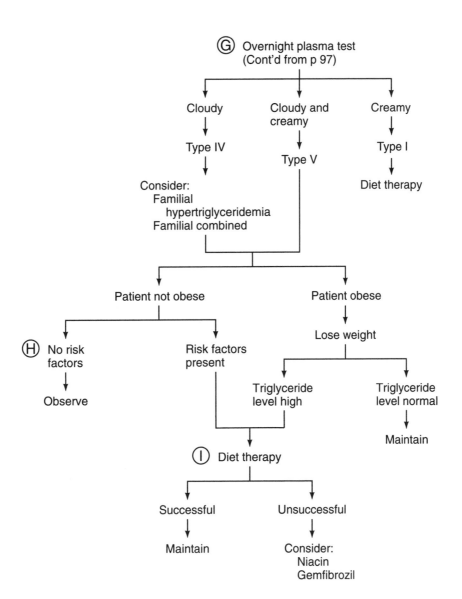

HYPOGLYCEMIA

Nancy A. Curosh, M.D.

Hypoglycemia occurs when there is decreased glucose production, increased glucose use, or a combination of both. Normally, hypoglycemia is prevented by neural and hormonal mechanisms. As blood sugar falls, there is increased sympathetic activity and release of catecholamines, which prevents further uptake of glucose by insulin-dependent tissues and stimulates hepatic gluconeogenesis. Counter-regulatory hormones such as glucagon, cortisol, and growth hormone are also released, which stimulate gluconeogenesis and lipolysis. The symptoms of hypoglycemia may be nonspecific and depend on the rate of fall and the severity of plasma glucose. The release of catecholamines may cause palpitations, sweating, anxiety, hunger, and tremulousness. If neuroglycopenia occurs, the patient may develop headache, confusion, lightheadedness, aberrant behavior, dysarthria, visual symptoms, seizures, and coma, and death may occur.

A. Documentation of hypoglycemia may be difficult but important because many patients will have symptoms of hypoglycemia but few are actually hypoglycemic. Hypoglycemia cannot be defined by precise quantitative measures. In normal healthy individuals, the plasma glucose level at which counter-regulatory hormones are released may vary from 50 to 70 mg/dl. In diabetic patients who are chronically hyperglycemic, a rapid drop of blood glucose may provoke symptoms even if their plasma glucose is well within the normal range for nondiabetics. In fasting healthy males, plasma glucose may be as low as 55 mg/dl, and in females it may be even lower, but they remain asymptomatic. Therefore, an arbitrary level of 50 mg/dl is used as a cutoff point to proceed with a detailed evaluation of hypoglycemia. A low glucose level must be documented in the laboratory using plasma or whole blood; fingersticks are inaccurate at low levels and are insufficient documentation of hypoglycemia. In addition to low blood sugar, the other conditions of Whipple's triad should be met: symptoms at the time of hypoglycemia and relief of symptoms with food. Relief should occur within minutes. If Whipple's triad is present, further investigation is warranted.

B. Often during a thorough history taking it is obvious that the hypoglycemia has exogenous causes, the most common being insulin or an oral hypoglycemic agent in diabetic patients. Alcohol can cause hypoglycemia, particularly in people who are drinking but not eating. If there is insufficient caloric intake, glycogen stores are depleted. If alcohol then inhibits gluconeogenesis, hypoglycemia may occur. Other drugs such as propranolol, aspirin, pentamidine, and the antimalarials may precipitate hypoglycemia.

C. By means of a detailed history, patients can usually be divided into two categories: those whose symptoms occur while fasting and those whose symptoms occur after eating. Patients with fasting hypoglycemia tend to notice symptoms just before meals or early in the morning after an overnight fast. Fasting hypoglycemia often results from organic causes and requires thorough investigation. In some cases it is difficult to document the hypoglycemia, especially if it occurs intermittently. In these cases the patient should be admitted for an observed fast. Whenever symptoms develop, blood should be drawn. If the plasma glucose is <50 mg/dl, further testing such as insulin and C-peptide levels should be analyzed simultaneously. The patient should also be given glucose to document relief of symptoms. Most patients with fasting hypoglycemia develop symptoms within 24 to 48 hours, but some may take up to 72 hours. If no low plasma glucose levels were recorded during a 72-hour fast, fasting hypoglycemia is very unlikely.

D. Insulinomas are often very small and difficult to locate. Consult with the surgeon before localization procedures. Although a CT scan is fairly benign, other localization techniques are invasive and many surgeons prefer intraoperative ultrasonography.

E. The cosyntropin stimulation test is used when primary adrenal insufficiency is suspected. A plasma cortisol level is drawn at baseline. Cosyntropin (synthetic adrenocorticotropic hormone), 0.25 mg, is given IV or IM. A second plasma cortisol level is obtained at 60 minutes. Normal stimulation is >7 µg/dl above the baseline cortisol or an absolute value of >18 µg/dl. A normal response excludes the diagnosis of primary adrenal insufficiency.

F. The cause of fasting hypoglycemia with suppressed insulin levels is often obvious. Liver disease, renal disease, and malnutrition are usually severe before hypoglycemia occurs. Nonpancreatic tumors are often very large. Other causes such as adrenal insufficiency, growth hormone deficiency, and hypothyroidism may be subtle and require further testing.

G. Postprandial hypoglycemia usually produces symptoms 2–4 hours after a meal. These patients frequently complain of hunger, palpitations, and tremulousness, which are promptly relieved with food. Patients rarely develop symptoms of neuroglycopenia. A small subset of these patients have undergone GI surgery and have abnormal food transit time. This can be corrected by changing meal patterns or sometimes by corrective surgery. However, most postprandial hypoglycemia is idiopathic. There is much controversy about the existence of this syndrome; this is reflected by its numerous names, including reactive, functional, idiopathic, and nonhypoglycemic hypoglycemia. Although commonly performed in the past, the oral glucose tolerance test usually is not indicated. Studies have shown that many healthy asymptomatic individuals have plasma glucose levels <50 mg/dl during an

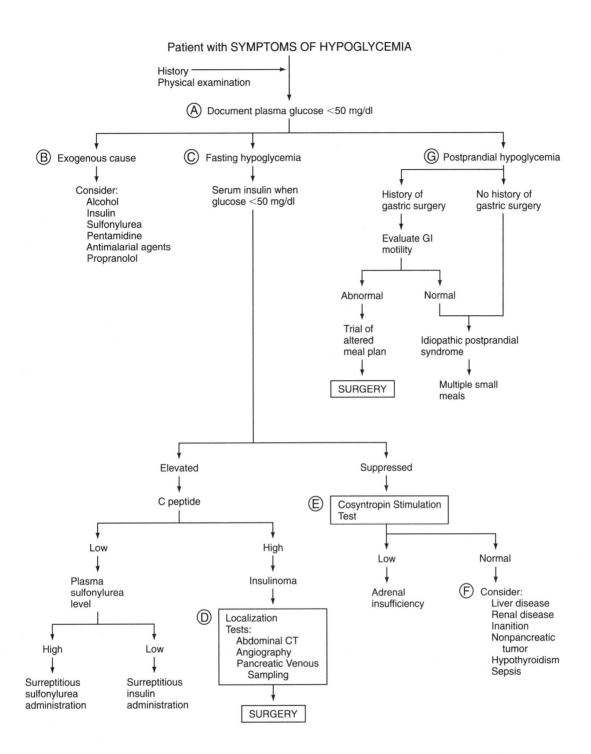

Patient with SYMPTOMS OF HYPOGLYCEMIA

History
Physical examination

Ⓐ Document plasma glucose <50 mg/dl

Ⓑ Exogenous cause

Consider:
  Alcohol
  Insulin
  Sulfonylurea
  Pentamidine
  Antimalarial agents
  Propranolol

Ⓒ Fasting hypoglycemia

Serum insulin when
glucose <50 mg/dl

Ⓖ Postprandial hypoglycemia

History of
gastric surgery

No history of
gastric surgery

Evaluate GI
motility

Abnormal

Normal

Trial of
altered
meal plan

SURGERY

Idiopathic postprandial
syndrome

Multiple small
meals

Elevated

C peptide

Low

High

Plasma
sulfonylurea
level

Insulinoma

Ⓓ Localization
Tests:
  Abdominal CT
  Angiography
  Pancreatic Venous
  Sampling

SURGERY

High

Low

Surreptitious
sulfonylurea
administration

Surreptitious
insulin
administration

Suppressed

Ⓔ Cosyntropin Stimulation
Test

Low

Normal

Adrenal
insufficiency

Ⓕ Consider:
  Liver disease
  Renal disease
  Inanition
  Nonpancreatic
    tumor
  Hypothyroidism
  Sepsis

oral glucose tolerance test. Therefore, this test has little meaning or diagnostic value. These patients are best treated with reassurance. They may try multiple small meals, but the high-protein, low-carbohydrate diet advocated in the past is not effective.

References

Comi RJ, Gorden P. Approach to hypoglycemia in adults. Compr Ther 1987; 13:38.

Lorenzi M. Hypoglycemia. In: Fitzgerald PA, ed. Handbook of clinical endocrinology. Chicago: Jones Medical Publications, 1986:410.

Malouf R, Brust JC. Hypoglycemia: causes, neurological manifestations, and outcome. Ann Neurol 1985; 17:421.

Service FJ. Hypoglycemias. West J Med 1991; 154:442.

Sherwin RS, Felig P. Hypoglycemia. In: Felig P, ed. Endocrinology and metabolism. 2nd ed. New York: McGraw-Hill, 1986:1179.

HYPERGLYCEMIA

Philip R. Orlander, M.D.
Thomas W. Boyden, M.D.

Insufficient insulin secretion coupled with insulin resistance may result in fasting or postprandial hyperglycemia. Criteria for the diagnosis of diabetes mellitus and other categories of glucose intolerance have been established by consensus of expert committees. A fasting serum glucose value >140 mg/dl (7.8 mmol/L) on several occasions, a 2-hour postprandial serum glucose >200 mg/dl (11.1 mmol/L), and/or random serum glucose values ≥200 mg/dl (11.1 mmol/L), along with classic symptoms of uncontrolled diabetes, establishes the diagnosis of diabetes, and no further testing is necessary. In special circumstances a 75-g oral glucose tolerance test can be performed. However, the results of this test are affected by age, diet, exercise, and intercurrent illness, and it must be performed fasting in the morning after 3 days of a high- carbohydrate diet. Screening for diabetes is currently recommended only during pregnancy.

A. Mild hyperglycemia is frequently asymptomatic and discovered inadvertently. Pertinent findings during the history include symptoms of polyuria, polydipsia, polyphagia, visual changes, weight changes, intercurrent illnesses, and mental status changes. Many patients with non-insulin–dependent diabetes mellitus (NIDDM) have first-degree relatives with the disease. Occasionally, evidence of end-organ damage may be found on initial presentation (funduscopic abnormalities, peripheral neuropathy, foot ulcers, peripheral vascular disease, or proteinuria).

B. Numerous medications may adversely affect carbohydrate tolerance. Glucocorticoids increase gluconeogenesis as well as impairing insulin action. Although the hyperglycemic state may resolve after withdrawal of glucocorticoids, diabetes persists in some patients at increased risk (those with obesity, those with a strong family history of diabetes, and certain ethnic groups such as Blacks and Hispanics).

C. Excess antagonistic counterregulatory hormones (glucagon, catecholamines, growth hormone, and cortisol) at times of illness may precipitate glucose intolerance. Gestational diabetes occurs only during pregnancy and resolves at delivery. Approximately 15–30% of women with a history of gestational diabetes subsequently develop NIDDM. Many endocrine disorders are associated with abnormal glucose tolerance: Cushing's syndrome, acromegaly, hyperthyroidism, pheochromocytoma, glucagonoma, and somatostatinoma. Other disease states affecting the pancreas include acute and chronic pancreatitis (secondary to alcohol), hemochromatosis, cystic fibrosis, and trauma.

D. Diabetes mellitus is conventionally divided into two major clinical syndromes: insulin-dependent (IDDM or type I), which makes up about 10–15% of diabetes, and non-insulin–dependent (NIDDM or type II), which makes up the remainder. There is a long list of certain secondary forms of diabetes: those previously mentioned as well as rare genetic conditions such as ataxia-telangiectasia and lipoatrophic syndromes. IDDM presents most frequently in young, thin, generally Caucasian populations and typically presents with diabetic ketoacidosis. IDDM is characterized by irreversible autoimmune destruction of the beta cells and is highly associated with certain HLA haplotypes (DQw8) and the presence of islet cell antibodies at onset. NIDDM is a heterogeneous syndrome characterized by detectable but insufficient glucose-stimulated insulin secretion and marked insulin resistance. Approximately 90% of individuals with NIDDM are obese and at least 40 years old. Maturity onset diabetes of the young (MODY) is a subset of NIDDM occurring in families with an autosomal dominant form of inheritance and presenting at <30 years of age. Many patients (especially blacks and Hispanics) are not easily classified by these clinical criteria. Measurement of serum insulin concentrations is not useful clinically for managing the patient with diabetes. Extremely elevated serum insulin levels are seen in severe insulin resistance associated with the skin lesion acanthosis nigricans. These are rare syndromes that may be associated with hyperandrogenism and defects in the insulin receptor (type A) or with autoimmune phenomenon and antibodies to the insulin receptor (type B).

E. The presence of serum ketone bodies indicates accelerated fatty acid oxidation due to severe insulin deficiency. Although diabetic ketoacidosis is a cardinal feature of IDDM, it is occasionally seen in patients with NIDDM who are subjected to severe stress (e.g., GI hemorrhage, myocardial infarction [MI], sepsis). The differential diagnosis includes alcoholic ketoacidosis and starvation ketosis. Nonketotic hyperosmolar states typically occur in patients with NIDDM who are elderly with multiple medical problems.

F. Acutely ill patients require immediate IV fluid resuscitation and parenteral insulin during evaluation for an underlying illness (i.e., infection). Patients suspected of having IDDM require life-long insulin therapy coordinated with a diet and exercise program to maintain ideal body weight. The initial therapy for obese patients with NIDDM is a weight-reducing diet and exercise regimen. Oral sulfonylurea or insulin may be also required to achieve euglycemia in selected individuals with NIDDM.

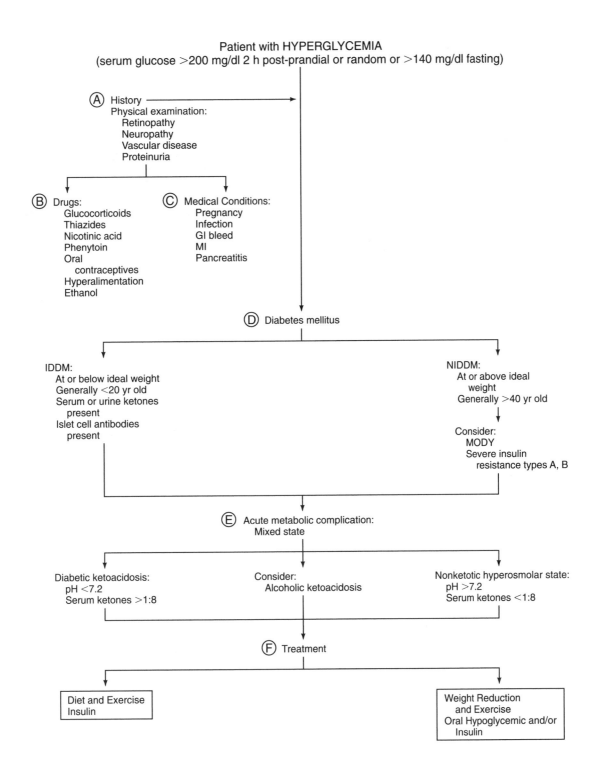

Patient with HYPERGLYCEMIA
(serum glucose >200 mg/dl 2 h post-prandial or random or >140 mg/dl fasting)

Ⓐ History
Physical examination:
    Retinopathy
    Neuropathy
    Vascular disease
    Proteinuria

Ⓑ Drugs:
    Glucocorticoids
    Thiazides
    Nicotinic acid
    Phenytoin
    Oral
      contraceptives
    Hyperalimentation
    Ethanol

Ⓒ Medical Conditions:
    Pregnancy
    Infection
    GI bleed
    MI
    Pancreatitis

Ⓓ Diabetes mellitus

IDDM:
    At or below ideal weight
    Generally <20 yr old
    Serum or urine ketones
      present
    Islet cell antibodies
      present

NIDDM:
    At or above ideal
      weight
    Generally >40 yr old

Consider:
    MODY
    Severe insulin
      resistance types A, B

Ⓔ Acute metabolic complication:
    Mixed state

Diabetic ketoacidosis:
    pH <7.2
    Serum ketones >1:8

Consider:
    Alcoholic ketoacidosis

Nonketotic hyperosmolar state:
    pH >7.2
    Serum ketones <1:8

Ⓕ Treatment

Diet and Exercise
Insulin

Weight Reduction
  and Exercise
Oral Hypoglycemic and/or
  Insulin

References

DeFronzo RA, Bonadonna RC, Ferraninni E. Pathogensis of NIDDM. Diabetes Care 1992; 15:318.

DeFronzo RA, Ferraninni E. Insulin resistance. Diabetes Care 1991; 14:173.

Eisenbarth GS. Type I diabetes mellitus: a chronic autoimmune disease. N Engl J Med 1986; 314:1360.

Genuth S. Insulin use in NIDDM. Diabetes Care 1990; 13:1240.

Kuhl C, Hornnes PJ, Andersen O. Etiology and pathophysiology of gestational diabetes mellitus. Diabetes 1985; 34(Suppl 2):66.

National Diabetes Data Group. Classification and diagnosis of diabetes mellitus and other categories of glucose intolerance. Diabetes 1979; 28:1039.

HYPOCALCEMIA

Philip R. Orlander, M.D.

A. The classic clinical signs of tetany may be associated with hypocalcemia, hypomagnesemia, hypokalemia, or alkalosis. Hypocalcemia enhances neuromuscular irritability, causing paresthesias, carpopedal spasm, and (if extreme) laryngeal spasm and seizures. The severity of symptoms depends on the rate of decrease of the calcium. Chronic hypocalcemia may show only signs of latent tetany (Chvostek's or Trousseau's sign), but the long-term consequences are substantial (lenticular cataracts, basal ganglion calcification, poor integuments, intestinal malabsorption, pseudotumor cerebri, psychiatric manifestations, and abnormal cardiac function). Hypoalbuminemia is associated with lower serum calcium concentrations but normal ionized calcium levels. Simple correction formulas adjusting for the serum albumin generally suffice in estimating ionized calcium if a direct measurement is not readily available. In pancreatitis, hypocalcemia results from a combination of saponification of calcium salts and impairment of parathyroid hormone (PTH) secretion due to the hypomagnesemia caused by alcohol abuse. Although cancer is much more commonly associated with hypercalcemia, patients with extensive osteoblastic metastases from prostate or breast rarely may present with hypocalcemia.

B. A low serum phosphate level generally indicates adequate parathyroid reserve. Direct attention to conditions that interfere with vitamin D metabolism, such as malabsorption states (sprue, short bowel, regional enteritis), hepatobiliary disease, anticonvulsant therapy, and vitamin D deficiency or resistance states. These conditions are associated with elevated PTH and alkaline phosphatase levels and low 25-hydroxyvitamin D levels. There may be evidence of metabolic bone disease.

C. A high serum phosphate level indicates PTH deficiency or resistance. Excessive phosphate intake or massive cell destruction (e.g., with chemotherapy or rhabdomyolysis) can substantially raise serum phosphate levels and thus lower serum calcium.

D. Renal insufficiency is a common cause of secondary hyperparathyroidism. An elevated calcium-phosphate product and low 1,25-dihydroxyvitamin D levels are commonly found.

E. Pseudohypoparathyroidism is a rare inherited condition involving a generalized impairment in G regulatory protein signal transduction, resulting in target tissue resistance to PTH as well as other hormones. Afflicted individuals are short and frequently have cognitive handicaps and musculoskeletal abnormalities, including a short fourth metacarpal. Several subtypes of this disorder are described and distinguished by the response of urinary cyclic AMP (cAMP) concentration to exogenous PTH infusion.

F. Idiopathic hypoparathyroidism is a rare condition that may be isolated, or associated with familial polyglandular endocrinopathy type II (mucocutaneous candidiasis, Addison's disease, hypoparathyroidism). It usually presents in childhood.

G. Head and neck surgery, primarily for thyroid or parathyroid diseases, can result in transient or sometimes permanent PTH deficiency due to parathyroid ischemia. Autotransplantation of the parathyroids at the time of surgery has decreased the incidence of this complication.

H. Hypomagnesemia is most commonly found in patients with a history of heavy alcohol abuse, malabsorption, intestinal tract diseases, or primary renal tubular defects or in patients receiving prolonged nutritional therapy that may have been lacking in magnesium (hyperalimentation). Certain drugs and antibiotics (diuretics, aminoglycosides, cisplatin, amphotericin B) may cause a renal loss of magnesium.

I. Treatment includes adequate replacement of calcium, magnesium, and vitamin D. IV calcium should be administered to symptomatic individuals. In conditions in which conversion of vitamin D to 1,25-vitamin D is perturbed (i.e., renal disease, vitamin D resistant rickets), replacement with calcitriol or a similar metabolite (dihydrotachysterol) is desirable. In other circumstances, vitamin D_2 (ergocalciferol) is less expensive, although the risk of prolonged hypercalcemia is higher.

References

Bell NH. Vitamin D—endocrine system. J Clin Invest 1985; 76:1.

Breslau NA. Calcium homeostasis. In: Griffin JE, Ojeda SR, eds. Textbook of endocrine physiology. New York: Oxford University Press, 1988:273.

Spiegel AM, Gierschik P, Levine MA, Downs RW. Clinical implications of guanine nucleotide-binding proteins as receptor-effector couplers. N Engl J Med 1985; 312:26.

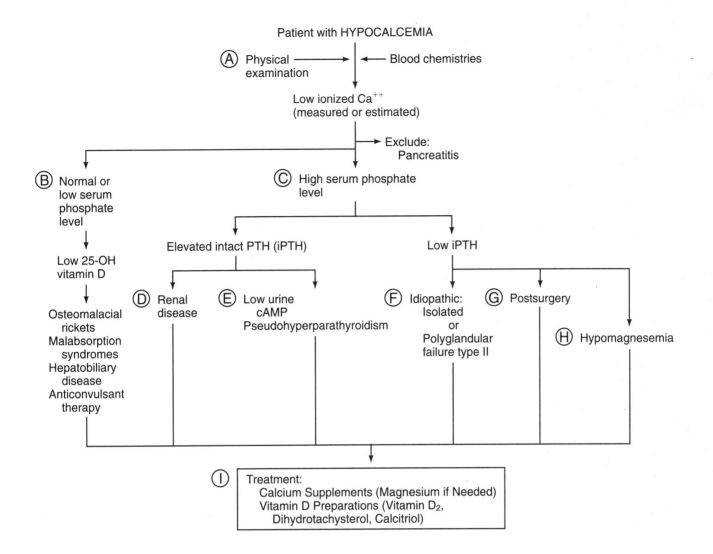

Patient with HYPOCALCEMIA

(A) Physical ⟶ ⟵ Blood chemistries
    examination

Low ionized Ca^{++}
(measured or estimated)

⟶ Exclude:
    Pancreatitis

(B) Normal or
    low serum
    phosphate
    level

(C) High serum phosphate
    level

Low 25-OH
vitamin D

Elevated intact PTH (iPTH)   Low iPTH

Osteomalacial
rickets
Malabsorption
syndromes
Hepatobiliary
disease
Anticonvulsant
therapy

(D) Renal
    disease

(E) Low urine
    cAMP
    Pseudohyperparathyroidism

(F) Idiopathic:
    Isolated
    or
    Polyglandular
    failure type II

(G) Postsurgery

(H) Hypomagnesemia

(I) Treatment:
    Calcium Supplements (Magnesium if Needed)
    Vitamin D Preparations (Vitamin D_2,
        Dihydrotachysterol, Calcitriol)

HYPERCALCEMIA

Philip R. Orlander, M.D.
Thomas W. Boyden, M.D.

A. The clinical presentation of hypercalcemia may range from severe dehydration, polyuria, and obtundation to a fortuitous discovery in an asymptomatic individual. Although there are many causes of hypercalcemia, the most likely diagnosis in an ambulatory population is hyperparathyroidism; malignancy is more common in a hospitalized population. Before an extensive evaluation is initiated, it is important to establish that the patient has persistent hypercalcemia. An estimate of ionized calcium is useful in excluding dehydration or increased protein binding (i.e., multiple myeloma). A careful medication history is essential, as several commonly used drugs can cause or exacerbate hypercalcemia (i.e., thiazide diuretics, calcium carbonate, vitamin A and D preparations, lithium, and antiestrogens in the treatment of breast carcinoma). Excessive use of calcium carbonate can result in a milk-alkali syndrome characterized by alkalosis, hypokalemia, hyperphosphatemia, hypercalcemia, and nephrocalcinosis. Strict immobilization may be associated with hypercalcemia only when there is concomitant accelerated bone resorption (i.e., children, severe trauma, or Paget's disease of bone). The physical examination will probably exclude several endocrine problems that may be associated with mild hypercalcemia (i.e., pheochromocytoma, Addison's disease, hyperthyroidism).

B. Multiphasic chemistry studies, CBC, and chest x-rays, although not diagnostic, may indicate the cause of the hypercalcemia. Hypercalcemia is seen in about 10–20% of patients with sarcoidosis, and rarely in other granulomatous diseases. The hypercalcemia is caused by production of 1,25-dihydroxyvitamin D by the alveolar macrophages. Low serum phosphate, elevated chloride, low bicarbonate, and elevated serum alkaline phosphatase levels are commonly seen in hyperparathyroidism. Acute renal failure can cause hypercalcemia, especially when accompanied by rhabdomyolysis.

C. The immunoradiometric assay for intact parathyroid hormone (iPTH) demonstrates elevated levels in most cases of PTH-related hypercalcemia and should replace the former assays.

D. Non-PTH–related hypercalcemia may be caused by excess production or ingestion of vitamin D, or by excess bone resorption (i.e., by a PTH-like substance). Hypercalcemia is a common finding in individuals with many types of malignancy. In most cases cancer has already been diagnosed, but occasionally hypercalcemia is noted while the tumor is still occult. Although extensive bone metastases may cause hypercalcemia, more commonly a humoral factor has been implicated: PTH-related protein in squamous cell carcinomas of the head, neck, lung, and genitourinary tract; prostaglandins, cytokines, and lymphokines in other tumors. A detailed history and physical examination (including careful breast, rectal, and pelvic examinations) along with cancer-detecting studies (mammography, bone scan, serum protein electrophoresis, urinalysis, stool for occult blood) are usually sufficient to exclude malignancy.

E. Familial hypocalciuric hypercalcemia is a rare disorder with an autosomal dominant inheritance pattern. The condition is characterized by elevated serum magnesium, normal PTH, and very low urinary calcium levels. The disease has a benign course and does not respond well to parathyroid surgery. It must be distinguished from other familial forms of hypercalcemia (multiple endocrine neoplasia [MEN] types I and II).

F. Primary hyperparathyroidism is a common disease of the elderly (prevalence 1/1000 with female predominance); >80% are caused by a single parathyroid adenoma. Most cases of hyperparathyroidism are discovered early, in routine blood chemistry studies, and it is now rare to see long-term complications such as osteitis fibrosa cystica, band keratopathy, or nephrocalcinosis. Preoperative evaluation (i.e., ultrasonography of the neck, nuclear medicine imaging, CT of the chest, venous sampling for iPTH) is useful only if the patient has undergone a previous unsuccessful neck exploration. Tertiary hyperparathyroidism may develop in individuals with prolonged parathyroid stimulation (due to renal insufficiency) who receive a functioning renal transplant. Surgery is indicated for those with evidence of osteitis fibrosa, reduced or falling cortical or trabecular bone mass, declining renal function, renal stones, mental status changes, pancreatitis, or serum calcium levels >12 mg/dl or in patients <50 years old. Removal of the adenoma is curative in >90% of individuals. Hyperplasia of all parathyroid glands is seen in MEN syndromes both I and II. A family history should be sought and the possibility of accompanying neoplasias (pheochromocytoma, medullary thyroid carcinoma) should be excluded before surgery. Parathyroid carcinoma is particularly rare and can be diagnosed with certainty only after metastases have been demonstrated.

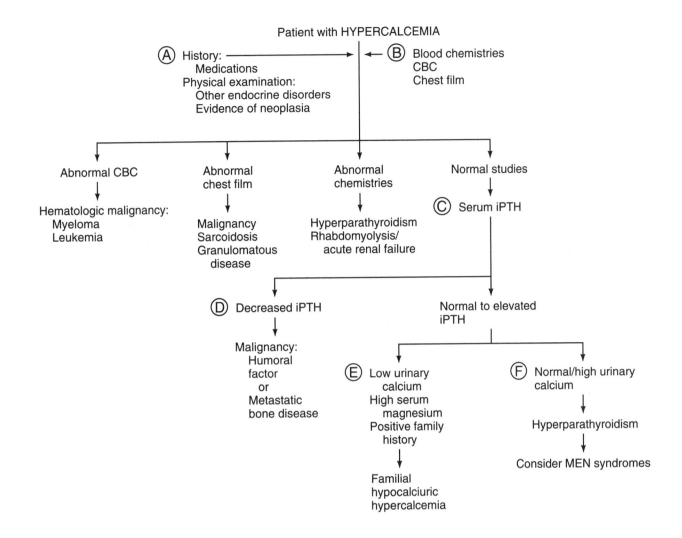

Patient with HYPERCALCEMIA

Ⓐ History:
Medications
Physical examination:
Other endocrine disorders
Evidence of neoplasia

Ⓑ Blood chemistries
CBC
Chest film

Abnormal CBC

Hematologic malignancy:
Myeloma
Leukemia

Abnormal chest film

Malignancy
Sarcoidosis
Granulomatous disease

Abnormal chemistries

Hyperparathyroidism
Rhabdomyolysis/ acute renal failure

Normal studies

Ⓒ Serum iPTH

Ⓓ Decreased iPTH

Malignancy:
Humoral factor
or
Metastatic bone disease

Normal to elevated iPTH

Ⓔ Low urinary calcium
High serum magnesium
Positive family history

Familial hypocalciuric hypercalcemia

Ⓕ Normal/high urinary calcium

Hyperparathyroidism

Consider MEN syndromes

References

Adams JS. Vitamin D metabolite mediated hypercalcemia. Endocrinol Metab Clin North Am 1989; 18:765.

Marx SJ, Spiegel AM, Levine MA, et al. Familial hypocalciuric hypercalcemia. N Engl J Med 1982; 307:416.

Potts JT. Management of asymptomatic hyperparathyroidism. J Clin Endocrinol Metab 1990; 70:1489.

Scholz DA, Purnell DC. Asymptomatic primary hyperparathyroidism: 10-year prospective study. Mayo Clin Proc 1981; 56:473.

Stewart AF, Broadus AE. Parathyroid hormone related proteins: coming of age in the 1990's. J Clin Endocrinol Metab 1990; 71:1410.

TESTS OF THYROID FUNCTION

Julie I. Rifkin, M.D.
Thomas W. Boyden, M.D.

The modern clinical laboratory offers several tests of thyroid function. The physician must be aware of the diagnostic accuracy and limitations of these tests. Abnormal test results must be interpreted with good clinical judgment. Thyroid function tests are not cost-effective as routine screens for thyroid disease.

Sensitive TSH (sTSH): A very useful test. Immunometric assays for TSH were introduced in the early 1980s. These assays generally make it possible to distinguish hyperthyroid from euthyroid patients. The sTSH is elevated in hypothyroidism. The sTSH assay has less cross reactivity with LH, FSH, and hCG. The normal range for an sTSH assay is approximately 0.4–6.2 μU/ml. The older nonsensitive radioimmunoassay (RIA) TSH assays have a range of 0–10 μU/ml.

Free Thyroxine Index (FTI): A useful calculation may soon be obsolete as new immunoassays for free thyroxine (FT_4) become available:

$$FTI = \text{total } T_4 \cdot \left[\frac{RT_3U = (\text{Resin } T_3 \text{ uptake of patient})}{\text{mean normal } RT_3U} \right]$$

This calculation "corrects" the total T_4 for protein-binding abnormalities. The FTI has several limitations. It is misleading in patients with familial and congenital thyroxine-binding protein disorders. Most importantly, the FTI is falsely low in euthyroid patients who are acutely ill.

Free Thyroxine (FT_4): FT_4 is the amount of non–protein-bound circulating thyroxine (about 0.03%). It is a better indicator of thyroid status than total T_4. Previously, measurement of FT_4 was difficult and time consuming (equilibrium dialysis). New two-step immunoassays are now available to measure FT_4 quickly and accurately and will probably replace the calculated FTI.

Triiodothyronine by RIA (T_3 RIA): Measures total T_3. Only useful in diagnosing T_3 toxicosis.

Thyroid Antimicrosomal (TMab) and Antithyroglobulin (TgAb) Antibodies: These antibodies may be elevated in Graves' disease and Hashimoto's thyroiditis. A patient may have Hashimoto's thyroiditis and no circulating antibodies. Positive antibodies are also found in portions of the general population and in patients with nonthyroidal illness.

24-hour Radioactive Iodine Uptake (RAIU): Measures of thyroid's ability to take up iodine. The test uses a tracer amount of ^{123}I or ^{131}I given orally. A gamma scintillation counter is used to measure the radioactivity over the thyroid at 4–6 hours and 24 hours after the dose. Normal percentage uptake varies widely. By itself, this test is not a very accurate test of thyroid function.

Thyroid Imaging – Radionuclide Scan (^{123}I or ^{99m}Tc pertechnetate): Does not produce a picture like a CT or MRI. Can provide information about gland/lobe contour. Identifies thyroid nodules as "hot" (functioning), "cold" (nonfunctioning), or "warm." Cannot be used to diagnose a nodule as benign or malignant.

References

Bethune JE. Interpretation of thyroid function tests. Dis Mon 1989; 35:543.

Klee GG, Hay ID. Sensitive thyrotropin assays; analytical and clinical performance criteria. Mayo Clin Proc 1988; 63:1123.

Santos ET, Mazzfeni EL. Thyroid function tests: guidelines for interpretation in common clinical disorders. Postgrad Med 1989; 85:333.

Surks MI, Chopra IJ, Marilish LN, et al. Committee on Nomenclature, American Thyroid Association: Association guidelines for use of laboratory tests in thyroid disorders. JAMA 1990; 263:1529.

HYPOTHYROIDISM

Julie I. Rifkin, M.D.
Thomas W. Boyden, M.D.

A. The most common cause of hypothyroidism in the United States is Hashimoto's (chronic) thyroiditis. Most, but not all, patients with Hashimoto's thyroiditis have a goiter. Serum thyroglobulin and microsomal antibody levels are elevated in most patients. Lymphoma of the thyroid may develop in glands with Hashimoto's thyroiditis. The hypothyroid phase of postpartum thyroiditis is usually transient; <5% develop permanent hypothyroidism.

B. Replacement therapy with L-thyroxine is conveniently and accurately monitored with the sTSH level. The pituitary requires 6–8 weeks to reach a new steady state after the start of thyroxine therapy or a change in the dosage. The sTSH should not be checked until steady state has been reached. The usual replacement dose of L-thyroxine is 0.05–0.2 mg/day with an average of 0.1–0.15 mg/day. When treating patients with thyroxine (replacement or suppression), the sTSH level should be kept within the euthyroid range. Older patients need less L-thyroxine than young patients to maintain euthyroidism.

C. The TRH stimulation test was initially used to confirm a diagnosis of hyperthyroidism, although the introduction of sensitive TSH assays has obviated the need for this test. At time zero, a TSH sample is drawn and then a 500-μg IV bolus of TRH is given; 30 minutes later a second TSH sample is drawn. In hyperthyroid patients there is no increment in TSH in the second sample (flat response). A normal response varies among different individuals, but in general it is an increment of 5–30 μU/ml and averages about 15 μU/ml. In patients with primary hypothyroidism the response is exaggerated. The TRH test is the only one available to distinguish secondary from tertiary hypothyroidism; however, the separation is not complete.

D. Patients with a normal FTI (FT_4), a slightly raised sTSH, and no clinical features of hypothyroidism may have subclinical hypothyroidism. In these patients thyroid failure does not always develop, and some appear to be in a stable compensated state. There are arguments for and against treating these patients.

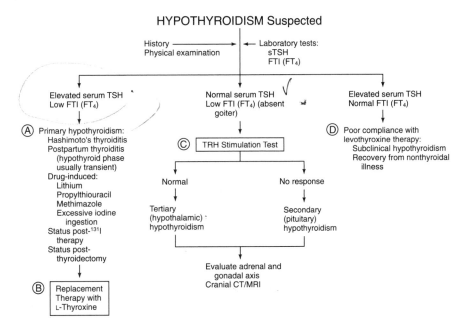

HYPOTHYROIDISM Suspected

References

Adlin EV, Maurer AH, Marks AD, Channick BJ. Bone mineral density in postmenopausal women treated with L-thyroxine. Am J Med 1991; 90:360.

Cooper DJL. Thyroid hormone treatment: new insights into an old therapy. JAMA 1989; 261:2694.

Cooper DS, Halpern R, Wood LC, et al. L-Thyroxine therapy in subclinical hypothyroidism. Ann Intern Med 1984; 101:18.

Hamburger JI, Kaplan MM. Hypothyroidism: don't treat patients who don't have it. Postgrad Med 1989; 86:67.

Hamburger JI, Miller JM, Kine SR. Lymphoma of the thyroid. Ann Intern Med 1983; 99:685.

Hennessey JV, Evaul JE, Tseng Y-I, et al. L-Thyroxine dosage: a re-evaluation of therapy with contemporary preparations. Ann Intern Med 1986; 105:11.

Nikolai TF, Turney SL, Roberts RCL. Postpartum lymphocytic thyroiditis. Arch Intern Med 1987; 147:221.

HYPERTHYROIDISM

Julie I. Rifkin, M.D.
Thomas W. Boyden, M.D.

The diagnosis of hyperthyroidism is suspected in patients with palpitations, nervousness, fatigue, and heat intolerance. These symptoms may be less pronounced or absent in older patients. Patients with atrial fibrillation should be evaluated for hyperthyroidism.

A. Graves' disease is an autoimmune disorder. Production of an antibody that stimulates the TSH receptor results in overproduction of thyroid hormones and goiter formation. Extrathyroidal complications include ophthalmopathy and pretibial myxedema.

B. There are several types of thyroiditis. Therapy depends on the cause of the disorder. Subacute and postpartum thyroiditis are usually transient. Chronic thyroiditis (Hashimoto's thyroiditis) is not usually associated with a painful gland, although there are reports of painful Hashimoto's thyroiditis. Although most (90–95%) thyroid adenomas do not cause hyperthyroidism, functioning adenomas may present with symptoms and signs of hyperthyroidism. This is most common in lesions >3 cm in diameter. Multinodular goiters are more likely to cause hyperthyroidism later in life. In younger patients, they are more likely to be asymptomatic or to present with symptoms of respiratory obstruction or dysphagia.

C. Most patients in the United States with Graves' disease are treated with [131]I. Remission rates with medical therapy are variable. Agranulocytosis is the major complication of antithyroid medications. Many patients with agranulocytosis are asymptomatic. Although it has not been standard practice, routine monitoring of WBC counts in these patients is indicated according to one study.

D. TSH-secreting pituitary adenomas are rare.

E. Increased serum levels of T_3 may occur in any disorder that causes hyperthyroidism. T_3 toxicosis is due to a prodominant hypersecretion of T_3 by the thyroid. The FTI and FT_4 are usually normal. Elevated T_3 may be the first indication of recurrent Graves' disease.

References

Cobler JL, William ME, Greenlan P. Thyrotoxicosis in institutionalized elderly patients with atrial fibrillation. Arch Intern Med 1984; 144:1758.

Gesundheit N, Petrick PA, Nisson M, et al. Thyrotropin secreting pituitary adenomas: clinical and biochemical heterogeneity. Ann Intern Med 1989; 111:827.

Hay ID. Thyroiditis: a clinical update. Mayo Clin Proc 1985; 60:836.

McDougall RI. Graves' disease—current concepts. Med Clin North Am 1991; 75:79.

Orgiazzi J. Management of Graves' hyperthyroidism. Endocrinol Metab Clin North Am 1987; 16:365.

Pharmakiotis AD, Tourkantonis AA. Isolated T_3 toxicosis. N Engl J Med 1980; 303:703.

Tajiri J, Noguchi S, Marakami T, et al. Anti-thyroid drug induced agranulocytosis: the usefulness of routine white blood cell count monitoring. Arch Intern Med 1990; 150:621.

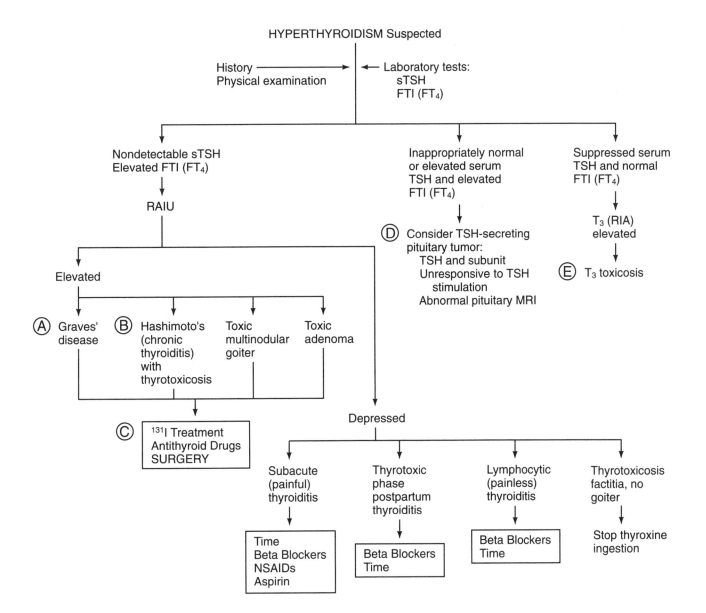

HYPERTHYROIDISM Suspected

History ———→ ←— Laboratory tests:
Physical examination   sTSH
                               FTI (FT$_4$)

Nondetectable sTSH
Elevated FTI (FT$_4$)

RAIU

Elevated

(A) Graves' disease
(B) Hashimoto's (chronic thyroiditis) with thyrotoxicosis
Toxic multinodular goiter
Toxic adenoma

(C) ^{131}I Treatment
Antithyroid Drugs
SURGERY

Inappropriately normal or elevated serum TSH and elevated FTI (FT$_4$)

(D) Consider TSH-secreting pituitary tumor:
TSH and subunit
Unresponsive to TSH stimulation
Abnormal pituitary MRI

Suppressed serum TSH and normal FTI (FT$_4$)

T$_3$ (RIA) elevated

(E) T$_3$ toxicosis

Depressed

Subacute (painful) thyroiditis

Time
Beta Blockers
NSAIDs
Aspirin

Thyrotoxic phase postpartum thyroiditis

Beta Blockers
Time

Lymphocytic (painless) thyroiditis

Beta Blockers
Time

Thyrotoxicosis factitia, no goiter

Stop thyroxine ingestion

GOITER

Julie I. Rifkin, M.D.
Thomas W. Boyden, M.D.

Nonimmunologic goiter formation generally occurs when there is impaired (partial or complete) production of thyroid hormone and compensatory TSH release. This type of goiter is often familial. The most common cause of immunologic goiter in the United States is Hashimoto's thyroiditis. Suppression therapy with L-thyroxine is often effective in reducing the size of a goiter due to Hashimoto's thyroiditis. Thyroxine therapy may slow or prevent further growth of nonimmunologic goiters that are presumed to be supported by TSH. Endemic goiter is essentially nonexistent in the United States. Depending on the cause of the goiter formation, a patient found to have a goiter may be euthyroid, hypothyroid, or hyperthyroid.

A. Iodine is the most important goitrogen in the American diet. Not all persons who ingest large quantities of iodine develop thyroid dysfunction. Thyroid hormone synthesis ceases when large quantities of iodide are transported into the thyroid (Wolff-Chaikoff effect). The normal thyroid "escapes" from the Wolff-Chaikoff effect and homeostasis resumes. The gland with an underlying defect in autoregulation fails to escape, and goiter ensues, with or without hypothyroidism. The gland with absent autoregulation increases thyroid hormone secretion when excess iodine is ingested. Increased hormone secretion leads to a hyperthyroid state (Jod-Basedow). The hyperthyroid state resolves when the source of excess iodine has been eliminated.

B. L-Thyroxine therapy must be administered cautiously in older individuals. A reasonable starting dose for an older individual or a patient with cardiac disease is 0.05 mg/day of L-thyroxine. Response to this dose may be assessed by sTSH measurement 6–8 weeks after the initiation of therapy, and increased if necessary at that time. Multinodular goiters may contain autonomously functioning nodules. Exogenous T_4 combined with autonomous production of T_4/T_3 can produce hyperthyroidism and lead to cardiovascular complications. The usual suppressive dose of L-thyroxine ranges from 0.1 to 0.15 mg/day. Larger (0.2 mg/day) or smaller (0.05 mg/day) doses may be required. Surgical therapy for goiter is rarely necessary. It is indicated when obstructive symptoms are present or the goiter is substernal.

References

Anderson PE, Hurley PR, Rosswick P. Conservative treatment and long term prophylactic thyroxine in the prevention of recurrence of multinodular goiter. Surg Gynecol Obstet 1990; 171:409-314.

Greenspan FS. The problem of the nodular goiter. Med Clin North Am 1991; 75:195.

Studee H, Peter HJ, Gerber H. Natural heterogeneity of thyroid cells: the basis for understanding thyroid function and nodular goiter growth. Endoc Rev 1989; 10:125.

Woeber KA. Iodine and thyroid disease. Med Clin North Am 1991; 75:169.

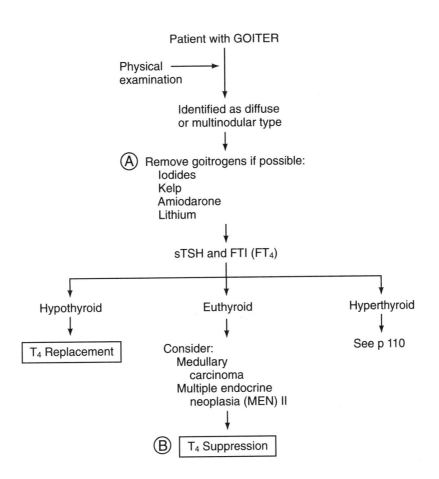

Patient with GOITER

Physical ——————▶
examination

Identified as diffuse
or multinodular type

(A) Remove goitrogens if possible:
    Iodides
    Kelp
    Amiodarone
    Lithium

sTSH and FTI (FT$_4$)

Hypothyroid   Euthyroid   Hyperthyroid

| T$_4$ Replacement |

Consider:
    Medullary
      carcinoma
    Multiple endocrine
      neoplasia (MEN) II

See p 110

(B) | T$_4$ Suppression |

THYROID NODULE

Julie I. Rifkin, M.D.
Thomas W. Boyden, M.D.

Thyroid nodules are common. They can be found in approximately 4% of the adult US population. They occur four times more frequently in females. Most thyroid nodules are benign. Conditions that may present as a thyroid nodule include thyroid cysts, parathyroid and thyroglossal duct cysts, a focal area of thyroiditis, a dominant portion of a multinodular gland, agenesis of a thyroid lobe, benign adenoma, and thyroid malignancies. Thyroid cysts are usually benign, but aspirated fluid should always be sent for cytologic analysis. Suspicion of thyroid malignancy is increased in a patient with a recent enlargement of a nodule, hoarseness or dysphagia, or a family history of medullary thyroid cancer (measure serum calcitonin). Suspicion of malignancy is heightened in young adults, men, and persons with a history of exposure to ionizing radiation.

A. Thin needle aspiration (TNA) or fine needle aspiration biopsy (FNAB) of thyroid nodules has been in use for over 40 years. It is an outpatient procedure that causes little discomfort to the patient and provides a cytologic tissue diagnosis.

B. Results of TNA are accurate about 96% of the time when reviewed by an experienced cytopathologist. A study with a 6-month follow-up found no significant difference in nodule size between thyroxine- and placebo-treated patients. Suppressive therapy with L-thyroxine is used by most endocrinologists for patients with benign thyroid nodules. A nodule that enlarges on suppressive therapy requires repeat biopsy.

C. Exogenous L-thyroxine given in replacement doses (0.05–0.2 mg/day) is given to suppress the thyroid's production of endogenous T_4 and T_3. This therapy is used in the euthyroid patient with a thyroid nodule. While the patient is on suppressive therapy, the sTSH should not fall below the normal range. During management of patients who have been treated for thyroid malignancy, however, more aggressive TSH suppression may be desirable, because growth of these neoplasms is often TSH dependent.

D. According to the Third National Cancer Survey, thyroid cancer accounts for 0.004% per year of cancer cases. The most common form of thyroid cancer is papillary carcinoma. With proper management, most of these patients are cured. Poor prognostic factors include age >40, male gender, primary lesion >4 cm, and extent of local invasion (node status does not correlate with outcome). The surgical procedure for treatment depends on the histologic type of the malignancy, the size of the primary tumor, and the extent of local disease. Pre- and postoperative serum thyroglobulin measurements are helpful. Postoperative ^{131}I therapy is useful in selected patients with papillary/follicular cancers after surgical management.

E. About 85% of follicular neoplasms are benign and 15% are malignant. Most of these lesions are identified as "cold" on thyroid scans, but some may be "hot."

References

Clark OH. TSH suppression of thyroid nodules and thyroid cancer. World J Surg 1981; 5:39.

Gharib H, James EM, Charboneade JW, et al. Suppressive therapy with levothyroxine for solitary thyroid nodules: a double-blind placebo controlled clinical study. N Engl J Med 1987; 317:70.

Golden AW. The indications for ablating normal thyroid tissue with ^{131}I in differentiated thyroid cancer. Clin Endocrinol 1985; 23:81.

Miller JM, Hamburger JI, Kim S. Diagnosis of thyroid nodules: use of fine-needle aspiration and needle biopsy. JAMA 1979; 241:481.

Schneider AB. Radiation-induced thyroid tumors. Endocrinol Metab Clin North Am 1990; 19:495.

Simpson WJ, et al. Papillary and follicular thyroid cancer: prognostic factors in 1578 patients. Am J Med 1987; 83:479.

Van Herle AJ, Rich P, Ljung BME, et al. The thyroid nodule. Ann Intern Med 1982; 96:221.

Patient with PALPABLE THYROID NODULE

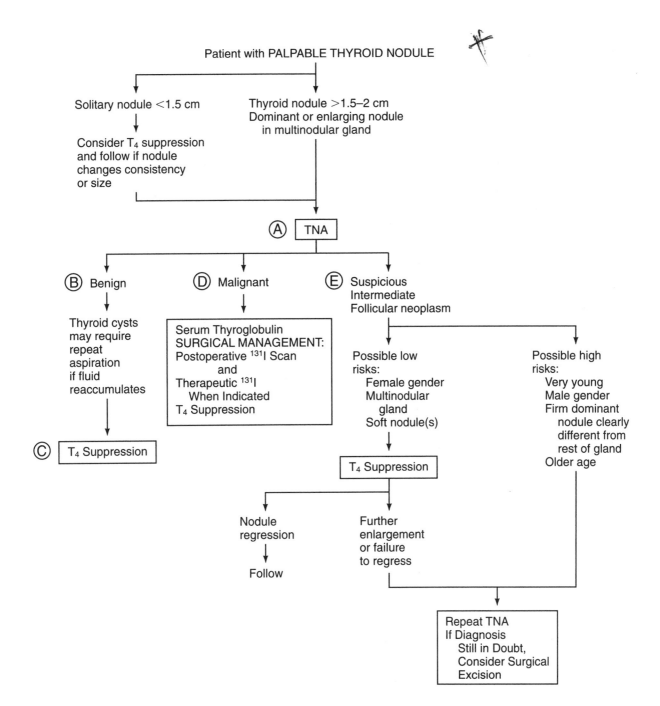

Solitary nodule <1.5 cm

Consider T₄ suppression and follow if nodule changes consistency or size

Thyroid nodule >1.5–2 cm
Dominant or enlarging nodule in multinodular gland

Ⓐ TNA

Ⓑ Benign

Thyroid cysts may require repeat aspiration if fluid reaccumulates

Ⓒ T₄ Suppression

Ⓓ Malignant

Serum Thyroglobulin
SURGICAL MANAGEMENT:
Postoperative ¹³¹I Scan
    and
Therapeutic ¹³¹I
    When Indicated
T₄ Suppression

Ⓔ Suspicious
Intermediate
Follicular neoplasm

Possible low risks:
    Female gender
    Multinodular gland
    Soft nodule(s)

T₄ Suppression

Nodule regression

Follow

Further enlargement or failure to regress

Possible high risks:
    Very young
    Male gender
    Firm dominant nodule clearly different from rest of gland
    Older age

Repeat TNA
If Diagnosis
    Still in Doubt,
    Consider Surgical
    Excision

PAINFUL THYROID

Nancy A. Curosh, M.D.

Any condition that causes very rapid growth of the thyroid may cause pain, because the thyroid is an encapsulated gland. Pain may be confined to the thyroid gland itself, but frequently radiates to the ears, jaw, or chest. Subacute thyroiditis is the classic disease causing severe thyroid pain. Acute suppurative thyroiditis and radiation thyroiditis are rare conditions that are often obvious on presentation. Hemorrhage into a cyst can be painful; it is usually suspected at physical examination and from its sudden onset. Common conditions that can cause very enlarged thyroids such as Graves' disease, Hashimoto's thyroiditis, and cancer may cause mild thyroid tenderness or pressure, but rarely cause pain because they develop less rapidly. Other nonthyroidal illnesses may cause neck pain, but the thyroid itself is not swollen or painful.

A. Rarely, treatment of hyperthyroidism with ^{131}I therapy can cause a painful thyroid clinically resembling subacute thyroiditis. Pain and swelling of the thyroid develops within 1–2 weeks of treatment and usually resolves within 3–4 weeks.

B. Acute suppurative thyroiditis is an inflammatory disease caused by bacterial, fungal, or parasitic infection of the thyroid. Since the discovery of antibiotics, this disease has become extremely rare. The thyroid itself is relatively resistant to infection, probably owing to its complete encapsulation, rich blood supply and lymphatic drainage, and high iodide content. Acute suppurative thyroiditis is usually preceded by an infection elsewhere in the body, most commonly an upper respiratory infection or pharyngitis. Many patients have a history of preexisting thyroid disease. Commonly, patients appear septic with fever, chills, tachycardia, and a painful swollen neck. Sore throat and dysphagia occur frequently. Laboratory evaluation reveals leukocytosis, but thyroid function tests and radioactive iodine uptake (RAIU) are normal. Fine needle aspiration (FNA) should be performed to identify the offending organism so that proper antibiotic therapy can be instituted. Surgical incision and drainage are sometimes required.

C. The RAIU test helps differentiate the types of hyperthyroidism. The patient ingests a small amount of radioactive iodine, and the percentage of iodine that is taken up by the thyroid gland at 24 hours is determined. In Graves' disease, in which the thyroid is actively producing thyroid hormone, the uptake is increased. In subacute thyroiditis, the uptake is decreased as the gland is damaged and unable to trap iodine and make thyroid hormone. The patient is hyperthyroid because of leakage of preformed hormone.

D. Subacute thyroiditis is a spontaneously remitting inflammatory disease of the thyroid that is most likely due to a viral infection. Infiltration of inflammatory cells leads to rapid thyroid swelling and pain. Because the thyroid gland is damaged, there is leakage of preformed thyroid hormone into the circulation, causing hyperthyroidism. However, since the gland is damaged, it temporarily is unable to take up iodine and make more thyroid hormone. This results in the low RAIU, which can help clarify the diagnosis. In most cases the diagnosis is obvious when the patient presents with rapid onset of a swollen tender thyroid gland without evidence of sepsis. In some cases, however, it may be difficult to differentiate subacute from acute thyroiditis, because fever and pain are common to both. Subacute thyroiditis also may be preceded by an upper respiratory infection. If one is in doubt clinically, some tests can be helpful. In subacute thyroiditis the WBC count is normal and, as mentioned, the patient is usually hyperthyroid with a low RAIU. A fine needle biopsy can confirm the diagnosis in difficult cases, but this is rarely necessary. Subacute thyroiditis is treated with salicylates for their anti-inflammatory action. In severe cases, corticosteroids may be needed. Beta blockers can be used during the initial hyperthyroid phase to decrease symptoms of hyperthyroidism. As the gland recovers, a transient hypothyroid phase may occur, but most people ultimately become euthyroid. Rarely, malignancies of the thyroid have presented with symptoms that mimic subacute thyroiditis. Therefore, if a patient fails to respond to the usual treatment, a biopsy should be performed to investigate for cancer.

E. Occasionally a patient presents with pain from a single thyroid nodule in an otherwise normal gland, or one prominent nodule in a multinodular gland. FNA should be performed. Possible causes include hemorrhage into a cyst, localized subacute thyroiditis, or (rarely) cancer.

F. A diffusely painful goiter in a euthyroid or hypothyroid patient is probably due to thyroid carcinoma or acute onset of Hashimoto's thyroiditis. Any condition that is suspicious for cancer, such as a rapidly growing gland or the development of hoarseness, should be investigated with a biopsy. Hashimoto's or chronic lymphocytic thyroiditis is an autoimmune disease that rarely causes thyroid pain. High titers of microsomal antibodies or thyroglobulin antibodies are frequently seen in Hashimoto's thyroiditis but are not specific. Caution is necessary because malignancies, especially lymphomas, may develop in patients with chronic lymphocytic thyroiditis. Therefore, if cancer seems unlikely and the presumptive diagnosis is Hashimoto's thyroiditis, a trial of thyroid hormone suppression and observation is indicated. However, a biopsy must be performed if the gland continues to enlarge.

Patient with PAINFUL THYROID

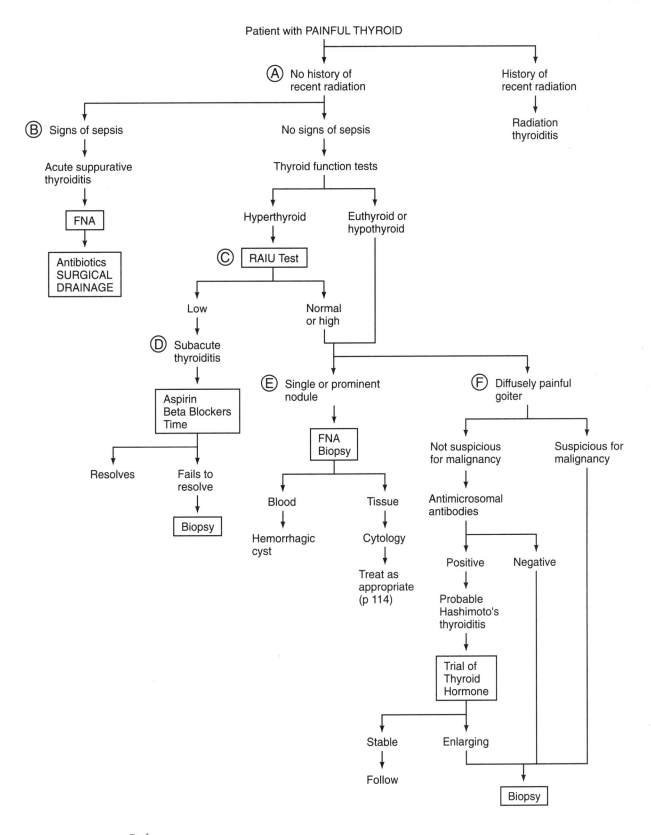

References

Hamburger JI. The various presentations of thyroiditis: diagnostic considerations. Ann Intern Med 1986; 104:219.

Hay ID. Thyroiditis: a clinical update. Mayo Clin Proc 1985; 60:836.

Rosen IB, Strawbridge HG, Walfish PG, Bain J. Malignant pseudothyroiditis: a new clinical entity. Am J Surg 1978; 136:445.

Szabo SM, Allen DB. Thyroiditis: differentiation of acute suppurative and subacute. Clin Pediatr 1989; 28:171.

THYROID FUNCTION TESTS IN NONTHYROIDAL ILLNESS

Julie I. Rifkin, M.D.

In hospitalized patients the incidence of true hypo- or hyperthyroidism is <1%. Clinical signs of thyroid disease may be masked in acutely ill patients. Conversely, some of the signs of severe illness mimic changes seen in thyroid diseases. Serum T_3 radioimmunoassay (RIA) is usually decreased in patients with nonthyroidal illness. The TSH response to TRH also is usually normal. It may be difficult to identify acutely ill patients with hypothalamic or pituitary disease. A sTSH above 20 μU/ml and low free T_4 (FT_4) is good evidence for primary thyroid failure.

A. The free thyroxine index (FTI) is frequently misleading because of drug-induced or disease-related binding protein abnormalities. The FT_4 is the preferred test for assessing the thyroxine level in this setting.

B. Up to 50% of acutely ill patients have a decrease in total T_4 and/or T_3. Both FT_4 and sTSH are usually normal. These findings provide good evidence that the patient is euthyroid.

C. During the acute phase of an illness, especially an acute psychiatric illness, a few patients have elevation of total T_4 and FT_4 and a normal sTSH. These patients may also display a flat response to TRH stimulation. Because these abnormalities resolve after a few weeks, great care must be taken in diagnosing an acutely psychotic patient as hyperthyroid. T_3 RIA is usually normal in these patients. Propranolol doses >320 mg/day, amiodarone, heparin, furosemide, and acute alcoholic hepatitis may all produce elevations of FT_4 with normal sTSH levels. In these situations, if there are no compelling clinical findings to indicate hyperthyroidism, it is best to simply repeat the tests in 2–3 weeks.

D. Patients with nephrotic syndrome may have mildly depressed FT_4 and normal sTSH. Glucocorticoids in stress doses acutely inhibit TSH secretion, and a small decrement in both sTSH and FT_4 may be observed. Dopamine infusions also cause acute suppression of TSH. In a truly hypothyroid patient receiving a dopamine infusion and/or stress doses of glucocorticoids, the TSH may be suppressed into the normal range.

E. Elevation of sTSH with normal FT_4 is found in patients recovering from a nonthyroidal illness. sTSH is usually less than 20 μU/ml, but rebound of up to 30 μU/ml may occur in patients recovering from severe sepsis. Slight elevations of TSH are commonly found in patients with chronic renal failure. Although the pathophysiology is unknown, these patients have a blunted TSH response to TRH.

References

Borst GL, Eil C, Birman KD. Euthyroid hyperthyroxinemia. Ann Intern Med 1983; 98:366.

Cavaliere RR. The effects of nonthyroid disease and drugs on thyroid function tests. Med Clin North Am 1991; 75:27.

Cavaliere RR, Pih-Rivers R. The effects of drugs on the distribution and metabolism of thyroid hormones. Pharmacol Rev 1981; 35:55.

Faber J, Kirkegaena C, Rasmassen B, et al. Pituitary-thyroid axis in critical illness. J Clin Endocrinol Metab 1987; 65:315.

Lim S, Fang V, Katz A, et al. Thyroid dysfunction in chronic renal failure: a study of the pituitary-thyroid axis and peripheral turnover kinetics of thyroxine and triiodothyronine. J Clin Invest 1977; 60:522.

Patient with ACUTE OR CHRONIC MEDICAL ILLNESS OR MAJOR SURGERY

(A) sTSH and FT$_4$

(B) Normal sTSH and normal FT$_4$

(C) Normal sTSH and normal to increased FT$_4$

(D) Normal to decreased sTSH and normal to decreased FT$_4$

(E) Normal to increased sTSH and normal FT$_4$

ADRENAL MASS

Nancy A. Curosh, M.D.

Abdominal CT has become commonplace, detecting incidental adrenal masses with increased frequency. The incidence has been estimated at 1–10% of patients having a high-resolution abdominal CT scan. In most cases the patient is asymptomatic. Autopsy series have found macroscopic adrenal nodules in 2–9% of patients. The history and physical examination in some cases may suggest a cause (evidence of adrenal hormone excess, discovery of a primary carcinoma that may have metastasized to the adrenal) and this should be pursued vigorously. Otherwise, complete diagnostic testing for every adrenal mass is not cost effective.

A. The likelihood of a pheochromocytoma in an incidentally discovered adrenal mass is low. However, because it is a potentially lethal condition that can have grave consequences if not diagnosed preoperatively, a high index of suspicion is necessary. Most patients with a pheochromocytoma have symptoms. The classic triad is headache, diaphoresis, and palpitations; the presence of two or more of these greatly increases the likelihood that the disease is present. New-onset hypertension; labile or severe hypertension; family history of multiple endocrine neoplasia (MEN) IIA or IIB; severe pressor responses to surgery, pregnancy, or anesthesia; and paradoxical responses to antihypertensive medications are all warning signs. Other symptoms occasionally seen with pheochromocytomas include pallor, paroxysms, anxiety, chest pain, weakness, and nausea.

B. In patients who are hypertensive at the time of sampling, a negative urine screening test makes a pheochromocytoma very unlikely. In patients who are normotensive or intermittently hypertensive, repeat testing may be necessary. The choice of screening and confirmation tests may depend on which assays are available at a particular laboratory. Usually the best screening tests are 24-hour urine collections for metanephrines or free catecholamines. Many medications and foods interfere with these assays. It is therefore essential to understand which assays are performed by a particular laboratory in order to prepare the patient adequately for collection and interpret the results correctly. In general, high-performance liquid chromatography methods are the most sensitive and reliable. The plasma norepinephrine level can also be a helpful diagnostic test, if available. For this test, strict guidelines must be followed in the collection and handling of the blood to avoid false-positive results.

C. MRI, meta-iodobenzylguanidine (MIBG), and selective venous sampling are all tests available to help localize a pheochromocytoma. If a pheochromocytoma is seen on CT, these tests are usually unnecessary. In some cases, especially in MEN syndromes, there may be multiple pheochromocytomas. If this is suspected, one of these additional tests may be useful.

D. Signs of female virilization include male-pattern baldness, deepening of the voice, clitorimegaly, increased strength, and increased libido. Male feminization may include decreased body hair, loss of muscle strength and mass, gynecomastia, and decreased libido.

E. Adrenal carcinomas are extremely rare and have a poor prognosis. Abdominal pain and a palpable mass are commonly present at the time of diagnosis. Hypokalemia is frequently seen. Excessive glucocorticoid, androgen, and mineralocorticoid hypersecretion has a rapid onset, and therefore the usual clinical features of hormonal excess may not have time to develop fully. Surgical resection is the treatment of choice if possible. Although surgical cure is rare because of frequent metastases, it at least reduces the tumor mass and the amount of steroid hypersecretion. Medical therapies include mitotane (o,p'-DDD), metyrapone, and aminoglutethimide.

F. Patients with Cushing's syndrome frequently have weight gain with truncal obesity, proximal muscle weakness, spontaneous ecchymoses, striae, and alterations in reproductive function (oligomenorrhea or amenorrhea in females; decreased libido or impotence in males). Hypertension is very common.

G. Aldosterone-secreting tumors are extremely rare, and the confirmatory tests are complicated and time consuming. If the patient is not hypertensive and does not spontaneously have hypokalemia, it is not cost effective to pursue this etiology. Serum potassium levels should be obtained with the patient on a normal to high sodium diet and off any potassium-altering medications.

References

Copeland PM. The incidentally discovered adrenal mass. Ann Intern Med 1983; 98:940.

Gross MD, Shapiro B, Bouffard JA, et al. Distinguishing benign from malignant euadrenal masses. Ann Intern Med 1988; 109:613.

Ross NS, Aron DC. Hormonal evaluation of the patient with an incidentally discovered adrenal mass. N Engl J Med 1990; 323:1401.

Stein PP, Black HR. A simplified diagnostic approach to pheochromocytoma: a review of the literature and report of one institution's experience. Medicine 1990; 70:46.

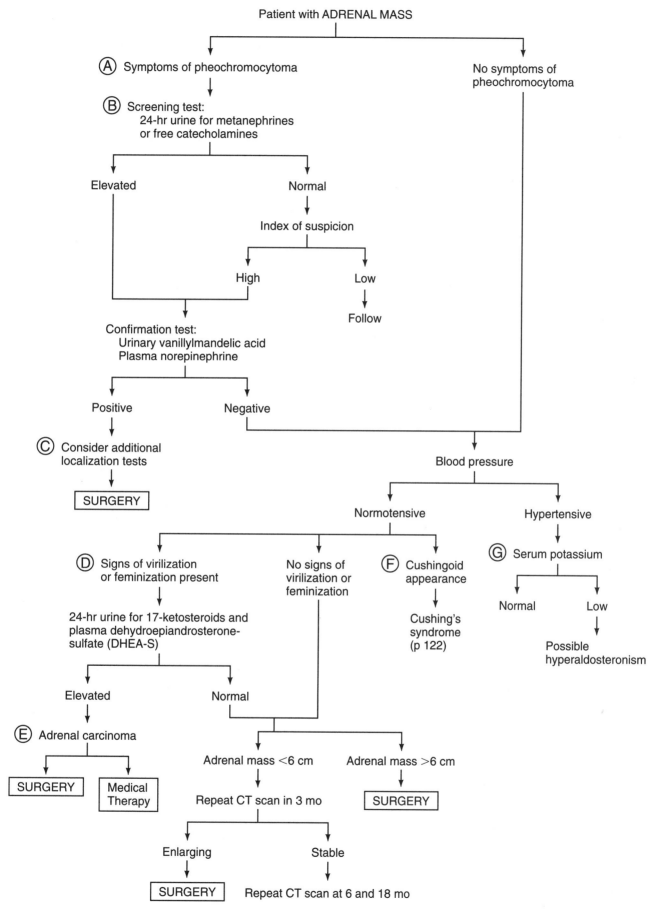

Patient with ADRENAL MASS

(A) Symptoms of pheochromocytoma

No symptoms of pheochromocytoma

(B) Screening test:
24-hr urine for metanephrines
or free catecholamines

Elevated

Normal

Index of suspicion

High

Low

Follow

Confirmation test:
Urinary vanillylmandelic acid
Plasma norepinephrine

Positive

Negative

(C) Consider additional
localization tests

Blood pressure

SURGERY

Normotensive

Hypertensive

(G) Serum potassium

(D) Signs of virilization
or feminization present

No signs of
virilization or
feminization

(F) Cushingoid
appearance

24-hr urine for 17-ketosteroids and
plasma dehydroepiandrosterone-
sulfate (DHEA-S)

Cushing's
syndrome
(p 122)

Normal

Low

Possible
hyperaldosteronism

Elevated

Normal

(E) Adrenal carcinoma

Adrenal mass <6 cm

Adrenal mass >6 cm

SURGERY

Medical
Therapy

Repeat CT scan in 3 mo

SURGERY

Enlarging

Stable

SURGERY

Repeat CT scan at 6 and 18 mo

CUSHING'S SYNDROME

Nancy A. Curosh, M.D.

Cushing's syndrome is caused by a chronic increase in circulating glucocorticoids. The most common cause is exogenous use of glucocorticoids in the treatment of other illnesses. Endogenous Cushing's syndrome can be caused by several different pathophysiologic mechanisms that all cause the adrenal glands to overproduce glucocorticoids. About 80% of cases of endogenous Cushing's syndrome are due to Cushing's disease, where the pituitary secretes excessive amounts of adrenocorticotropic hormone (ACTH). Ectopic ACTH producing tumors and adrenal adenomas each occur about 10% of the time. Rare causes include adrenal carcinoma, bilateral nodular adrenal hyperplasia, and corticotropin releasing hormone (CRH)-secreting tumors. Cushing's disease is more common in females than in males, but the other forms of Cushing's syndrome have an equal sex frequency. The clinical signs and symptoms of Cushing's syndrome are protean and are modified by the amount and duration of cortisol excess. Common manifestations include central obesity, hypertension, thin skin with easy bruising, purple striae, hirsutism, oligomenorrhea in females or decreased libido in males, proximal muscle weakness, osteoporosis, glucose intolerance, and depression or psychosis. It is often difficult to distinguish Cushing's syndrome from Cushingoid obesity, as many symptoms are common to both. The following may be seen with Cushing's syndrome but usually are not seen with Cushingoid obesity: objective weakness, striae >1 cm in diameter, hypokalemia, spontaneous bruising, and osteoporosis.

A. Urinary free cortisol confirms the diagnosis of cortisol excess. Low-dose dexamethasone suppression tests are made to rule out Cushing's syndrome; an abnormal test does not establish the diagnosis. There are two low-dose suppression tests. In the overnight dexamethasone suppression test, 1 mg dexamethasone is given orally at midnight. A plasma cortisol level is drawn at 8 AM. If the cortisol is <5 μg/dl, Cushing's syndrome is excluded. The Liddle low-dose test is performed by giving 0.5 mg dexamethasone every 6 hours for 2 days. Plasma cortisol, urinary 17-hydroxycorticosteroid, or urine-free cortisol is obtained each day. Cushing's syndrome is excluded if suppression occurs.

B. Suppression may not occur if the patient failed to take the dexamethasone, was on medication(s) that may have interfered with the test (estrogen, dilantin, phenobarbital, rifampin), or was under stress. Depressed patients frequently have elevated cortisol production rates and fail to suppress with low-dose dexamethasone. However, they do not have the stigmata of Cushing's syndrome. Occasionally, alcoholics appear floridly Cushingoid and may fail to suppress during the low-dose test. These manifestations usually disappear within days of abstinence. The cortisol response to an insulin tolerance test may be useful in differentiating true Cushing's syndrome, where cortisol does not rise with hypoglycemia, from the depressed or alcoholic patient, where a normal cortisol increase occurs. This test may be dangerous and warrants adequate precautions.

C. High-dose dexamethasone suppression testing can be done by two methods. The traditional Liddle test consists of 2 mg dexamethasone every 6 hours for 2–3 days. Plasma cortisol, urinary 17-hydroxycorticosteroid, or urine-free cortisol levels are obtained at baseline and each day. A 50% reduction from baseline indicates pituitary disease. The alternative test is an 8-mg overnight dexamethasone suppression test. Cushing's disease responds to suppression, resulting in an 8 AM plasma cortisol <50% of baseline.

D. The plasma ACTH level is very helpful in differentiating ectopic tumors, where ACTH is high, from adrenal tumors, where it is suppressed. Unfortunately, ACTH radioimmunoassays are not available in all areas, and strict guidelines as to collection times and methods and handling of the specimen must be adhered to for an accurate test. If this is not available, localization procedures usually aid in the diagnosis.

E. Most patients with ectopic ACTH have known malignancies. Oat cell carcinoma is the most common; others include bronchial adenomas or carcinoids, pheochromocytomas, thymic carcinoids, pancreatic islet cell tumors, and medullary carcinomas of the thyroid. In some cases, because of rapid progression of the disease, the classic characteristics of Cushing's syndrome may not be present. Spontaneous hypokalemia may be a diagnostic clue. Several cases have been reported where the malignant tumor secretes CRH instead of ACTH.

F. Cushing's disease is usually caused by very small pituitary adenomas. If these are seen on CT or MRI, this may help confirm the diagnosis. In most cases, however, the scans are normal. Additional confirmatory tests can be performed as deemed necessary. These include bilateral inferior petrosal sinus catheterization or exaggerated responses to metyrapone, ACTH, or CRH. Cushing's disease is best treated with transsphenoidal pituitary surgery. Bilateral adrenalectomy is an alternative choice, but 10–15% of patients may develop Nelson's syndrome: hyperpigmentation and increasing size of the pituitary tumor, which may invade locally.

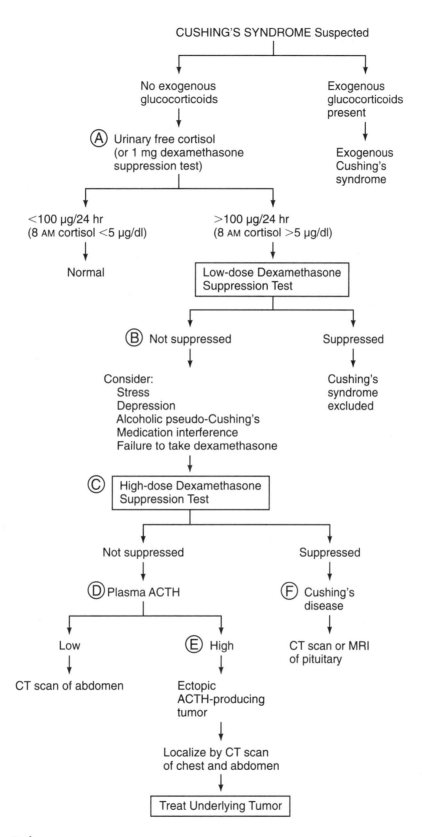

CUSHING'S SYNDROME Suspected

No exogenous glucocorticoids

Exogenous glucocorticoids present

Exogenous Cushing's syndrome

Ⓐ Urinary free cortisol (or 1 mg dexamethasone suppression test)

<100 μg/24 hr (8 AM cortisol <5 μg/dl)

Normal

>100 μg/24 hr (8 AM cortisol >5 μg/dl)

Low-dose Dexamethasone Suppression Test

Ⓑ Not suppressed

Suppressed

Consider:
Stress
Depression
Alcoholic pseudo-Cushing's
Medication interference
Failure to take dexamethasone

Cushing's syndrome excluded

Ⓒ High-dose Dexamethasone Suppression Test

Not suppressed

Suppressed

Ⓓ Plasma ACTH

Ⓕ Cushing's disease

Low

Ⓔ High

CT scan or MRI of pituitary

CT scan of abdomen

Ectopic ACTH-producing tumor

Localize by CT scan of chest and abdomen

Treat Underlying Tumor

References

Carpenter PC. Diagnostic evaluation of Cushing's syndrome. Endocrinol Metab Clin North Am 1988; 17:445.

Felicetta JV. Cushing's syndrome: how to pinpoint and treat the underlying cause. Postgrad Med 1989; 86:79.

Flack MR, Oldfield EH, Cutler GB, et al. Urine free cortisol in the high dose dexamethasone suppression test for the differential diagnosis of the Cushing syndrome. Ann Intern Med 1992; 116:211.

Kaye TB, Crapo L. The Cushing syndrome: an update on diagnostic tests. Ann Intern Med 1990; 112:434.

PITUITARY TUMOR

Philip R. Orlander, M.D.

A. Suspect a pituitary tumor if there is evidence of either hormonal excess or deficiency, or if symptoms suggest compression of surrounding brain structures. Incidental abnormalities of the pituitary may be noted during an evaluation for head injury or other common neurologic complaints. Pituitary abnormalities should be considered in women with complaints of infertility. Pituitary adenomas that are completely within the sella turcica (<1 cm) are considered microadenomas and present primarily with hormone excess syndromes. Macroadenomas may expand in a suprasellar direction, causing neuroanatomic manifestations such as headache, bitemporal hemianopsia, cranial nerve abnormalities, CSF rhinorrhea, and hypothalamic dysregulation. Formal visual field tests should be performed by an ophthalmologist. In patients with abrupt onset of severe headache, change in mental status, and evidence of hormone deficiency, consider the rare syndrome of pituitary apoplexy with hemorrhage into a macroadenoma.

B. Prolactinomas are the most common pituitary tumors. They generally present as microadenomas in women with symptoms of infertility, menstrual irregularities, or galactorrhea, whereas men present with larger lesions accompanied by impotence and symptoms of mass effect. The differential diagnosis of hyperprolactinemia includes numerous medications (e.g., phenothiazines, narcotics, estrogens, reserpine), hypothyroidism, renal disease, cirrhosis, chest wall or breast disease, pregnancy, and hypothalamic disease affecting the pituitary stalk. The clinical suspicion of acromegaly can be confirmed with an elevated serum growth hormone (GH) level that does not suppress normally after an oral 100-g glucose load or an elevated serum insulin-like growth factor level (IGF-I). The diagnosis of pituitary-dependent Cushing's disease requires consistent evidence of hypercortisolism (elevated urinary-free cortisol and inadequate suppression after dexamethasone) and a normal to high adrenocorticotropic hormone (ACTH) level (to exclude an adrenal source). A dose of 1 mg of dexamethasone given PO at bedtime should suppress the morning cortisol to <5 μg/dl. Stress, intercurrent illness, and depression may invalidate this screening test; a 24-hour urine collection for free cortisol is a useful adjunctive test. Further dynamic testing with higher doses of dexamethasone and imaging studies should be performed only in patients who fail to suppress. Petrosal sinus drainage for ACTH is useful in ruling out an ectopic syndrome (e.g., bronchial carcinoid). Rare thyrotropin (TSH) secreting tumors can produce hyperthyroidism. Gonadotrophin secreting tumors are generally large and present primarily with neurologic complaints.

C. In adults suspected of having pituitary disease, a morning serum cortisol level <20 μg/dl, or borderline to low values of thyroid or gonadal hormones, should initiate formal pituitary testing. This can be accomplished by an infusion of hypothalamic releasing factors (thyrotropin releasing hormone [TRH], gonadotropin releasing hormone [GnRH], corticotropin releasing hormone [CRH]) and insulin, and requires special expertise. The posterior pituitary can be evaluated with a water deprivation test. Most pituitary lesions do not cause hypopituitarism. Primary empty sella is a defect in the diaphragm of the sella and is rarely associated with any hormone abnormality. Large pituitary adenomas, craniopharyngiomas, and other tumors and infiltrating diseases of the hypothalamus and pituitary can be associated with panhypopituitarism (anterior and posterior pituitary). Diabetes insipidus may be the presenting complaint. Patients with untreated primary hypothyroidism or gonadal failure (Turner's or Klinefelter's syndrome) may be found to have an enlarged sella.

D. MRI of the pituitary has replaced older techniques such as lateral skull radiography and tomography of the sella, but CT imaging is still useful if MRI is not available. The optic chiasm and pituitary stalk are easily demonstrated. In a high percentage of patients with Cushing's disease there is no detectable lesion in the pituitary on MRI. Autopsy studies demonstrate that pituitary microadenomas are not uncommon, and abnormal scans in the absence of hormonal abnormality or mass effect may not require therapy.

E. Rapid responses to medical therapy with marked tumor shrinkage have been noted in patients with prolactinomas and, less often, in those with acromegaly. Unfortunately, tumor re-expansion is generally seen after discontinuation of treatment, and maintenance therapy is usually necessary. Replacement of all target organ hormones is essential in patients with pituitary deficiency. Intranasal desmopressin (DDAVP) is the treatment of choice for diabetes insipidus. Most pituitary lesions can be reached by a transsphenoidal approach. Macroadenomas may require additional radiation therapy, and the risk of hypopituitarism is high.

References

Cardosa ER, Peterson EW. Pituitary apoplexy: a review. Neurosurgery 1984; 14:363.

Kaye TB, Crapo L. The Cushing syndrome; an update on diagnostic tests. Ann Intern Med 1990; 112:435.

Klibanski A, Zervas NT. Diagnosis and management of hormone secreting pituitary adenomas. N Engl J Med 1991; 324:822.

Liuzzi A, Dallabonzana D, Oppizzi G, et al. Low doses of dopamine agonists in the long-term treatment of macroprolactinomas. N Engl J Med 1985; 313:656.

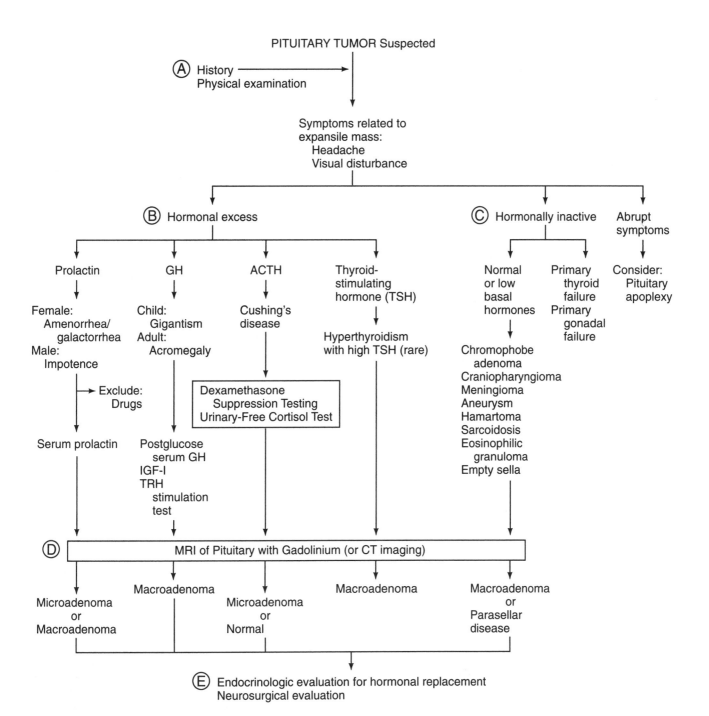

PITUITARY TUMOR Suspected

(A) History
Physical examination

Symptoms related to
expansile mass:
Headache
Visual disturbance

(B) Hormonal excess

(C) Hormonally inactive

Abrupt symptoms

Prolactin

GH

ACTH

Thyroid-stimulating hormone (TSH)

Normal or low basal hormones

Primary thyroid failure
Primary gonadal failure

Consider: Pituitary apoplexy

Female: Amenorrhea/ galactorrhea
Male: Impotence

Child: Gigantism
Adult: Acromegaly

Cushing's disease

Hyperthyroidism with high TSH (rare)

Chromophobe adenoma
Craniopharyngioma
Meningioma
Aneurysm
Hamartoma
Sarcoidosis
Eosinophilic granuloma
Empty sella

→ Exclude: Drugs

Dexamethasone Suppression Testing Urinary-Free Cortisol Test

Serum prolactin

Postglucose serum GH
IGF-I
TRH stimulation test

(D) MRI of Pituitary with Gadolinium (or CT imaging)

Microadenoma or Macroadenoma

Macroadenoma

Microadenoma or Normal

Macroadenoma

Macroadenoma or Parasellar disease

(E) Endocrinologic evaluation for hormonal replacement
Neurosurgical evaluation

SECONDARY AMENORRHEA

Nancy A. Curosh, M.D.

Secondary amenorrhea is arbitrarily defined as the absence of menses for 6 months or the equivalent of three previous cycle intervals, whichever is longer, in women who previously had menses. Physiologic amenorrheas such as pregnancy, the immediate postpartum state, lactation, and the menopause should be excluded. It is helpful to consider secondary amenorrhea as an abnormality in one of four areas: the outflow tract, including the uterus, cervix, and vagina; the ovaries; the anterior pituitary; and the hypothalamus. Take a careful history, including questions concerning menstrual history, surgical procedures, medication use, changes in weight or diet, exercise patterns, and medical illnesses. On physical examination, pay attention to body habitus, secondary sexual characteristics, evidence of androgen excess, galactorrhea, visual fields, evidence of endocrinopathies, and a thorough pelvic examination. If localizing signs or symptoms are found, the investigation can be channeled as appropriate.

A. Approximately 20% of cases of secondary amenorrhea are due to hyperprolactinemia. Although galactorrhea may indicate this diagnosis, its absence is not reassuring, and all patients should be screened with a serum prolactin level. A number of physiologic and pharmacologic events can alter prolactin levels. Elevation can occur from any stress, physical or emotional. In fact, the stress of a blood draw may increase the level slightly. Levels should not be drawn after a recent breast examination, as breast stimulation can increase prolactin. Prolactin can also be increased by many medications, including oral contraceptives, estrogens, phenothiazines, tricyclic antidepressants, metoclopramide, and benzodiazepines. The prolactin is usually <100 ng/ml if due to one of these causes. If levels remain elevated after excluding these, further investigation is needed.

B. The progestin challenge test is used to assess the endogenous estrogen level and the competence of the outflow tract; 10 mg medroxyprogesterone acetate (Provera) is given PO for 5 days. Withdrawal bleeding should occur within 2 days to 2 weeks if there is a sufficient estrogen level and a competent outflow tract. Any amount of bleeding is considered a positive test, but very mild spotting implies marginal estrogen levels, and periodic re-evaluation is wise. The presence of estrogen suggests that the major components of the hypothalamic, pituitary, ovarian, and uterine pathways are at least minimally functioning. The diagnosis of anovulation is made. Management of anovulation depends on whether the patient currently desires pregnancy or contraception. Because chronic unopposed estrogen can induce endometrial hyperplasia, endometrial shedding should be induced on a regular basis.

C. If there is no withdrawal bleeding after a progestin challenge, there is either an outflow tract problem or insufficient estrogen. An estrogen-progestin challenge test can help differentiate between these two problems. Orally active estrogen is given to stimulate endometrial proliferation. An appropriate dose is 2.5 mg of conjugated estrogens daily for 21–25 days. A progestational agent (10 mg Provera) is given for the last 5–10 days to induce withdrawal. If no withdrawal bleeding occurs, there is a problem with the outflow tract, such as Asherman's syndrome or active endometritis. In a patient with a normal pelvic examination and no history of pelvic infections or trauma, including curettage, the estrogen-progestin challenge test may be eliminated.

D. Hypothalamic amenorrhea is the most common cause of secondary amenorrhea, occurring in approximately 60% of cases. It is most likely due to a defect in the pattern of pulsatile gonadotropin releasing hormone (GnRH) secretion. Hypothalamic amenorrhea is a diagnosis of exclusion, but there are clearly groups where this occurs frequently, such as in patients with anorexia nervosa, strenuous exercisers, and patients under stress. If possible, the precipitating circumstances should be dealt with and eliminated. Often, reassurance and time is all that is necessary. These patients should be followed closely to ensure that nothing has been overlooked. Estrogen replacement should be considered if the amenorrhea is not resolved in a reasonable time. If fertility is desired, clomiphene, Pergonal, and GnRH are often effective.

E. If luteinizing hormone (LH) and follicle stimulating hormone (FSH) are high, ovarian failure is the most likely explanation. Patients <age 35 should undergo karyotyping. If a Y chromosome is found, the chance of a gonadal malignancy is greatly increased. In rare circumstances, LH and FSH are elevated but the ovaries contain follicles. However, in most cases, if the gonadotropins are elevated, the diagnosis of premature ovarian failure can be made. Premature ovarian failure can be due to autoimmune disease, and this should be considered and investigated as deemed appropriate. If there are no contraindications, hormonal replacement therapy should be used in premature ovarian failure to avoid the long-term sequelae of estrogen deficiency.

F. Hyperprolactinemia warrants a CT or MRI scan of the head. Various tumors such as craniopharyngiomas and meningiomas may cause hyperprolactinemia, but pituitary adenomas are the most common. Bromocriptine, radiation therapy, or neurosurgery is a therapeutic option for pituitary adenomas, depending on the

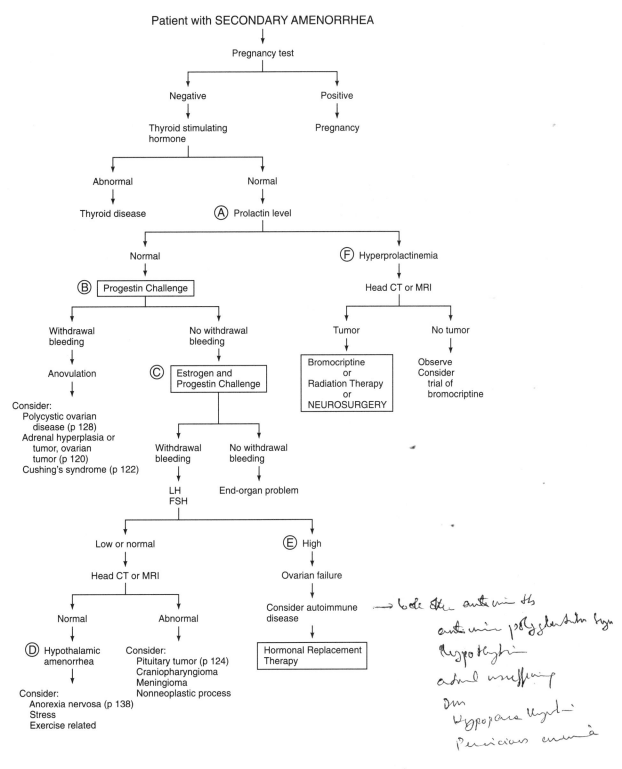

Patient with SECONDARY AMENORRHEA

Pregnancy test

- Negative → Thyroid stimulating hormone
  - Abnormal → Thyroid disease
  - Normal → (A) Prolactin level
    - Normal → (B) Progestin Challenge
      - Withdrawal bleeding → Anovulation
        - Consider:
          Polycystic ovarian disease (p 128)
          Adrenal hyperplasia or tumor, ovarian tumor (p 120)
          Cushing's syndrome (p 122)
      - No withdrawal bleeding → (C) Estrogen and Progestin Challenge
        - Withdrawal bleeding → LH FSH
          - Low or normal → Head CT or MRI
            - Normal → (D) Hypothalamic amenorrhea
              - Consider:
                Anorexia nervosa (p 138)
                Stress
                Exercise related
            - Abnormal → Consider:
              Pituitary tumor (p 124)
              Craniopharyngioma
              Meningioma
              Nonneoplastic process
          - (E) High → Ovarian failure
            - Consider autoimmune disease
            - Hormonal Replacement Therapy
        - No withdrawal bleeding → End-organ problem
    - (F) Hyperprolactinemia → Head CT or MRI
      - Tumor → Bromocriptine or Radiation Therapy or NEUROSURGERY
      - No tumor → Observe Consider trial of bromocriptine
- Positive → Pregnancy

References

Malo JW, Bezdicek BJ. Secondary amenorrhea: a protocol for pinpointing the underlying cause. Postgrad Med 1986; 79:86.

Scommegna A, Carson SA. Secondary amenorrhea and the menopause. In: Gold JJ, Josimovich JB, eds. Gynecologic endocrinology. 4th ed. New York: Plenum, 1987:369.

Speroff L, ed. Clinical gynecologic endocrinology and infertility. 4th ed. Baltimore: Williams & Wilkins, 1989:165.

size and extension of the tumor and the presence of symptoms. Excellent results are usually obtained with bromocriptine. Frequently, no tumor is found and careful observation is warranted. A trial of bromocriptine can be considered, particularly if fertility is desired.

127

HIRSUTISM

Nancy A. Curosh, M.D.

Hirsutism is the presence of excessive coarse terminal hair in a male-pattern growth distribution such as on the face, chest, abdomen, lower back, and thighs. This is due to increased androgen production. Hirsutism must be distinguished from hypertrichosis, which is an excess of thin vellus hair in a nonsexual hair distribution. The amount of vellus hair is highly dependent on patients' racial and family background. Hair density is usually highest in Caucasian women and lowest in blacks and Asians. An increase in vellus hair can also be caused by some metabolic disorders such as anorexia nervosa, porphyria cutanea tarda, and hypothyroidism.

A. Certain drugs may cause hirsutism, including phenytoin, anabolic steroids, diazoxide, minoxidil, and cyclosporine. Virilization is not present except in some cases of anabolic steroid use.

B. Signs of virilization include male-pattern baldness, deepening of the voice, clitorimegaly, increasing strength, loss of breast tissue, and increasing libido. Benign causes of hirsutism frequently begin gradually around the time of puberty. Hirsutism that has a rapid onset or that begins in childhood or after menopause is compatible with an ovarian or adrenal tumor.

C. Dehydroepiandrosterone sulfate (DHEA-S) values >700 µg/dl are usually due to an adrenal tumor. These are very rare and about half are palpable at the time of diagnosis. If an abdominal CT scan does not show a tumor, adrenal hyperplasia should be considered, because this rarely can show very elevated DHEA-S levels.

D. The virilizing forms of congenital adrenal hyperplasia are the 11-hydroxylase, 21-hydroxylase, and 3β-hydroxysteroid dehydrogenase deficiencies. By far the most common is the 21-hydroxylase–deficient form. The classic forms are usually discovered in childhood, but the attenuated or late onset forms may first be discovered in adulthood during investigation of hirsutism or virilization. In these patients, the early-morning 17-hydroxyprogesterone level is usually elevated. By measuring specific precursor to product ratios, the exact deficiency can be discovered. In mild cases, ACTH stimulation may be necessary to exaggerate these differences. If the patient has only mild hirsutism, it may not be cost efficient to elucidate the exact cause. These patients usually respond to the same treatment as is given to idiopathic hirsutism.

E. If there is gradual onset of the hirsutism, usually beginning around the time of puberty, and if there is no evidence of virilization, a careful menstrual history is helpful. Patients who have irregular menses must be investigated for hypothyroidism and prolactinomas. If these are excluded, the most likely diagnosis is polycystic ovarian disease. This classically consists of obesity, anovulation, and hyperandrogenemia, but the clinical presentation varies widely. The anovulation may be expressed as oligomenorrhea, amenorrhea, dysfunctional uterine bleeding, or infertility. The hyperandrogenemia may be asymptomatic or may present as hirsutism or acne. Obesity is seen in fewer than half of the patients. Ovarian size can be determined by pelvic examination or ultrasonography, but is not always a helpful parameter for diagnosis. Classically, polycystic ovaries are two to five times enlarged with 20 or more follicles, but this does not occur in all patients. Many patients have normal ovarian structures. Polycystic ovarian disease appears primarily to be a functional rather than anatomic abnormality. It is usually associated with a strong family history and may be inherited in an autosomal dominant pattern. Testosterone often is moderately elevated. The luteinizing hormone to follicle stimulating hormone ratio (LH/FSH) is >2 in 80% of cases. However, in most circumstances the diagnosis can be achieved without these laboratory values. If the menses are regular, polycystic ovarian disease is still possible but less likely, and the aforementioned laboratory tests may be helpful. If polycystic ovarian disease seems improbable, the diagnosis of idiopathic hirsutism is made. Idiopathic hirsutism is the term used to describe patients with hirsutism for which a distinct etiology cannot be found. Most patients have regular menses, but irregular menses may occur. If intensively studied, a cause may be discovered in many of these women, but this is not cost effective and would most likely not change their therapeutic options. Treatment of hirsutism due to polycystic ovarian disease or idiopathic hirsutism is often the same. Options include mechanical treatments such as bleaching, shaving, or electrolysis; or drug therapy such as low-dose glucocorticoids, oral contraceptives, or antiandrogens.

References

Barnes R, Rosenfield RL. The polycystic ovary syndrome: pathogenesis and treatment. Ann Intern Med 1989; 110:386.

Ehrmann DA, Rosenfield RL. An endocrinologic approach to the patient with hirsutism. J Clin Endocrinol Metab 1990; 71:1.

Rittmaster RS, Loriaux DL. Hirsutism. Ann Intern Med 1987; 106:95.

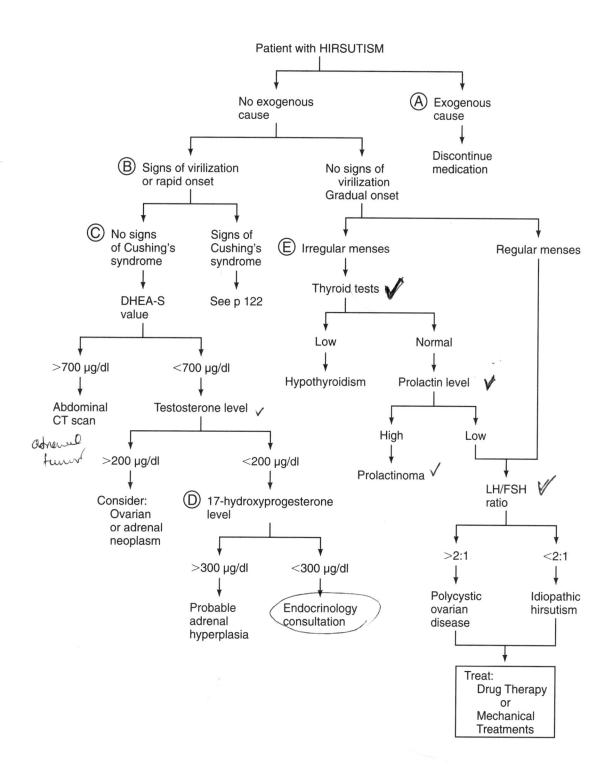

Patient with HIRSUTISM

No exogenous cause   (A) Exogenous cause

↓ Discontinue medication

(B) Signs of virilization or rapid onset

No signs of virilization Gradual onset

(C) No signs of Cushing's syndrome

Signs of Cushing's syndrome

↓ DHEA-S value

See p 122

>700 µg/dl
Abdominal CT scan
adrenal tumor

<700 µg/dl
Testosterone level ✓

>200 µg/dl
Consider: Ovarian or adrenal neoplasm

<200 µg/dl
(D) 17-hydroxyprogesterone level

>300 µg/dl
Probable adrenal hyperplasia

<300 µg/dl
Endocrinology consultation

(E) Irregular menses
↓ Thyroid tests ✓

Regular menses

Low → Hypothyroidism

Normal → Prolactin level ✓

High → Prolactinoma ✓

Low

LH/FSH ratio ✓

>2:1
Polycystic ovarian disease

<2:1
Idiopathic hirsutism

Treat: Drug Therapy or Mechanical Treatments

GYNECOMASTIA

Nancy A. Curosh, M.D.
Thomas W. Boyden, M.D.

Gynecomastia is a glandular enlargement of the male breast with a simultaneous increase in surrounding connective tissue. The breasts are sensitive to hormonal influences, and gynecomastia can occur as a result of an excess of stimulatory hormones such as estrogens, a decrease in inhibitory hormones such as androgens, or an imbalance between stimulatory and inhibitory hormones. Gynecomastia is not a rare finding when careful examination is performed. Frequently, the patient is unaware of its presence, but it is sometimes quite painful.

A. Numerous drugs have been associated with gynecomastia (Table 1) and their mechanisms of action are varied. Estrogens directly stimulate the breasts. Androgens are converted to estrogens. Cytotoxic agents damage the testes, causing primary hypogonadism. Cimetidine blocks androgen receptors. Alcohol lowers serum testosterone levels and may increase estrogen levels because of augmented peripheral conversion of androgens to estrogen. Some drugs increase prolactin levels and cause a hypogonadal state. In many drugs the mechanism of action is unknown.

B. After World War II many former prisoners of war developed gynecomastia after they were renourished. This has also been observed in patients recovering from any prolonged illness in which they had lost considerable weight. This refeeding gynecomastia usually resolves in months to 2 years.

C. Gynecomastia can occur in a wide range of illnesses. Patients with liver disease, especially cirrhosis, develop gynecomastia because of an estrogen excess; there is increased production of estrogen from circulating precursors, and elevated levels of sex hormone binding globulin decrease free testosterone. Hyperthyroidism also causes gynecomastia because of increased estrogen levels. Adrenal diseases can cause gynecomastia, since cortisol excess inhibits testosterone production. Prolactin excess also works through this mechanism. Patients with chronic renal disease often develop gynecomastia soon after beginning hemodialysis, probably because of a refeeding phenomenon caused by their improved well-being and appetite. Patients on dialysis also often have low serum testosterone, elevated luteinizing hormone (LH), an increased estrogen to androgen ratio, and mildly increased prolactin. Pulmonary and cardiac diseases and AIDS are other illnesses sometimes associated with gynecomastia.

D. A careful breast examination is necessary to distinguish gynecomastia from a breast carcinoma. Gynecomastia relates to subareolar glandular tissue. To be sure it is glandular and not adipose tissue, compare the tissue with the adipose tissue of the anterior axillary fold. Gynecomastia is often asymptomatic and may be unilateral. Fixed, indurated, irregular, or firm areas suggest breast carcinoma. Mammography or ultrasonography may be useful in this situation, but if any doubt remains, biopsy is indicated.

E. A normal adult testis measures 3.5–5.5 cm in length and 2.1–3.2 cm in width. With a Prader orchidometer, the volume should be 20–30 ml. Eunuchoidal proportions are present if the arm span is >2 cm longer than the patient's height and the floor-to-pubis length is 2 cm greater than the pubis-to-crown distance. Eunuchoidal proportions frequently are seen in patients who were hypogonadal before puberty.

F. Gynecomastia is common at certain stages in life. Neonates frequently have gynecomastia because of high levels of estrogen in the placental-fetal circulation. During puberty gynecomastia can be found in 40–60% of boys. This may be due to an increase in plasma estrogens compared with androgens. Likewise, gynecomastia is common in men >65 years of age, probably because of varying degrees of testicular failure. If these patients are asymptomatic, observation may be all that is necessary.

G. A low testosterone level with a high LH level indicates testicular failure. Klinefelter's syndrome is a male genetic disorder in which there is an extra X chromosome. Patients have a eunuchoidal appearance and small testes. Eighty-five percent of patients with Klinefelter's syndrome have gynecomastia. It is important to differentiate Klinefelter's syndrome from other causes of testicular failure such as trauma, orchitis, and damage from radiation or chemotherapy. Unlike most other conditions causing gynecomastia, Klinefelter's syndrome is associated with an increased incidence of breast cancer, and therefore closer observation is needed. If suspected, Klinefelter's syndrome can be confirmed by a buccal smear or chromosomal karyotyping.

TABLE 1 Some Drugs Associated with Gynecomastia

Alcohol	Ketoconazole
Androgens	Marijuana
Calcium channel blockers	Methyldopa
Cimetidine	Phenytoin
Cytotoxic drugs	Reserpine
Digitalis	Spironolactone
Estrogens	Tricyclic antidepressants
Isoniazid	

Male Patient with BREAST ENLARGEMENT

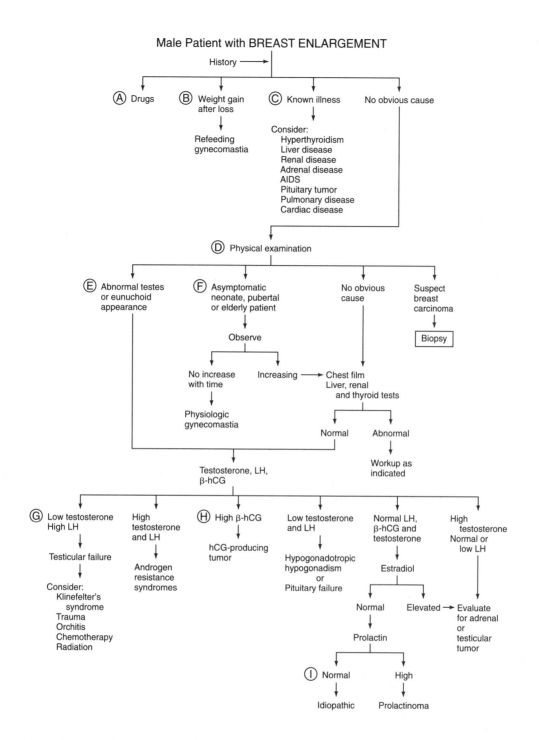

H. A serum beta—human chorionic gonadotropin (β-hCG) radioimmunoassay is recommended, since urinary pregnancy tests, which also measure hCG, are not sufficiently sensitive. Elevated hCG indicates a tumor. A variety of malignant testicular tissues produce hCG, and these may be suggested by an asymmetrically enlarged testis. However, nontesticular tumors such as some pulmonary, gastric, and pancreatic tumors may also secrete hCG. A careful search must be made to locate these tumors.

I. In a significant number of patients, no definite cause of gynecomastia is found after thorough investigation. These patients should receive periodic followup.

References

Carlson HE. Gynecomastia. N Engl J Med 1980; 303:795.

Couderc LJ, Clauvel JP. HIV-infection-induced gynecomastia. Ann Intern Med 1987; 107:257.

Leung AKC. Gynecomastia. Am Fam Physician 1989; 39:215.

Lucas LM, Kumar KL, Smith DL. Gynecomastia: a worrisome problem for the patient. Postgrad Med 1987; 82:73.

Santen RJ. The testis. In: Felig P,. ed. Endocrinology and metabolism. 2nd ed. New York: McGraw-Hill, 1987: 886.

GASTROENTEROLOGY

ACUTE ABDOMINAL PAIN

Steven Palley, M.D.

Evaluation of acute abdominal pain remains a difficult task in clinical medicine. The internist addressing the patient with acute abdominal pain ideally should eliminate medical causes and recognize the proper setting for surgical consultation. There should be a low threshold in general, for involving surgical expertise. History and physical examination are the critical elements in evaluation. Admission for evaluation is common and should be considered for acute pain without obvious surgical indication that persists for 6 hours.

A. A careful history can narrow the differential diagnosis. Age and sex are important considerations. Mesenteric adenitis occurs in younger persons, while vascular and neoplastic disease occurs in the elderly. In a sexually active female, consider ectopic pregnancy or pelvic inflammatory disease. Medical history can reveal previous peptic ulcer disease, gallstones, diverticular disease, inflammatory bowel disease, and abdominal surgery. Medication history can disclose corticosteroids or immunosuppressants. Coexisting medical conditions such as diabetes mellitus can affect the presentation. The onset and character of the pain is important. A sudden onset of intense, localized, "somatic" pain should suggest peritonitis, as in perforation of bowel or ulcer. Crescendo-decrescendo "visceral" pain or colic is more characteristic of bowel, cystic duct, or ureteral obstruction. An evolving pain pattern, visceral at first and later somatic, may suggest appendicitis, cholecystitis, or strangulated bowel. Disproportionate pain compared with a lesser physical finding occurs with ischemia. Characteristic radiation patterns are noted with cholecystitis, pancreatitis, and appendicitis.

B. Observe the patient before the examination. Visceral pain usually causes restlessness; parietal pain increases with movement. Auscultate the abdomen for bruits, rubs, and bowel sounds. Palpation should begin away from the site of pain. Involuntary guarding or rebound tenderness, especially with light percussion, implies parietal peritonitis. Deeper palpation can search for organomegaly or masses. Perform rectal and pelvic examinations.

C. A hemodynamically unstable patient with possible intra-abdominal hemorrhage may require immediate laparotomy. The acutely ill patient with hypotension, high fever, leukocytosis, and a suggestive physical examination (involuntary guarding, rigidity, increasing severe tenderness) should also undergo immediate surgical evaluation. Suspected bowel ischemia with acidosis, fever, and evidence of hypovolemia should also be evaluated surgically, as should the patient with evidence of perforation by plain radiography, contrast

study, or paracentesis. Resuscitation is critical both before and during further evaluation, including possible ventilatory support, IV access and fluids, nasogastric suction, oxygen, and urinary output monitoring, as well as frequent checks on vital signs and preliminary laboratory tests. Ideally, important medical causes of acute pain can be ruled out before surgery with urinalysis, electrocardiography, and chest films.

D. The more stable patient should be closely observed. Medical causes of acute abdominal pain can be ruled out, although the list can be extensive. The more common causes are acute pneumonitis, especially lower lobe; pyelonephritis; hepatitis; and mesenteric adenitis. Collagen vascular disease can cause perforation. Multiple metabolic disorders, including diabetic ketoacidosis, Addisonian crisis, uremia, and acute intermittent porphyria, can lead to abdominal pain. A history of chronic liver disease with ascites may suggest spontaneous bacterial peritonitis.

E. Certain patients may present with a discrepancy between severity of disease and physical finding. These include those who are elderly, malnourished, obese, immunosuppressed, or on steroids; early postoperative patients; those with mental status changes; and paraplegics.

F. Laboratory evaluation should include Hgb/HCt, WBC count, differential, electrolytes, blood gases, amylase, liver tests, coagulation times, urinalysis, and possible stool studies. Supine and upright abdominal films may suggest obstruction, ischemia, perforation, biliary calculi, or intra-abdominal abscess. Angiography is useful for suspected hemorrhage or ischemia. Contrast studies are useful for suspected perforation. Ultrasonography and CT imaging can demonstrate pancreatitis, abscess, retroperitoneal mass, or dilated biliary tree.

G. Close observation may disclose an evolutionary pattern to the abdominal pain syndrome. If acute pain persists >6 hours, obtain a surgical consultation if this has not already been requested.

References

Boey JH. Acute abdomen. In: Way LW, ed. Current surgical diagnosis and treatment. Norwalk, CT: Appleton & Lange, 1988:393.

Fulenwider JT, McGarity WC. Evaluation of acute abdominal pain in adults. In: Conn R, ed. Current diagnosis 7. Philadelphia: WB Saunders, 1985:31.

Thomson JH, Jones PF. Active observation in acute abdominal pain. Am J Surg 1986; 2:522.

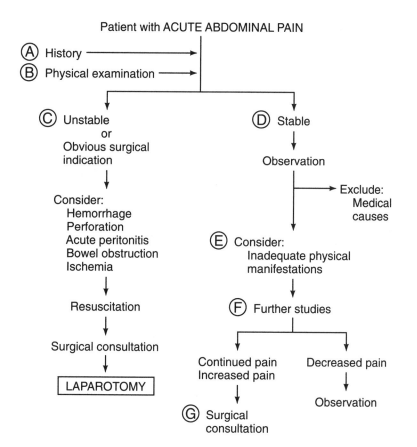

Patient with ACUTE ABDOMINAL PAIN

(A) History

(B) Physical examination

(C) Unstable
or
Obvious surgical
indication

Consider:
Hemorrhage
Perforation
Acute peritonitis
Bowel obstruction
Ischemia

Resuscitation

Surgical consultation

LAPAROTOMY

(D) Stable

Observation

Exclude:
Medical
causes

(E) Consider:
Inadequate physical
manifestations

(F) Further studies

Continued pain
Increased pain

Decreased pain

Observation

(G) Surgical
consultation

CHRONIC ABDOMINAL PAIN

Lee J. Hixson, M.D.

A. Postprandial pain suggests peptic ulceration, pancreatitis, biliary obstruction, partial small bowel obstruction, irritable bowel syndrome, lactose intolerance, or chronic mesenteric insufficiency. Pain that is diminished by bending forward suggests pancreatic cancer, chronic pancreatitis, or an abdominal aortic aneurysm. Most patients with truly chronic recurrent abdominal pain are, after exhaustive evaluation, labeled with a "functional" disorder such as irritable bowel syndrome or nonulcer dyspepsia.

B. Screening laboratory tests should generally include a CBC with differential, liver biochemistries (bilirubin, transaminases, alkaline phosphatase), and amylase. Additional appropriate tests frequently include a full chemistry panel, urinalysis, stool analysis (microscopic for leukocytes, ova, and parasites), and abdominal radiography to detect such conditions as stones, bowel obstruction, visceral displacement or enlargement, and calcification.

C. Pain originating in the abdominal wall is superficial and exacerbated by movement or touch. It is often attributed to costochondritis when localized to the upper abdomen over the xiphoid or costal margin. Pain associated with recently healed lesions may indicate nerve entrapment or regeneration with neuroma formation. Radicular pain across the abdomen may also be worse with movement and be caused by irritation of the spinal nerve root from disc and vertebral body disease, a meningeal tumor, tabes dorsalis secondary to syphilis or diabetes, or postherpetic neuralgia. Abdominal wall and radicular pain can usually be obliterated by blocking the intercostal or paravertebral nerves.

D. If pain has a pelvic source, consider ovarian and uterine cysts and tumors, chronic pelvic inflammatory disease, and endometriosis.

E. The following metabolic disorders may be associated with abdominal pain: porphyria, hyper- and hypothyroidism, adrenal insufficiency, hypercalcemia, familial Mediterranean fever, hereditary angioedema, diabetic neuropathy, and carcinoid syndrome.

F. Chronic narcotic use may result in the narcotic bowel syndrome with pain presumably secondary to bowel spasm. Dilantin, NSAIDs, and other agents may be associated with pain.

G. "Functional" pain is a diagnosis of exclusion. The pain may be severe, well localized, or diffuse, and rarely awakens the patient from sleep. Irritable bowel syndrome is classically associated with altered bowel habits, constipation alternating with diarrhea. Pain relief with defecation, mucus in the stool, and a sensation of incomplete evacuation are typical.

H. Chronic mesenteric ischemia is an uncommon clinical diagnosis characterized by postprandial pain and weight loss. Mesenteric vasculitis is usually associated with signs and symptoms of concurrent involvement in other organ systems outside the abdomen.

I. Pain originating from the liver results from distention of the hepatic capsule, which may be secondary to hepatic congestion, inflammation, infiltration, or tumor/cyst growth.

J. Colonic tumors and diverticulosis usually are not painful but may become so with bowel perforation or obstruction. Diverticulosis may be associated with marked hypertrophy and thickening of the bowel wall, which on occasion may produce left lower quadrant pain with constipation.

References

Rogers M, Cerda JJ. The narcotic bowel syndrome. J Clin Gastroenterol 1989; 11:132.

Schuster MM. Irritable bowel syndrome. In: Sleisenger MH, Fordtran JS, eds. Gastrointestinal disease. 4th ed. Philadelphia: WB Saunders, 1989:1402.

Snapper I. Extra-abdominal causes of abdominal pain. Am J Gastroenterol 1982; 77:795.

Trnka Y, Warfield CA. Chronic abdominal pain. Hosp Pract 1984; 19:201.

Patient with CHRONIC ABDOMINAL PAIN

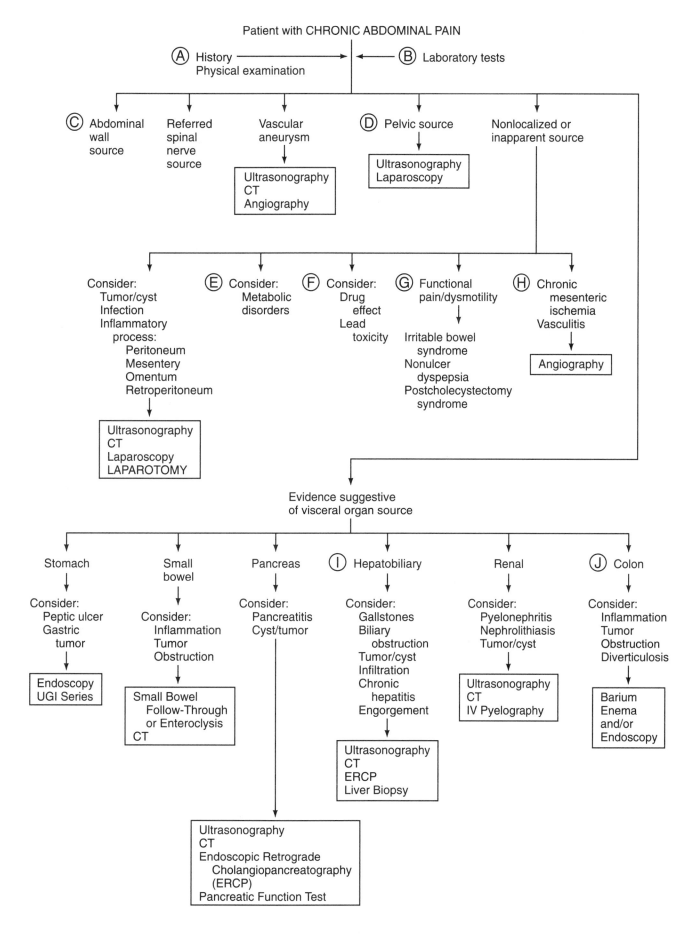

Ⓐ History
Physical examination

Ⓑ Laboratory tests

Ⓒ Abdominal wall source

Referred spinal nerve source

Vascular aneurysm

Ⓓ Pelvic source

Nonlocalized or inapparent source

Ultrasonography
CT
Angiography

Ultrasonography
Laparoscopy

Consider:
Tumor/cyst
Infection
Inflammatory process:
Peritoneum
Mesentery
Omentum
Retroperitoneum

Ultrasonography
CT
Laparoscopy
LAPAROTOMY

Ⓔ Consider:
Metabolic disorders

Ⓕ Consider:
Drug effect
Lead toxicity

Ⓖ Functional pain/dysmotility

Irritable bowel syndrome
Nonulcer dyspepsia
Postcholecystectomy syndrome

Ⓗ Chronic mesenteric ischemia
Vasculitis

Angiography

Evidence suggestive of visceral organ source

Stomach

Small bowel

Pancreas

Ⓘ Hepatobiliary

Renal

Ⓙ Colon

Consider:
Peptic ulcer
Gastric tumor

Consider:
Inflammation
Tumor
Obstruction

Consider:
Pancreatitis
Cyst/tumor

Consider:
Gallstones
Biliary obstruction
Tumor/cyst
Infiltration
Chronic hepatitis
Engorgement

Consider:
Pyelonephritis
Nephrolithiasis
Tumor/cyst

Consider:
Inflammation
Tumor
Obstruction
Diverticulosis

Endoscopy
UGI Series

Small Bowel Follow-Through or Enteroclysis
CT

Ultrasonography
CT
ERCP
Liver Biopsy

Ultrasonography
CT
IV Pyelography

Barium Enema and/or Endoscopy

Ultrasonography
CT
Endoscopic Retrograde Cholangiopancreatography (ERCP)
Pancreatic Function Test

NAUSEA AND VOMITING

Steven Palley, M.D.

Nausea, though a common symptom, is difficult to define precisely. Vomiting is a complex, well-coordinated act with neurologic pathways that are described, at least in part. Vomiting needs to be distinguished from regurgitation in which gastric or esophageal contents are returned to the pharynx by pressure differentials. Regurgitation can occur with gastroesophageal reflux disease, esophageal stricture, achalasia, and Zenker's diverticulum.

A. The history may reveal the possibility of pregnancy, a family history of similar disorder, drug intake, or psychiatric abnormality. The characteristics of the vomiting episode are relatively nonspecific. A large volume of emesis or emesis of food ingested more than 12 hours previously suggests organic causes. A succussion splash, skin changes or Raynaud's phenomenon, orthostatic hypotension, or neurologic finding may suggest the cause. A plain abdominal film is inexpensive and easy and may contribute information.

B. Nausea and vomiting of acute onset (<1 week) should prompt a different work-up from that of a long-standing complaint. Historical considerations are important. A careful drug history may disclose opiates, anticholinergics, beta agonists, erythromycin, or chemotherapeutics. Drug toxicity such as from digoxin should be considered. Acute vestibular causes such as motion sickness and acute labyrinthitis are possible. Viral gastroenteritis is a common cause. Visceral pain syndromes causing acute nausea include myocardial infarction, pancreatitis, renal colic, and biliary colic.

C. Chronic nausea and vomiting is commonly related to structural lesions affecting the upper GI tract. Pregnancy should be ruled out in appropriate patients. Perform upper endoscopy to evaluate mucosal lesions, peptic ulcer disease, a deformed pylorus, or other gastric outlet obstruction. If the examination is unhelpful or there is a suggestion of an extrinsic process, perform an upper GI contrast study. Extrinsic lesions should be further evaluated with ultrasonography or CT of the abdomen.

D. If the above examinations are negative, perform a thorough neurological and vestibular evaluation. Psychiatric screening can be useful. Further evaluation for collagen vascular disease or endocrine disorder should be considered. If the above evaluations are unhelpful, offer a therapeutic trial with a promotility agent such as metoclopramide.

E. If the therapeutic trial is unsuccessful, further evaluation is warranted. Perform a radionuclide gastric emptying study and evaluate solid and liquid emptying. This may document a gastric emptying disorder but unfortunately cannot determine the cause. This may suffice in the appropriate setting, such as long-standing diabetes mellitus, autonomic insufficiency, or progressive systemic sclerosis.

F. In severe, persistent, unexplained nausea and vomiting, further evaluation may be warranted. The patient should show evidence of functional impairment or nutritional deficit. Evaluation at a specialized gastric motility center can determine the type of motility disorder and may suggest a specific intervention such as antrectomy for distal gastric motility disorder. Exploratory laparotomy with full-thickness small bowel biopsy can sometimes yield a diagnosis.

References

Feldman M. Nausea and vomiting. In: Sleisenger MH, Fordtran JS, eds. Gastrointestinal disease. 4th ed. Philadelphia: WB Saunders, 1989:222.

Hanson JS, McCallum RW. The diagnosis and management of nausea and vomiting: a review. Am J Gastroenterol 1985; 80:210.

Malagelada JR, Camilleri M. Unexplained vomiting: a diagnostic challenge. Ann Intern Med 1984; 101:211.

Patient with NAUSEA AND VOMITING

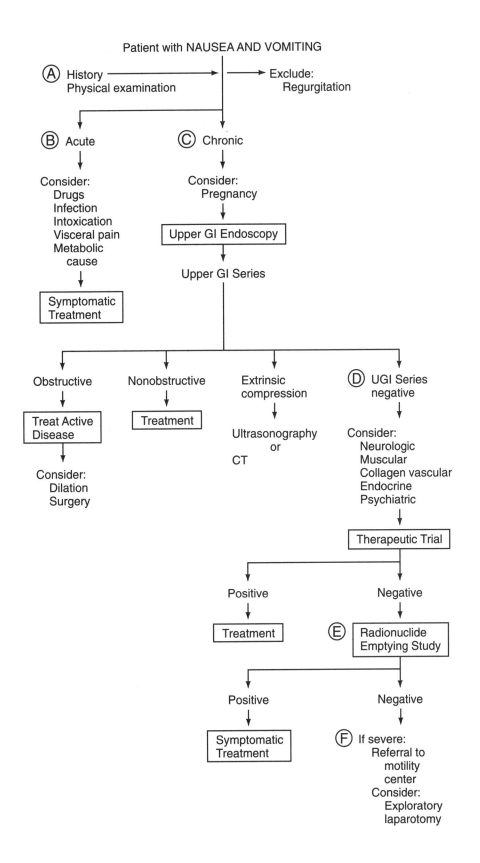

Ⓐ History ——————→ Exclude:
Physical examination   Regurgitation

Ⓑ Acute   Ⓒ Chronic

Consider: Consider:
  Drugs   Pregnancy
  Infection
  Intoxication   Upper GI Endoscopy
  Visceral pain
  Metabolic   Upper GI Series
    cause

Symptomatic
Treatment

Obstructive   Nonobstructive   Extrinsic   Ⓓ UGI Series
                                 compression   negative

Treat Active   Treatment   Ultrasonography Consider:
Disease   or   Neurologic
                                 CT   Muscular
Consider: Collagen vascular
  Dilation   Endocrine
  Surgery   Psychiatric

                                                 Therapeutic Trial

                          Positive   Negative

                          Treatment   Ⓔ Radionuclide
                                                Emptying Study

                          Positive   Negative

                          Symptomatic   Ⓕ If severe:
                          Treatment   Referral to
                                                   motility
                                                   center
                                                 Consider:
                                                   Exploratory
                                                   laparotomy

ANOREXIA

M. Angelo Trujillo, M.D.

A. Anorexia (loss of appetite) is often clinically difficult to differentiate from pure weight loss. The diagnostic considerations and work-up usually are the same for both clinical problems. Perform a careful history and physical examination, including medication history, social history, and psychological screening examination. The causes of anorexia and weight loss may be divided into five major groups: (1) medical conditions, (2) psychological conditions, (3) social factors, (4) age-related factors, and (5) anorexia nervosa and related eating disorders.

B. A medication profile on patients with anorexia is of utmost importance, since it can identify an easily treated cause. Medications as listed are commonly associated with anorexia, especially in elderly patients.

C. Perform a head CT or MRI scan in patients who have anorexia with suspected CNS disease. Symptoms of visual disturbance, headaches, or signs of increased intracranial pressure (e.g., papilledema or cranial nerve involvement) should alert one to a potential CNS cause. Consider CNS tumors, especially hypothalamic tumors.

D. Several GI disorders can cause anorexia and/or weight loss. Malabsorption syndromes can mimic eating disorders (e.g., parasitic diseases, inflammatory bowel disease, celiac sprue, pancreatic insufficiency). Laboratory findings that can help differentiate organic disease from eating disorders are leukocytosis, steatorrhea, fever, hematochezia, and histologic or radiographic findings typical of certain GI disease states. Malignancy involving the GI tract can cause weight loss by several mechanisms: oral cavity pain or swallowing difficulty, esophageal obstruction or motility problems, gastric outlet obstruction, bowel obstruction, biliary disease, pancreatitis, and abdominal pain. Distant metastases of GI malignancies can also produce anorexia or weight loss by several mechanisms.

E. Social and cultural factors play an important role in the attitudes and behaviors of eating and body image. These factors are important components in the complex etiology of eating disorders. Other factors, such as difficulty with food acquisition and social isolation, can be important in some patients, especially the elderly.

F. Dementia and depression may cause significant weight loss. These are more commonly seen in the elderly and are very important considerations, since these disorders are potentially treatable. All cases of depression should be treated and reversible causes for dementia sought. Alcoholism is a common cause of anorexia or weight loss. Obtain a careful alcohol and drug abuse history in all cases.

G. Normal physiologic changes in the elderly may cause anorexia and weight loss. Hypogeusia (diminished sense of taste) and decreased olfactory function may result in food being less desirable. Visual and hearing problems may interfere with the usual mealtime socialization and may cause social isolation. Visual disorders and other physical disabilities may interfere with food preparation.

H. Anorexia nervosa and bulimia nervosa are eating disorders that affect 1–4% of women, being much more common in women. These disorders are usually diagnosed in the second or third decades, but reports of diagnosis in persons in their thirties or forties are increasing. Anorexia nervosa and bulimia nervosa result from complex interactions of physiologic, psychological, and sociocultural dysfunction. Diagnostic criteria for these eating disorders used by most authors are those found in the DSM-III-R of the American Psychiatric Association. Patient history should reveal intense fear of fatness, disturbed perception of body image, and an obsessional desire to lose weight. Patients with bulimia nervosa classically have binge eating commonly associated with self-induced vomiting, abuse of cathartics or diuretics, and fear of loss of control over eating. Treatment of these disorders is complex and should follow a team approach, with a primary care physician managing medical care and coordinating treatment by psychiatric/psychologic and nutritional consultants. Many medical complications may result from eating disorders; treatment of these should have priority.

References

Bo-Linn GW. Obesity, anorexia nervosa, bulimia, and other eating disorders. In: Sleisenger MH, Fordtran JS, eds. Gastrointestinal disease. 4th ed. Philadelphia: WB Saunders, 1989:173.

Comerci GD. Medical complications of anorexia nervosa and bulimia nervosa. Med Clin North Am 1990; 74:1293.

Morley JE. Anorexia in older patients: its meaning and management. Geriatrics 1990; 45:59, 65.

Olsen-Noll EG, Bosworth MF. Anorexia and weight loss in the elderly. Postgrad Med 1989; 15:140.

Patient with ANOREXIA

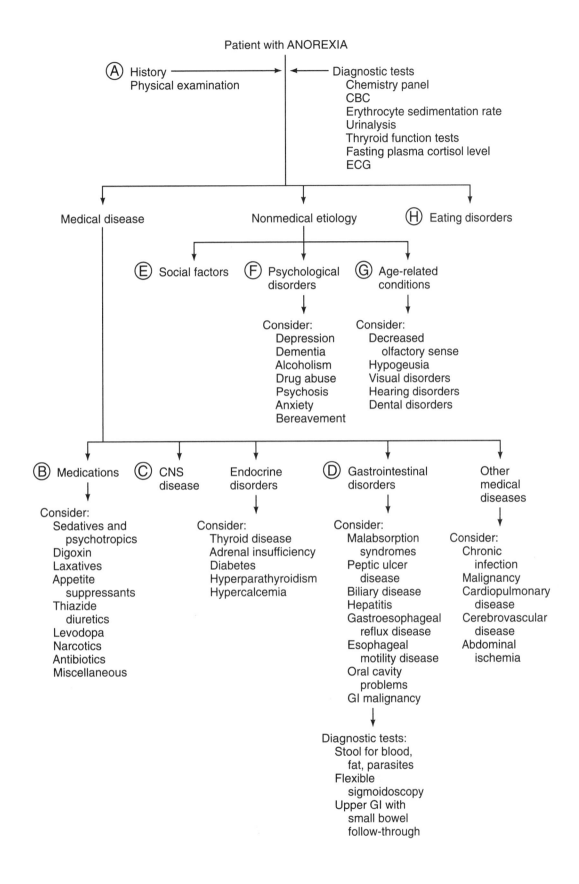

(A) History ——→ ←—— Diagnostic tests
Physical examination   Chemistry panel
                              CBC
                              Erythrocyte sedimentation rate
                              Urinalysis
                              Thryroid function tests
                              Fasting plasma cortisol level
                              ECG

Medical disease   Nonmedical etiology   (H) Eating disorders

                    (E) Social factors   (F) Psychological   (G) Age-related
                                             disorders   conditions

                                          Consider: Consider:
                                            Depression   Decreased
                                            Dementia   olfactory sense
                                            Alcoholism   Hypogeusia
                                            Drug abuse   Visual disorders
                                            Psychosis   Hearing disorders
                                            Anxiety   Dental disorders
                                            Bereavement

(B) Medications (C) CNS   Endocrine   (D) Gastrointestinal   Other
                     disease   disorders   disorders   medical
                                                                    diseases

Consider: Consider: Consider: Consider:
  Sedatives and   Thyroid disease   Malabsorption   Chronic
    psychotropics   Adrenal insufficiency syndromes   infection
  Digoxin   Diabetes   Peptic ulcer   Malignancy
  Laxatives   Hyperparathyroidism disease   Cardiopulmonary
  Appetite   Hypercalcemia   Biliary disease   disease
    suppressants   Hepatitis   Cerebrovascular
  Thiazide   Gastroesophageal   disease
    diuretics   reflux disease   Abdominal
  Levodopa   Esophageal   ischemia
  Narcotics   motility disease
  Antibiotics   Oral cavity
  Miscellaneous   problems
                                                   GI malignancy

                                                  Diagnostic tests:
                                                    Stool for blood,
                                                      fat, parasites
                                                    Flexible
                                                      sigmoidoscopy
                                                    Upper GI with
                                                      small bowel
                                                      follow-through

DYSPHAGIA

Philip E. Jaffe, M.D.

A. Dysphagia consists of a sense that there is impairment in the act of swallowing. It can result from (1) abnormalities in preparing and delivering the food bolus from the mouth to the esophagus (transfer dysphagia), (2) structural abnormalities of the esophagus (rings, webs, strictures, tumor masses, infection, or inflammation) or of adjacent structures (mediastinal masses or enlargement of the left atrium), or (3) motility abnormalities of the esophagus (achalasia, esophageal spasm, nutcracker esophagus, nonspecific motility disorders). Depending on the characteristics of the symptoms (dysphagia to solids, mechanical obstruction versus liquids, motility disorder), chronicity of complaints, and age of the patient, one may suspect a specific cause. However, esophagogastroduodenoscopy (EGD) should be performed in virtually all patients with this complaint. In rare cases when there is a compelling temporal relationship to a recent cerebrovascular accident (CVA) or progressive neurologic disease (amyotrophic lateral sclerosis, Parkinson's disease, myasthenia gravis) and a history suggestive of transfer dysphagia, or if the patient has scleroderma, the work-up may begin with barium esophagography. Because of the relative insensitivity of barium esophagography in detecting mucosal abnormalities, including early esophageal cancers, esophagoscopy is the preferred means of initial evaluation. This is especially true in immunocompromised patients in whom fungal or viral esophagitis is suspected.

B. When an etiology is determined on EGD, a specific treatment plan is usually undertaken. Dilate strictures, rings and webs using either rubber or plastic bougies or balloon catheters through an endoscope. Concurrent antireflux measures and antiacid treatment in the case of peptic strictures are imperative. Occasionally, severe reflux disease may cause dysphagia without anatomic obstruction. There are many options in treating esophageal cancer, including dilatation, chemotherapy, surgery, radiation therapy, laser, tumor probe, alcohol injection, and stenting. Their application depends on the extent and location of disease as well as the condition of the patient.

C. With a normal EGD, a motility disturbance of the esophagus should be suspected. Here again history is usually helpful, but esophageal manometry is necessary to differentiate achalasia from the other motility disorders, as the treatment differs radically. If the history suggests transfer dysphagia, cine or video esophagography should precede manometry.

D. Abnormalities in the preparation and passage of the food bolus from the tongue to the pharynx and then into the esophagus (transfer dysphagia) are most commonly seen with acute CVAs or progressive neurologic disorders (see section A). The dysfunction may slowly resolve over weeks after a CVA, and temporary nasogastric feeding supplementation may be necessary. In many cases the abnormality persists and endoscopic or surgical gastrostomy offers the best palliation. For patients who have progressive neurologic disorders with transfer dysphagia, referral to a speech pathologist who works with them to determine the optimal consistency of foods and ideal head and neck positioning to facilitate swallowing is useful. However, many patients ultimately require a gastrostomy.

E. Abnormalities in esophageal peristalsis and lower esophageal sphincter (LES) pressure and coordination with peristalsis are known as motility disorders. Measurement of the esophageal intraluminal pressures via manometry may define (1) achalasia — aperistalsis of the esophageal body and incomplete LES relations; (2) diffuse esophageal spasm — intermittent, simultaneous contraction in >10% of swallows; (3) nutcracker esophagus — high-amplitude esophageal contractions; and (4) nonspecific motility disorder — nontransmitted, triple-peaked or simultaneous contractions or low-amplitude contractions that do not fit into other defined disturbances. The association of chest pain with dysphagia often suggests a motility disorder and is frequently a more disturbing symptom to the patient. The use of edrophonium during manometry may precipitate these symptoms and manometric findings. Treatment of achalasia usually requires fluoroscopically guided balloon dilatation. Good results are seen in 60–95% of patients; the procedure is complicated by perforation in 2–4%. Surgical myotomy is now generally reserved for those who fail balloon dilatation. Other measures, including serial bougienage, nitrates, and calcium channel blockers, are effective but offer only temporary relief of symptoms. For patients with diffuse esophageal spasm, nutcracker esophagus, or nonspecific motility disorders, drugs that decrease esophageal contractility (nitrate or calcium channel blockers) may be of value.

F. If esophagoscopy and manometry are normal and symptoms persist, consider an extrinsic esophageal mass or adjacent structure partially obstructing the esophagus. In this case, barium esophagography may be superior to esophagoscopy. Mediastinal tumors, left atrial enlargement, and osteophytes from cervical degenerative joint disease are the most common causes.

G. In a significant number of patients the evaluation yields no diagnosis. It is important to be sure the patient truly has dysphagia, as some may misinterpret the sense that something is constantly stuck in the upper neck region ("globus") as dysphagia. In the remaining patients the symptoms may be related to

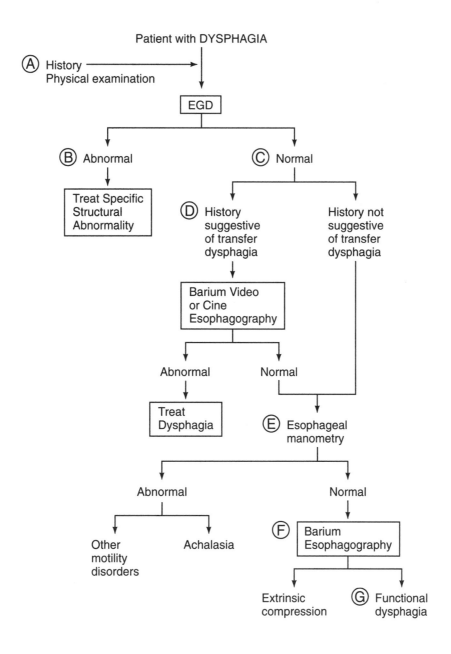

Patient with DYSPHAGIA

(A) History ——————→
Physical examination

EGD

(B) Abnormal

Treat Specific
Structural
Abnormality

(C) Normal

(D) History
suggestive
of transfer
dysphagia

History not
suggestive
of transfer
dysphagia

Barium Video
or Cine
Esophagography

Abnormal

Treat
Dysphagia

Normal

(E) Esophageal
manometry

Abnormal

Other
motility
disorders

Achalasia

Normal

(F) Barium
Esophagography

Extrinsic
compression

(G) Functional
dysphagia

emotional or psychiatric disorders or may be part of a more complex functional GI disorder (e.g., anorexia nervosa).

References

Bonavina L, et al. Drug-induced esophageal strictures. Ann Surg 1987; 206:173.

Clouse R, et al. Psychiatric illness and contraction abnormalities of the esophagus. N Engl J Med 309:1337.

Gelfand M, Botoman V. Esophageal motility disorders: a clinical overview. Am J Gastroenterol 1987; 82:181.

Patterson D, et al. Natural history of benign esophageal strictures treated by dilation. Gastroenterology 1983; 346.

Triadafilopoulous G. Nonobstructive dysphagia in reflux esophagitis. Am J Gastroenterol 1989; 84:614.

HEARTBURN

Richard E. Sampliner, M.D.

A. Heartburn is the leading symptom of gastroesophageal reflux disease (GERD). It is a substernal sensation of burning that radiates orad and usually reflects the presence of acid in the esophagus.

B. Lifestyle modifications that can ameliorate the symptom of heartburn include weight loss, elevation of the head of the bed, avoidance of tight clothing around the waist, avoidance of eating 2 hours before reclining, and avoiding foods and medications that lower the lower esophageal sphincter pressure. When lifestyle modifications are accompanied by conventional dose twice-daily H_2-receptor antagonist (H_2RA) therapy, most patients have symptomatic resolution.

C. Step-down treatment indicates the need to define the lowest level of therapy that will provide symptom relief. This may include only lifestyle modifications or perhaps these plus a nocturnal dose of H_2RA.

D. The alarm symptoms and signs of GERD include dysphagia (difficulty swallowing), weight loss, and anemia. These findings warrant immediate endoscopy to look for complications that need prompt attention, such as esophageal stricture, esophageal ulcer, and cancer.

E. Upper GI endoscopy plays an essential role in the evaluation of patients with heartburn. It helps identify the subgroup of patients with erosive esophagitis who will ultimately develop the inflammatory complications of GERD. The 40–50% of patients with chronic reflux symptoms who have erosive esophagitis are subject to the complications of esophageal ulcer, esophageal stricture, and ultimately Barrett's esophagus—a metaplastic change in the esophageal epithelium that can proceed to adenocarcinoma of the esophagus.

F. In patients lacking endoscopic esophagitis in whom the diagnosis of GERD needs to be confirmed, the next step is 24-hour pH monitoring to document abnormal esophageal acid exposure.

G. More intensive medical therapy involves raising the dose of H_2RA, adding additional measures such as promotility agents or mucosal defense agents, or using a proton pump inhibitor.

H. Because proton pump inhibitors are currently approved only for 2 months of use, patients should be stepped down to twice-daily H_2RA maintenance therapy. Because of the high frequency of recurrence of erosive esophagitis, maintenance therapy should be full dose.

I. Surgery is a viable option for patients who either have failed medical therapy or choose surgery instead of a chronic medical regimen. The procedure of fundoplication has been standardized sufficiently and has a high enough success rate to be an acceptable therapeutic option.

References

Hetzel DJ, Dent J, Reed WD, et al. Healing and relapse of severe peptic esophagitis after treatment with omeprazole. Gastroenterology 1988; 95:903.

Richter JE, Castell DO. Gastroesophageal reflux, pathogenesis, diagnosis, and therapy. Ann Intern Med 1982; 97:93.

Schindlbeck NE, Heinrich C, Konig A, et al. Optimal thresholds, sensitivity, and specificity of long-term pH-metry for the detection of gastroesophageal reflux disease. Gastroenterology 1987; 93:85.

Sontag SJ. The medical management of reflux esophagitis: role of antacids and acid inhibition. Gastroenterol Clin North Am 1990; 19:683.

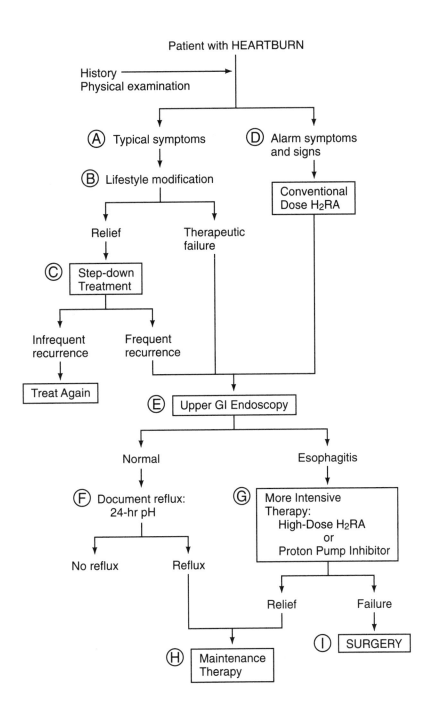

Patient with HEARTBURN

History ──────→
Physical examination

Ⓐ Typical symptoms   Ⓓ Alarm symptoms and signs

Ⓑ Lifestyle modification

Conventional Dose H₂RA

Relief   Therapeutic failure

Ⓒ Step-down Treatment

Infrequent recurrence   Frequent recurrence

Treat Again

Ⓔ Upper GI Endoscopy

Normal   Esophagitis

Ⓕ Document reflux: 24-hr pH

Ⓖ More Intensive Therapy: High-Dose H₂RA or Proton Pump Inhibitor

No reflux   Reflux   Relief   Failure

Ⓘ SURGERY

Ⓗ Maintenance Therapy

NONCARDIAC CHEST PAIN

M. Brian Fennerty, M.D.

A. Chest pain causes anxiety because of the possibility of cardiac disease. Coronary disease should be excluded before investigating esophageal causes of chest pain. Although microvascular angina is possible with normal coronary arteries, this is probably unusual. Over 600,000 patients a year undergo cardiac catheterization, and one third of these have normal coronary arteries. Thus, 150,000+ patients per year may require evaluation for noncardiac chest pain. Esophageal disorders may cause the cardiac-type chest pain in up to 50% of these patients. Associated symptoms of dysphagia, odynophagia, or heartburn are suggestive of an esophageal source, but are frequently absent.

B. Endoscopy is used initially to exclude structural or mucosal abnormalities such as erosive esophagitis, esophageal strictures/tumors, achalasia, hiatal hernia, and gastric ulcers. Although the diagnostic yield is low, this remains an important test for excluding complicated esophageal disease.

C. Thirty-five to 50% of patients with normal coronary arteries and cardiac chest pain have gastroesophageal reflux disease (GERD). This may or may not be manifested by erosive esophagitis. Thus a normal endoscopic result does not exclude reflux, and reflux may cause cardiac-type chest pain without symptoms of dysphagia or heartburn. In addition, acid perfusion of the esophagus not only lowers the threshold for myocardial ischemia but may induce this condition. The most sensitive test for documenting GERD is 24-hour ambulatory pH monitoring, which allows for correlation of chest pain events with reflux events. An etiologic association can be assumed if cardiac type chest pain is temporally related to reflux. Unfortunately, pH monitoring is not widely available.

D. Motility disorders of the esophagus account for cardiac type chest pain in 5–38% of patients evaluated in noncardiac chest pain series. Manometry measures the pressure and function of the lower esophageal sphincter and the motility of the esophageal body. Most motility abnormalities are intermittent and may be missed during manometry. In addition, the motility abnormality infrequently is accompanied by chest pain during the study. Nutcracker esophagus is the most common motility disorder diagnosed in chest pain patients (up to 30%), followed by nonspecific motility disorders (20–30%), diffuse esophageal spasm (DES) (5–10%), and achalasia (2–3%). Unless chest pain occurs with the observed motility disturbance, causation cannot be assumed.

E. If motility testing is nonspecific or nondiagnostic, provocative testing may be done at this time. Provocative testing is based on the hypothesis that the esophagus is hypersensitive to normal or physiologic stimuli and that chest pain is simply an altered or heightened perception of these stimuli. Most patients with noncardiac chest pain have personality traits similar to irritable bowel syndrome patients (i.e., they are anxious, depressed, hypochondriacal, and neurotic), and one third meet diagnostic criteria for panic disorder. Provocative tests include perfusing the distal esophagus with acid (Bernstein test), IV infusion of a cholinergic agent (Tensilar), or inflation of a balloon in the esophagus (balloon distention). Reproduction of the cardiac-type pain is diagnostic of an esophageal source of the pain.

References

Browning TH. Diagnosis of chest pain of esophageal origin: a guideline of the Patient Care Committee of the American Gastrointestinal Organization. Dig Dis Sci 1990; 35:289.

Cannon RO, Cattau LE, Yokshe PN, et al. Coronary flow reserve, esophageal motility, and chest pain in patients with angiographically normal coronary arteries. Amer J Med 1990; 88:217.

Katz PO, Dalton CB, Richter JE, et al. Esophageal testing of patients with noncardiac chest pain or dysphagia: results of three years' experience with 1161 patients. Ann Intern Med 1987; 106:593.

Lieberman D. Noncardiac chest pain: there's often an esophageal cause. Postgrad Med 1989; 86:207.

Richter JE, Bradley LA, Castell DO. Esophageal chest pain: current controversies in pathogenesis, diagnosis and therapy. Ann Intern Med 1989; 100:66.

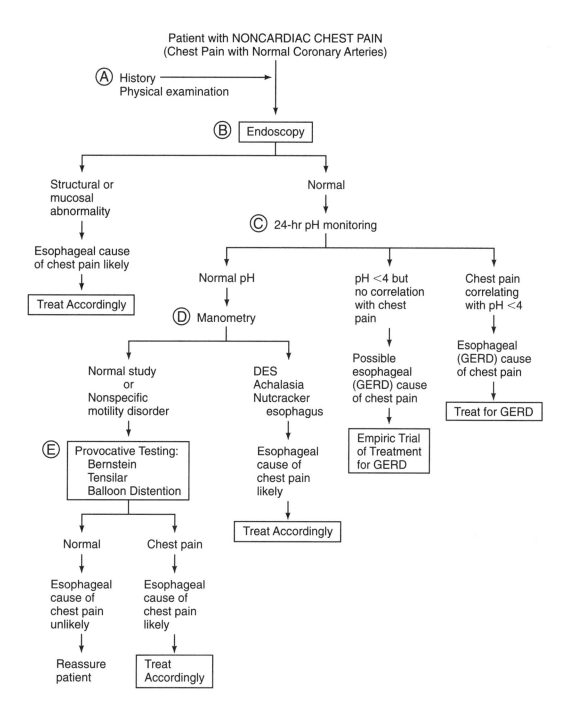

Patient with NONCARDIAC CHEST PAIN
(Chest Pain with Normal Coronary Arteries)

Ⓐ History
Physical examination

Ⓑ Endoscopy

Structural or mucosal abnormality

Esophageal cause of chest pain likely

Treat Accordingly

Normal

Ⓒ 24-hr pH monitoring

Normal pH

Ⓓ Manometry

Normal study or Nonspecific motility disorder

Ⓔ Provocative Testing:
Bernstein
Tensilar
Balloon Distention

Normal

Esophageal cause of chest pain unlikely

Reassure patient

Chest pain

Esophageal cause of chest pain likely

Treat Accordingly

DES
Achalasia
Nutcracker esophagus

Esophageal cause of chest pain likely

Treat Accordingly

pH <4 but no correlation with chest pain

Possible esophageal (GERD) cause of chest pain

Empiric Trial of Treatment for GERD

Chest pain correlating with pH <4

Esophageal (GERD) cause of chest pain

Treat for GERD

BELCHING

Gregory L. Eastwood, M.D.

A. Belching, burping, and eructation have roughly the same meaning and refer to the passage of gas from the stomach or esophagus through the mouth. In some patients, belching is the only symptom. In others, belching may be accompanied by abdominal discomfort, chest pain, or the passage of excess flatus. All people swallow air in variable amounts and all people belch from time to time.

B. Most patients who complain of belching swallow excess amounts of air. In fact, they may unwittingly take air into the esophagus before each belch that then is eructated. This practice may be associated with psychological stress or is thought by some patients to relieve other abdominal symptoms. Some patients may improve simply by being made aware of the cause of belching and reassurance that they are otherwise well. Avoidance of gum chewing and carbonated beverages is also helpful.

C. Occasionally, belching is a sign of organic disease. If the gastric outlet is obstructed partially by peptic disease or carcinoma, swallowed air cannot pass into the bowel and eructation may develop, sometimes accompanied by abdominal pain and vomiting. For unexplained reasons, patients who have symptomatic gallstones may complain of belching. Finally, belching of feculent-smelling gas may indicate prolonged gastric stasis or a gastrocolic fistula that has developed from a carcinoma of the stomach or transverse colon.

D. Upper GI x-ray series or upper GI endoscopy evaluate the stomach for partial gastric outlet obstruction and rarely may indicate a gastrocolic fistula complicating a gastric carcinoma. In general, because gastric outlet obstruction or a carcinoma that is large enough to erode into the colon is likely to be diagnosed by an upper GI x-ray series, that study is the appropriate first step in the diagnostic evaluation of belching. However, in some patients with peptic disease who have a small ulcer or have erosions and gastritis, the upper GI x-ray series may be nondiagnostic. In these, an upper GI endoscopy may be necessary to confirm the diagnosis.

E. The diagnosis of gallstones can be made either by ultrasonography of the upper abdomen or by oral cholecystography. The ultrasound study is more convenient for the patient, costs about the same as oral cholecystography, and is more accurate. However, if the clinical suspicion of gallstones remains high after a negative ultrasound examination, oral cholecystography should be ordered.

F. Perform a barium enema if the patient belches foul-smelling gas and if the question of a gastrocolic fistula remains after a nondiagnostic upper GI x-ray series or endoscopy.

References

Eastwood GL, Avunduk C. Intestinal gas. In: Manual of gastroenterology. Diagnosis and therapy. Boston: Little, Brown, 1988:177.

Levitt MD, Bond JH. Intestinal gas. In: Sleisenger MH, Fordtran JS, eds. Gastrointestinal disease. 4th ed. Philadelphia: WB Saunders, 1989:257.

BELCHING Patient

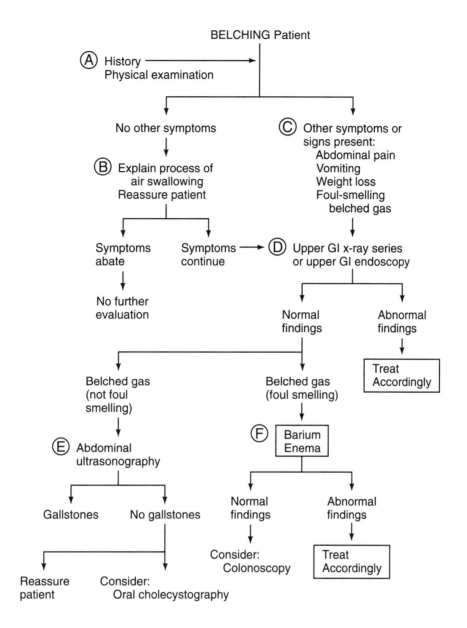

Ⓐ History ——————→
Physical examination

No other symptoms

Ⓒ Other symptoms or
signs present:
Abdominal pain
Vomiting
Weight loss
Foul-smelling
belched gas

Ⓑ Explain process of
air swallowing
Reassure patient

Symptoms
abate

Symptoms ——→
continue

Ⓓ Upper GI x-ray series
or upper GI endoscopy

No further
evaluation

Normal
findings

Abnormal
findings

Treat
Accordingly

Belched gas
(not foul
smelling)

Belched gas
(foul smelling)

Ⓔ Abdominal
ultrasonography

Ⓕ Barium
Enema

Gallstones

No gallstones

Normal
findings

Abnormal
findings

Reassure
patient

Consider:
Oral cholecystography

Consider:
Colonoscopy

Treat
Accordingly

DYSPEPSIA

Lee J. Hixson, M.D.

Dyspepsia may be defined as episodic or persistent abdominal symptoms, often related to eating, which are attributed to disorders of the proximal digestive tract. Symptoms may include upper abdominal discomfort, postprandial fullness, early satiety, anorexia, belching, bloating, nausea with or without vomiting, and heartburn with or without regurgitation. Overall, 20% of dyspeptic patients harbor a peptic ulcer and <1% have cancer. In ≥50% of patients there remains no pathologic diagnosis after a complete evaluation describing functional, nonulcer, or essential dyspepsia.

A. Consider eosinophilic gastroenteritis, Crohn's disease, sarcoidosis, and infections (syphilis and mycobacteria). Much debate centers over whether *Helicobacter pylori* colonization may cause dyspepsia when not associated with ulceration.

B. Functional dyspeptic symptoms frequently overlap with those of irritable bowel syndrome and are commonly associated with features suggestive of psychiatric disease. Historical risk factors suggesting an "organic" process include dysphagia, weight loss, GI bleeding, onset of symptoms after age 50, male sex, active smoking, previous ulcer history, pain that interrupts sleep, and vomiting.

C. Lactose intolerance secondary to acquired lactase deficiency may cause dyspepsia without diarrhea. Specific food allergy is rare.

D. Disruption of normal motility within the proximal GI tract may result in dysphagia, regurgitation, nausea, vomiting, and abdominal pain. Intrinsic disease of smooth muscle and the enteric and/or autonomic nervous systems, drug effect, metabolic and electrolyte derangements, and paraneoplastic syndromes may impair normal gut motility.

E. Examination should assess for GI blood loss, jaundice, an abdominal mass, presence of succussion splash over the stomach (suggestive of retained fluid), organomegaly, and signs of malabsorption.

F. Screening laboratory tests should include CBC, general (including liver) biochemistries, and amylase. Additional studies may include stool inspection with suspected malabsorption or parasitosis, abdominal radiography (for obstruction, mass effect, calcification), and ECG.

G. An empiric trial of H_2-receptor antagonists for presumed peptic disease is often warranted before radiographic or endoscopic testing if the clinical scenario suggests an uncomplicated course. Response of symptoms is not specific for peptic disease, since functional dyspepsia may also be ameliorated. Persistent symptoms after 7–10 days or recurrence after completion of therapy warrant a more aggressive diagnostic evaluation. Endoscopy is more sensitive than radiography in detecting a mucosal process and allows procurement of mucosal biopsies.

H. Perform manometry of the proximal GI tract by placing a multiport catheter connected with pressure transducers into the appropriate viscus lumen, and recording pressure fluctuation over time as a reflection of periodic peristaltic contractions. Dysmotility may be characterized by lack of or disorganized peristalsis, abnormal contraction configuration, and abnormal motor response to stimuli.

References

American College of Physicians. Endoscopy in the evaluation of dyspepsia. Ann Intern Med 1985; 102:266.

Barbara L, Camilleri M, Corinaldesi R, et al. Definition and investigation of dyspepsia. Dig Dis Sci 1989; 34:1272.

Dobrilla G, Comberlato M, Steele A, Vallaperta P. Drug treatment of functional dyspepsia. J Clin Gastroenterol 1989; 11:169.

Talley NJ, Phillips SF. Non-ulcer dyspepsia: potential causes and pathophysiology. Ann Intern Med 1988; 108:865.

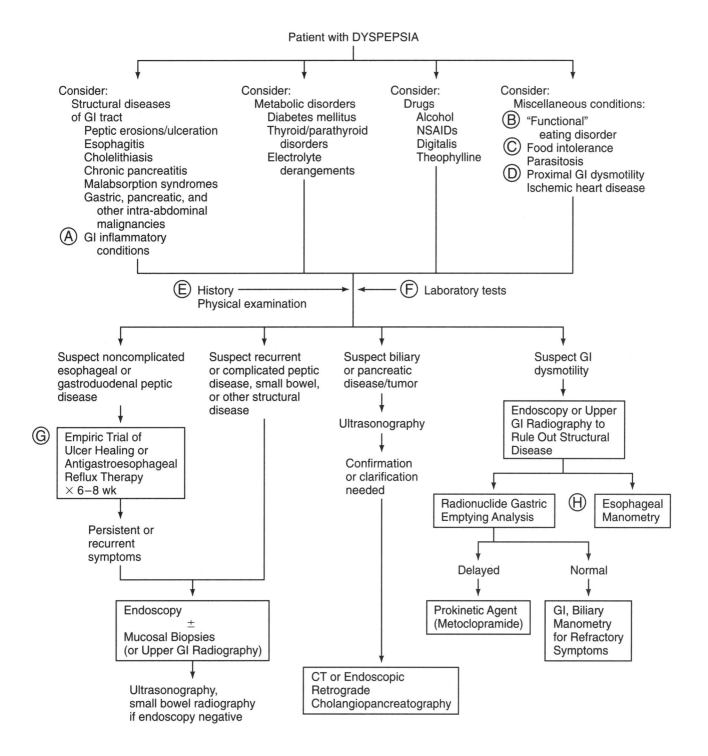

Patient with DYSPEPSIA

Consider:
Structural diseases
of GI tract
Peptic erosions/ulceration
Esophagitis
Cholelithiasis
Chronic pancreatitis
Malabsorption syndromes
Gastric, pancreatic, and
other intra-abdominal
malignancies
Ⓐ GI inflammatory
conditions

Consider:
Metabolic disorders
Diabetes mellitus
Thyroid/parathyroid
disorders
Electrolyte
derangements

Consider:
Drugs
Alcohol
NSAIDs
Digitalis
Theophylline

Consider:
Miscellaneous conditions:
Ⓑ "Functional"
eating disorder
Ⓒ Food intolerance
Parasitosis
Ⓓ Proximal GI dysmotility
Ischemic heart disease

Ⓔ History
Physical examination

Ⓕ Laboratory tests

Suspect noncomplicated
esophageal or
gastroduodenal peptic
disease

Suspect recurrent
or complicated peptic
disease, small bowel,
or other structural
disease

Suspect biliary
or pancreatic
disease/tumor

Suspect GI
dysmotility

Ⓖ Empiric Trial of
Ulcer Healing or
Antigastroesophageal
Reflux Therapy
× 6–8 wk

Persistent or
recurrent
symptoms

Endoscopy
±
Mucosal Biopsies
(or Upper GI Radiography)

Ultrasonography,
small bowel radiography
if endoscopy negative

Ultrasonography

Confirmation
or clarification
needed

CT or Endoscopic
Retrograde
Cholangiopancreatography

Endoscopy or Upper
GI Radiography to
Rule Out Structural
Disease

Radionuclide Gastric
Emptying Analysis

Ⓗ Esophageal
Manometry

Delayed

Normal

Prokinetic Agent
(Metoclopramide)

GI, Biliary
Manometry
for Refractory
Symptoms

JAUNDICE

Richard E. Sampliner, M.D.

A. Clinical evaluation of jaundice consists of history, physical examination, and laboratory tests focused on highlighting medication exposures and diseases that may cause impaired bile flow. The diagnosis may be apparent in a patient taking a medication known to cause a cholestatic drug reaction. In contrast, some patients may have many factors that could lead to jaundice. A complete battery of liver tests, including aminotransferases, alkaline phosphatase, albumin, globulin, and prothrombin time, may point the way toward a clinical diagnosis. An "obstructive" pattern with elevated bilirubin, markedly elevated alkaline phosphatase, and moderately elevated aminotransferase levels may suggest obstruction but can also be seen with infiltrative liver disease. These overlapping patterns in laboratory tests necessitate a more elaborate work-up as detailed in the tree.

B. An inadequate ultrasound study may result from patient obesity or excess abdominal gas. It is also necessary to calibrate the local ultrasonography, because ultrasound is a more operator-dependent imaging technique than CT. If the ultrasound study is technically inadequate or equivocal, abdominal CT may help clarify the issue.

C. When the clinical evaluation suggests an intrahepatic process, the inciting agent (alcohol or a medication) should be discontinued. If within the next 2 weeks there is an appropriate resolution of laboratory abnormalities, the work-up may be complete. However, if there is no resolution, a liver biopsy is essential to define the cause of jaundice.

D. When extrahepatic obstruction is suspected on the basis of the clinical evaluation, and even if an imaging procedure reveals a nondilated biliary system, direct visualization of the common bile duct is essential. As many as 10% of patients in whom jaundice is diagnosed have a nondilated system in spite of extrahepatic obstruction being documented.

E. Percutaneous transhepatic cholangiography (PTC) is used if ERCP has been unsuccessful in demonstrating the biliary tree. ERCP is used as the first procedure because it affords an opportunity to visualize the pancreatic duct and has a lower risk in a patient with ascites or coagulopathy.

F. Therapy proceeds on the basis of the ductal abnormality defined by direct visualization. The former distinction of "medical" and "surgical" jaundice no longer exists. With the possibility of intervening by means of therapeutic endoscopy or therapeutic radiology, what was formerly only possible by surgery can now be accomplished by nonsurgical techniques. Malignant obstruction can be bypassed by placement of either a retrograde or a percutaneous stent. The common bile duct can be cleared of gallstones by means of retrograde sphincterotomy.

References

Frank BV. Clinical evaluation of jaundice. JAMA 1989; 262:3031.

Hawes RH, Cotten PB, Vallon AG. Follow-up 6–11 years after duodenoscopic sphincterotomy for stones in patients with prior cholecystectomy. Gastroenterology 1990; 98:1008.

Matzen P, Malchow-Moller A, Brun B, et al. Ultrasonography, computer tomography, cholescintigraphy in suspected obstructive jaundice — a prospective comparative study. Gastroenterology 1983; 84:1492.

O'Connor KW, Snodgrass PJ, Swonder JE, et al. A blinded prospective study comparing four current non-invasive approaches in the differential diagnosis of medical vs. surgical jaundice. Gastroenterology 1983; 84:1498.

Venu R, Geenen JE, Toouli J, et al. Endoscopic retrograde cholangiopancreatography, diagnosis of cholelithiasis in patients with normal gallbladder x-ray and ultrasound studies. JAMA: 1983; 249:758.

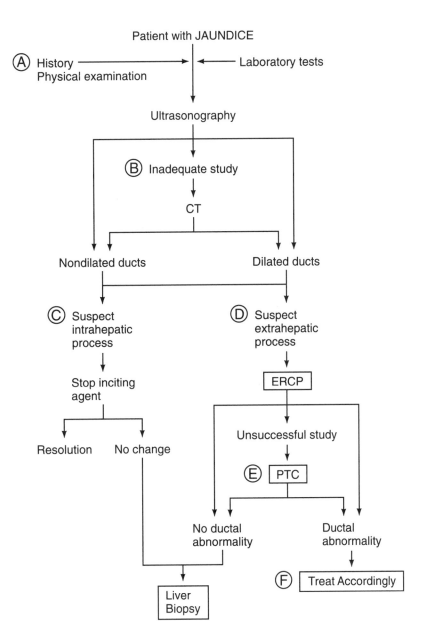

Patient with JAUNDICE

(A) History ⟶ ⟵ Laboratory tests
Physical examination

Ultrasonography

(B) Inadequate study

CT

Nondilated ducts   Dilated ducts

(C) Suspect   (D) Suspect
intrahepatic   extrahepatic
process   process

Stop inciting   ERCP
agent

Resolution   No change   Unsuccessful study

(E) PTC

No ductal   Ductal
abnormality   abnormality

Liver   (F) Treat Accordingly
Biopsy

ASCITES

Richard E. Sampliner, M.D.

A. Perform paracentesis in any patient with ascites. A good reason needs to be found not to perform a paracentesis. New ascites should be evaluated diagnostically to determine the cause. In a patient with decompensated liver disease who has been hospitalized with ascites, a paracentesis is essential to rule out spontaneous bacterial peritonitis. The database obtained at the time of paracentesis includes WBC count, differential, total protein, albumin, culture, sensitivity, and amylase. The serum-ascites albumin gradient should be calculated; i.e., the albumin level in the ascites is subtracted from that in the serum.

B. When the serum albumin minus the ascites albumin is <1.1, this represents low-gradient ascites. This implies an exudative process due to something other than just portal hypertension.

C. If a specific diagnosis is not evident after the results of culture and cytology, abdominal CT is appropriate to seek intra-abdominal malignancy or abscess. The final possible evaluation short of an exploratory laparotomy is laparoscopy, which can examine and sample the peritoneal and hepatic surfaces for potential malignant or infectious processes.

D. High-gradient ascites (serum albumin minus ascites albumin >1.1), indicates portal hypertension.

E. Once ascites due to portal hypertension has been established, therapy can be initiated. Its aggressiveness needs to be tempered by the patient's renal function, electrolyte balance, and level of encephalopathy. A stable patient can be treated vigorously with diuretics or large-volume paracentesis as long as careful daily monitoring is performed. Follow-up should include observations on weight, peripheral edema, mental status, volume compensation, electrolytes, and renal function.

F. An absolute polymorphonuclear count >250 is the most sensitive rapid way of detecting bacterial peritonitis. Because of the high frequency of spontaneous bacterial peritonitis in patients hospitalized with cirrhosis and ascites, it is essential to evaluate ascites and treat early with appropriate antibiotics.

G. The only way to recognize the pancreas as the source of ascites is to determine the amylase level. The ascitic amylase is usually a multiple of the serum amylase in a pancreatic process. Chronic pancreatic ascites may present clinically very similarly to decompensated liver disease.

References

Mauer K, Manzione NC. Usefulness of serum-ascites albumin difference in separating transudative from exudative ascites. Dig Dis Sci 1988; 33:1208.

Pockros PJ, Reynolds TB. Rapid diuresis in patients with ascites from chronic liver disease: the importance of peripheral edema. Gastroenterology 1986; 90:1827.

Quintero E, Gines P, Arroyo V, et al. Paracentesis vs. diuretics in the treatment of cirrhotics with tense ascites. Lancet 1985; I:611.

Runyan B. Hoefs JC, Morgan TR. Ascitic fluid analysis and malignancy-related ascites. Hepatology 1988; 8:1104.

Tito L, Gines P, Arroyo V, et al. Total paracentesis associated with intravenous albumin management of patients with cirrhosis and ascites. Gastroenterology 1990; 98:146.

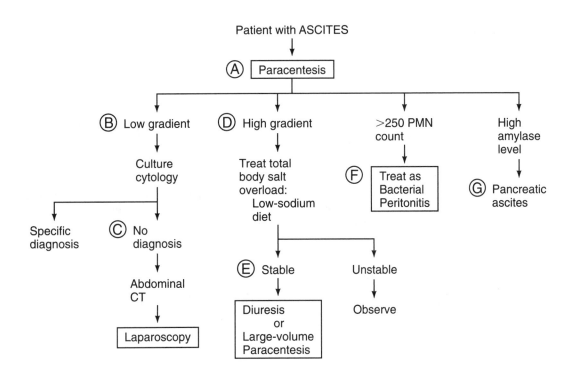

Patient with ASCITES

Ⓐ Paracentesis

Ⓑ Low gradient

Culture
cytology

Specific
diagnosis

Ⓒ No
diagnosis

Abdominal
CT

Laparoscopy

Ⓓ High gradient

Treat total
body salt
overload:
Low-sodium
diet

Ⓔ Stable

Diuresis
or
Large-volume
Paracentesis

Unstable

Observe

>250 PMN
count

Ⓕ Treat as
Bacterial
Peritonitis

High
amylase
level

Ⓖ Pancreatic
ascites

BILIARY COLIC

Philip E. Jaffe, M.D.

Biliary colic refers to abdominal pain caused by sudden obstruction of the cystic or common bile duct (CBD). This generally occurs in the right upper quadrant or epigastrium, lasts 15 minutes to 4 hours, comes on suddenly, and may be severe, requiring narcotics for pain relief. Gallstone disease is by far the most common etiology, although biliary parasites, clots, or tumor may cause a similar picture. The pain may be confused with peptic ulcer disease, pancreatitis, urinary calculi, diverticulitis, or functional bowel disease.

A. The initial history taking should attempt to elicit the location, duration, and character of pain as described above. Nausea and vomiting are frequently associated with pain. There usually is a history of less severe episodes. An association with fatty meals is often touted as a reliable sign but has not been proved. Murphy's sign, or involuntary cessation of inspiration while the right upper quadrant is being palpated secondary to pain, is seen commonly with cholecystitis but is not specific. Right upper quadrant tenderness is common, and peritoneal signs may be elicited with more severe attacks. The WBC count is generally normal or mildly elevated. Bilirubin or aminotransferase levels are mildly elevated in many patients, but normal in nearly 60%. Amylase and urine should be checked to exclude pancreatitis (with or without biliary disease) and nephrolithiasis.

B. Abdominal ultrasonography should detect gallstones with about 95% sensitivity. It is less valuable in detecting common bile duct stones (15–25% sensitivity) and should reveal CBD dilation in about three fourths of patients with CBD obstruction. Other causes of abdominal pain that may mimic biliary colic, e.g., pancreatitis and nephrolithiasis, may also be detected.

C. Occasionally, patients with a good history for biliary colic but no gallstones on ultrasound study may be found to have gallstones on oral cholecystography. This technique, combined with administration of cholecystokinin, also gives information about the contractile function of the gallbladder. However, oral cholecystography has limited value in centers with high-quality ultrasonography.

D. The absence of gallstones should suggest another etiology such as peptic ulcer disease, functional bowel disease, or sphincter of Oddi dysfunction. Upper GI endoscopy is a safe, reliable test to exclude ulcer disease and should be performed in the right clinical setting. If liver tests are abnormal, this may be bypassed and direct evaluation of the biliary tract with endoscopic retrograde cholangiopancreatography (ERCP) and/or biliary manometry performed.

E. A history compatible with biliary colic along with elevated bilirubin and/or alkaline phosphatase levels and no detectable gallbladder disease suggests the possibility of CBD pathology. Perform ERCP in these patients to exclude choledocholithiasis, tumors, parasites, and biliary dyskinesia. Perform delayed images of the bile ducts in patients in whom no anatomic obstruction is seen on ERCP. Persistence of contrast in the bile ducts at 45 minutes suggests sphincter of Oddi dysfunction, and sphincterotomy is warranted in the proper clinical setting. Biliary manometry, where available, is useful in defining specific sphincter of Oddi disorders that may be responsive to sphincterotomy.

F. When gallstones are detected on ultrasonography, consider the possibility of common bile duct stones. Markedly elevated alkaline phosphatase and/or bilirubin levels or a dilated common bile duct are suggestive and ERCP should be performed where available. Alternatively, if an open cholecystectomy is planned and the patient is a good surgical candidate, perform intraoperative cholangiography to evaluate this. If a laparoscopic cholecystectomy is planned and if choledocholithiasis is suspected, perform ERCP preoperatively.

G. If there is nothing to suggest CBD pathology, treatment should be aimed at removing the stones. In otherwise healthy patients, cholecystectomy (either open or laparoscopic) is now a relatively safe procedure. In the elderly or infirm, alternatives include oral dissolution therapy, shock wave lithotripsy, or the use of direct dissolution agents (e.g., methyl-tert-butyl ether) in centers where these techniques are available. In patients in whom sphincterotomy has been performed for removal of CBD stones, and who have cholelithiasis, relatively few (about 10%) go on to require cholecystectomy for subsequent cholecystitis. Thus, in patients in this unique situation, with multiple comorbid conditions that may limit their life expectancy and increase the hazards of cholecystectomy, observation without cholecystectomy or gallstone dissolution is a reasonable alternative.

References

Anclaux M, et al. Prospective study of clinical and biological features of symptomatic choledocholithiasis. Dig Dis Sci 1986; 31:449.

Davidson B, et al. Endoscopic sphincterotomy for common bile duct calculi in patients with gall bladders in situ considered unfit for surgery. Gut 1988; 29:114.

Einstein D, et al. Insensitivity of sonography in the detection of choledocholithiasis. Am J Roentgenol 1984; 142:725.

Geenen J, et al. The efficacy of endoscopic sphincterotomy after cholecystectomy in patients with sphincter-of Oddi dysfunction. N Engl J Med 1989; 320:82.

Marton K, Doubilet P. How to image the gallbladder in suspected cholecystitis. Ann Intern Med 1988; 109:722.

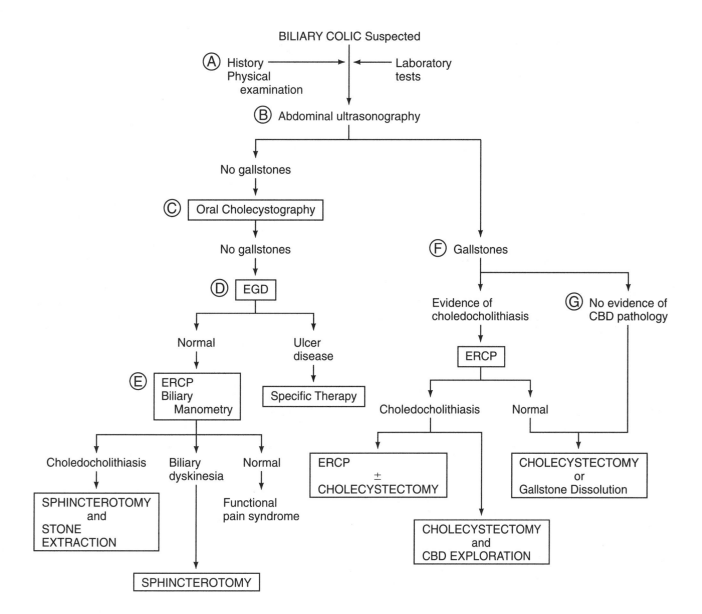

BILIARY COLIC Suspected

Ⓐ History — Physical examination ← Laboratory tests

Ⓑ Abdominal ultrasonography

No gallstones

Ⓒ Oral Cholecystography

No gallstones

Ⓓ EGD

Normal

Ⓔ ERCP Biliary Manometry

Choledocholithiasis

SPHINCTEROTOMY and STONE EXTRACTION

Biliary dyskinesia

Normal

Functional pain syndrome

SPHINCTEROTOMY

Ulcer disease

Specific Therapy

Ⓕ Gallstones

Evidence of choledocholithiasis

ERCP

Choledocholithiasis

ERCP ± CHOLECYSTECTOMY

CHOLECYSTECTOMY and CBD EXPLORATION

Normal

Ⓖ No evidence of CBD pathology

CHOLECYSTECTOMY or Gallstone Dissolution

GASTROINTESTINAL BLEEDING

Gregory L. Eastwood, M.D.

The principles of acute management of active GI bleeding are the same in almost all patients, although diagnostic tests vary depending on the presumed site of bleeding (Table 1). In an emergency (i.e., active bleeding), the usual orderly sequence of history taking, physical examination, diagnostic evaluation, and treatment is altered to meet immediate demands. In patients who are acutely ill, prompt resuscitative measures may be necessary.

A. Melena, or black stool, may develop with as little as 50 ml of blood loss per day. Although melena usually signifies bleeding from the upper GI tract, it can result from a source as low as the proximal colon. Brisker rates of bleeding may appear as red blood per rectum (hematochezia) or vomiting of blood (hematemesis). Hematemesis of either frank red blood or "coffee-ground" material usually signifies an upper GI tract source, but can result from swallowed blood from the respiratory tract. Hematochezia is usually a sign of lower GI tract bleeding, although it may result from profuse upper GI bleeding (e.g., from esophageal varices or an eroded artery in the base of an ulcer).

Advanced age worsens the prognosis. The patient's age also makes some diagnoses more or less likely. The differential diagnosis of acute lower GI bleeding in patients >60 years of age includes ischemic colitis, colon carcinoma, arteriovenous malformation, and diverticulosis; none of these is a serious consideration in a 25-year-old patient. Bleeding from inflammatory bowel disease or a Meckel's diverticulum is more likely in a child or young adult.

Recent ingestion of aspirin, other NSAIDs, or alcohol predisposes to gastric mucosal injury. Aspirin also interferes with platelet adhesion; thus, bleeding lesions in patients who take aspirin are less likely to clot.

The number of associated medical conditions is directly related to increasing risk of death in acute GI bleeding. Patients with liver disease are at risk for esophageal varices. Although upper GI bleeding in patients with esophageal varices is most likely to be from the varices, other sources must be considered.

Bleeding from a Mallory-Weiss mucosal tear at the esophagogastric junction is traditionally associated with repeated vomiting or retching before the onset of hematemesis. However, such a history is obtained in fewer than one third of patients. The diagnosis must be made by endoscopy. Patients with an aortoenteric fistula typically have massive hematemesis or hematochezia. The bleeding may stop abruptly; if it recurs, it is often fatal. Most fistulas occur in patients who have had aortic grafts, developing between the graft on the aorta and the adjacent portion of the GI tract. They also may develop between unoperated aneurysms and the GI tract. Promptly arrange upper endoscopy for any older patient with massive GI bleeding that stops abruptly, particularly if there is a history of aneurysm or aneurysm repair. Endoscopy rarely identifies the fistula, but if it identifies no other source of bleeding, emergency surgery should be considered.

CT of the abdomen may show a leaking aneurysm or fistula and thus helps in the decision of whether to operate. Nonocclusive ischemic vascular disease of the bowel typically occurs in patients >60 years of age who have a cardiovascular condition (e.g., congestive heart failure, arrhythmia) that predisposes to transient reduction in bowel perfusion. Also, aortic aneurysm repair places a patient at risk for ischemic colitis because of interruption of inferior mesenteric artery blood flow in the absence of adequate collateral circulation. Patients with ischemic colitis characteristically have an abrupt onset of moderate lower

TABLE 1. Diagnostic Considerations in Gastrointestinal Bleeding

Upper GI Bleeding	Lower GI Bleeding
Nose or pharyngeal bleeding	Hemorrhoids
Hemoptysis	Anal fissure
Esophageal rupture (Boerhaave's syndrome)	Inflammatory bowel disease (Crohn's disease, ulcerative colitis)
Esophagogastric mucosal tear (Mallory-Weiss syndrome)	
Inflammation and erosions (esophagitis, gastritis, duodenitis)	Neoplasm (carcinoma or polyps)
Peptic ulcer of esophagus, stomach, or duodenum or surgical anastomosis	Angiodysplasia
	Diverticulosis
Varices of esophagus, stomach, or duodenum	Antibiotic-associated colitis
	Radiation colitis
Neoplasm (carcinoma, lymphoma, leiomyosarcoma, polyps)	Amyloidosis
	Meckel's diverticulum
Hemobilia	Vascular-enteric fistula
Vascular-enteric fistula (usually from aortic aneurysm or graft)	Brisk bleeding from an upper GI source

(Continued on page 158)

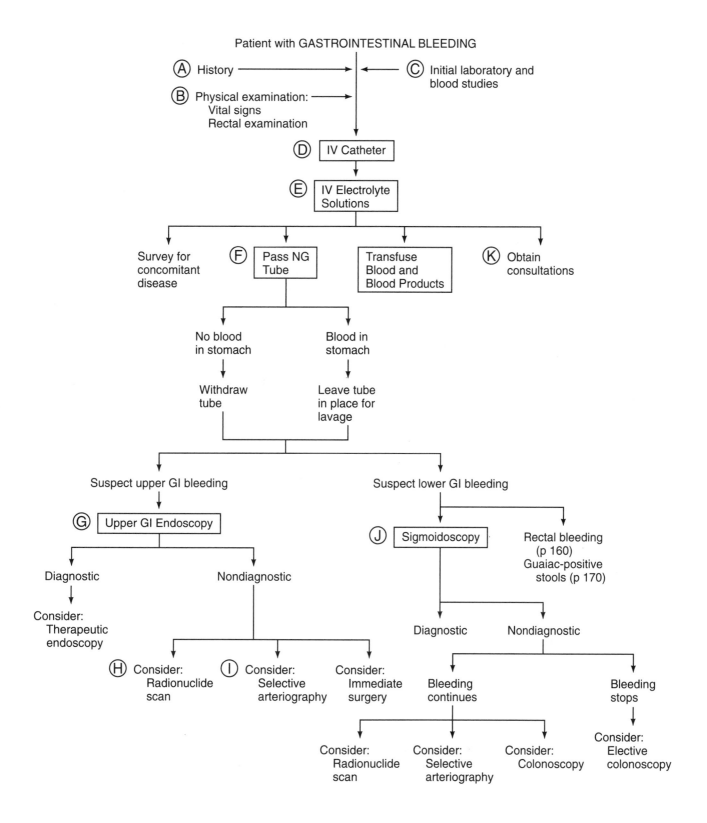

Patient with GASTROINTESTINAL BLEEDING

(A) History

(C) Initial laboratory and blood studies

(B) Physical examination:
Vital signs
Rectal examination

(D) IV Catheter

(E) IV Electrolyte Solutions

Survey for concomitant disease

(F) Pass NG Tube

Transfuse Blood and Blood Products

(K) Obtain consultations

No blood in stomach

Blood in stomach

Withdraw tube

Leave tube in place for lavage

Suspect upper GI bleeding

Suspect lower GI bleeding

(G) Upper GI Endoscopy

(J) Sigmoidoscopy

Rectal bleeding (p 160)
Guaiac-positive stools (p 170)

Diagnostic

Nondiagnostic

Diagnostic

Nondiagnostic

Consider:
Therapeutic endoscopy

(H) Consider:
Radionuclide scan

(I) Consider:
Selective arteriography

Consider:
Immediate surgery

Bleeding continues

Bleeding stops

Consider:
Radionuclide scan

Consider:
Selective arteriography

Consider:
Colonoscopy

Consider:
Elective colonoscopy

abdominal pain with bloody stool. In most patients the course is self-limited, with spontaneous recovery in several days. A few patients develop bowel infarction and peritonitis and require surgical intervention.

GI bleeding may develop from the acute effects of irradiation on the gut or may occur months to years after irradiation. The latter is a form of ischemic colitis that is accelerated by the perivascular inflammation that results from the effects of irradiation.

B. Cardiac output and blood pressure (BP) fall and pulse rate increases in response to acute blood loss. Under conditions of severe volume loss, postural compensation of BP and pulse are inadequate. If pulse rate increases >20 beats/min and systolic BP drops >10 mm Hg when the patient stands, blood loss is probably >1 L. However, age, cardiovascular status, and rate of blood loss influence the development of these postural signs. Blood loss and peripheral vasoconstriction may result in coolness of the extremities and pallor of the conjunctivae, mucous membranes, nailbeds, and palmar creases. Rectal examination provides direct access to the GI tract and should not be omitted, even when upper GI bleeding appears obvious. As indicated previously, red blood per rectum usually signifies lower GI bleeding, whereas melena may indicate an upper GI source. If the patient has vomited blood or coffee-ground material, yet the stool is brown or even negative for occult blood, the bleeding may have been of brief duration. Occult blood in the stool can be detected with as little as 15 ml of blood loss per day. Stools may remain positive for occult blood for nearly 2 weeks after an acute loss of ≥1000 ml of blood from an upper GI source.

C. Initial laboratory studies should include CBC, electrolytes, BUN, creatinine, glucose, calcium, phosphate, magnesium, and blood typing. Blood gases should be monitored in severely ill patients. Hemoglobin and hematocrit usually are low and may have some relation to blood loss. However, some patients bleed so rapidly that the blood volume has insufficient time to equilibrate, and hemoglobin and hematocrit are normal or only slightly reduced. In acutely bleeding patients, changes in BP and pulse and direct evidence of continued bleeding via nasogastric (NG) tube or per rectum are better indicators of the need to administer electrolyte solutions and replace blood. Assess clotting status by means of platelet count, prothrombin time, and partial thromboplastin time. Prompt correction of any clotting defect is crucial. Extensive blood transfusion dilutes platelets and clotting factors, especially factors V and VII. This can be treated by infusion of platelets and fresh frozen plasma as needed. Many patients who bleed while taking therapeutic anticoagulants do so from a clinically significant lesion. Thus, it is important to evaluate these patients for GI pathology in addition to correcting the clotting status. An elevation in WBC count can be associated with acute GI bleeding but usually is not >15,000/mm³. Do not attribute leukocytosis to acute blood loss without first considering sources of infection. Elevated BUN in a patient whose BUN has recently been normal or whose creatinine is normal suggests an upper GI source if the site of bleeding is not initially apparent. The rise in BUN can result from digestion of blood in the small intestine and absorption of nitrogenous products. However, hypovolemia due to acute blood loss of either upper or lower GI origin can also raise BUN. In patients with marginal liver function, the increased protein load from blood in the gut may induce or aggravate hepatic encephalopathy. Thus, gastric lavage and control of bleeding are of particular importance in these patients.

D. Promptly insert a large-bore IV catheter into a peripheral vein. In a profusely bleeding patient, two or more IV catheters may be needed to provide adequate blood replacement. In an acute emergency in which a peripheral vein is not available, establish venous access via a jugular, subclavian, or femoral vein. A CVP or Swan-Ganz catheter may be necessary to evaluate the effects of volume replacement and the need for continued infusion of blood, particularly in elderly patients or those with cardiovascular disease.

E. Rapidly infuse normal saline until blood is available for transfusion. In actively bleeding patients who have excess body sodium (e.g., those with ascites or peripheral edema), restoration of hemodynamic stability should take precedence over other considerations. Thus, if blood is not yet available for transfusion, infuse saline without regard to the sodium balance. If bleeding is less severe, infuse hypotonic sodium solutions until blood arrives.

F. Pass an NG tube in patients with a history of melena or hematemesis. Blood from an esophageal or gastric source will pool in the stomach, and in >90% of bleeding duodenal ulcers the blood refluxes back across the pyloric channel into the stomach. If the aspirate is clear or clears promptly with lavage, the NG tube may be removed. If there is a large amount of blood or retained material, lavage the stomach with a large-bore sump tube (20–24 Fr) or an Ewald tube. Removal of gastric contents facilitates subsequent endoscopy and decompresses the stomach. Because the NG tube is uncomfortable for the patient, predisposes to gastroesophageal reflux and pulmonary aspiration, and may irritate the esophageal and gastric mucosa, it should be removed when it is no longer fulfilling a purpose.

G. Endoscopic diagnosis of a specific bleeding site may dictate a specific treatment regimen. Further, identification of the so-called stigmata of recent hemorrhage (SRH) within an ulcer crater has prognostic and therapeutic implications. SRH include a protruding visible vessel, an adherent clot, a black eschar, and actual oozing or spurting of blood. Patients with SRH are more likely to have uncontrolled or recurrent bleeding and to require therapeutic endoscopy or surgery. The treatment of bleeding lesions through the endoscope has become widely available through a variety of methods, including thermal electrocoagulation, laser photocoagulation, injection of ethanol or hypertonic solutions, and injection sclerosis of esophageal varices.

H. Scanning the abdomen after IV injection of sulfur colloid or ^{99}Tc-labeled RBCs may indicate the bleeding site. A positive scan may lead to more definitive diagnostic or therapeutic procedures. The radionuclide scan appears to be more sensitive than selective arteriography in detecting active bleeding because a positive scan requires a lower rate of bleeding (0.1 ml/min vs. 0.5–1.0 ml/min). However, the radionuclide scan is less specific than arteriography in locating the site of bleeding.

I. Selective arteriography of the celiac axis, the superior or inferior mesenteric artery, or their branches can be both diagnostic and therapeutic. A focal extravasation of dye usually indicates an arterial bleeding source. A diffuse blush in the stomach area may be found in hemorrhagic gastritis. During the venous phase of the study, esophageal, gastric, or intestinal varices may be seen, although actual variceal bleeding cannot be detected. Angiodysplastic lesions and vascular tumors can be suspected by their angiographic appearance. Bleeding from arterial lesions may be controlled by injecting autologous clot or small pieces of gel foam. Variceal bleeding has been treated by infusion of vasopressin, 0.1–0.5 U/min, into the superior mesenteric artery to diminish mesenteric blood flow and reduce portal venous pressure. Venous infusion of nitroglycerin should be given simultaneously with vasopressin in patients at risk for ischemic cardiovascular disease.

J. Sigmoidoscopy using either a rigid or a flexible instrument should be performed early in the evaluation of acute lower GI bleeding. The role of emergency colonoscopy is somewhat controversial because the diagnostic value of the procedure is limited by blood and stool. Cleanse the colon with osmotically balanced electrolyte solution, administered orally or by NG tube; this enhances the diagnostic capability of colonoscopy.

K. The management of acute GI bleeding involves a team of health care workers. Specific diagnostic studies usually require the skills of a gastroenterologist or a radiologist. The surgeon, when consulted early, may offer valuable assistance in managing the patient and is in a better position to make a decision regarding operative intervention should the need arise later.

References

Bornman PC, Theodorou NA, Shuttleworth RD, et al. Importance of hypovolaemic shock and endoscopic signs in predicting recurrent haemorrhage from peptic ulceration: a prospective evaluation. Br Med J 1985; 291:245.

Daniel WA Jr, Egan S. The quantity of blood required to produce a tarry stool. JAMA 1939; 113:2232.

Fleischer D. Endoscopic control of upper gastrointestinal bleeding. J Clin Gastroenterol 1990; 12(Suppl 2):S41.

Graham DY, Schwartz JT. The spectrum of the Mallory-Weiss tear. Medicine 1978; 57:3007.

Johnston JH. Endoscopic risk factors for bleeding peptic ulcer. Gastrointest Endosc 1990; 36:S16.

Luk GD, Bynum TE, Hendrix TR. Gastric aspiration in localization of gastrointestinal hemorrhage. JAMA 1979; 241:576.

Proceedings of the Consensus Conference on Therapeutic Endoscopy in Bleeding Ulcers. Gastrointest Endosc 1990; Sept-Oct Suppl.

Steffes BC, O'Leary JP. Primary aortoduodenal fistula: a case report and review of the literature. Am Surg 1980; 46:121.

Storey DW, Bown SG, Swain CP, et al. Endoscopic prediction of recurrent bleeding in peptic ulcers. N Engl J Med 1981; 305:915.

Sutton FM. Upper gastrointestinal bleeding in patients with esophageal varices. Am J Med 1987; 83:273.

RECTAL BLEEDING

Steven Palley, M.D.

Visible blood per rectum is referred to as hematochezia. It can present as blood-streaked stool, bright red blood, or maroon liquid stool.

A. The primary assessment determines bleeding severity. Rapid blood loss is suggested by hemodynamic alterations. Resting tachycardia (rate >100) or systolic hypotension (systolic blood pressure <100) suggest a 20–30% decrease in blood volume. Orthostatic hypotension suggests a 10–20% decrease. Hematocrit determination is misleading in the face of acute bleeding. History can be significant in the setting of peptic ulcer disease, vascular grafts, inflammatory bowel disease, weight loss or change of stool caliber, hemorrhoidal disease, or acute diarrheal illness. Physical examination may disclose abdominal or rectal mass or hemorrhoids. Anoscopy should always be performed with the initial assessment.

B. In the absence of evidence of severe bleeding, the work-up can proceed electively. If there is a history of hematochezia but not active bleeding, further evaluation is influenced by risk of colorectal carcinoma. A patient <40 years of age without a strong family history of colorectal carcinoma, previous colorectal neoplasm, or long-standing ulcerative colitis should undergo sigmoidoscopy with air contrast barium enema if negative. Other patients should undergo colonoscopy.

C. A patient with evidence of active bleeding should undergo urgent sigmoidoscopy in an attempt to identify the bleeding source while it is still active. Distal lesions such as anorectal disease, left-sided neoplasia, rectal ulceration, ulcerative proctitis, or infectious colitis can be visualized. An active bleeding site precludes further evaluation. If no actively bleeding site is noted, prepare the patient for colonoscopy. A negative examination should lead to enteroclysis.

D. The differential diagnosis for severe rectal bleeding is similar to that for milder bleeding. However, upper GI sources must be included and can account for about 10% of severe hematochezia. The distribution of diagnoses varies with the method of evaluation in various series. In an endoscopic series, bleeding angiodysplasia was diagnosed in 30%, diverticular bleed in 17%, and neoplasm in 11%.

E. Patients thought to have a severe bleed should be resuscitated in an ICU setting. Adequate IV access is essential. Perform nasogastric tube placement and lavage in all patients. Further evaluation depends on the stability of the patient. The rare patient who cannot be stabilized should be rushed for emergent laparotomy. If the situation permits, preoperative or intraoperative angiography can be performed.

F. Patients who can be stabilized should undergo a limited sigmoidoscopy with retroflexion examinations of the anorectal region. They should receive a rapid bowel prep (purge) and then undergo colonoscopy. In most instances an upper endoscopy should precede the colonoscopic examination. If the degree of bleeding obscures the field or if colonoscopy is negative, perform a tagged RBC scan, with angiography if positive.

G. A negative evaluation should be followed with small bowel enteroclysis study. Although its yield is small, it can be as high as 20% if it follows adequate upper and lower GI evaluation.

H. Finally, if all previous evaluation is nondiagnostic and the patient has repeated episodes of severe hematochezia, consider provocative testing. Administer anticoagulants, thrombolytics, or vasodilators, with angiographic and surgical back-up, to encourage bleeding with immediate diagnosis and treatment.

References

Jensen DM, Machicado GA. Diagnosis and treatment of severe hematochezia. Gastro 1988; 95:1569.

Koval G, et al. Aggressive angiographic diagnosis in acute lower gastrointestinal hemorrhage. Dig Dis Sci 1987; 32:248.

Rex DK, et al. Enteroclysis in the evaluation of suspected small intestinal bleeding. Gastro 1989; 97:58.

Schrock TR. Colonoscopic diagnosis and treatment of lower gastrointestinal bleeding. Surg Clin North Am 1989; 69:1309.

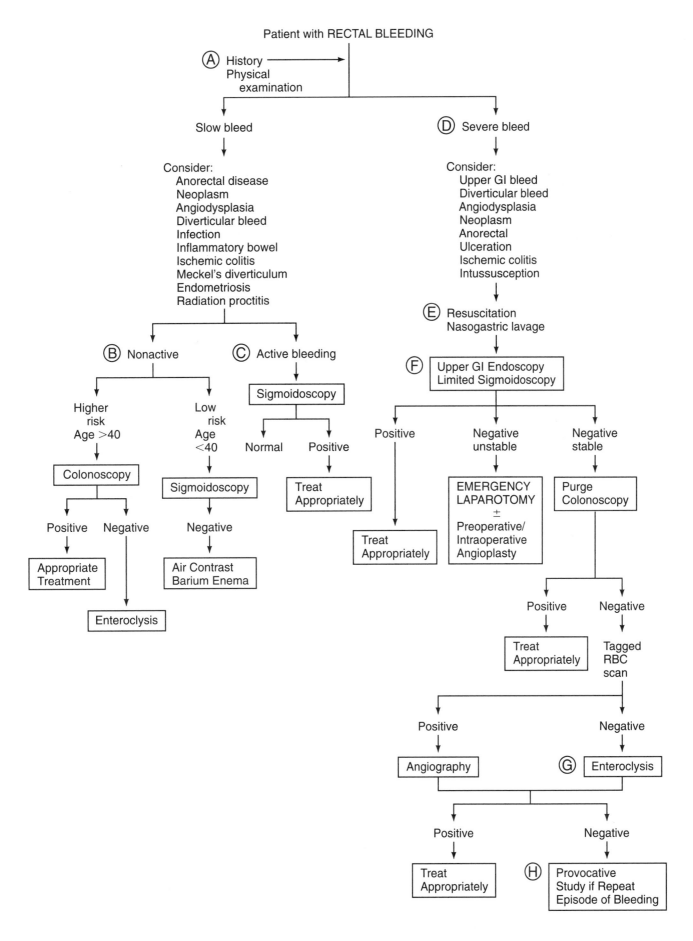

Patient with RECTAL BLEEDING

Ⓐ History
Physical
examination

Slow bleed

Consider:
Anorectal disease
Neoplasm
Angiodysplasia
Diverticular bleed
Infection
Inflammatory bowel
Ischemic colitis
Meckel's diverticulum
Endometriosis
Radiation proctitis

Ⓑ Nonactive

Ⓒ Active bleeding

Higher
risk
Age >40

Low
risk
Age
<40

Colonoscopy

Sigmoidoscopy

Normal   Positive

Positive   Negative

Negative

Appropriate
Treatment

Air Contrast
Barium Enema

Treat
Appropriately

Enteroclysis

Ⓓ Severe bleed

Consider:
Upper GI bleed
Diverticular bleed
Angiodysplasia
Neoplasm
Anorectal
Ulceration
Ischemic colitis
Intussusception

Ⓔ Resuscitation
Nasogastric lavage

Ⓕ Upper GI Endoscopy
Limited Sigmoidoscopy

Positive   Negative
unstable

Negative
stable

Treat
Appropriately

EMERGENCY
LAPAROTOMY
±
Preoperative/
Intraoperative
Angioplasty

Purge
Colonoscopy

Positive   Negative

Treat
Appropriately

Tagged
RBC
scan

Positive   Negative

Angiography   Ⓖ Enteroclysis

Positive   Negative

Treat
Appropriately

Ⓗ Provocative
Study if Repeat
Episode of Bleeding

161

ACUTE DIARRHEA

M. Brian Fennerty, M.D.

A. Diarrhea is one of the most common complaints resulting in visits to a physician. The history and physical (including rectal examination) are critical in determining who needs further diagnostic evaluation and in selecting appropriate therapy. Important questions to ask are length of illness, volume of stool, presence of blood or pus in stool, and symptoms of systemic illness such as fever, anorexia, weight loss, and volume depletion. Most patients should not undergo further evaluation at this time but be treated symptomatically. However, the presence of systemic symptoms dictates that the stool be more closely evaluated for evidence of invasive infection or inflammatory bowel disease (IBD).

B. The simplest test that can be performed in the office to evaluate inflammatory changes of the bowel mucosa is to inspect by microscopy a fecal sample for WBCs/RBCs. The presence of either of these implies infection with invasive organisms and/or IBD.

C. To evaluate infection by an invasive bacterial organism, a stool culture is necessary. Most clinical laboratories routinely test for *Shigella, Salmonella,* and *Campylobacter* spp. If travel or other historical features suggest others, more specific testing for *Amoeba,* *Yersinia* spp. or *Clostridium difficile,* and others may be necessary.

D. In patients with WBCs/RBCs in the stool and a negative culture, or those without inflammatory cells but continued diarrhea, perform flexible sigmoidoscopy to evaluate the presence of IBD, which may be present even if the mucosa is grossly normal appearing. Thus, a biopsy is helpful to detect minimal mucosal changes. In addition, the histologic appearance in the setting of gross inflammatory changes can help differentiate acute infectious self-limited colitis from IBD. A biopsy should generally be performed irrespective of gross findings.

E. In patients with negative cultures and sigmoidoscopy but continued diarrhea, further evaluation may be required.

References

Fedorak R. Antidiarrheal therapy. Dig Dis Sci 1987; 32:195.

Harris JC, DuPont HL, Hornick RB. Fecal leukocytes in diarrheal illness. Ann Intern Med 1972; 76:697.

Plotkin G. Gastroenteritis: etiology, pathophysiology and clinical manifestations. Medicine 1979; 58:95.

Patient with ACUTE DIARRHEA

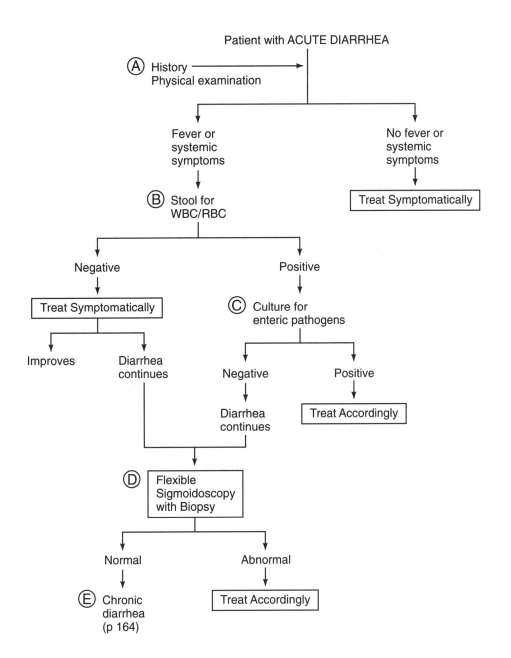

(A) History
Physical examination

Fever or systemic symptoms

No fever or systemic symptoms

Treat Symptomatically

(B) Stool for WBC/RBC

Negative

Treat Symptomatically

Improves

Diarrhea continues

Positive

(C) Culture for enteric pathogens

Negative

Diarrhea continues

Positive

Treat Accordingly

(D) Flexible Sigmoidoscopy with Biopsy

Normal

(E) Chronic diarrhea (p 164)

Abnormal

Treat Accordingly

CHRONIC DIARRHEA

Lee J. Hixson, M.D.

Diarrhea is best defined as an increase in stool weight and liquidity. Normal stool weight for a western diet is <200 g/day. Chronicity is defined as diarrhea lasting >3 weeks.

A. Most intestinal bacterial infections resolve spontaneously within 1–2 weeks, although symptoms occasionally persist for 2–3 months. Giardiasis and amebiasis may result in chronic symptoms, as can most helminthic infestations. Infectious diarrhea in the setting of AIDS is most commonly secondary to cryptosporidiosis, microsporidiosis, and *Mycobacterium avium-intracellulare*. Bacterial overgrowth within the small intestine, usually secondary to disorders that promote intestinal stasis or recirculation of enteric contents, causes diarrhea by several potential mechanisms.

B. Hydroxylated fatty acids and bile acids that are not absorbed by the small intestine stimulate electrolyte and H_2O secretion by the colonic mucosa. Malabsorbed carbohydrates exert an osmotic force within the bowel lumen, leading to excessive fecal H_2O losses.

C. Irritable bowel syndrome (IBS) is classically characterized by alternating diarrhea and constipation, although a subset of patients present with mainly loose stools. Fecal output in IBS has been reported to range up to 400 g/day.

D. A variety of commonly used drugs, including ethanol, antihypertensive agents, H_2-receptor antagonists, antacids, and digoxin, can cause diarrhea. Surreptitious laxative and diuretic abuse accounts for a significant percentage of patients with chronic diarrhea of unknown cause. Fecal impaction may present with frequent small-volume, liquid stools secondary to an "overflow" secretory response by the colon attributed to high intraluminal hydrostatic pressure.

E. Bloody diarrhea suggests inflammatory bowel disease (IBD), ischemia, radiation damage, or certain infections which do (cholera, giardiasis, and cryptosporidiosis do not cause bleeding). Additional historical features to note are recent foreign travel (increased risk of infectious diarrhea), sexual exposure ("gay bowel syndrome"), drug history including recent antibiotic use (increased risk of *Clostridium difficile* infection), surgical history (for dumping syndrome, and ileal resection that promotes bile acid and fat malabsorption), and a history of associated arthritis (suggestive of IBD, certain bacterial infections, and Whipple's disease, and after intestinal bypass surgery).

F. Examine a wet mount of fresh stool and saline for ova, parasites, and meat fibers. Multiple samples may need to be examined to detect parasitosis. Fecal leukocytes, indicative of intestinal inflammation, are best seen with methylene blue, Wright's, or Gram's stains. Excessive stool fat is determined with a Sudan stain. A low fecal pH suggests carbohydrate malabsorption. A fecal osmotic gap (serum Osm $-2 \times$ {fecal [Na] + [K]}) >150 confirms that an unmeasured osmotic agent is present. Stool water that turns red after alkalinization confirms the presence of phenolphthalein, a stimulant laxative.

G. Inspection of the rectal and left colon mucosa frequently detects changes secondary to inflammatory disorders. Despite normal-appearing mucosa at sigmoidoscopy, mucosal biopsies may suggest Crohn's disease and microscopic and collagenous colitis.

H. Colonoscopy is more sensitive than barium enema in detecting mucosal disease and allows procurement of mucosal biopsies. The terminal ileum may also be inspected in most patients.

I. An imaging study of the abdomen may demonstrate evidence suggestive of an inflammatory or neoplastic process involving the intestines, mesentery, and other abdominal viscera that may promote diarrhea.

J. Chronic secretory diarrhea may be associated with a variety of endocrine tumors, including gastrinomas and vipomas (usually arising in the pancreas), medullary thyroid carcinoma, carcinoid syndrome, and pheochromocytoma. Hyperthyroidism is typically associated with hyperdefecation without increased stool liquidity.

References

Fine KD, Drejs GH, Fordtran JS. Diarrhea. In: Sleisenger MH, Fordtran JS, eds. Gastrointestinal disease. 4th ed. Philadelphia: WB Saunders, 1989:290.

Kirsh M. Bacterial overgrowth. Am J Gastroenterol 1990; 85:231.

Morris AI, Turnberg LA. Surreptitious laxative abuse. Gastroenterology 1979; 77:780.

Read NW, Krejs GH, Read MG, et al. Chronic diarrhea of unknown origin. Gastroenterology 1980; 78:264.

Shian YF, Feldman GM, Resnick MA, Coff PM. Stool electrolyte and osmolality measurements in the evaluation of diarrheal disorders. Ann Intern Med 1985; 102:773.

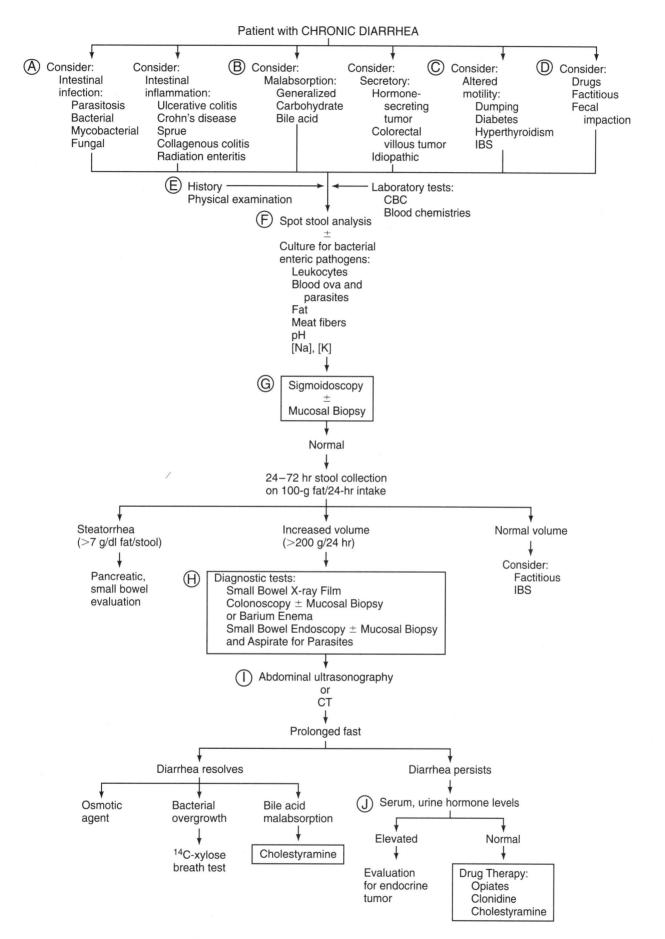

Patient with CHRONIC DIARRHEA

Ⓐ Consider:
Intestinal
infection:
Parasitosis
Bacterial
Mycobacterial
Fungal

Consider:
Intestinal
inflammation:
Ulcerative colitis
Crohn's disease
Sprue
Collagenous colitis
Radiation enteritis

Ⓑ Consider:
Malabsorption:
Generalized
Carbohydrate
Bile acid

Consider:
Secretory:
Hormone-
secreting
tumor
Colorectal
villous tumor
Idiopathic

Ⓒ Consider:
Altered
motility:
Dumping
Diabetes
Hyperthyroidism
IBS

Ⓓ Consider:
Drugs
Factitious
Fecal
impaction

Ⓔ History
Physical examination

Laboratory tests:
CBC
Blood chemistries

Ⓕ Spot stool analysis
±
Culture for bacterial
enteric pathogens:
Leukocytes
Blood ova and
parasites
Fat
Meat fibers
pH
[Na], [K]

Ⓖ Sigmoidoscopy
±
Mucosal Biopsy

Normal

24–72 hr stool collection
on 100-g fat/24-hr intake

Steatorrhea
(>7 g/dl fat/stool)

Pancreatic,
small bowel
evaluation

Increased volume
(>200 g/24 hr)

Ⓗ Diagnostic tests:
Small Bowel X-ray Film
Colonoscopy ± Mucosal Biopsy
or Barium Enema
Small Bowel Endoscopy ± Mucosal Biopsy
and Aspirate for Parasites

Normal volume

Consider:
Factitious
IBS

Ⓘ Abdominal ultrasonography
or
CT

Prolonged fast

Diarrhea resolves

Osmotic
agent

Bacterial
overgrowth

14C-xylose
breath test

Bile acid
malabsorption

Cholestyramine

Diarrhea persists

Ⓙ Serum, urine hormone levels

Elevated

Evaluation
for endocrine
tumor

Normal

Drug Therapy:
Opiates
Clonidine
Cholestyramine

165

CONSTIPATION

Philip E. Jaffe, M.D.

A. In Western society, adults average three bowel movements per week. There is significant variation in normals, and stool frequency varies depending on age, sex, diet, culture, and geography. History should be directed toward defining the character, chronicity, and severity of patients' complaints. New onset of decreased stool frequency in older patients requires exclusion of an obstructing colonic lesion by flexible sigmoidoscopy and barium enema, unless there is rectal bleeding or a strong family history of colorectal neoplasia suggesting colonoscopy as the initial study. In patients with more chronic complaints and in younger age groups, Hirschsprung's disease, irritable bowel syndrome, colorectal motility disorders, and anorectal processes (fissures, abscesses, thrombosed hemorrhoids) are more common. The use of medications, including antidepressants, calcium channel blockers, sedatives, opiate analgesics, aluminum antacids, and oral iron supplements, should be discontinued. The presence of systemic diseases, including diabetes mellitus, multiple sclerosis, and scleroderma or CREST syndrome, should be evaluated. Perform a physical examination, including rectal examination and anoscopy, in all patients. Look for physical signs of hypothyroidism, hypercalcemia, Parkinson's disease, and autonomic neuropathy. Check serum Ca^{++} and thyroid stimulating hormone (TSH) levels. In many cases simple dietary changes and discontinuation of offending medication cause symptoms to abate; however, persistent symptoms warrant exclusion of an obstructing colorectal mass.

B. Flexible sigmoidoscopy and barium enema exclude an obstructing colorectal lesion in most patients. If Hemoccult-positive stools or rectal bleeding accompany complaints of constipation, colonoscopy is indicated as the initial diagnostic procedure. The finding of a neoplastic polyp on flexible sigmoidoscopy also warrants colonoscopy because of the greater incidence of a proximal colonic polyp and/or cancer.

C. The finding of an obstructing colonic mass, usually adenocarcinoma, generally requires surgical intervention to prevent complete obstruction. In selected cases when there is metastatic disease or the patient is a poor surgical candidate, effective palliation with laser photocoagulation via endoscopy may be achieved.

D. Anorectal disorders, including fissures, thrombosed hemorrhoids, and perirectal abscesses, may all lead to constipation by causing avoidance of defecation because of pain. This in turn may worsen the underlying condition. Conservative measures, including stool-bulking agents, local anesthetics, and sitz baths, are preferred unless symptoms persist or an abscess develops requiring surgery.

E. In patients with chronic constipation and normal imaging studies of the colon and rectum, a radiopaque marker study is useful in confirming the presence of a transit problem and helps to better define the cause. The number of markers present in each segment of the large bowel on any given day after ingestion of markers is determined by radiography and compared with normals. Not infrequently, marker evacuation is normal and the "constipation" is either misinterpreted or misrepresented by the patient. The finding of normal marker transit may encourage a concerned patient by presenting objective evidence that the problem is one of perception. Those with persistence of markers in the rectosigmoid region should be evaluated for an anorectal motility disorder as described in section H. Those who have persistence of markers throughout the colon are said to have colonic inertia. Bulking agents and osmotic agents are advocated in this condition, but they have not definitively been proven to work.

F. A significant percentage of patients complaining of constipation have normal colonic transit times as measured by marker studies. In some the feeling of "constipation" may reflect their expectations relative to their upbringing or cultural norms; most probably have a variant of the irritable bowel syndrome. Empiric treatment generally begins with a bulking agent, a high-fiber diet, and increased fluid intake. Some patients require the addition of osmotic agents such as lactulose or milk of magnesia. Avoid chronic use of stimulant or irritant laxatives, as this may precipitate the development of colonic hypomotility and dilatation (cathartic colon).

G. The finding of colonic dilatation, on barium enema suggests the possibility of neurologic impairment of the colon (e.g., Hirschsprung's disease), an anorectal motility disorder, chronic cathartic use, or colonic pseudo-obstruction. Rectal biopsy in children is useful in diagnosing Hirschsprung's disease (absence of neurons in the rectum). The finding of melanosis coli, either endoscopically or by biopsy, is diagnostic of chronic abuse of anthraquinone laxatives (e.g., cascara or senna).

H. Anorectal motility studies using catheters that measure pressures within the rectum and across the anal sphincter are useful in excluding Hirschsprung's disease or anorectal motility disorders in patients with colonic dilatation and no clear etiology on biopsy. In addition, if significant numbers of markers remain in the rectosigmoid when transit is measured, an anorectal motility study is indicated. Specific treatment for anorectal motility disorders depends on the specific cause, but include biofeedback training, bulking agents, and occasionally surgery.

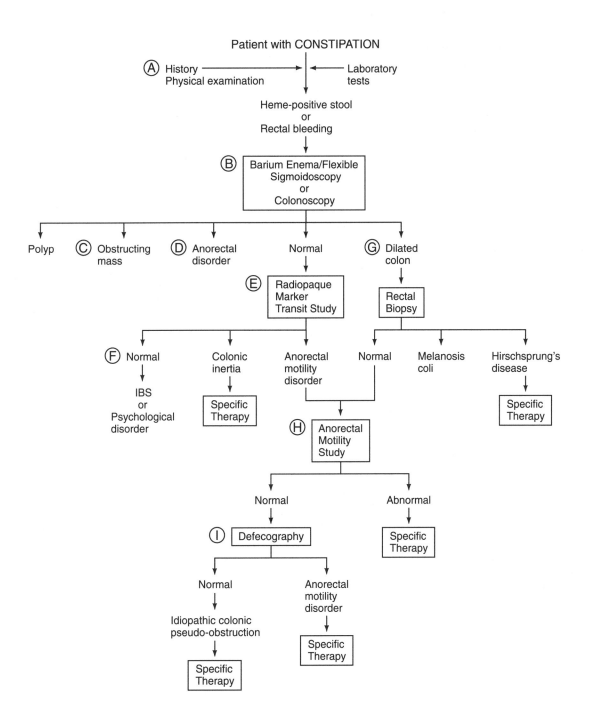

Patient with CONSTIPATION

(A) History — Physical examination → ← Laboratory tests

Heme-positive stool
or
Rectal bleeding

(B) Barium Enema/Flexible Sigmoidoscopy or Colonoscopy

Polyp   (C) Obstructing mass   (D) Anorectal disorder   Normal   (G) Dilated colon

(E) Radiopaque Marker Transit Study

Rectal Biopsy

(F) Normal   Colonic inertia   Anorectal motility disorder   Normal   Melanosis coli   Hirschsprung's disease

IBS or Psychological disorder   Specific Therapy

(H) Anorectal Motility Study

Specific Therapy

Normal   Abnormal

(I) Defecography   Specific Therapy

Normal   Anorectal motility disorder

Idiopathic colonic pseudo-obstruction   Specific Therapy

Specific Therapy

I. When further anatomic definition of the anorectal abnormality is required, perform defecography using barium paste or other synthetic radiopaque substances that simulate the characteristics of stool. By doing so, abnormalities in the perineal descent during defecation and complications of chronic constipation and straining, including rectal prolapse and rectocele, may be detected. Those with chronic constipation and colonic dilatation with normal anatomic studies, biopsy, and anorectal motility are said to have chronic idiopathic colonic pseudo-obstruction. In the past this was frequently treated by colectomy and ileostomy. However, up to 50% develop subsequent small bowel obstruction, and surgery is now considered only after a long therapeutic trial of more conservative measures.

References

Kamm M, et al. Outcome of colectomy for severe idiopathic constipation. Gut 1989; 969.

Read N, Timms J. Defecation and the pathophysiology of constipation. Clin Gastroenterol 1986; 15:937.

Reynolds J, et al. Chronic severe constipation: prospective motility studies in 25 consecutive patients. Gastroenterology 1987; 92:414.

Schuster M. Evaluation and treatment of constipation. Pract Gastroenterol 1986; 10:15.

ANORECTAL PAIN

M. Angelo Trujillo, M.D.

A. Anorectal pain has several potential causes, including local and nonlocal disease processes. A careful history and physical examination, including neurologic, anoscopic, and pelvic examinations, are important in the search for an etiology, which may range from an easily treated condition to a life-threatening one. Important considerations in the history are associated symptoms and reported signs (e.g., fever, rectal bleeding, vaginal discharge, hematuria, neurologic dysfunction). Rapid onset of symptoms, sexual practices, and any history of inflammatory bowel disease should also be noted.

B. Careful inspection, along with digital and anoscopic examinations, reveals most local causes of anorectal pain, but further evaluation with rectosigmoidoscopy may be necessary. This also provides a means for obtaining biopsy specimens for culture and histology. Rectal bleeding, mucous discharge, diarrhea, and anorectal pain suggest proctitis due to infection or other inflammatory causes.

C. A pelvic examination and consideration of pelvic ultrasonography or CT scan are important in the diagnosis of conditions that may cause referred pain to the anus and rectum. Most of these conditions have a common pathway of irritation of the pudendal nerves that supply sensory innervation to the anus and rectum. Cervical and vaginal cultures plus urinalysis with culture are necessary when considering pelvic inflammatory disease, prostatitis, or nephrolithiasis. IV pyelography should also be considered if the clinical picture is otherwise consistent with nephrolithiasis.

D. The diagnosis of proctalgia fugax rests on the history and the exclusion of other pelvic or anorectal abnormality. It is a benign condition of unknown cause characterized by paroxysmal anorectal pain of varying severity and sudden onset. Coccygodynia consists of throbbing or aching pain in the coccygeal region. Organic causes include fracture of the coccyx and traumatic arthritis of the sacrococcygeal joint. A functional coccygodynia also exists. Coccygeal tenderness associated with spasm of surrounding muscles are common findings on physical examination. Tension myalgia of the pelvic floor describes a syndrome of chronic vague discomfort in the rectum, pelvis, or lower back in patients without any other definable cause of pain. Pain is typically constant. Some authorities believe that the pain may be related to poor posture, generalized deconditioning, and possible psychological disorders. Chronic idiopathic anal pain has features that overlap with the other chronic pain syndromes.

E. There are several neurologic causes of anorectal pain. Associated neurologic signs and symptoms, pain characteristics, onset of pain, and spinal pathology are important factors in considering a neurologic cause for rectal pain. After a careful neurologic examination the procedures listed will be helpful in diagnosis of a specific neurologic disorder. Formal neurology consultation is recommended.

F. Pain may originate in sacral spinal cord segments or sacral nerve roots. Neoplasm, abscess, or inflammatory processes of the conus medullaris may present with pain. Associated loss of bowel or bladder function often occurs.

G. Entrapment of the sacral nerve roots of the cauda equina may occur secondary to inflammatory reactions in the CSF, or they may be compressed by tumor, abscess, or lumbosacral disc herniation.

H. The sacral plexus is located against the posterior pelvic wall. The plexus may be compressed by tumor or enlarged lymph nodes. Consider CT or MRI of the sacral spine and pelvis.

I. Spinal subarachnoid hemorrhage is a rare cause of rectal pain. This is most commonly the result of vascular malformation rupture, but it may also be associated with trauma, anticoagulant therapy, blood dyscrasias, or tumor. Ependymoma is the most common tumor associated with spinal subarachnoid hemorrhage. In patients with sudden onset of rectal pain associated with back pain, headache, stiff neck, and fever, consider spinal subarachnoid hemorrhage.

References

Lieberman DA. Common anorectal disorders. Ann Intern Med 1984; 101:837.

Peery WH. Proctalgia fugax: a clinical enigma. South Med J 1988; 81:621.

Rappaport B, Emsellem HA, Shesser R, et al. An unusual case of proctalgia. Ann Emerg Med 1990; 19:201.

Schrock TR. Examination of the anorectum, rigid sigmoidoscopy, flexible sigmoidoscopy, and disease of the anorectum. In: Sleisenger MH, Fordtran JS, eds. Gastrointestinal Disease. 4th ed. Philadelphia: WB Saunders, 1989:1570.

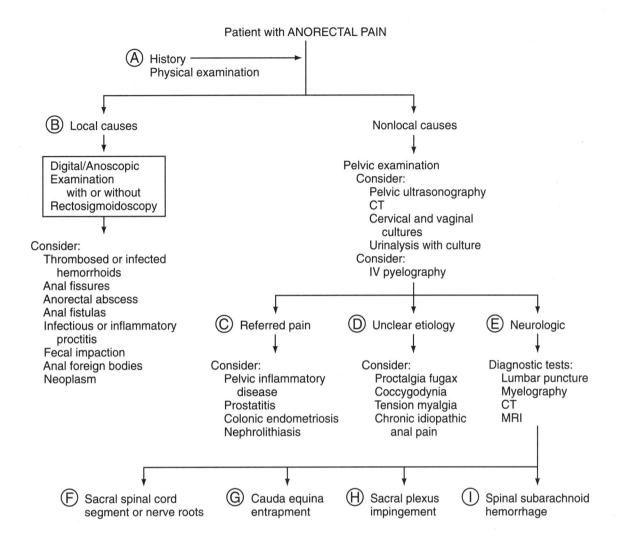

Patient with ANORECTAL PAIN

(A) History
Physical examination

(B) Local causes

Digital/Anoscopic
Examination
    with or without
Rectosigmoidoscopy

Consider:
    Thrombosed or infected
        hemorrhoids
    Anal fissures
    Anorectal abscess
    Anal fistulas
    Infectious or inflammatory
        proctitis
    Fecal impaction
    Anal foreign bodies
    Neoplasm

Nonlocal causes

Pelvic examination
    Consider:
        Pelvic ultrasonography
        CT
        Cervical and vaginal
            cultures
        Urinalysis with culture
    Consider:
        IV pyelography

(C) Referred pain

Consider:
    Pelvic inflammatory
        disease
    Prostatitis
    Colonic endometriosis
    Nephrolithiasis

(D) Unclear etiology

Consider:
    Proctalgia fugax
    Coccygodynia
    Tension myalgia
    Chronic idiopathic
        anal pain

(E) Neurologic

Diagnostic tests:
    Lumbar puncture
    Myelography
    CT
    MRI

(F) Sacral spinal cord
    segment or nerve roots

(G) Cauda equina
    entrapment

(H) Sacral plexus
    impingement

(I) Spinal subarachnoid
    hemorrhage

GUAIAC-POSITIVE STOOLS

M. Brian Fennerty, M.D.

Colon cancer will affect 6% of us during our lifetime. Each year in the United States there are over 140,000 new cases and 60,000 deaths from colorectal carcinoma. Accumulating evidence suggests that screening patients for colorectal neoplasia may either prevent colorectal cancer by detecting individuals with colon polyps that may evolve into carcinoma, or allow detection of colorectal cancer at a presymptomatic earlier stage, making curative therapy more likely. At present this screening strategy consists of (1) testing stool for the presence of hemoglobin, most commonly using guaiac-impregnated cards; and (2) directly observing the distal colon by sigmoidoscopic examinations.

A. The clinical utility of a positive Hemoccult test obtained at the time of digital rectal examination has not been adequately validated. Despite the absence of data regarding accuracy in detecting neoplastic disease, this is a widely accepted and practiced clinical test. It has been estimated that false-positive rates up to 25% occur with fecal occult blood testing (FOBT) on digital rectal examination. Until the specificity of FOBT by digital rectal examination is clarified, it is recommended that patients undergo FOBT only on spontaneously evacuated stools.

B. Patients should be sent home with guaiac cards and educated regarding diet and medicines while providing stool samples. Any one of six samples testing positive should be further evaluated. The test is positive in 4–6% of asymptomatic patients tested, but only 5–10% of these have colorectal cancer and 20–30% have colon polyps; thus, 60–75% are false-positive results. In addition, 30–50% of patients with proven colon cancer have a false-negative test. Therefore, a positive test results in further evaluation in many patients without disease, and a negative test does not exclude disease.

C. For evaluating a patient with a positive fecal occult test, two strategies are available: (1) flexible sigmoidoscopy and air contrast barium enema or (2) colonoscopy. The first is cheaper, but any positive finding (e.g., polyp or cancer) necessitates colonoscopy. Additionally, the first strategy alone misses 10% of cancers and 20% of large polyps. Therefore, colonoscopy is the preferred means of evaluation when available. It also may provide the most cost-effective strategy under certain conditions.

D. If symptoms dictate or if there is iron deficiency, a normal colonoscopy indicates that a further search for GI blood loss from the upper gut is indicated. Esophagogastroduodenoscopy (EGD) should be performed to evaluate the presence of upper GI structural lesions (ulcer, inflammation, tumors, arteriovenous malformations [AVMs]).

E. Although small bowel tumors, or Crohn's disease of the small bowel, unusually present with heme-positive stools, a negative endoscopic examination of colon and upper GI tract should prompt evaluation of the small bowel, preferably by enteroclysis or if this is not available, a small bowel follow-through. However, neither of these tests will detect small mucosal lesions such as AVM or small tumors.

F. If stools remain guaiac positive, consider invasive studies such as angiography or small bowel enteroscopy (not routinely available). These may permit visualization of small vascular lesions or tumors undetectable by other means.

G. If a colon cancer or large "cherry"-red polyp is found, this may be presumed to be the cause of bleeding and may be treated endoscopically or surgically. Similarly, the presence of mucosal inflammation (i.e., colitis) is also presumably the source. However, the presence of AVMs or diverticula is not sufficient to exclude either proximal source.

References

Barry MJ, Mulley AG, Richter JM. Effect of workup strategy on the cost-effectiveness of fecal occult blood screening for colorectal cancer. Gastroenterology 1987; 93:301.

Fleisher DE, Goldberg SB, Browning TH, et al. Detection and surveillance of colorectal cancer. JAMA 1989; 261:580.

Knight KK, Fielding JE, Battista R. Occult blood screening for colorectal cancer. JAMA 1989; 261:587.

Simon JB. Occult blood screening for colorectal carcinoma: a critical review. Gastroenterology 1985; 88:820.

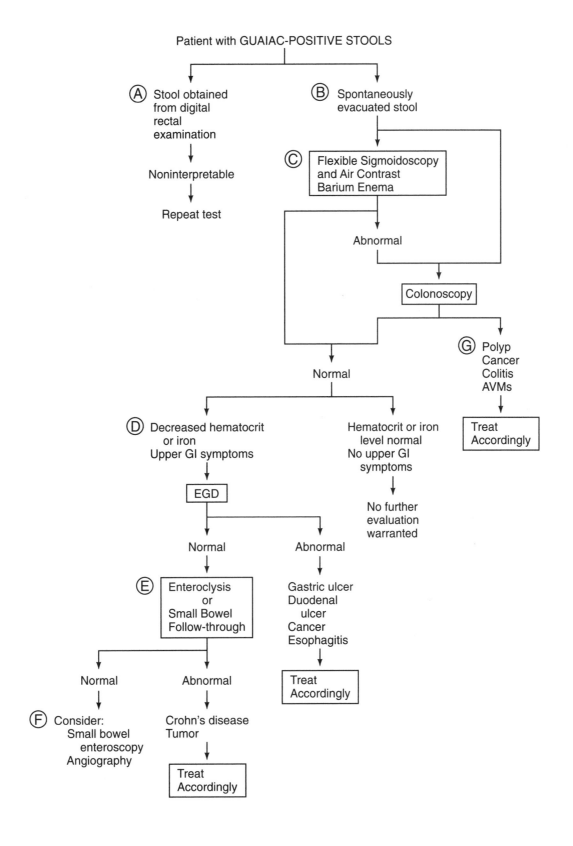

Patient with GUAIAC-POSITIVE STOOLS

(A) Stool obtained from digital rectal examination

Noninterpretable

Repeat test

(B) Spontaneously evacuated stool

(C) Flexible Sigmoidoscopy and Air Contrast Barium Enema

Abnormal

Colonoscopy

Normal

(G) Polyp Cancer Colitis AVMs

Treat Accordingly

(D) Decreased hematocrit or iron Upper GI symptoms

EGD

Normal

Abnormal

Hematocrit or iron level normal No upper GI symptoms

No further evaluation warranted

(E) Enteroclysis or Small Bowel Follow-through

Gastric ulcer Duodenal ulcer Cancer Esophagitis

Treat Accordingly

Normal

Abnormal

(F) Consider: Small bowel enteroscopy Angiography

Crohn's disease Tumor

Treat Accordingly

FLATULENCE

Gregory L. Eastwood, M.D.

A. Flatulence refers to the passage of excess intestinal gas per rectum or the feeling that excessive gas is in the abdomen. Many patients complain of bloating, meaning that the abdomen becomes uncomfortably distended, usually after eating. Often, bloating is attributed to excessive intestinal gas. However, the perception that the passage of flatus or the amount of intestinal gas is excessive may be inaccurate, as it may not actually be due to an abnormal amount of intestinal gas. Patients who complain of excessive flatus or of abdominal pain due to gas sometimes have disorders of gut motility and a heightened pain response to intestinal gas, rather than excess intestinal gas. Some patients who complain of abdominal pain and bloating do have demonstrable disorders, such as peptic disease, gallbladder disease, Crohn's disease, or recurrent bowel obstruction. If, in addition to complaints of gaseousness, the patient has loss of weight, localized abdominal pain, vomiting, or blood in the stool, the suspicion of an organic GI disorder is increased.

B. Bacterial action on dietary substrates produces gas. Some patients can identify certain foods that aggravate the symptoms. A common offender is lactose, which causes excess intestinal gas production, cramps, and diarrhea in lactase-deficient individuals. Elimination of milk and milk products, legumes, cabbage, and similar foods may be effective in alleviating symptoms.

C. Perform sigmoidoscopy and a barium enema to look for anorectal disease and colonic disorders. Reflux into the terminal ileum may identify Crohn's disease.

D. Upper GI and small bowel x-ray series may identify Crohn's disease of the small intestine, recurrent small bowel obstruction, or other disorders of the upper GI tract. Ultrasonography of the abdomen and pelvis may identify gallstones or an extraintestinal mass.

E. High-fiber bulking agents or so-called antispasmodics, such as dicyclomine, may be useful in patients who have no demonstrable treatable disorder or in whom a specific food has not been implicated. However, bulking agents, because they contain nondigestible substrates, may cause increased flatus. In some patients, stress reduction therapy may be helpful.

References

Eastwood GL, Avunduk C. Intestinal gas. In: Manual of gastroenterology. Diagnosis and therapy. Boston: Little, Brown, 1988:177.

Lasser RB, Bond JH, Levitt MD. The role of intestinal gas in functional abdominal pain. N Engl J Med 1975; 293:524.

Levitt MD. Volume and composition of human intestinal gas determined by means of an intestinal washout technic. N Engl J Med 1971; 284:1394.

Levitt MD, Bond JH. Intestinal gas. In: Sleisenger MH, Fordtran JS, eds. Gastrointestinal disease. 4th ed. Philadelphia: WB Saunders, 1989:257.

Levitt MD, et al. Studies of a flatulent patient. N Engl J Med 1976; 295:260.

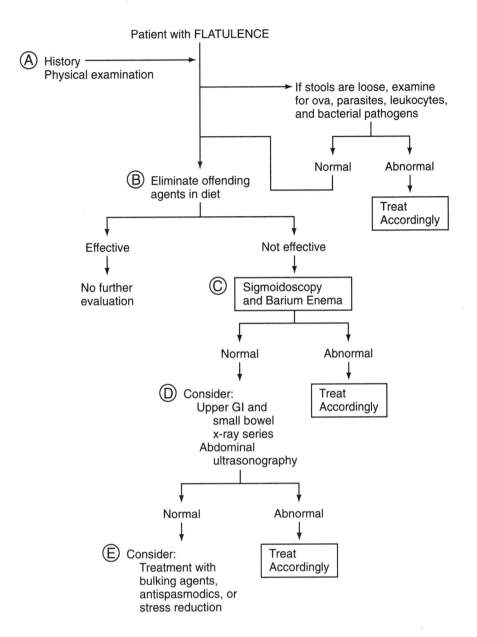

Patient with FLATULENCE

Ⓐ History
Physical examination

If stools are loose, examine
for ova, parasites, leukocytes,
and bacterial pathogens

Normal   Abnormal

Treat
Accordingly

Ⓑ Eliminate offending
agents in diet

Effective   Not effective

No further
evaluation

Ⓒ Sigmoidoscopy
and Barium Enema

Normal   Abnormal

Treat
Accordingly

Ⓓ Consider:
Upper GI and
small bowel
x-ray series
Abdominal
ultrasonography

Normal   Abnormal

Treat
Accordingly

Ⓔ Consider:
Treatment with
bulking agents,
antispasmodics, or
stress reduction

FECAL INCONTINENCE

Philip E. Jaffe, M.D.

A. A history of rectal trauma, surgery, or infections often provides clues to the cause of incontinence. A temporal relation to systemic neuromuscular conditions, cerebrovascular accidents, or diabetes is also helpful. Diarrhea or tenesmus and urgency may suggest inflammatory proctitis. On physical examination, exclude perirectal disease, including fissures, hemorrhoids, abscesses, and prolapse. Perform a thorough digital examination and try to define sphincter laxity, puborectalis integrity, and the presence of masses. This also excludes rectal impaction, a common cause of incontinence.

B. Perform proctoscopy with a flexible endoscope to exclude a distal rectal mass or proctitis. However, it is unusual for these to cause incontinence as an isolated symptom. The finding of ulcerative proctitis warrants a full colonoscopic examination to determine the extent and better define the etiology.

C. Anorectal manometry with a balloon-tipped, water-infused catheter will define resting and squeeze sphincter pressures, the threshold for rectal sensation to distention, and the threshold for internal sphincter relaxation on rectal distention. It also occasionally helps determine abnormalities in rectal compliance. Higher than normal sensory thresholds are seen commonly in diabetics with incontinence and may respond to bulking agents, opioid antidiarrheal agents, and biofeedback when available. Those with traumatic disruption of the anal sphincter (e.g., through a childbirth injury or after hemorrhoidal surgery) should be considered if conservative measures fail and low pressures are documented manometrically.

D. When available, defecography can define abnormalities in the anorectal angle during defecation. This frequently correlates with weakness of the puborectalis and pelvic floor, and in selected patients may respond to surgical repair when conservative measures fail.

E. Diseases of the rectum, including inflammatory proctitis, ischemia, and radiation proctitis, can lead to decreased rectal compliance and incontinence. Infusion of saline into the rectum and simultaneous measurement of rectal pressure associated with leakage can define this condition. If the condition is severe enough and refractory to opioids, fecal diversion with a colostomy may be the only alternative in selected patients.

References

Schiller L. Fecal Incontinence. Clin Gastroenterol 1986; 15:687.

Schiller L, et al. Pathogenesis of fecal incontinence in diabetes mellitus. N Engl J Med 1982; 307:1666.

Wald A. Fecal Incontinence: effects of non-surgical treatment. Postgrad Med 1986; 80:123.

Wald A. Disorders of defecation and fecal incontinence. Cleve Clin J Med 1989; 56:491.

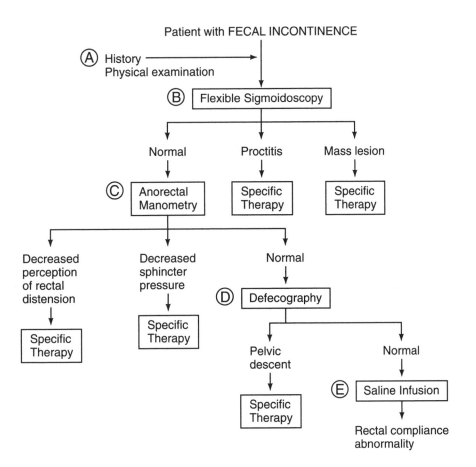

Patient with FECAL INCONTINENCE

Ⓐ History
Physical examination

Ⓑ Flexible Sigmoidoscopy

Normal

Proctitis

Mass lesion

Ⓒ Anorectal Manometry

Specific Therapy

Specific Therapy

Decreased perception of rectal distension

Decreased sphincter pressure

Normal

Specific Therapy

Specific Therapy

Ⓓ Defecography

Pelvic descent

Normal

Specific Therapy

Ⓔ Saline Infusion

Rectal compliance abnormality

ASYMPTOMATIC INCREASED TRANSAMINASES

Steven Palley, M.D.

The increase in asymptomatic patients being evaluated for increased transaminase (TA) levels is related to the proliferation of automated chemistry panel use and the use of alanine aminotransferase (ALT) as a surrogate marker at blood donation centers.

A. Historical considerations are important. Patients with clear histories of ethanol intake should be asked to refrain and present for a repeat blood test. Many prescription drugs and some over-the-counter drugs can lead to elevated TA levels and should also be stopped as a trial. A history of other hepatotoxin exposure should be sought. Diabetes mellitus can lead to hepatic steatosis. A history of exposure to viral agents should include any IV drug abuse, transfusion, and homosexual contact. HIV risk should be assessed also. Asymptomatic HIV-positive patients require no further work-up for elevated TA. A family history of hemochromatosis and Wilson's disease may be sought.

B. Physical examination may reveal evidence consistent with chronic liver disease, including spider angiomata, palmar erythema, hepatomegaly, or splenomegaly. Ethanol use is suggested by enlarged parotids. A degree of obesity is significant for a diagnosis of fatty liver.

C. The first evaluation should be a repeat TA determination along with a liver test panel, including alkaline phosphatase, total bilirubin, prothrombin time, and albumin and globulin levels. A cholestatic picture should prompt abdominal ultrasound examination. Progressive elevation of TA requires further evaluation. An elevated aspartate aminotransferase (AST)/ALT ratio suggests alcoholic liver disease, and the patient should be questioned further.

D. The intensity of follow-up depends on the level of TA elevation. Low-level elevations should be followed up at 2- to 3-month intervals. Moderate-range elevations should lead to an etiologic battery of laboratory tests and repeat enzymes at 1- to 2-monthly intervals. The etiologic panel includes iron-binding capacity and ferritin for hemochromatosis, ceruloplasmin for Wilson's disease, alpha-1-antitrypsin levels, ANA and anti-smooth muscle antibody for autoimmune chronic active hepatitis, and viral serology for hepatitis B and C. Higher elevations should be followed closely with 2- to 4-weekly levels of enzymes. An etiologic battery should be sent. A progressive rise in TA should prompt early liver biopsy.

E. At 6 months, if TA levels have decreased to normal, resolving hepatitis is the likely diagnosis and liver biopsy is not necessary. Laboratory tests should be repeated every 6–12 months. Persistent low-grade elevations ($<2\times$ normal) should prompt an etiologic panel, if not already done, and a liver biopsy should be considered. Higher elevations at this time should lead to a liver biopsy in the hope of histologic diagnosis. When pre- and postbiopsy diagnoses are compared, biopsy can change treatment in about 10% of patients and change the diagnosis in a higher percentage.

References

Friedman LS, et al. Evaluation of blood donors with elevated serum alanine aminotransferase. Ann Intern Med 1987; 107:137.

Hultcranz R, et al. Liver investigation in 149 asymptomatic patients with moderately elevated activities of serum aminotransferases. Scand J Gastroenterol 1986; 21:109.

Sampliner RE, et al. The persistence and significance of elevated alanine aminotransferase levels in blood donors. Transfusion 1985; 25:102.

Sherman KE. Alanine aminotransferase in clinical practice. Arch Intern Med 1991; 151:260.

Van Ness MM, Diehl AM. Is liver biopsy useful in the evaluation of patients with chronically elevated liver enzymes? Ann Intern Med 1989; 111:473.

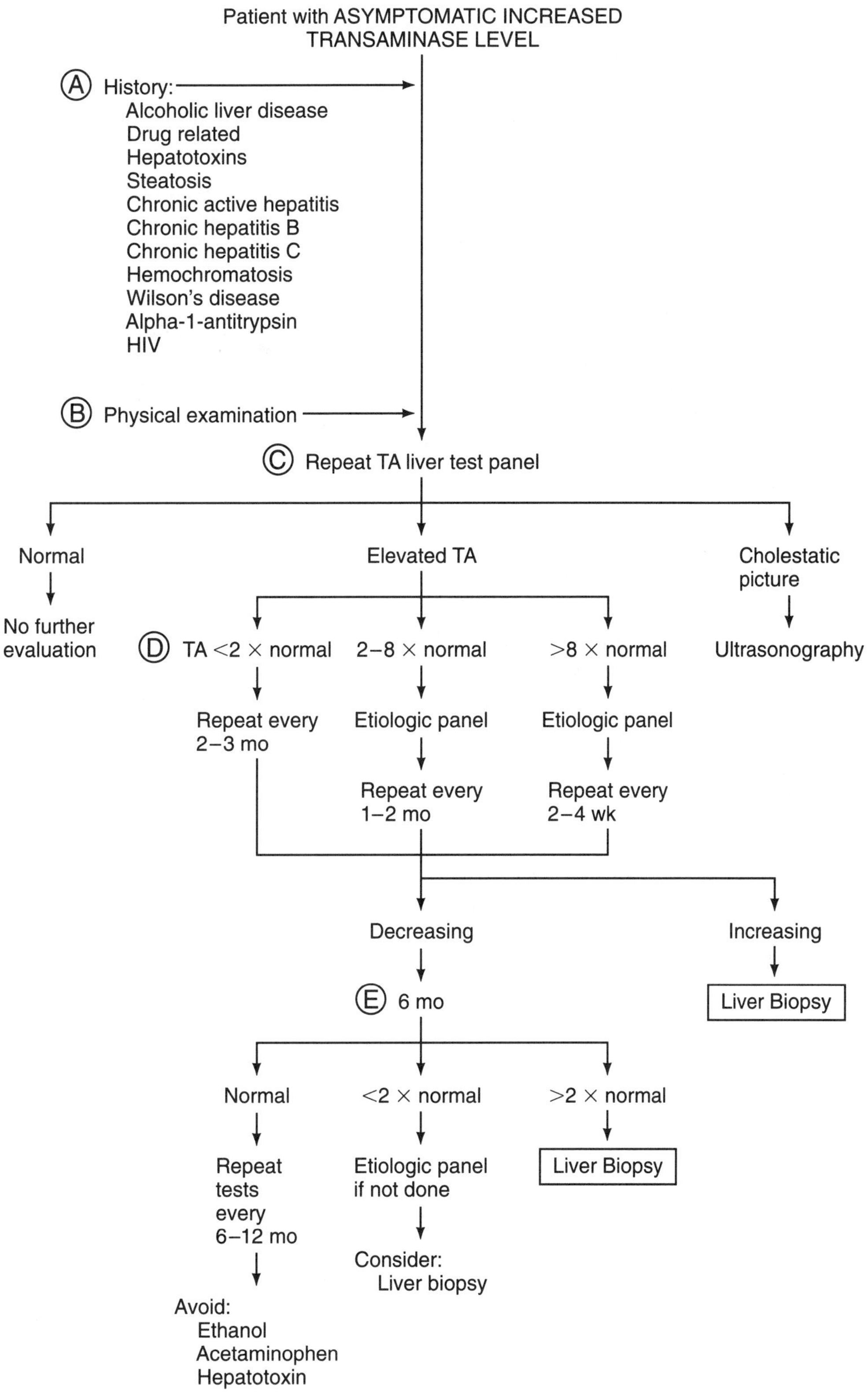

Patient with ASYMPTOMATIC INCREASED
TRANSAMINASE LEVEL

(A) History:
    Alcoholic liver disease
    Drug related
    Hepatotoxins
    Steatosis
    Chronic active hepatitis
    Chronic hepatitis B
    Chronic hepatitis C
    Hemochromatosis
    Wilson's disease
    Alpha-1-antitrypsin
    HIV

(B) Physical examination

(C) Repeat TA liver test panel

Normal → No further evaluation

Elevated TA

(D) TA <2 × normal → Repeat every 2–3 mo

2–8 × normal → Etiologic panel → Repeat every 1–2 mo

>8 × normal → Etiologic panel → Repeat every 2–4 wk

Cholestatic picture → Ultrasonography

Decreasing

Increasing → Liver Biopsy

(E) 6 mo

Normal → Repeat tests every 6–12 mo → Avoid: Ethanol, Acetaminophen, Hepatotoxin

<2 × normal → Etiologic panel if not done → Consider: Liver biopsy

>2 × normal → Liver Biopsy

ELEVATED SERUM IRON

M. Brian Fennerty, M.D.

A. Hemochromatosis is an inherited autosomal recessive disorder characterized by excessive GI absorption of iron and progressive iron deposition in parenchymal organs. The gene frequency in the population is 0.06%. Clinical characteristics include lethargy, weight loss, increased skin pigmentation, loss of libido, abdominal pain, joint pain, diabetes, hepatomegaly, testicular atrophy, and arthropathy. Asymptomatic hemochromatosis patients with increased serum iron must be differentiated from patients with iron overload secondary to alcoholic liver disease, hemolytic anemias, and medicinal iron. The family history may be indicative of liver disease.

B. The serum iron is a poor screening test to detect idiopathic hemochromatosis (IHC) because false-positive results occur in those ingesting iron, alcoholic patients, and heterozygotes of the hemochromatosis allele. However, calculating the transferrin saturation from the serum iron and the iron-binding capacity proves to have a sensitivity of >90% (for saturation >60%). Unfortunately as many as 24% of people (many heterozygotes) with normal iron stores also have saturation in this range. The serum ferritin reflects total body iron, and an increase in ferritin usually reflects increased body stores. When combined, increased transferrin saturation and elevated ferritin have a sensitivity of 94%.

C. The diagnosis of IHC requires direct documentation of excess iron in the liver. In addition, quantifying the amount of iron and liver damage has important treatment and prognostic implications. Hepatic iron concentrations in normals are 300–800 μg/g dry weight. In those with hemochromatosis, the hepatic iron concentration is usually >10,000 μg/g dry weight. Presymptomatic patients with hemochromatosis may occasionally have iron concentrations that overlap with those with alcoholic liver disease.

D. To differentiate alcoholic siderosis from hemochromatosis, Bassett and colleagues compared hepatic iron concentration in predominantly young homozygous hemochromatosis patients with that in patients with alcoholic liver disease. Hepatic iron index (HII) was calculated by converting μg of dry weight to μmols (μg/56 = μmols) and then dividing by the patient's age. This group discovered that all homozygous patients had an HII >2.0, and all ALD and heterozygotes had HII <2.0. This value appears to be the most discriminating test available to diagnose IHC.

References

Bassett ML, Halliday JW, Powell LW. Genetic hemochromatosis. Semin Liver Dis 1984; 4:217.

Bassett ML, Halliday JW, Powell LW. Value of hepatic iron measurements in early hemochromatosis and determination of the critical iron level associated with fibrosis. Hepatology 1986; 6:24.

Dadone MM, Kushner JP, Edwards CQ, et al. Hereditary hemochromatosis: analysis of laboratory expression of the disease by gene type in 18 pedigrees. Am J Clin Pathol 1982; 78:196.

Edwards CQ, Griffen LM, Goldgar D, et al. Prevalence of hemochromatosis among 11,065 presumably healthy blood donors. N Engl J Med 1988; 318:1355.

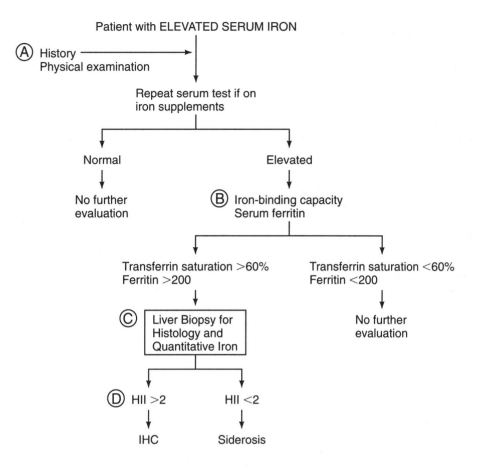

Patient with ELEVATED SERUM IRON

(A) History
Physical examination

Repeat serum test if on
iron supplements

Normal

Elevated

No further
evaluation

(B) Iron-binding capacity
Serum ferritin

Transferrin saturation >60%
Ferritin >200

Transferrin saturation <60%
Ferritin <200

No further
evaluation

(C) Liver Biopsy for
Histology and
Quantitative Iron

(D) HII >2

HII <2

IHC

Siderosis

ELEVATED SERUM AMYLASE

M. Angelo Trujillo, M.D.

A. Amylase is an enzyme with a molecular weight of 55,000 daltons that hydrolyses starch. The pancreas and salivary glands contain very high concentrations of amylase. It is also produced by a number of organs in lower concentrations. Approximately 35–45% of normal serum amylase is of pancreatic origin. Amylase has a serum half-life of 1–2 hours. Approximately 20% of circulating amylase is excreted in the urine; the remainder is catabolized at an unknown site. Increased serum amylase is most commonly caused by pancreatitis, but hyperamylasemia may be associated with several other nonpancreatic disorders with similar clinical presentations.

B. In acute pancreatitis serum amylase rises within 24–48 hours of the acute onset of pancreatitis. Levels return to normal within 3–5 days in most cases. A normal serum amylase level is occasionally seen in acute pancreatitis. This may represent early pancreatitis, after a transient rise and fall of amylase, extensive pancreatic necrosis with inability to produce amylase, or cases of acute exacerbation of chronic pancreatitis in which the gland cannot produce amylase. Serum amylase may also be normal when pancreatitis is associated with hypertriglyceridemia. In this case, a urinary amylase measurement usually shows a marked elevation. Cholelithiasis, ethanol, and idiopathic causes are responsible for approximately 90% of all cases of acute pancreatitis. Commonly used drugs known to cause pancreatitis include ethanol, hydrochlorothiazide, furosemide, sulfonamides, tetracyclines, estrogens, valproate, and azathioprine. A serum amylase level >3 times the upper limit of normal is consistent with pancreatitis. Other abdominal processes usually do not cause amylase levels >2–2.5 times the upper limit of normal, with the exception of salivary gland disease and gut perforation or infarction.

C. In acute pancreatitis with persistent elevated serum amylase levels, complications of acute pancreatitis as listed should be considered. Abdominal CT is useful in identifying pseudocysts, abscesses, ascites, and some tumors. Consider endoscopic retrograde cholangiopancreatography (ERCP) in pancreatitis of biliary origin or idiopathic pancreatitis.

D. In a patient with epigastric pain and elevated serum amylase, causes other than acute pancreatitis need to be ruled out. In cases of perforated peptic ulcer, peritoneal absorption of upper GI contents results in elevated serum amylase. The patient usually has a more abrupt onset of pain and more peritoneal irritation. Several other nonpancreatic conditions listed also present with more pronounced signs of peritonitis, and most need surgical intervention.

E. The elevation of serum amylase in renal insufficiency is usually modest, seldom >2 times the upper limit of normal. Macroamylasemia is a condition in which the major portion of serum amylase is bound to IgA. These macromolecular aggregates cannot undergo glomerular filtration; thus, the urine amylase level is low or normal. The amylase-creatinine clearance ratio (ACR) is calculated as follows:

$$ACR = \frac{A\ (urine) \times CR\ (serum)}{A\ (serum) \times CR\ (urine)} \times 100$$

where A = amylase concentration and CR = creatinine concentration In macroamylasemia, the ACR is abnormally low (usually <0.2%).

F. After the common causes have been considered, more obscure causes should be sought. Isoamylase measurements may be helpful. Elevated serum amylase secondary to lung disease or certain tumors is commonly of the salivary or s-isoenzyme.

References

Jensen DM, Rayse VL, Newell J, et al. Use of amylase isoenzymes in laboratory evaluation of hyperamylasemia. Dig Dis Sci 1987; 32:561.

Salt WB, Schenker S. Amylase—its significance: a review of the literature. Medicine 1976; 55:269.

Soergel KH. Acute pancreatitis. In: Sleisenger MH, Fordtram JS, eds. Gastrointestinal disease. 4th ed. Philadelphia: WB Saunders, 1989:1814.

Tietz NW, Huang Wx Yx, Rauh DF, Shuey DF. Laboratory tests in the differential diagnosis of hyperamylasemia. Clin Chem 1986; 32:301.

Toskes PP. Biochemical tests in pancreatic disease. Curr Op Gastro 1991; 7:709.

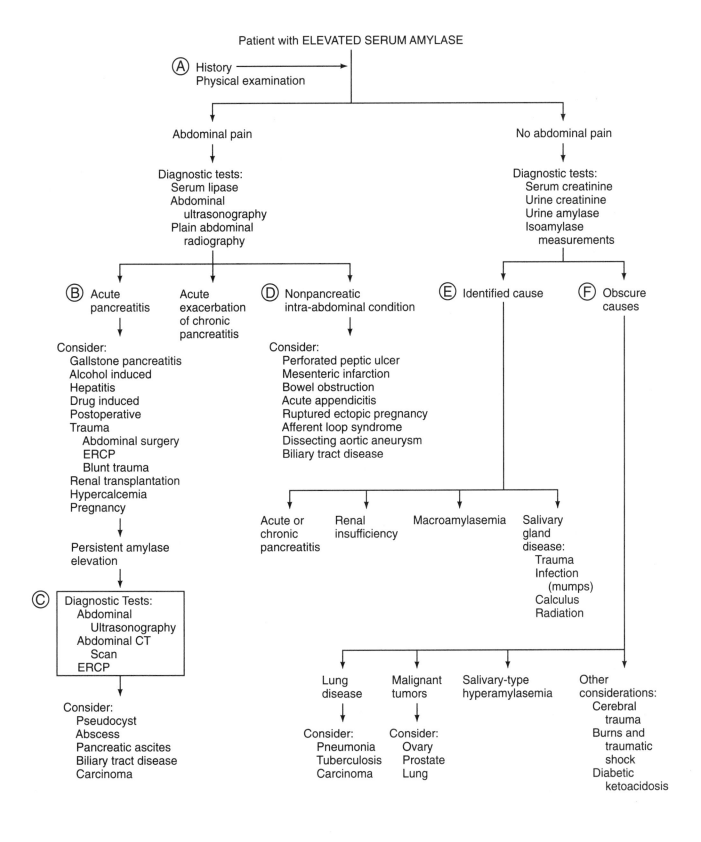

Patient with ELEVATED SERUM AMYLASE

Ⓐ History
Physical examination

Abdominal pain

Diagnostic tests:
Serum lipase
Abdominal
ultrasonography
Plain abdominal
radiography

Ⓑ Acute
pancreatitis

Acute
exacerbation
of chronic
pancreatitis

Ⓓ Nonpancreatic
intra-abdominal condition

Consider:
Gallstone pancreatitis
Alcohol induced
Hepatitis
Drug induced
Postoperative
Trauma
Abdominal surgery
ERCP
Blunt trauma
Renal transplantation
Hypercalcemia
Pregnancy

Persistent amylase
elevation

Ⓒ Diagnostic Tests:
Abdominal
Ultrasonography
Abdominal CT
Scan
ERCP

Consider:
Pseudocyst
Abscess
Pancreatic ascites
Biliary tract disease
Carcinoma

Consider:
Perforated peptic ulcer
Mesenteric infarction
Bowel obstruction
Acute appendicitis
Ruptured ectopic pregnancy
Afferent loop syndrome
Dissecting aortic aneurysm
Biliary tract disease

No abdominal pain

Diagnostic tests:
Serum creatinine
Urine creatinine
Urine amylase
Isoamylase
measurements

Ⓔ Identified cause

Ⓕ Obscure
causes

Acute or
chronic
pancreatitis

Renal
insufficiency

Macroamylasemia

Salivary
gland
disease:
Trauma
Infection
(mumps)
Calculus
Radiation

Lung
disease

Malignant
tumors

Salivary-type
hyperamylasemia

Other
considerations:
Cerebral
trauma
Burns and
traumatic
shock
Diabetic
ketoacidosis

Consider:
Pneumonia
Tuberculosis
Carcinoma

Consider:
Ovary
Prostate
Lung

HEMATOLOGY/ONCOLOGY

ANEMIA

Raymond Taetle, M.D.

A. The general evaluation of anemia includes an initial evaluation of volume status. If there are clinical signs of intravascular volume depletion, such as orthostatic hypotension, RBC and plasma loss may be present. Correction of intravascular volume status by appropriate blood product support is required before evaluation for anemia.

B. The initial evaluation of the pathophysiology of anemia is performed by clinically assessing effective RBC production. The normal steady-state reticulocyte production is approximately $100,000/mm^3$ and the maximum production approximately $400,000/mm^3$. Under extreme stress, reticulocytes may be released from marrow early, and even higher levels of apparent production achieved. These figures may be used as guides to interpret whether RBC production is increased or decreased.

C. When production is increased and the patient is anemic, this is presumptive evidence of increased RBC destruction (hemolysis). The hemolysis may be intravascular or predominantly extravascular. In either case, haptoglobin, the major plasma heme-binding protein, will be depressed. In intravascular hemolysis, free hemoglobin (Hb) may be present in plasma, and Fe in renal tubule cells (urinary hemosiderin). Coombs' test is used to distinguish immune and nonimmune origins of hemolysis. A positive direct Coombs' test indicates antibody or complement on the RBC cell surface. Only certain IgG isotypes react with macrophage Fc receptors; thus, a positive Coombs' test may be present without causing increased RBC destruction.

D. If the spleen is palpable and thus clinically enlarged, hypersplenism cannot be ruled out as the cause of RBC destruction. This can occur secondary to other processes that themselves lead to anemia, such as the ineffective erythropoiesis accompanying thalassemia, and hemolysis due to abnormal Hb, such as sickle cell disease.

E. If hypersplenism is unlikely, hemolysis may be due to mechanical trauma or congenital enzyme or Hb defects within the RBC. Microangiopathic hemolytic anemia (MAHA) results from RBC trauma from fibrin strands in small vessels (thrombotic thrombocytopenic purpura, hemolytic-uremic syndrome) or, more rarely, prosthetic heart valves. Enzymatic defects can be drug dependent, such as in G6PD deficiency, or constitutive, such as in pyruvate kinase deficiency. Abnormal Hb, such as sickle globin, and membrane defects (hereditary spherocytosis) can also cause hemolysis.

Acquired causes of hemolysis include the excess complement sensitivity acquired in paroxysmal nocturnal hemoglobinuria (PNH) and infections such as malaria.

F. When RBC production is decreased or normal in the face of anemia (normal production with a reduced RBC mass constitutes depressed production), guidance as to the origin of the anemia may be provided by RBC size obtained through automated cell counting. Microcytic anemias generally involve processes in which Hb or heme synthesis is impaired. Thalassemia minor is a common cause of mild microcytic anemia. Major thalassemias cause more severe anemia and are often accompanied by organomegaly and/or skeletal abnormalities due to marrow expansion. Anemia of chronic disease can be microcytic and shows reduced serum Fe, reduced total iron-binding capacity (TIBC), and increased serum ferritin. In contrast, Fe deficiency is characterized by reduced serum Fe, increased TIBC, and reduced serum ferritin.

G. In normocytic anemias, anemia of chronic disease is considered in the appropriate clinical settings when the aforementioned laboratory findings are present. If anemia of chronic disease is not present, a bone marrow test is indicated to rule out a marrow defect in RBC production due to aplasia, processes replacing the marrow (myelophthisic anemia), or malnutrition. Protein calorie malnutrition causes anemia in disorders such as anorexia nervosa. Other metabolic disorders also cause severe anemia, including uremia. The primary defect in most uremic patients is a relative lack of the erythroid-stimulating hormone erythropoietin. The Fe status of these patients depends on their transfusion and medication histories.

H. Macrocytic anemias are due to either vitamin deficiencies or primary processes involving the marrow. Vitamin B_{12} deficiency may be due to pernicious anemia or secondary to other causes of B_{12} malabsorption, but is almost never due to dietary deficiency. In recent years, many early cases of B_{12} deficiency are detected early by serum B_{12} assays and confirmatory tests (increased methylmalonic acid or homocysteine). Folate deficiency is usually due to diet alone or diet in combination with ethanol ingestion. Some drugs also impair folate absorption (phenytoin) or metabolism (trimethoprim).

I. When folate and B_{12} levels are normal, macrocytic anemias are usually due to myelodysplasia or to unusual congenital dyserythropoietic anemias (types I, II, or III).

Patient with ANEMIA (DECREASED RBC MASS)

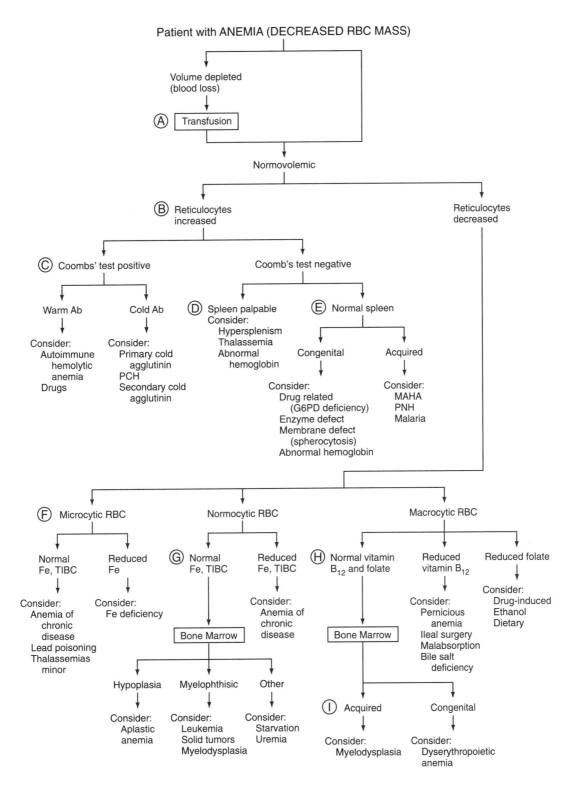

Reference

Johnson RA, Roodman GD. Hematologic manifestations of malignancy. Dis Mon 1989; 35:726.

Nissenson AR, et al. Recombinant erythropoietin and renal anemia: molecular biology, clinical efficacy, and nervous system effects. Ann Intern Med 1991; 114:402.

Rapaport S. Introduction to hematology. Philadelphia: JB Lippincott, 1987:10.

Rose PE, Clark AJB. Haematology of the haemolytic uraemic syndrome. Blood Rev 1898; 3:136.

Stabler SP, et al. Clinical spectrum and diagnosis of cobalamin deficiency. Blood 1990; 76:871.

Yip R, Dallman PR. The roles of inflammation and iron deficiency as causes of anemia. Am J Clin Nutr 1988; 48:1295.

POLYCYTHEMIA

Raymond Taetle, M.D.

A. Increased plasma hemoglobin (Hb) does not necessarily mean an elevated total body RBC mass. If repeat determinations confirm an increased plasma Hb, RBC mass and plasma volume should be determined using radiolabeled RBC and albumin.

B. Increased RBC mass indicates "true" polycythemia vera. An increase in plasma Hb attributed to a normal or high normal RBC mass and reduced plasma volume is termed "spurious" polycythemia. In the past, many cases of spurious polycythemia resulted from treatment with diuretics for hypertension. Although such patients do not have an expanded RBC mass, the decreased ratio of plasma to RBC in blood results in unfavorable rheology. Spurious polycythemia is associated with a high incidence of morbid arterial thrombotic events. Discontinue diuretics and substitute other forms of treatment, or evaluate the patient to delineate other possible causes of the decreased plasma volume.

C. If the RBC mass is elevated, test arterial blood gases for Hb O_2 saturation. When saturation is <90%, hypoxia may be causing increased erythropoietin production and secondary polycythemia. In some patients, hypoxia occurs only at night, but this is sufficient to elevate erythropoietin levels and cause polycythemia. Nighttime blood gas or oximeter readings may clarify this problem. Regardless of the cause, elevation of Hb levels to above normal is generally considered to result in unfavorable rheology for O_2 delivery. Supplemental O_2 should be provided if indicated to lower the erythropoietin stimulus. Right-to-left cardiac shunts can also cause decreased blood O_2 content and polycythemia, but usually present in childhood.

D. When plasma erythropoietin levels are increased in the absence of hypoxia, consider localized hypoxia within the kidney or impaired O_2 delivery. Renal cysts and tumors can cause compression of intrarenal vessels and local hypoxia, leading to increased renal elaboration of erythropoietin. Ultrasonography or CT of the kidneys is usually diagnostic, but in occasional patients arteriography is necessary. Certain rare tumors can also produce erythropoietin, such as hepatomas or cerebellar hemangiomas. Rarely, uterine fibromas have also been associated with this finding. Secondary polycythemia can occur with normal erythropoietin levels in chronic hypoxia or oxyhemoglobin desaturation. During the initial response to hypoxia, erythropoietin levels are elevated, but once steady-state erythrocytosis is achieved, the erythropoietin levels required to maintain an elevated Hb level may fall within the normal assay range.

E. Abnormal Hb levels that result in reduced O_2 unloading in tissues also cause tissue hypoxia and increased erythropoietin production. The most common cause is probably increased carboxyhemoglobin levels due to CO_2 in cigarette smoke. Carboxyhemoglobin levels >6% can cause increased Hb levels. Unusual congenital Hb levels also release O_2 poorly and cause polycythemia. Both result in a shift in the oxyhemoglobin dissociation curve and an increased O_2 concentration at which 50% O_2 delivery (P-50) occurs.

F. Patients with normal plasma erythropoietin levels and increased RBC mass have "autonomous erythropoiesis," usually polycythemia vera (PV). In many cases, the diagnosis remains unconfirmed. The Polycythemia Vera Study Group (PVSG) proposed criteria for diagnosis of PV. In concept, these criteria are based on clinical findings indicating a multilineage myeloproliferative disorder. A normal arterial O_2 saturation is assumed, since in the presence of hypoxia, increased erythropoiesis can never be definitively described as autonomous. An increased RBC mass is also required. If these findings are noted in a patient with a palpable spleen (major criteria), the diagnosis of PV is established. If a palpable spleen is absent, an increased RBC mass in the presence of persistently increased leukocyte alkaline phosphatase (LAP), platelet, or WBC counts or evidence of increased WBC turnover is accepted. Both the elevated vitamin B_{12} level and elevated B_{12}-binding capacity (transcobalamin) result from increased WBC membrane turnover, and are thus indirect indices of increased WBC proliferation. The major criteria of increased RBC mass and two of these minor criteria are considered diagnostic. However, many patients presenting with PV do not meet such criteria. Some present after GI bleeding and may have initially reduced Hb levels. Others may lack the full diagnostic criteria, but require therapy because of the unfavorable rheologic effects of polycythemia. Presenting symptoms of polycythemia are nonspecific and reflect increased blood viscosity. These include headaches, plethora, and fatigue. Occasional patients present with major thrombotic events such as stroke or myocardial infarction, and some with bleeding manifestations. Such patients should not undergo surgery until polycythemia has been corrected. For reasons that have not been fully elucidated, polycythemia per se results in a bleeding diathesis. Platelet dysfunction may exacerbate this problem in PV but is usually normal at initial presentation. PV is managed with phlebotomy to reduce Hb levels to normal. Patients treated with phlebotomy alone show an increased incidence of thrombotic events early in the disease

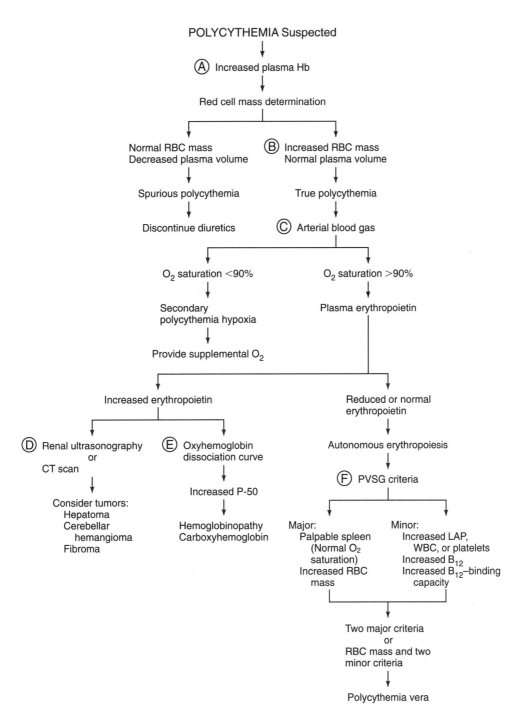

POLYCYTHEMIA Suspected

Ⓐ Increased plasma Hb

Red cell mass determination

Normal RBC mass   Ⓑ Increased RBC mass
Decreased plasma volume   Normal plasma volume

Spurious polycythemia   True polycythemia

Discontinue diuretics   Ⓒ Arterial blood gas

O₂ saturation <90%   O₂ saturation >90%

Secondary   Plasma erythropoietin
polycythemia hypoxia

Provide supplemental O₂

Increased erythropoietin   Reduced or normal
                                   erythropoietin

Ⓓ Renal ultrasonography   Ⓔ Oxyhemoglobin   Autonomous erythropoiesis
   or   dissociation curve
   CT scan   Ⓕ PVSG criteria
                              Increased P-50

Consider tumors: Major: Minor:
Hepatoma   Hemoglobinopathy   Palpable spleen   Increased LAP,
Cerebellar   Carboxyhemoglobin (Normal O₂   WBC, or platelets
  hemangioma   saturation)   Increased B₁₂
Fibroma   Increased RBC   Increased B₁₂–binding
                                                  mass   capacity

                                                 Two major criteria
                                                 or
                                                 RBC mass and two
                                                 minor criteria

                                                 Polycythemia vera

course. The addition of alkylating agents to phlebotomy reduces thrombotic events but results in increased late transformation to acute leukemia. In recent years the antimetabolite hydroxyurea has been used instead of alkylating agents. No controlled trials have examined the effects of hydroxyurea on the natural history of PV, but retrospective studies suggest that it does not increase leukemia transformation. Recently, a new agent with profound effects on platelet production, angrelide, has been used to control elevated platelet counts in PV and other myeloproliferative disorders, but experience with this agent is limited.

References

Golde DW, et al. Polycythemia: mechanisms and management. Ann Intern Med 1981; 95:71.

Kaplan ME, et al. Long-term management of polycythemia vera with hydroxyurea: a progress report. Semin Hematol 1986; 23:167.

Nissenson AR, et al. Recombinant human erythropoietin and renal anemia: molecular biology, clinical efficacy, and nervous system effects. Ann Intern Med 1991; 114:402.

Silverstein MN, et al. Angrelide: a new drug for treating thrombocytosis. N Engl J Med 1988; 318:1292.

Wasserman LR. Polycythemia vera study group: a historical perspective. Semin Hematol 1986; 23:183.

LEUKOCYTOSIS

Robert M. Rifkin, M.D.

Increases in the number of circulating leukocytes may represent either a primary disorder of WBC production or a secondary response to an underlying disease. Leukocytosis should be defined in terms of population normal values for age. Abnormal elevations in the mature neutrophil count represent the most common cause of leukocytosis.

A. Neutrophilia is best defined as an elevation in the absolute neutrophil count by >2 standard deviations above the mean value for normal individuals.

B. Initially, laboratory error should be excluded as the cause of neutrophilia. With the advent of electronic blood cell counting, human error has virtually been eliminated. Blood counts that do not make sense in the context of clinical history must be repeated. Factitious leukocytosis may result from blood sampling problems (inadequate anticoagulant). In this instance, the WBC count is rarely increased by >10% and is accompanied by a spurious thrombocytopenia. In cryoglobulinemia, a temperature-dependent increase in the WBC and platelet counts occurs when various sizes of precipitated cryoglobulin particles begin to clump.

C. The work-up of neutrophilia begins with a thorough history and physical examination to search for an underlying disease state. Neutrophilia commonly results from an acute or chronic inflammatory process. A bone marrow examination often provides little useful information except in certain patients in whom direct invasion of the bone marrow is suspected. Bone marrow biopsy and culture may be helpful when chronic infections (fungal or mycobacterial) are suspected. In the asymptomatic patient with very mild neutrophilia, remember that the WBC count in 2.5% of the general population must be >2 standard deviations above the mean. Since regulation of the neutrophil count is genetically controlled, examination of siblings and family members is often helpful in these difficult cases.

D. Neutrophilia is best classified as either acute or chronic. In normal individuals the neutrophil count varies diurnally with the serum cortisol level; both levels peak in the late afternoon. Neutrophil counts also rise slightly after meals, with postural changes, and with emotional stimuli. These changes are not sufficient to cause a significant change in the total WBC count.

E. Acute neutrophilia may result from a wide variety of physical and emotional stimuli, including cold, heat, exercise, seizures, pain, labor, surgery, panic, and rage. Many localized and systemic bacterial, mycotic, and viral infections may result in acute neutrophilia. Inflammation and tissue necrosis from burns, electrical shocks, trauma, gout, collagen vascular disease, and activation of complement frequently are responsible for rises in the neutrophil count. Epinephrine, endotoxin, corticosteroids, venoms, and vaccines are not infrequent causes of leukocytosis. Finally, the newly released colony stimulating factors (G-CSF and GM-CSF) also elicit a striking acute neutrophilia.

F. Chronic neutrophilia may result from persistence of any of the infections that cause acute neutrophilia. Long-standing inflammatory states, including rheumatoid arthritis, gout, vasculitis, myositis, colitis, dermatitis, periodontitis, and drug reactions, may produce puzzling chronic neutrophilia. Nonhematologic malignancies are often associated with chronic neutrophilia. These include carcinomas of the stomach, lung, breast, kidney, liver, pancreas, and uterus. Lymphomas (Hodgkin's and non-Hodgkin's), brain tumors, melanoma, and myeloma are rare causes of neutrophilia. Certain metabolic diseases, including eclampsia, thyroid storm, and excess corticosteroid states, regularly produce neutrophilia. Benign hematologic disorders may also cause chronic neutrophilia. These include rebound from agranulocytosis or therapy for megaloblastic anemia, chronic hemolysis, asplenia, and chronic idiopathic leukocytosis. Malignant hematologic diseases such as chronic myelogenous leukemia and other myeloproliferative disorders must also be considered as causes of the chronic neutrophilia. The neutrophil alkaline phosphatase score is elevated in infectious causes of neutrophilia, variable in myeloproliferative states, and depressed in chronic myelogenous leukemia. Down syndrome and familial hyperleukocytosis are rare causes of chronic neutrophilia.

References

Appelbaum FR. The clinical use of hematopoietic growth factors. Semin Hematol 1989; 26:(3 Suppl 3):7.

Coates T, Baehner R. Leukocytosis and leukopenia. In: Hoffman R, Benz EJ, Shattil SJ, et al, eds. Hematology: basic principles and practice. New York: Churchill Livingstone, 1991:552.

Dale DC. Neutrophilia. In: Williams WJ, Beutler E, Erslev AJ, Lichtman MA, eds. Hematology. 4th ed. New York: McGraw-Hill, 1990:816.

Jandl JH. Blood—textbook of hematology. Boston: Little, Brown, 1987:441.

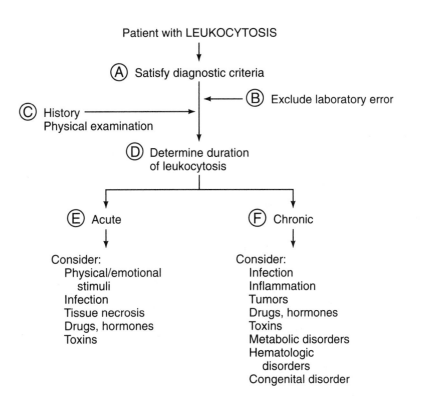

Patient with LEUKOCYTOSIS

Ⓐ Satisfy diagnostic criteria

Ⓑ Exclude laboratory error

Ⓒ History
Physical examination

Ⓓ Determine duration
of leukocytosis

Ⓔ Acute

Consider:
   Physical/emotional
      stimuli
   Infection
   Tissue necrosis
   Drugs, hormones
   Toxins

Ⓕ Chronic

Consider:
   Infection
   Inflammation
   Tumors
   Drugs, hormones
   Toxins
   Metabolic disorders
   Hematologic
      disorders
   Congenital disorder

LEUKOPENIA

William H. Kreisle, M.D.
Manuel Modiano, M.D.

In adults, leukopenia is defined as a total WBC count <3700 cells/mm^3. Most cases are due to absolute neutropenia (<2500 cells/mm^3); rare cases are secondary to absolute lymphopenia (<1000 cells/mm^3).

A. Initial evaluation should include a thorough history and physical examination. Special attention should be given to the use of drugs and the presence of adenopathy, splenomegaly, ecchymoses, petechiae, and signs of infection. CBC, differential, and platelet counts are essential to determine absolute neutrophil and lymphocyte counts and to rule out any accompanying anemia or thrombocytopenia. The blood smear provides important information concerning RBC and WBC morphology. The results of these tests frequently lead to specific diagnoses.

B. Neutropenic patients usually present with signs and symptoms of infection that are often life threatening. Fever in the absence of localizing signs of infection is common. After obtaining cultures, start broad-spectrum antibiotics immediately.

C. Isolated neutropenia and pancytopenia can occur with many commonly used noncytotoxic drugs (e.g., penicillins, sulfonamides, phenothiazines, diuretics), alkylating agents, antimetabolites, and other neoplastic agents. If physical examination and laboratory tests are negative for a neoplastic or hematologic disorder, stop the drug and observe the patient with frequent blood counts. Perform a bone marrow biopsy and aspirate if the neutropenia fails to resolve in 5–7 days or if blood counts continue to decline.

D. Disorders leading to splenomegaly with splenic sequestration can cause neutropenia, but there is usually associated thrombocytopenia. Differential diagnosis includes cirrhosis, sarcoidosis, glycogen storage diseases, and other uncommon conditions.

E. If the bone marrow result is unremarkable and there is no evidence of splenomegaly or an autoimmune disorder, consider rare chronic neutropenic states.

Observe the patient with serial blood counts to document the neutropenic pattern.

F. Most cases of neutropenia are associated with anemia and/or thrombocytopenia. Unless a drug is strongly suspected as the cause, perform a bone marrow biopsy and aspirate to rule out a primary hematologic disorder that requires prompt treatment.

G. If the only bone marrow abnormality is the absence of mature granulocytes, this suggests maturation arrest or autoimmune destruction. Perform a work-up for an autoimmune disorder. If available, an antineutrophil antibody assay can be helpful.

H. Infections that can cause neutropenia with anemia and/or thrombocytopenia include viruses (Epstein-Barr, cytomegalovirus, HIV, hepatitis, measles); bacteria (severe; gram-negative and gram-positive organisms); *Mycobacterium*, typhoid fever, malaria; and fungi. Bone marrow should be cultured as part of an extensive work-up for infection.

I. Lymphopenia without associated neutropenia is uncommon. Most cases are secondary to drugs (e.g., steroids), radiation injury, or renal failure. Some viral infections, particularly HIV, can also cause absolute lymphopenia.

References

Dale DC. Neutrophil disorders: benign, quantitative abnormalities of neutrophils. In: Williams WJ, ed. Hematology. 4th ed. New York: McGraw-Hill, 1990:807.

Logue GL, Schimm DS. Autoimmune granulocytopenia. Annu Rev Med 1980; 31:191.

Murphy MF, Metcalf P, et al. Incidence and mechanism of neutropenia and thrombocytopenia in patients with human immunodeficiency virus infection. Br J Haematol 1987; 66:337.

Vincent PC. Drug-induced aplastic anemia and agranulocytosis. Incidence and mechanisms. Drugs 1986; 31:52.

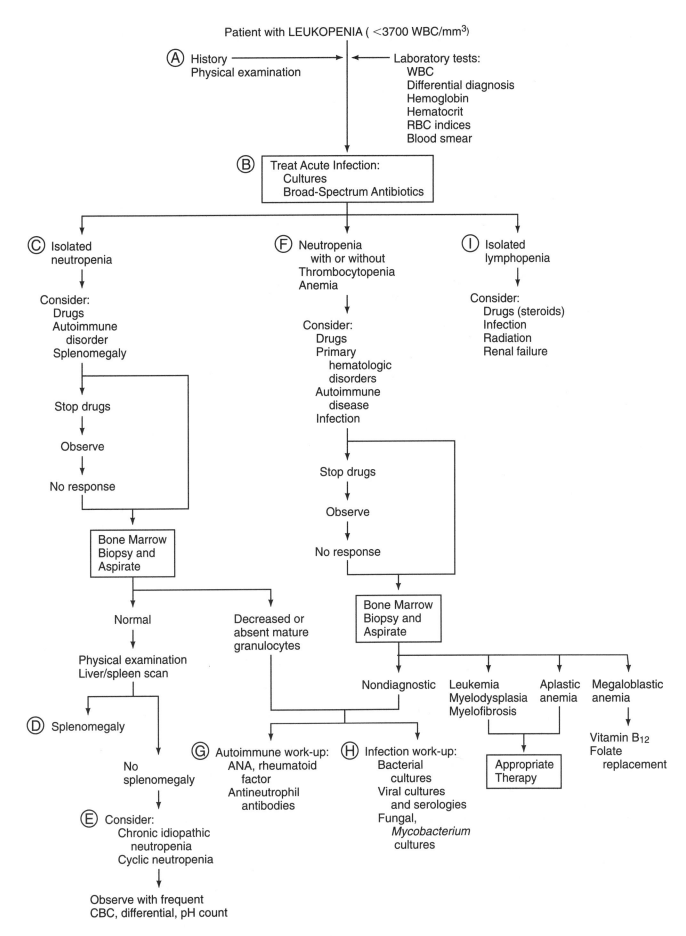

Patient with LEUKOPENIA (<3700 WBC/mm³)

Ⓐ History ——————→ ←—— Laboratory tests:
Physical examination | WBC
| Differential diagnosis
| Hemoglobin
| Hematocrit
| RBC indices
| Blood smear

Ⓑ Treat Acute Infection:
Cultures
Broad-Spectrum Antibiotics

Ⓒ Isolated   Ⓕ Neutropenia   Ⓘ Isolated
neutropenia   with or without   lymphopenia
Thrombocytopenia
Anemia

Consider: Consider: Consider:
Drugs   Drugs   Drugs (steroids)
Autoimmune   Primary   Infection
disorder   hematologic   Radiation
Splenomegaly   disorders   Renal failure
Autoimmune
disease
Infection

Stop drugs   Stop drugs

Observe   Observe

No response   No response

Bone Marrow
Biopsy and
Aspirate   Bone Marrow
Biopsy and
Aspirate

Normal   Decreased or
absent mature
granulocytes

Physical examination   Nondiagnostic   Leukemia   Aplastic   Megaloblastic
Liver/spleen scan   Myelodysplasia anemia   anemia
Myelofibrosis

Ⓓ Splenomegaly   Vitamin B₁₂
Folate
replacement

No   Ⓖ Autoimmune work-up: Ⓗ Infection work-up: Appropriate
splenomegaly   ANA, rheumatoid   Bacterial   Therapy
factor   cultures
Antineutrophil   Viral cultures
Ⓔ Consider: antibodies   and serologies
Chronic idiopathic   Fungal,
neutropenia   Mycobacterium
Cyclic neutropenia   cultures

Observe with frequent
CBC, differential, pH count

DISSEMINATED INTRAVASCULAR COAGULATION

Raymond Taetle, M.D.

A. A wide variety of diseases, infections, and circulatory abnormalities initiate diffuse clotting within vessels. In many cases this may occur through tissue factor activation of the extrinsic clotting pathways, but other mechanisms are possible. These reactions share a common pathophysiology resulting from continuous clotting activation, consumption of clotting factors and platelets, and lysis of the generated fibrin. The clinical manifestations of disseminated intravascular coagulation (DIC) vary from diffuse hemorrhagic diathesis to clotting, depending on the balance between clot generation, consumption, and clot lysis. This algorithm considers the evaluation of acute DIC resulting in a diffuse hemorrhagic diathesis (more than three bleeding sites). However, clotting within vessels is extremely important in the pathogenesis of this syndrome. Even in acute DIC when most clinical manifestations are due to hemorrhage, substantial organ damage may occur from microvascular thrombosis. In settings such as advanced metastatic adenocarcinoma, patients may present with veno-occlusive or, more rarely, arterial occlusive disease. This chronic DIC (Trousseau's syndrome) results from slow, continuous activation of clotting, presumably from tissue factor elaboration by tumor. Classically, these patients present with migratory superficial thrombophlebitis, but have varying degrees of thrombocytopenia and circulating fibrin split products (FDP) in plasma. However, excessive bleeding may occur when patients are challenged by surgery or ulcer disease. This chronic form of DIC is mentioned below and may be accompanied by microangiopathic hemolytic anemia (MAHA). In contrast to the situation displayed in the algorithm, such patients may have short in vitro prothrombin (PT) and partial thromboplastin (PTT) times. This results from activated clotting factors in plasma causing rapid activation of clotting in vitro. It is sometimes very difficult to obtain blood from such patients, since clotting occurs in the syringe or tube before calcium chelation can render plasma unclottable.

B. Most patients with DIC are seen in the setting of diffuse bleeding from venipuncture and other sites. Initial evaluation is directed at defining the origin of the hemorrhagic diathesis. Initial screening tests consist of PT, PTT, and platelets. If these tests are normal, bleeding must result from excessive activation of plasmin clot lysis, or from platelet dysfunction. Deficiencies of alpha$_2$-antiplasmin can cause a lifelong hemorrhagic diathesis. Recently, acquired cases of selective alpha$_2$-antiplasmin deficiency have been described. In the future, other acquired deficiencies of clot lysis will be documented. Platelet abnormalities are indicated by an abnormal bleeding time and/or abnormal platelet in vitro function.

C. A dramatic, isolated increase in PT sufficient to cause diffuse bleeding indicates an abnormality in the extrinsic pathway. A quick screen for the presence of inhibitors can be performed by mixing patient plasma 1:1 with normal, pooled plasma and repeating the test. Correction (usually to within 1.5 seconds) indicates clotting factor deficiency. Failure to correct the PT suggests an acquired inhibitor of coagulation. Such inhibitors are uncommonly detected by the PT, but large quantities of heparin can cause this finding. Much more common are factor deficiencies due to liver disease or vitamin K deficiency. Less commonly, surreptitious ingestion of coumarin or previously undetected congenital clotting factor deficiencies may be considered.

D. The differential diagnosis for a prolonged PTT is similar, except that this test is much more sensitive to the presence of inhibitors. The most common source of this finding is heparin administration. However, acquired inhibitors of coagulation factors such as factor VIII can cause severe bleeding. PTT is generally less affected by liver disease and vitamin K deficiency than PT.

E. Decreased platelets alone can cause severe bleeding, usually mucocutaneous. Myelophthisic processes or aplasia can cause severe thrombocytopenia but are usually obvious from other blood findings. The peripheral blood smear should be examined for fragmented RBC (MAHA) to rule out thrombotic thrombocytopenic purpura (TTP) or hemolytic uremic syndrome (HUS). MAHA may also occur in DIC but is accompanied by prolonged clotting times and increased FDP, findings usually absent in TTP. A normal peripheral smear and short clotting times may suggest chronic DIC. A normal smear or one with large platelets suggests immune thrombocytopenia, which can be confirmed by assays for specific antiplatelet antibodies.

F. When both PT and PTT are significantly prolonged and the platelet count is depressed, DIC is strongly indicated. When the platelet count is normal, consider a primary abnormality in fibrinogen.

G. DIC is confirmed by detecting products of fibrin degradation in plasma. These tests include immunologic assays for FDP and new assays for fibrin that has been crosslinked by factor XIII and then subjected to plasmin lysis. These D-D dimer fragments are highly specific for clot lysis and correlate closely with other FDP measurements. Immunologic assays for FDP are highly sensitive; the D-D dimer test has a lower sensitivity but greater specificity. Optimal sensitivity and specificity is achieved by using FDP assays as screens and confirming DIC with D-D dimer assays.

DISSEMINATED INTRAVASCULAR COAGULATION Suspected

A. Diffuse hemorrhagic diathesis

B. Normal PT, PTT, platelets
→ Clot lysis
→ Consider: Clot lysis abnormality, Platelet abnormality

C. Increased PT
→ 1:1 PT
- Normal → Factor assays → Factor deficiency → Consider: Congenital Vitamin K deficiency, Coumarin ingestion, Liver disease
- Abnormal → Inhibitor → Consider: Heparin antibody

D. Increased PTT
→ 1:1 PTT
- Normal → Factor assays → Factor deficiency → Consider: Congenital Vitamin K deficiency
- Abnormal → Inhibitor → Consider: Heparin antibody

E. Decreased platelets (p 198)
→ Blood smear
- MAHA → TTP HUS
- RBC normal → Consider: Chronic DIC → Platelet antibody → ITP

F. Increased PT, PTT
→ Platelet count
- Decreased → G. FDP, Fibrinogen, thrombin time → DIC
- Normal → H. Fibrinogen, thrombin time, FDP → Consider: Abnormal fibrinogen, Primary fibrinolysis, Snake bite, Severe liver disease

The protamine paracoagulation phenomenon (3P) test measures the presence of fibrin monomer that has been generated in plasma but inhibited from clotting by the presence of high-molecular-weight FDP. This test is also highly specific for continuous, activated clotting and lysis. Because of clotting factor consumption during DIC, factor VIII levels are usually depressed and may be used as a confirmatory test. However, factor VIII is an acute-phase reactant and may be near-normal in the early stages of DIC. The continuous fibrin generation results in secondary activation of plasmin and the generation of FDP. Consumption and clotting factor destruction also consumes anticoagulant proteins, such as antithrombin (AT) III and protein C. ATIII levels are useful as a confirmatory test for DIC, and the depression in ATIII may play an important role in microthrombosis. Transfusions of ATIII have been reported to ameliorate the clinical manifestations of DIC, but experience with this therapy is limited. Treatment of DIC is directed at eliminating the underlying disease. Without correction of the inciting process, other interventions are unlikely to affect patient outcome significantly.

H. When PT and PTT are abnormal and platelet counts are normal, fibrinogen levels and thrombin time should be assessed. Reduced levels of factors VII, V, X, and fibrinogen, with normal factor VIII levels, suggest severe liver disease. Rarely, plasmin is activated without initiation of clotting. This "primary fibrinolysis" may be seen in patients with liver disease and some tumors. Fibrinogen and fibrin are consumed and FDP thus generated, but other clotting factor levels are normal. However, because clotting is not initiated, fibrin will not be crosslinked and the D-D dimer assay should also be normal. Certain snake venoms also contain materials that lyse fibrinogen without initiating DIC. (Note that DIC can also occur with some snake envenomation.) If fibrinogen levels are normal or FDP absent, and the thrombin time is either long or short, fibrinogen levels may be abnormal.

References

Bick RL. Disseminated intravascular coagulation and related syndromes. Semin Thromb Hemost 1988; 14:299.

Meehan J, et al. Diagnosis of disseminated intravascular coagulation. Am J Clin Pathol 1989; 91:280.

Pinzon R, et al. Pancreatic carcinoma and Trousseau's syndrome: experience at a large cancer center. J Clin Oncol 1986; 4:509.

Wilde JT, et al. Plasma D-dimer levels and their relationship to serum fibrinogen/fibrin degradation products in hypercoagulable states. Br J Haematol 1989; 71:65.

DEEP VENOUS THROMBOSIS

Guillermo Gonzalez-Osete, M.D.
Manuel Modiano, M.D.

Deep venous thrombosis (DVT) is caused by intravascular deposits of predominantly fibrin, RBCs, platelets, and WBC components, accumulating in a vein and producing obstruction to venous outflow, vessel wall inflammation, or both. The clinical manifestations depend on the severity of these inflammatory processes. Often the initial sign is a pulmonary embolus (PE).

A. Detailed history taking should look for previous episodes and for inherited disorders of protein C and S deficiency or antithrombin (AT) III deficiency. With such deficiencies there is a strong family history of recurrent DVT or PE that presents at an early age; >80% of patients with protein C deficiency have had an episode of DVT or PE by age 40. Patients with AT III deficiency have a similar presentation and also may have a history of failure to be anticoagulated with heparin. Obtain a complete drug and medication history, including use of estrogen or oral contraceptives. A history of frequent abortions with a prolonged partial thromboplastin time (PTT) should make one suspect a lupus anticoagulant. This is also present in some collagen vascular diseases such as systemic lupus erythematosus (p 194). Surgery that requires >30 min and certain surgical procedures (orthopedics; those involving trauma to lower limbs, e.g., knee surgery; urologic; gynecologic) are associated with increased incidence of DVT. Other risk factors are trauma, pregnancy, puerperium, congestive heart failure (CHF), myocardial infarction, cerebrovascular accidents, extremity paralysis, malignancy (especially of prostate or pancreas), obesity, varicose veins, immobilization, use of estrogens, and age. All of these may increase the risk of DVT by stasis and/or increased activation of coagulation.

B. Pain is present in approximately 50% of patients with DVT. Swelling and tenderness to compression are also found in 75% of patients. The clinical diagnosis of DVT is not accurate. Thrombosis does not always produce complete obstruction or inflammation. In 30% of patients who present with pain and swelling, there is proven DVT. The classic Homan sign (discomfort in the calf muscles on forced dorsiflexion of the foot) is not sensitive. It is noted in 33% of patients with positive venography and 50% with negative venography. Unilateral swelling associated with discoloration is an important sign that should alert one to the diagnosis.

C. The differential diagnosis includes ruptured Baker's cyst, muscle tear, cramp, hematoma, arthritis, bone disease, varicose veins, and postphlebitic syndrome. If no cause is apparent, consider noninvasive screening.

D. When the history and physical examination suggest DVT, ancillary tests such as noninvasive impedance plethysmography and duplex ultrasound or invasive tests such as ^{125}I and contrast xenography will corroborate the diagnosis. Laboratory tests should include platelet count, prothrombin time (PT), and PTT.

E. Noninvasive diagnostic tests available are impedance plethysmography (IPG) and duplex ultrasonography (D-US). IPG is good for detecting proximal vein thrombosis and/or recurrent DVT but is insensitive for detecting nonobstructive proximal thrombosis and calf vein thrombosis. Its sensitivity is 83–93%; its specificity is 83–90%. It must be repeated serially to increase its sensitivity. False-positive results may occur with CHF, postoperative leg swelling, excessive leg tension, or external compression. D-US (sensitivity, 95%; specificity, 98%) is the ideal method of screening patients with suspected DVT. It is good for detecting proximal but not calf vein thrombosis. Calf vein thrombosis usually requires no treatment other than bed rest and elevation of the extremity. In 20–30% of cases, however, the thrombus may extend into the popliteal vein, and full anticoagulation is required because of the increased incidence of PE. Extension into the popliteal system is often missed on initial noninvasive tests, but may be seen if the examination is repeated after 3–5 days.

F. Iodine-125 with fibrinogen detects only altered blood flow, so nonoccluding thrombi may be missed. It detects calf vein thrombosis in 90% of cases and proximal vein thrombosis in 60–80%. Fibrinogen carries with it the risks of using any blood product, including allergic reactions and transmittal of infections. It is contraindicated in iodine allergy, pregnancy, and lactation. The combined approach of ^{125}I and IPG was positive in 81 of 86 patients with positive venograms; both tests were negative in 104 of 114 patients who had a negative venogram. This is a useful approach if DVT is suspected clinically and ^{125}I is inconclusive. Venography is the gold standard but is invasive, is not always available, and may not visualize the deep venous system. It may itself cause a DVT.

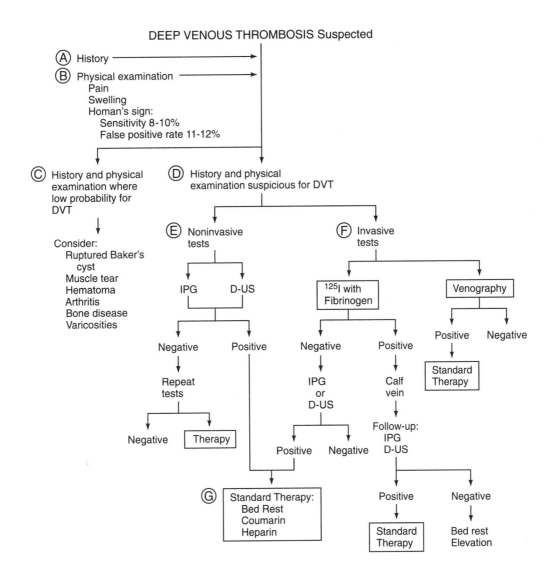

DEEP VENOUS THROMBOSIS Suspected

Ⓐ History

Ⓑ Physical examination
    Pain
    Swelling
    Homan's sign:
        Sensitivity 8-10%
        False positive rate 11-12%

Ⓒ History and physical examination where low probability for DVT

Consider:
    Ruptured Baker's cyst
    Muscle tear
    Hematoma
    Arthritis
    Bone disease
    Varicosities

Ⓓ History and physical examination suspicious for DVT

Ⓔ Noninvasive tests — IPG, D-US
  Negative → Repeat tests → Negative / Therapy
  Positive → Standard Therapy

Ⓕ Invasive tests — ^{125}I with Fibrinogen, Venography
  ^{125}I with Fibrinogen:
    Negative → IPG or D-US → Positive / Negative
    Positive → Calf vein → Follow-up: IPG, D-US → Positive → Standard Therapy / Negative → Bed rest, Elevation
  Venography:
    Positive → Standard Therapy / Negative

Ⓖ Standard Therapy:
    Bed Rest
    Coumarin
    Heparin

G. If the diagnosis is confirmed, begin treatment. Standard treatment includes IV or subcutaneous heparin, oral anticoagulants, bed rest, and extremity elevation. Patients with protein C deficiency may have skin necrosis and increased sensitivity to coumarin. Start therapy with IV heparin bolus, 1000–5000 U, followed by continuous infusion of heparin, approximately 1000 U/hr or 800–10,000 U subcutaneous heparin over 6–8 hr. Monitor activated PTT at 6 hr and thereafter until stabilized at 1.5–2 times control values. Obtain a baseline platelet count and monitor every 3 days while the patient is on heparin. Begin warfarin sodium on the first day by instituting the estimated daily maintenance dose (5–10 mg). Maintain PT at 1.3–1.5 times control. It usually takes 72–96 hr for the PT to reach this range, and heparin should be continued until the PT is at this level. Treatment should last at least 12 weeks. Patients with factor deficiency should be treated indefinitely.

References

Carter C, Gent M, Leclerc J. Epidemiology of venous thrombosis. In: Colman RW, Hirsh J, Marder, Salzman, eds. Hemostasis and thrombosis. 2nd ed. Philadelphia: JB Lippincott, 1987:1185.

Hull RD, Hirsh J. Natural history and clinical features of venous thrombosis. In: Colman RW, Hirsh J, Marder, Salzman, eds. Hemostasis and thrombosis. 2nd ed. Philadelphia: JB Lippincott, 1987:1208.

Hull RD, Secker-Walker R, Hirsh J. Diagnosis of deep vein thrombosis. In: Colman RW, Hirsh J, Marder, Salzman, eds. Hemostasis and thrombosis. 2nd ed. Philadelphia: JB Lippincott, 1987:1220.

Hull RD, et al. Heparin for 5 days as compared with 10 days in the initial treatment of proximal venous thrombosis. N Engl J Med 1990; 322:1260.

Hyers T, Hull RD, Weg J. Antithrombotic therapy for venous thromboembolic disease. Chest 1989; 95:37s.

White R, McGahan JP, Daschbach M, Hartling RP. Diagnosis of deep vein thrombosis using duplex ultrasound. Ann Intern Med 1989; 111:297.

COAGULATION ABNORMALITIES

Manuel Modiano, M.D.

A. Blood coagulation represents conversion of the soluble extended plasma protein fibrinogen into an insoluble fibrillar polymer, fibrin. It is the end result of complex serial reactions involving procoagulant proteins that circulate in plasma as inert precursors until converted sequentially by specific chain reactions to their active forms. Factors are numbered not by the order in which they become activated, but by the order in which they were discovered. The partial thromboplastin time (PTT) measures the intrinsic pathway of coagulation, including the final common pathway, and the conversion of fibrinogen to fibrin. The test is very sensitive to deficiencies of factors XII, XI, IX, and VII and somewhat less so to deficiencies of factors V and X, prothrombin (factor II), and fibrinogen (factor I).

B. When confronted with a prolonged clotting time, first take a careful history, including previous bleeding or bruising, spontaneously or after surgery or trauma. A family history of bleeding and a complete list of medications being taken (prescription or not) are essential. Confirm that platelets are normal by count and bleeding time (if not, see p 198).

C. Patients with a history of bleeding disorders often know the etiologic factors and corrective measures taken in the past. If so, correct the situation as before (if possible, check with patients' regular physician for dose and type of factor correction) or refer them to a hematologist.

D. When the cause is unknown or when there is no history of bleeding, first confirm the abnormality of the coagulation times, especially if there has been no previous bleeding with trauma or major surgery. Again, a detailed history, including medications, and a full physical examination are essential.

E. When repeating the test, it is useful to perform mixing studies in which the patient's plasma and serum are combined in an equal mixture with that from a normal control.

F. When coagulation times do not correct with mixing studies, it is usually because inhibitors are present.

Factor inhibition may be chemical, as with the presence of heparin or protamine, or immune. The acquired anticoagulants may appear in persons who do not have hemophilia or other hereditary disorders of coagulation and who have never received factor replacement therapy. Most of these anticoagulants are autoantibodies directed against specific factors, the most common of which are autoantibodies against factor VIII. These latter may arise during or after pregnancy, in autoimmune disorders (including systemic lupus erythematosus [SLE]), during allergic reactions to drugs, or in otherwise healthy persons. The presence of autoantibodies after one pregnancy is not predictive of complications in future pregnancies. They usually disappear within 12–18 months and tend never to reappear. Treatment of bleeding may require corticosteroids and, at times, factor VIII. Hematology consultation is recommended. Inhibitors to factors V, IX, and XIII have also been described.

G. The lupus anticoagulant is a misleading term: it rarely if ever interferes with hemostasis, most patients with a lupus anticoagulant do not have SLE, and only 5–10% of patients with SLE have the anticoagulant. This anticoagulant is manifested clinically by repeated thrombotic episodes. Lupus anticoagulant antibody appears to enhance platelet adhesiveness and to suppress prostacyclin synthesis by vascular tissue. This action leads to platelet adhesion to endothelium, vascular obstruction, and finally thrombosis. Look for lupus anticoagulant activity in all patients with unexplained thrombotic complications or repeated fetal loss. Suppression of antibody levels with prednisone, combined with aspirin inhibition of platelet cyclooxygenase, appears to diminish thrombotic episodes; if started early in pregnancy it may also reduce fetal loss in women at risk. Hematology consultation is advised.

H. When coagulation times correct with mixing studies, the problem is most likely a deficiency of one of the coagulation factors.

(Continued on page 196)

Patient with ABNORMAL COAGULATION TESTS

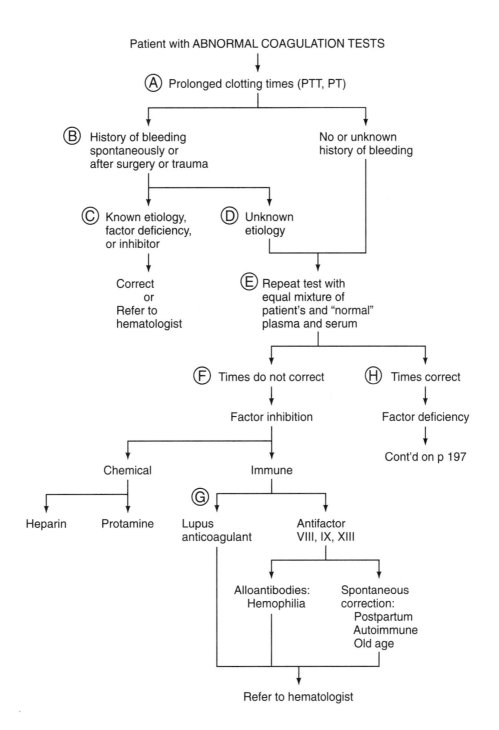

Ⓐ Prolonged clotting times (PTT, PT)

Ⓑ History of bleeding spontaneously or after surgery or trauma

No or unknown history of bleeding

Ⓒ Known etiology, factor deficiency, or inhibitor

Ⓓ Unknown etiology

Correct
or
Refer to hematologist

Ⓔ Repeat test with equal mixture of patient's and "normal" plasma and serum

Ⓕ Times do not correct

Ⓗ Times correct

Factor inhibition

Factor deficiency

Cont'd on p 197

Chemical

Immune

Heparin

Protamine

Ⓖ Lupus anticoagulant

Antifactor VIII, IX, XIII

Alloantibodies: Hemophilia

Spontaneous correction:
Postpartum
Autoimmune
Old age

Refer to hematologist

I. To determine which factors are deficient, quantify the fibrinogen. When fibrinogen levels are normal, elevation of the PTT is usually due to a deficiency of those factors active in the intrinsic coagulation cascade: VII, IX, XI, or XII. Abnormalities in both prothrombin time (PT) and PTT are usually secondary to either a single factor deficiency (prothrombin, factor V, or factor X) or multiple factor deficiencies, usually of the prothrombin (extrinsic) system. If the PT is abnormal and PTT normal, factor VII (extrinsic cascade) deficiency is the usual cause. In these cases, hematology consultation is strongly recommended.

J. When fibrinogen is low, the diagnosis is probably afibrinogenemia and/or multiple factor deficiencies, most often secondary to severe malnutrition, consumptive disorders, or liver disease. This can often be treated with vitamin K.

K. Often, coagulation times correct with plasma but not with serum, or vice versa. This is an extremely useful diagnostic finding. When the PTT corrects with serum but not with plasma, factor IX deficiency is present. Hemophilia B (Christmas disease) is an X-linked hemorrhagic disorder of variable severity caused by a hereditary deficiency in factor IX activity. Hemophilia B is clinically indistinguishable from hemophilia A (factor VIII). Emergency factor replacement can be effected with fresh frozen plasma (FFP), exchange plasmapheresis, or factor IX concentrate (the treatment of choice). The patient should be followed with or by a hematologist.

L. Complete correction of both PTT and PT with serum, not plasma, is due to a deficiency of Factor X.

M. Correction of PTT by plasma, not serum, indicates factor VII deficiency, which is responsible for bleeding in patients with "classic" hemophilia A or von Willebrand's disease. Hemophilia A is a lifelong bleeding disorder transmitted by a faulty gene on the X chromosome; thus, only males are affected clinically, whereas females are carriers. It is the most common severe coagulation disorder. Treatment should be coordinated with an experienced hematologist, but emergency replacement can be done with FFP, cryoprecipitate, or factor VIII concentrates. von Willebrand's disease is the most common and most heterogeneous of heritable defects of coagulation. It arises from qualitative or quantitative deficiency of the adhesive glycoprotein von Willebrand's factor (vWF), a secretory product of endothelial cells and megakaryocytes that is required for platelet adhesion and for stabilization of plasma factor VIII. vWF is controlled by chromosome 12. Discussion of the types and treatment of von Willebrand's disease is beyond the scope of this chapter. Initial treatment can be with DDAVP, which stimulates release of endogenous factor VIII and vWF into the circulation. However, be careful not to treat pseudo-von Willebrand's disease.

N. Factor V deficiency is characterized by correction of PTT and PT with plasma, but not with serum.

References

Ey FS, Goodnight SH. Bleeding disorders in cancer. Semin Oncol 1990; 17:187.

Jandl JH. Disorders of coagulation. In: Blood: textbook of hematology. Boston: Little, Brown, 1987:1095.

Levine M, Hirsh J. The diagnosis and treatment of thrombosis in the cancer patient. Semin Oncol 1990; 17:160.

Patterson WP. Coagulation and cancer: an overview. Semin Oncol 1990; 17:137.

Patterson WP, Caldwell CW, Doll DC. Hyperviscosity syndromes and coagulopathies. Semin Oncol 1990; 17:210.

Patterson WP, Ringenberg QS. The pathophysiology of thrombosis in cancer. Semin Oncol 1990; 17:140.

Rapaport S. Preoperative hemostatic evaluation: which tests, if any? Blood 1983; 61:229.

Schaffer AI. The hypercoagulable states. Ann Intern Med 1985; 102:814.

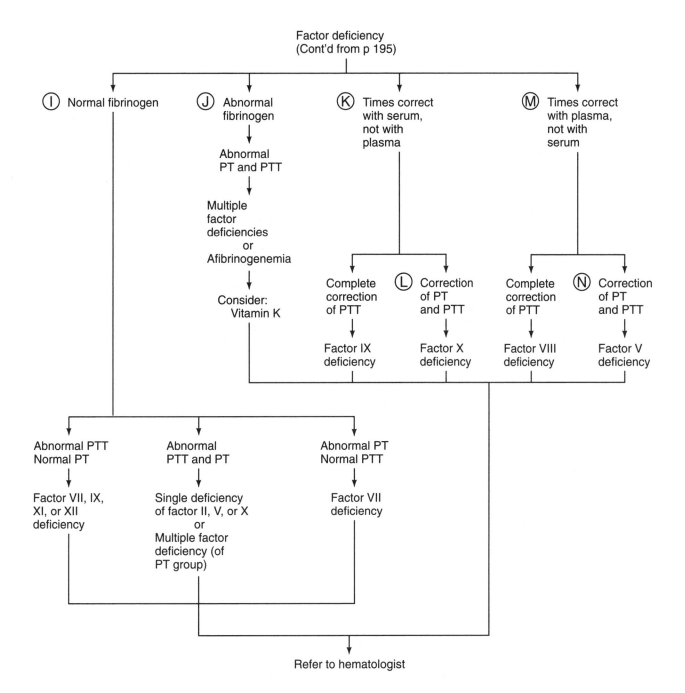

Factor deficiency
(Cont'd from p 195)

(I) Normal fibrinogen

(J) Abnormal fibrinogen
→ Abnormal PT and PTT
→ Multiple factor deficiencies
or
Afibrinogenemia
→ Consider: Vitamin K

(K) Times correct with serum, not with plasma

Complete correction of PTT → Factor IX deficiency

(L) Correction of PT and PTT → Factor X deficiency

(M) Times correct with plasma, not with serum

Complete correction of PTT → Factor VIII deficiency

(N) Correction of PT and PTT → Factor V deficiency

Abnormal PTT
Normal PT
→ Factor VII, IX, XI, or XII deficiency

Abnormal PTT and PT
→ Single deficiency of factor II, V, or X
or
Multiple factor deficiency (of PT group)

Abnormal PT
Normal PTT
→ Factor VII deficiency

Refer to hematologist

TRANSFUSION THERAPY: PLATELETS

June Clements, M.D.
Douglas Huestis, M.D.

Platelet concentrates (PCs) are obtained either from a unit of whole blood (random-donor unit, RDP) or by apheresis (single-donor apheresis unit, SDP). One SDP provides about the same number of platelets as seven RDPs. Platelets are appropriate for transfusion in situations of significant bleeding with a dangerously low platelet count. The risk of serious hemorrhage is low with a platelet count >20,000/μl. Some authors do not advocate transfusions until counts fall below 15,000 or even 10,000/μl. Platelet counts of 60,000-70,000/μl may be necessary for biopsy and/or surgery.

The dosage of PCs depends on the patient's size and clinical disorder. In adults, one RDP should increase the platelet count by 5000-10,000/μl. The dose is one RDP per 10 kg body weight, or one SDP. A 1-hour post-transfusion platelet count is important to assess the response. The following formula provides a corrected count increment:

$$\frac{\text{absolute platelet count increment} \times \text{body surface area (m}^2)}{\text{no. of platelets transfused} \times 10^{11}}$$

A poor response to transfused platelets may be due to alloimmunization, infection, sepsis, drugs, or splenomegaly. Repeated platelet transfusions may necessitate SDPs, which reduce exposure to platelet antigens and decrease the rate of alloimmunization. Previous transfusions and pregnancy may stimulate HLA and antiplatelet antibodies, in which case HLA-matched platelets may be necessary. Leukocyte filters seem to decrease HLA immunization. ABO-incompatible platelets may have a shortened blood survival. It is worth trying ABO-compatible PC for type 0 patients whose counts are refractory to unselected PC.

A. With spontaneous or excessive bleeding and a normal platelet count, suspect functional platelet disorder or factor deficiency. Use appropriate laboratory tests to differentiate between these two. If abnormal platelet function is suspected, examine a blood smear to assess platelet morphology. This may aid in the diagnosis of a hereditary platelet disorder. In such disorders, transfuse filtered SDP to decrease alloimmunization. Platelet transfusions are ineffective in uremic patients.

B. Platelet transfusions are often necessary to control bleeding in patients with decreased platelet production. Start with a dose of one RDP per 10 kg. In patients who may require long-term treatment, such as aplastic anemia, leukemia, and transplantation patients, use SDP units with leukocyte filters to decrease alloimmunization.

C. Transfused platelets usually have a short survival in patients with increased platelet destruction. Treat the underlying cause of the thrombocytopenia. However, with life-threatening bleeding or anticipated surgery, give platelet transfusions. Begin with one RDP per 10 kg or one SDP and follow up according to clinical and platelet response. Do not give PCs in thrombotic thrombocytopenic purpura (TTP) and hemolytic uremic syndrome (HUS).

References

Bishop JF, McGrath K, Wolf MM, et al. Clinical factors influencing the efficacy of pooled platelet transfusions. Blood 1988; 71:383.

Bolan CD, Alving BM. Pharmacologic agents in management of bleeding disorders. Transfusion 1990; 30:541.

George JM, Shattil SJ. The clinical importance of acquired abnormalities of platelet function. N Engl J Med 1991; 324:27.

Harker LA, Malposs TW, Branson HE, et al. Mechanism of abnormal bleeding in patients undergoing cardiopulmonary bypass: acquired transient platelet dysfunction associated with selective oc-granule release. Blood 1980; 56:324.

Kaplan BS, Proesmans W. Hemolytic uremic syndrome of childhood and its variants. Semin Hematol 1987; 24:148.

Welborn JL, Emrich P, Acevedo M. Rapid improvement of thrombotic thrombocytopenic purpura with vencresline and plasmapheresis. Am J Hematol 1990; 35:18.

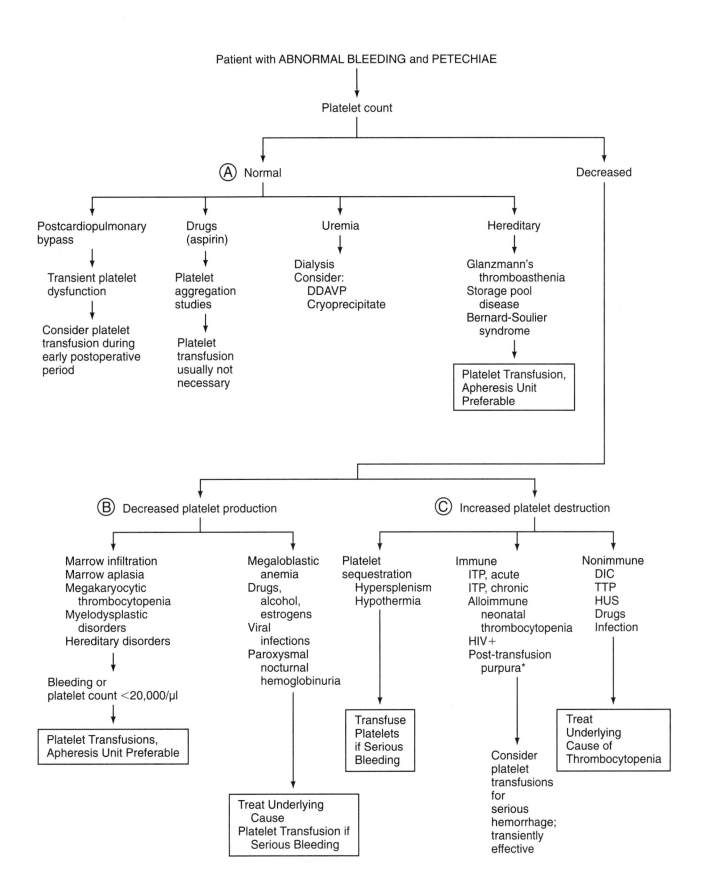

Patient with ABNORMAL BLEEDING and PETECHIAE

Platelet count

Ⓐ Normal

Decreased

Postcardiopulmonary bypass

Transient platelet dysfunction

Consider platelet transfusion during early postoperative period

Drugs (aspirin)

Platelet aggregation studies

Platelet transfusion usually not necessary

Uremia

Dialysis
Consider:
DDAVP
Cryoprecipitate

Hereditary

Glanzmann's thromboasthenia
Storage pool disease
Bernard-Soulier syndrome

Platelet Transfusion, Apheresis Unit Preferable

Ⓑ Decreased platelet production

Marrow infiltration
Marrow aplasia
Megakaryocytic thrombocytopenia
Myelodysplastic disorders
Hereditary disorders

Bleeding or platelet count <20,000/μl

Platelet Transfusions, Apheresis Unit Preferable

Megaloblastic anemia
Drugs, alcohol, estrogens
Viral infections
Paroxysmal nocturnal hemoglobinuria

Treat Underlying Cause
Platelet Transfusion if Serious Bleeding

Ⓒ Increased platelet destruction

Platelet sequestration
Hypersplenism
Hypothermia

Transfuse Platelets if Serious Bleeding

Immune
ITP, acute
ITP, chronic
Alloimmune neonatal thrombocytopenia
HIV+
Post-transfusion purpura*

Consider platelet transfusions for serious hemorrhage; transiently effective

Nonimmune
DIC
TTP
HUS
Drugs
Infection

Treat Underlying Cause of Thrombocytopenia

*Platelet transfusion ineffective.

TRANSFUSION THERAPY: RED BLOOD CELLS

June Clements, M.D.
Douglas Huestis, M.D.

Red blood cells (RBCs) are prepared from a collection of whole blood by removal of plasma. This leaves 250–350 ml RBCs with a hematocrit of 70–75%, containing about 2×10^9 leukocytes. The maximum storage time is 42 days at 1–6° C.

Transfuse RBCs to increase oxygen-carrying capacity or to replace acute blood loss. One unit should increase the hemoglobin in an adult 1 g/dl or increase the hematocrit by 3%. For immunocompromised patients, irradiated RBCs can prevent transfusion-associated graft-versus-host disease. Directed-donor components from first-degree relatives should also be irradiated regardless of the recipient's immune status (see p 204).

The removal of leukocytes by passage through special filters inhibits HLA alloimmunization for patients who will need future platelet support or transplantation. Leukocyte filters can reduce transfused white cells by 99–99.9%. Leukocyte filters also prevent febrile reactions and possibly transfusion-transmitted cytomegalovirus (CMV) infection.

A. Acute hemorrhage due to trauma or GI bleeding may require transfusion of RBCs along with crystalloid solutions.

B. Anemia is not in itself a reason to transfuse RBCs. In patients with chronic anemia, hemoglobins of 6–7 g/dl may be well tolerated. If the patient has clinical signs and symptoms not amenable to specific therapy, transfuse RBCs. Patients with chronic renal failure may respond to erythropoietin therapy. In patients with asymptomatic anemia, investigate and treat the cause. In patients with hemolytic anemia, investigate the cause and treat accordingly. In hereditary hemolytic conditions such as hereditary spherocytosis, splenectomy may be advantageous.

C. Premature infants with compromised pulmonary function may need a hematocrit >40% for adequate oxygen-carrying capacity. Also, in transfusing these infants, consider using either CMV-negative blood components or leukocyte filters.

D. For elective surgery, autologous transfusions (the patient's own blood) are increasingly popular, largely because of increased public awareness of transfusion-associated diseases. Several units of autologous blood can be drawn in the weeks before surgery. Donor restrictions are not as stringent as for homologous blood donations. If the surgery is delayed, give the patient's older units back and draw new ones for surgery ("leapfrogging"). Operative blood salvage techniques involve collection of blood lost during surgery (if the surgical field is sterile) and its return to the patient during or after the procedure.

References

Anderson KC, Weinstein HJ. Transfusion-associated graft versus host disease. N Engl J Med 1990; 323:315.

Eslev AJ. Erythropoietin. N Engl J Med 1991; 324:1339.

Grindon AJ, Tomasulo PS, Bergin JJ, et al. The hospital transfusion committee. JAMA 1985; 253:540.

Snyder EL. Clinical use of white cell-poor blood components (editorial). Transfusion 1989; 29:568.

Zuck TF, Carey PM. Autologous transfusion practice. Vox Sang 1990; 58:234.

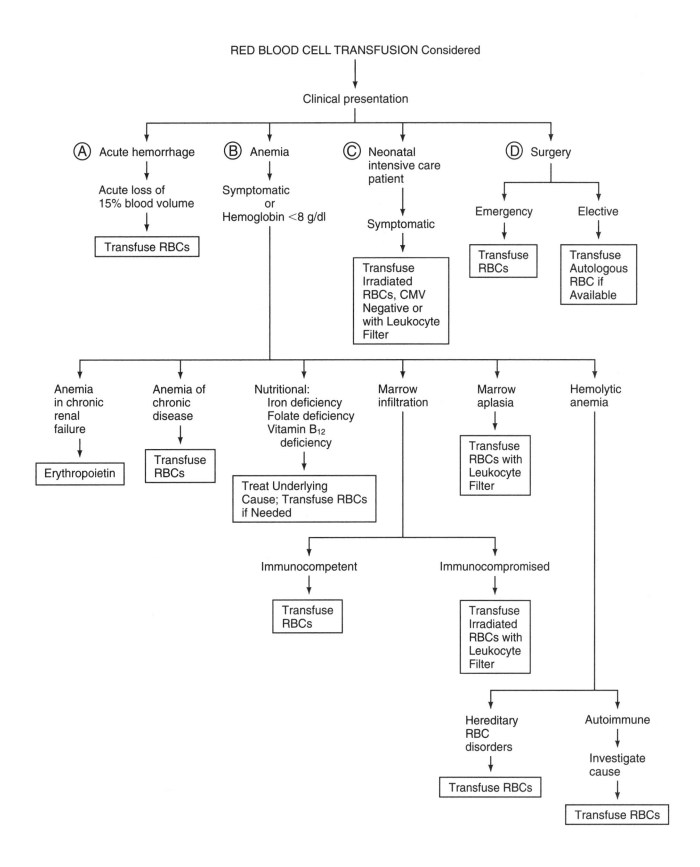

RED BLOOD CELL TRANSFUSION Considered

Clinical presentation

Ⓐ Acute hemorrhage

Acute loss of 15% blood volume

Transfuse RBCs

Ⓑ Anemia

Symptomatic or Hemoglobin <8 g/dl

Ⓒ Neonatal intensive care patient

Symptomatic

Transfuse Irradiated RBCs, CMV Negative or with Leukocyte Filter

Ⓓ Surgery

Emergency

Transfuse RBCs

Elective

Transfuse Autologous RBC if Available

Anemia in chronic renal failure

Erythropoietin

Anemia of chronic disease

Transfuse RBCs

Nutritional: Iron deficiency Folate deficiency Vitamin B$_{12}$ deficiency

Treat Underlying Cause; Transfuse RBCs if Needed

Marrow infiltration

Marrow aplasia

Transfuse RBCs with Leukocyte Filter

Hemolytic anemia

Immunocompetent

Transfuse RBCs

Immunocompromised

Transfuse Irradiated RBCs with Leukocyte Filter

Hereditary RBC disorders

Transfuse RBCs

Autoimmune

Investigate cause

Transfuse RBCs

TRANSFUSION THERAPY: GRANULOCYTES

June Clements, M.D.
Douglas Huestis, M.D.

Granulocytes are collected by leukapheresis and stored at room temperature. Each concentrate should contain at least 10^{10} granulocytes for a minimal dose of 1.4×10^8/kg for a 70-kg person, which approximates 10% of the daily neutrophil production in a noninfected person. Donors premedicated with corticosteroids provide more neutrophils. Perform transfusion of granulocytes as soon as possible after collection, at least within the first 24 hours.

A. One indication for granulocyte transfusion is an absolute neutrophil count <500/μl in an infected patient. If the count is >1000/μl, granulocyte transfusions are not useful except for abnormal neutrophil function (e.g., chronic granulomatous disease).

B. In neutropenic patients, local or systemic infection justifies granulocyte transfusions, particularly in gram-negative sepsis. However, granulocytes are not useful for fungal infections and may cause complications in persons taking amphotericin B. Prophylactic granulocyte transfusions are not appropriate in uninfected neutropenic patients, since adverse effects are likely to exceed the benefits. For example, alloimmunization may compromise future effectiveness of granulocytes, platelets, and bone marrow transplantation. Patients with transient neutropenia and normal bone marrow production are not candidates for granulocyte transfusions. Give appropriate antibiotics to such patients. Patients who are persistently neutropenic with decreased bone marrow production may respond to therapeutic granulocyte transfusions. This is particularly effective in neonatal sepsis with neutropenia and decreased bone marrow reserve.

C. Transfuse granulocytes with caution. A concentrate of granulocytes contains 15–50 ml RBCs and therefore *should be ABO compatible* with the recipient. If not ABO compatible, the RBCs should be removed from the concentrate. Possible adverse reactions include fever, transient hypotension, pulmonary infiltrates, graft-versus-host disease, and various infections (e.g., cytomegalovirus, hepatitis, HIV). In adults, give a trial of antibiotics first if the patient is stable. If there is no improvement, give granulocytes. An adult dose is one concentrate every 24 hours.

D. If neutrophil dysfunction is suspected, neutrophil function studies may be helpful to characterize any deficiency. Give antibiotics if bacterial infection is present. If there is no improvement, transfuse granulocytes.

References

Dutcher JP. The potential benefit of granulocyte transfusion therapy. Cancer Invest 1989; 7:457.

Huestis DW, Bove JR, Case J. Practical blood transfusion. 4th ed. Boston: Little, Brown, 1988:337.

Menitove JE, Abrams RA. Granulocyte transfusions in neutropenic patients. Crit Rev Oncol Hematol 1987; 7:89.

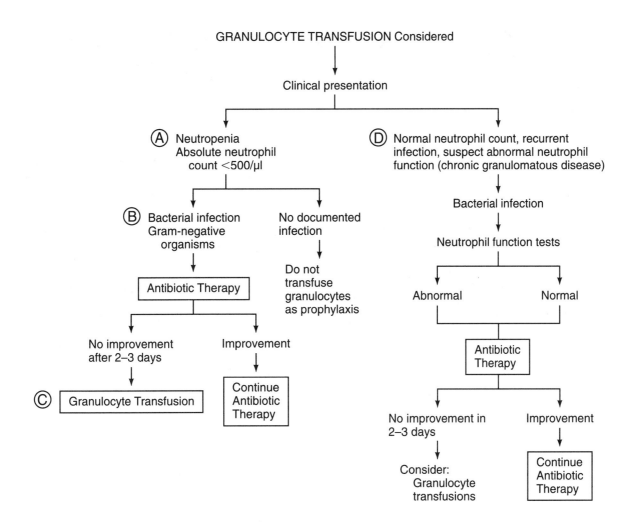

GRANULOCYTE TRANSFUSION Considered

Clinical presentation

Ⓐ Neutropenia
Absolute neutrophil
count <500/µl

Ⓑ Bacterial infection
Gram-negative
organisms

Antibiotic Therapy

No improvement
after 2–3 days

Ⓒ Granulocyte Transfusion

Improvement

Continue
Antibiotic
Therapy

No documented
infection

Do not
transfuse
granulocytes
as prophylaxis

Ⓓ Normal neutrophil count, recurrent
infection, suspect abnormal neutrophil
function (chronic granulomatous disease)

Bacterial infection

Neutrophil function tests

Abnormal   Normal

Antibiotic
Therapy

No improvement in
2–3 days

Consider:
Granulocyte
transfusions

Improvement

Continue
Antibiotic
Therapy

TRANSFUSION REACTIONS AND COMPLICATIONS

June Clements, M.D.
Douglas Huestis, M.D.

Transfusion can cause numerous adverse effects. Besides an immediate reaction to various blood components, there are also infectious complications. These include viral hepatitis (90% due to hepatitis C), cytomegalovirus, malaria, syphilis, and HIV. Current screening methods minimize the transmission of such infections. If any adverse reactions occur, stop the transfusion and notify the responsible physician and the blood bank. Recheck the identification of blood and patient at once. Draw a new blood sample and send it with the remaining blood component to the blood bank. The laboratory examines the patient's pre- and post-transfusion serum for evidence of hemolysis, checks the blood types, and does a direct antiglobulin test on the post-transfusion sample.

A. Fever during transfusion may indicate a febrile nonhemolytic reaction, bacterial contamination, noncardiogenic pulmonary edema, or a hemolytic reaction or may be coincidental. A febrile nonhemolytic reaction is defined as a rise in temperature of 1° C or more. Most occur in previously transfused patients or multiparous women and are probably caused by leukocyte antibodies in the recipient. Febrile reactions can be treated by antipyretics and prevented by leukocyte filters. Bacterial contamination causes sudden high fever, chills, and shock, requiring emergency therapy. Fever and chills may also signify a hemolytic transfusion reaction, usually caused by ABO discrepancies. These reactions may be fatal. A hemolytic transfusion reaction can be due to either intravascular (most often ABO incompatibility) or extravascular (e.g., Rh and other antibodies) RBC destruction. In any case, stop the transfusion and start supportive care immediately.

B. Allergic reactions usually involve itching, hives, and erythema, without fever, caused by reaction to plasma proteins. Stop the transfusion. If the reaction is mild, give an antihistamine. If the hives resolve, the transfusion may be continued. Anaphylactic reactions occasionally occur in IgA-deficient persons.

C. Elderly patients of small body size and those with underlying cardiopulmonary disease sometimes develop congestive heart failure because of volume overload. Symptomatic treatment is usually enough, but occasionally phlebotomy is necessary. Give subsequent transfusions slowly and consider concomitant diuresis.

D. Delayed hemolytic transfusion reaction is generally due to an anamnestic antibody response to certain transfused red cell antigens. This does not usually require clinical support, but the cause of decreasing hemoglobin needs to be identified. Post-transfusion purpura, caused by an antiplatelet antibody response, is rare. Give supportive care and control any bleeding.

References

Brubaker DB. Clinical significance of white cell antibodies in febrile nonhemolytic transfusion reactions. Transfusion 1990; 30:733.

Sazama K. Reports of 355 transfusion-associated deaths: 1976 through 1985. Transfusion 1990; 30:583.

Seeger W, Schneider V, Kreusler B, et al. Reproduction of transfusion-related acute lung injury in an ex vivo lung model. Blood 1990; 76:1438.

Walker RH. Technical manual. Arlington, VA: American Association of Blood Banks, 1990.

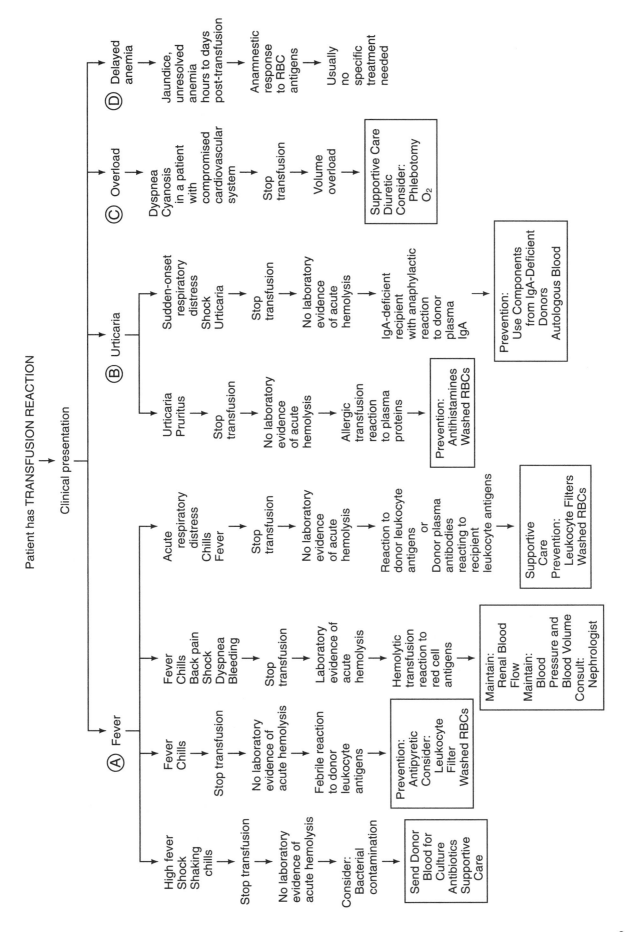

Patient has TRANSFUSION REACTION

Clinical presentation

A Fever

High fever
Shock
Shaking
chills
→ Stop transfusion → No laboratory evidence of acute hemolysis → Consider: Bacterial contamination → [Send Donor Blood for Culture Antibiotics Supportive Care]

Fever
Chills
→ Stop transfusion → No laboratory evidence of acute hemolysis → Febrile reaction to donor leukocyte antigens → [Prevention: Antipyretic Consider: Leukocyte Filter Washed RBCs]

Fever
Chills
Back pain
Shock
Dyspnea
Bleeding
→ Stop transfusion → Laboratory evidence of acute hemolysis → Hemolytic transfusion reaction to red cell antigens → [Maintain: Renal Blood Flow Maintain: Blood Pressure and Blood Volume Consult: Nephrologist]

Acute respiratory distress
Chills
Fever
→ Stop transfusion → No laboratory evidence of acute hemolysis → Reaction to donor leukocyte antigens or Donor plasma antibodies reacting to recipient leukocyte antigens → [Supportive Care Prevention: Leukocyte Filters Washed RBCs]

B Urticaria

Urticaria
Pruritus
→ Stop transfusion → No laboratory evidence of acute hemolysis → Allergic transfusion reaction to plasma proteins → [Prevention: Antihistamines Washed RBCs]

Sudden-onset respiratory distress
Shock
Urticaria
→ Stop transfusion → No laboratory evidence of acute hemolysis → IgA-deficient recipient with anaphylactic reaction to donor plasma IgA → [Prevention: Use Components from IgA-Deficient Donors Autologous Blood]

C Overload

Dyspnea
Cyanosis
in a patient with compromised cardiovascular system
→ Stop transfusion → Volume overload → [Supportive Care Diuretic Consider: Phlebotomy O₂]

D Delayed anemia

Jaundice, unresolved anemia hours to days post-transfusion → Anamnestic response to RBC antigens → Usually no specific treatment needed

205

HODGKIN'S DISEASE

Carol S. Portlock, M.D.

Hodgkin's disease typically presents with progressive, nontender, rubbery lymphadenopathy in supraclavicular, cervical, axillary, or occasionally inguinal regions. Most commonly, patients are 15–35 years of age. Mediastinal adenopathy may be detected incidentally or may lead to symptoms of cough and/or shortness of breath.

A. The diagnosis is usually made on lymph node biopsy; extranodal sites may be confirmatory. The pathology should be reviewed by an expert hematopathologist to rule out benign causes or non-Hodgkin's lymphoma.

B. The following baseline studies are performed in all patients to assess clinical stages: (1) complete blood count, platelet count; (2) ESR; (3) liver enzymes; (4) serum alkaline phosphatase; (5) renal function tests; (6) chest roentgenogram (Fig. 1); (7) CT of chest, abdomen, and pelvis; (8) lymphography (Fig. 2); and (9) bone marrow biopsy.

C. Consider staging laparotomy in any patient who would be a candidate for radiation therapy (i.e., patients with clinically localized disease).

D. Radiation therapy is employed only in patients who have been pathologically staged, including staging laparotomy. Radiation therapy usually includes mantle and para-aortic fields with doses of 3500–4400 rad.

E. Since systemic chemotherapy is indicated in all patients with large mediastinal masses and in those with stages IIIB, IVA, and IVB, no staging laparotomy is performed. Treatment is based on clinical staging only.

F. Combination chemotherapy is indicated in all clinically staged patients as well as those who have been pathologically staged and found to have advanced disease. Four-drug regimens (mechlorethamine, oncovin, procarbazine, and prednisone [MOPP] or adriamycin, bleomycin, vinblastine, and dacarbazine [ABVD]) or eight-drug (MOPP and ABVD) programs are often used.

G. Radiation therapy is often given during or after combination chemotherapy in high-risk patients. All patients with large mediastinal masses ($>0.3\times$ the transverse chest diameter) should receive combined modality therapy.

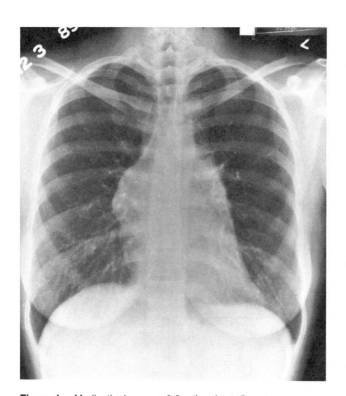

Figure 1 Mediastinal mass $>0.3\times$ the chest diameter.

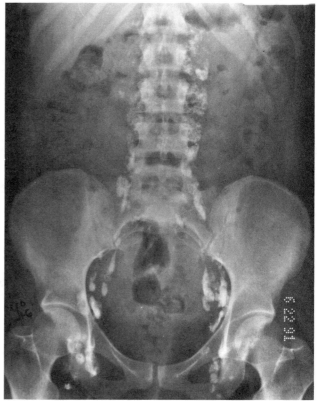

Figure 2 Abnormal lymphogram in a patient with Hodgkin's disease.

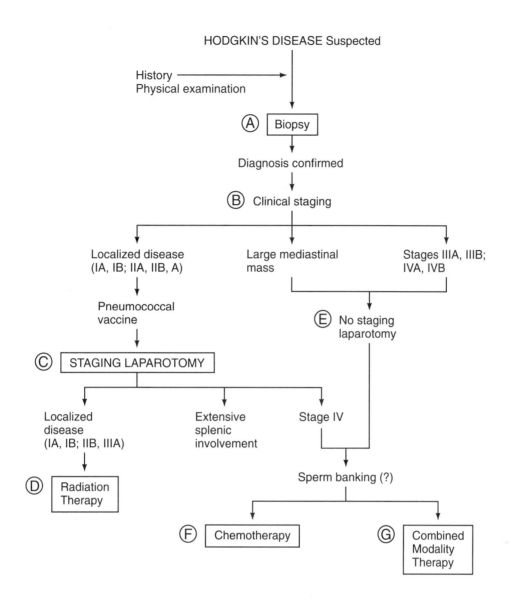

HODGKIN'S DISEASE Suspected

History ───────→
Physical examination

Ⓐ Biopsy

Diagnosis confirmed

Ⓑ Clinical staging

Localized disease
(IA, IB; IIA, IIB, A)

Large mediastinal
mass

Stages IIIA, IIIB;
IVA, IVB

Pneumococcal
vaccine

Ⓔ No staging
laparotomy

Ⓒ STAGING LAPAROTOMY

Localized
disease
(IA, IB; IIB, IIIA)

Extensive
splenic
involvement

Stage IV

Ⓓ Radiation
Therapy

Sperm banking (?)

Ⓕ Chemotherapy

Ⓖ Combined
Modality
Therapy

References

Banks PM. The pathology of Hodgkin's disease. Semin Oncol 1990; 17:683.

DeVita VT Jr, Hubbard SM, Longo DL. Treatment of Hodgkin's disease. J Natl Cancer Inst Monogr 1990; 10:19.

Hoppe RT. Radiation therapy in the management of Hodgkin's disease. Semin Oncol 1990; 17:704.

Leibenhaut MH, Hoppe RT, Efron B. Prognostic indicators of laparotomy findings in clinical stage I–II supradiaphragmatic Hodgkin's disease. J Clin Oncol 1989; 7:81.

Lister TA, Crowther D. Staging for Hodgkin's disease. Semin Oncol 1990; 17:696.

Longo DL. The use of chemotherapy in the treatment of Hodgkin's disease. Semin Oncol 1990; 17:71.

CHRONIC MYELOGENOUS LEUKEMIA

Robert M. Rifkin, M.D.

Chronic myelogenous leukemia (CML) accounts for about 25% of adult leukemia with an incidence of 1 case per 100,000 persons per year. The incidence peaks during the 5th–6th decades of life, but CML may occur at any age. Currently, the causative factors remain a mystery. Manifestations of CML relate to the unrestrained proliferation of granulocytes. Classically, the disease pursues a triphasic course. The chronic phase, which usually lasts 3–5 years, features mild constitutional symptoms that vanish with therapy. The Philadelphia chromosome −t(9;22) is present in >90% of patients in the chronic phase of CML. CML next evolves into an accelerated phase that becomes resistant to drug therapy. The final or acute phase (blast crisis) resembles acute myelogenous leukemia. It exhibits a complex karyotype and pursues a course identical to that of acute myelogenous leukemia, and this blast crisis is refractory to treatment.

A. Most patients with CML present in the chronic phase with lethargy, symptoms of anemia, or splenomegaly. Sweating and moderate weight loss are common, but fever is rare in the chronic phase. The most common physical finding at diagnosis is splenomegaly (85% of patients). The size of the spleen usually correlates with the duration of the disease. Hepatomegaly may be noted in 50% of patients. A few patients present with adenopathy in the chronic phase. As the disease transforms, fever, night sweats, weight loss, and bone pain often occur. There may also be rapid development of generalized lymphadenopathy or subcutaneous nodules. Rarely, patients may present de novo in blast crisis.

B. The leukocyte count is usually 75,000–300,000/μl but may be >500,000/μl. Thrombocytosis is observed in about one-third of cases. Anemia is usually a feature of untreated CML. The observed leukocytosis displays the full spectrum of maturing myeloid cells. Basophilia and eosinophilia are commonly seen. Nucleated RBCs may also be present and help to define the leukoerythroblastic reaction characteristic of CML.

C. Increased levels of serum uric acid occur in untreated CML but seldom cause problems. Neutrophil alkaline phosphatase (NAP) is usually decreased in CML. The NAP score can be useful as a diagnostic test, since it is usually elevated in other myeloproliferative disorders and stress.

D. Bone marrow is hypercellular due to granulocytic hyperplasia with an M:E ratio often >25:1. Mitotic figures are easily observed and megakaryocyte numbers are often increased with dysplasia. The most commonly observed cell in the bone marrow is the myelocyte. Sea-blue histiocytes resembling Gaucher cells are also present. Marrow fibrosis may be evident and is a poor prognostic feature. In the accelerated phase, ≥20% blasts plus promyelocytes are observed, and in the acute phase, ≥30% blasts plus promyelocytes are observed in the blood or bone marrow.

E. Once the diagnosis is established, explain the course of the disease to the patient and discuss an overall therapeutic strategy. The initial objective of therapy is to alleviate symptoms and prevent complications. This can be accomplished with hydroxyurea, busulfan, or alpha-interferon. Soon after diagnosis, review with younger patients the possibility of treatment with curative intent using bone marrow transplantation (BMT).

F. In patients <50 years of age with a histocompatible sibling, allogeneic BMT within 12 months of diagnosis is the preferred treatment. If a sibling donor is not available, begin therapy with hydroxyurea to control the leukocytosis. Alpha-interferon should then be used in an attempt to induce a hematologic response (normalization of the peripheral blood counts) and a cytogenetic response (suppression of the Philadelphia chromosome). This generally requires 6–12 months of therapy. If a cytogenetic remission is achieved, continue interferon therapy. If no remission is observed, consider a matched-unrelated or autologous BMT.

G. Management of the patient with the acute phase must be individualized. If a lymphoblastic transformation is identified (positive tdT), vincristine and prednisone therapy have a 60% initial response rate. If a myeloid transformation is identified (negative tdT), it usually does not respond to this treatment, and results with conventional leukemia treatment regimens have been dismal. Investigational therapy is therefore suggested.

CHRONIC MYELOGENOUS LEUKEMIA Suspected

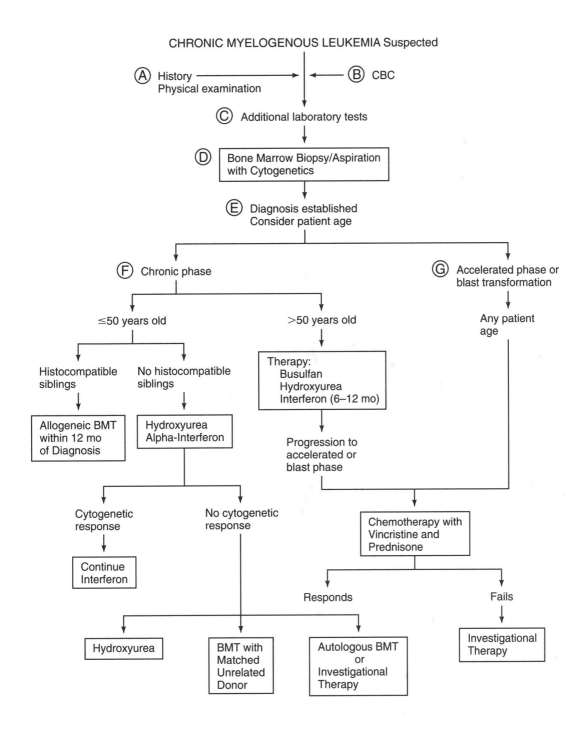

References

Beatty PG, Ash R, Hows JM, McGlave PB. The use of unrelated bone marrow donors in the treatment of patients with chronic myelogenous leukemia: experience of four marrow transplant centers. Bone Marrow Transplant 1989; 4:287.

Sandberg AA. Chromosomes and causation of human cancer and leukemia: XL. The Ph¹ and other translocations in CML. Cancer 1980; 46:2221.

Segel GB, Simon W, Lichtman MA. Variables influencing the timing of marrow transplantation in patients with chronic myelogenous leukemia. Blood 1986; 68:1055.

Talpaz M, Kurzrock R, Kantarjian HM, Gutterman JU. Recent advances in the therapy of chronic myelogenous leukemia. In: DeVita VT, Hellman S, Rosenberg SA, eds. Important advances in oncology: 1988. Philadelphia: JB Lippincott, 1988:297.

Thomas ED, Clift RA, Fefer A, et al. Marrow transplantation for the treatment of chronic myelogenous leukemia. Ann Intern Med 1986; 104:155.

Young JL, Percy CL, Asire AJ, et al. Cancer incidence and mortality in the United States, 1973–77. National Cancer Institute Monograph, No. 57, Bethesda, MD. NCI, Surveillance, Epidemiology, and End Results Program, 1978.

ABNORMAL SERUM PROTEIN ELECTROPHORESIS

Antonio C. Buzaid, M.D.

Monoclonal gammopathy is defined as the presence of a monoclonal protein (M protein) in the serum or urine. It may consist of one or more of the immunoglobulins, a heavy chain and/or a light chain. Monoclonal gammopathy may be seen in a variety of diseases, both benign and malignant.

A. The focus of the initial work-up is to quantitate and better characterize the abnormal protein present and determine whether there is evidence of a coexisting disorder. The bone survey and marrow examination are especially helpful in excluding multiple myeloma.

B. Patients with elevated IgG, A, D, or E may have a solitary or extramedullary plasmacytoma, multiple myeloma, amyloidosis, or a monoclonal gammopathy of unknown significance (MGUS). Patients with elevated IgM have MGUS, Waldenström's macroglobulinemia, or another lymphoproliferative disorder. The listed screening examinations guide the diagnosis. Statistically, most patients with a monoclonal gammopathy have MGUS. Of the 873 cases of monoclonal gammopathy evaluated at Mayo Clinic up to 1988, 64 % had MGUS and 16% had multiple myeloma. Less common diagnoses were amyloidosis (8%), non-Hodgkin's lymphoma (6%), chronic lymphocytic leukemia (2%), solitary or extramedullary plasmacytoma (2%), and Waldenström's macroglobulinemia (2%).

C. Solitary plasmacytoma occasionally presents with a monoclonal gammopathy, although most cases show no M-component in either serum or urine. The diagnosis is based on histologic evidence of a tumor consisting of plasma cells, identical to those seen in multiple myeloma, and confined to a single bone site. Radiotherapy is the treatment of choice. Although 50% of the patients will be alive at 10 years, the disease-free survival is only 20% because most patients develop multiple myeloma. Accordingly, follow-up with serum protein electrophoresis (SPEP), immunoelectrophoresis (IEP), and urine protein electrophoresis (UPEP) is indicated in all patients after completion of radiotherapy.

D. Extramedullary plasmacytoma is a plasma cell tumor that arises outside the bone marrow, most frequently in the upper respiratory tract, including the nasal cavity and sinuses, nasopharynx, and larynx. As in solitary plasmacytoma, most patients do not have a detectable M-component in either serum or urine. The diagnosis is based on the finding of a plasma cell tumor in an extramedullary site, the absence of multiple myeloma in the bone marrow, and no lytic lesions in the bone survey. Treatment consists of radiotherapy, which is curative in >50% of patients.

E. The presence of multiple lytic lesions, >10% plasma cell in the bone marrow, a serum M-component ≥3 g/dl, and the presence of light chain in the urine (usually >1 g in 24 hours) suggests multiple myeloma. Chemotherapy with melphalan-based regimens results in a median survival of 2–3 years. Carefully monitor patients for evidence of the most common complications of this disease: hypercalcemia, infection, and renal failure.

F. MGUS indicates the presence of an M-component in patients without multiple myeloma, solitary plasmacytoma, extramedullary plasmacytoma, amyloidosis, macroglobulinemia, or other lymphoproliferative disorders. MGUS is characterized by an M-component <3 g/dl, normal CBC, absence of hypercalcemia, and no lytic lesions on bone survey. More important, over a long period the M-component must remain stable and no additional abnormalities must develop. The incidence of MGUS increases with age, reaching approximately 10% in patients >80 years old. In a large series of 240 patients with MGUS, the concentration of the M-component was 0.3–3.2 g/dl (median 1.7 g/dl). IEP revealed IgG in 74%, IgA in 10%, and IgM in 16 % of patients. Approximately 6% of patients had a urinary monoclonal gammopathy. The number of plasma cells in the bone marrow was 1–10% (median 3%). Multiple myeloma, amyloidosis, macroglobulinemia, or other lymphoproliferative processes developed in 22% of the patients, with an actuarial rate of 17% at 10 years and 33% at 20 years. Most patients (68%) developed multiple myeloma 2–21 years from the diagnosis of MGUS, indicating that such patients must be followed indefinitely.

G. The presenting manifestations of primary amyloidosis include weakness, weight loss, ankle edema, dyspnea, paresthesias, light-headedness, syncope, peripheral neuropathy, carpal tunnel syndrome, congestive heart failure, periorbital purpura, arthralgia, orthostatic hypotension, macroglossia, and diarrhea with malabsorption syndrome. Although rectal biopsy has been the classic method of establishing the diagnosis of amyloidosis, a recent study has shown that abdominal fat aspiration, using a 19-gauge needle, can yield positive results in >70% of patients. There is no established treatment for primary amyloidosis.

H. Patients with an elevated IgM (often <2 g/dl) and peripheral adenopathy frequently have an underlying B-cell neoplasm. A lymph node biopsy should be obtained to exclude non-Hodgkin's lymphoma and chronic lymphocytic leukemia. In a series of 430 patients with IgM MGUS diagnosed at Mayo Clinic in 1956–1978, 17% developed lymphoma. The median duration from presentation with MGUS until the diagnosis of the lymphoma was 4 years (range 0.4–22 years).

Patient with MONOCLONAL GAMMOPATHY

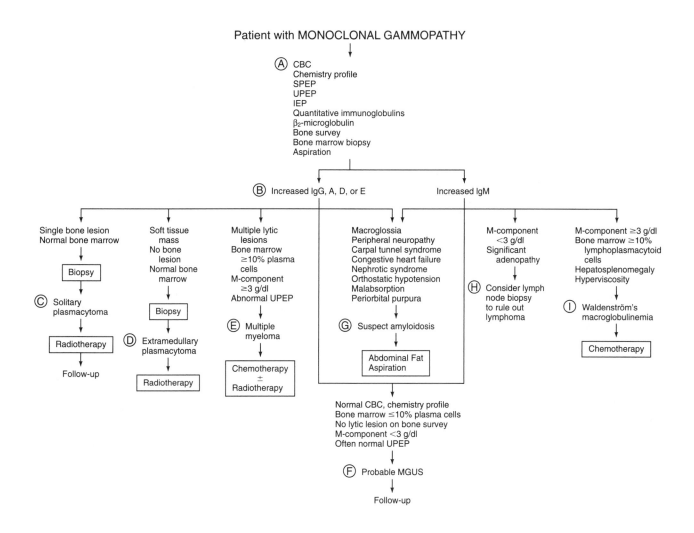

Ⓐ CBC
Chemistry profile
SPEP
UPEP
IEP
Quantitative immunoglobulins
β₂-microglobulin
Bone survey
Bone marrow biopsy
Aspiration

Ⓑ Increased IgG, A, D, or E   Increased IgM

Single bone lesion
Normal bone marrow
↓
Biopsy
↓
Ⓒ Solitary plasmacytoma
↓
Radiotherapy
↓
Follow-up

Soft tissue mass
No bone lesion
Normal bone marrow
↓
Biopsy
↓
Ⓓ Extramedullary plasmacytoma
↓
Radiotherapy

Multiple lytic lesions
Bone marrow ≥10% plasma cells
M-component ≥3 g/dl
Abnormal UPEP
↓
Ⓔ Multiple myeloma
↓
Chemotherapy ± Radiotherapy

Macroglossia
Peripheral neuropathy
Carpal tunnel syndrome
Congestive heart failure
Nephrotic syndrome
Orthostatic hypotension
Malabsorption
Periorbital purpura
↓
Ⓖ Suspect amyloidosis
↓
Abdominal Fat Aspiration

M-component <3 g/dl
Significant adenopathy
↓
Ⓗ Consider lymph node biopsy to rule out lymphoma

M-component ≥3 g/dl
Bone marrow ≥10% lymphoplasmacytoid cells
Hepatosplenomegaly
Hyperviscosity
↓
Ⓘ Waldenström's macroglobulinemia
↓
Chemotherapy

Normal CBC, chemistry profile
Bone marrow ≤10% plasma cells
No lytic lesion on bone survey
M-component <3 g/dl
Often normal UPEP
↓
Ⓕ Probable MGUS
↓
Follow-up

I.   Waldenström's macroglobulinemia is a rare disease (one seventh as common as myeloma) and is the result of an uncontrolled proliferation of lymphocytes and plasma cells in which a large monoclonal IgM is produced. The presenting signs and symptoms include weakness, fatigue, bleeding (especially oozing from the oronasal area), blurred vision, dyspnea, weight loss, paresthesias, retinal lesions ("sausage" formation), hepatosplenomegaly, and lymphadenopathy. IgM levels often exceed 3 g/dl. Chlorambucil is the chemotherapy drug of choice. The median survival is approximately 5 years.

References

Barlogie B, Epstein J, Selvanayagam P, Alexanian R. Plasma cell myeloma—new biological insights and advances in therapy. Blood 1989; 73:865.

Knowling MA, Harwood AR, Bergsagel DE. Comparison of extramedullary plasmacytomas with solitary and multiple plasma cell tumors of bone. J Clin Oncol 1983; 1:255.

Kyle RA. Diagnosis and management of multiple myeloma and related disorders. Prog Hematol 1986; 14:257.

Kyle RA, Greipp PR, O'Fallon WM. Primary systemic amyloidosis: multivariate analysis for prognostic factors in 168 cases. Blood 1986; 68:220.

BREAST MASS

Laurie L. Fajardo, M.D.

Breast cancer is the most frequent malignancy and the second leading cause of cancer-related death among American women. The most effective means for diagnosing early breast cancer is screening mammography in combination with physical examination. Nonpalpable breast lesions (detectable only by mammography) may represent small, early, and potentially curable cancers. Mammography does not always provide a specific diagnosis of benignancy or malignancy. Over 1 million breast biopsies are performed in the United States annually; 11–36% of biopsies performed for mammographically identified nonpalpable abnormalities are positive. The use of percutaneous fine needle aspiration (FNA) biopsy for palpable breast masses, or mammography guided stereotactic FNA biopsy for nonpalpable masses, may reduce the expense and morbidity associated with the diagnostic work-up of breast lesions, and decrease the number of benign breast biopsies performed. (See also Gynecomastia, p 130.)

A. Diagnostic mammography is indicated (1) for breast signs or symptoms (pain, mass, discharge, thickening, skin or nipple retraction, nipple eczema), (2) before breast surgery (biopsy, augmentation, reduction), (3) as routine follow-up of a patient with previous breast cancer (all remaining breast tissue), and (4) for metastatic cancer of unknown primary site. Preoperative mammography is performed (1) to characterize a lesion as obviously benign (lipoma, oil cyst, calcified fibroadenoma) or malignant (to plan the surgical approach), (2) to determine the size and extent of the lesion for adequate excision and treatment selection (especially important in a patient for whom conservative surgery and irradiation are being considered, since multicentric disease in the affected breast is a contraindication to this procedure), (3) to detect additional lesions in the ipsilateral or contralateral breast, and (4) to obtain a baseline for comparison with follow-up mammography. It is important to recognize that mammograms may be negative even when breast cancer is obviously present. Thus, a negative mammogram does not replace the need for biopsy of a palpable mass.

B. For palpable breast masses, percutaneous FNA or core needle biopsy can be performed with local anesthesia. To evaluate nonpalpable masses, FNA and core needle biopsy can be guided with stereotactic mammography images. The accuracy of these procedures is >90%. If needle biopsy shows a breast mass to be benign, conservative follow-up with physical examination and mammography can be instituted, obviating the need for further surgical intervention. If a needle biopsy is positive, surgical excision can be planned to

cure or stage the patient with a single surgical procedure.

C. When breast malignancy is confirmed histologically, a routine outpatient work-up to exclude distant metastasis is indicated. Complete physical examination, complete blood counts (CBC), liver function tests (LFTs), and chest radiography are routinely performed. A preoperative bone scan is indicated only if the patient has symptoms that are suspicious for bony metastasis. CT of the liver is indicated only if the LFTs are abnormal. The AJC-UICC staging system for breast cancer has been modified recently. Clinical staging includes careful inspection and palpation of the skin, breast, and lymph nodes (axillary, supraclavicular, and cervical) as well as pathologic examination of the breast or other tissues to establish the diagnosis of breast carcinoma. Pathologic staging includes data used for clinical staging, surgical resection, and a pathologic examination of the primary carcinoma. Pathologic staging can now be performed if the primary tumor is removed with no growth tumor in the margins and, in addition, if at least the lowest level (1) of axillary lymph nodes is resected, rather than all three levels.

D. Surgical treatment has recently focused on preserving the breast, yet successfully treating the cancer. Modified radical mastectomy is the preferred surgical procedure because it is now accepted that radical mastectomy confers no survival advantage.

E. Conservative therapy is an increasingly accepted alternative to mastectomy for the treatment of early breast cancer. It may include lumpectomy (complete removal of the primary tissue with a 0.5–1.0 cm margin of normal-appearing tumor) or segmental mastectomy (quadrantectomy). Limited axillary dissection is necessary to stage the malignancy adequately, and postoperative radiation therapy is usually indicated if the primary tumor is invasive. There are contraindications to conservative therapy, including multiple foci of carcinoma in situ. The therapy should be chosen by the patient after a thorough explanation of the advantages and disadvantages of each option.

F. After pathologic staging is completed, consultations with the radiation oncologist and medical oncologists are necessary to determine whether local radiation therapy or adjuvant systemic chemotherapy is indicated. Systemic adjuvant chemotherapy may also include hormonal (estrogen receptor antagonist) therapy.

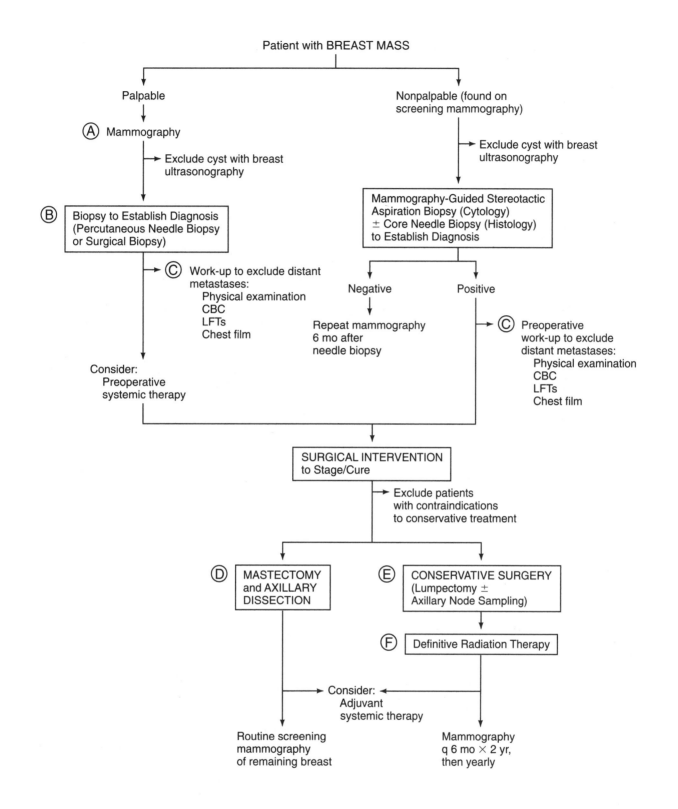

Patient with BREAST MASS

Palpable

Ⓐ Mammography

→ Exclude cyst with breast ultrasonography

Ⓑ Biopsy to Establish Diagnosis (Percutaneous Needle Biopsy or Surgical Biopsy)

→ Ⓒ Work-up to exclude distant metastases:
Physical examination
CBC
LFTs
Chest film

Consider:
Preoperative systemic therapy

Nonpalpable (found on screening mammography)

→ Exclude cyst with breast ultrasonography

Mammography-Guided Stereotactic Aspiration Biopsy (Cytology) ± Core Needle Biopsy (Histology) to Establish Diagnosis

Negative

Repeat mammography 6 mo after needle biopsy

Positive

→ Ⓒ Preoperative work-up to exclude distant metastases:
Physical examination
CBC
LFTs
Chest film

SURGICAL INTERVENTION to Stage/Cure

→ Exclude patients with contraindications to conservative treatment

Ⓓ MASTECTOMY and AXILLARY DISSECTION

Ⓔ CONSERVATIVE SURGERY (Lumpectomy ± Axillary Node Sampling)

Ⓕ Definitive Radiation Therapy

Consider:
Adjuvant systemic therapy

Routine screening mammography of remaining breast

Mammography q 6 mo × 2 yr, then yearly

References

American Joint Committee on Cancer. Manual for staging of cancer. 4th ed. Philadelphia: JB Lippincott, 1992.

Bigelow R, Smith R, Goodman PA, Wilson GS. Needle localization of nonpalpable breast masses. Arch Surg 1985; 120:565.

Fajardo LL, Davis JR, Wiens JL, Trego DC. Mammography-guided stereotactic fine needle aspiration cytology of nonpalpable breast lesions: prospective comparison with surgical biopsy results. AJR 1990; 155:977.

Howard J. Using mammography for cancer control: an unrealized potential. CA 1987; 37:33.

Silverberg E, Borring CC, Squires TS. Cancer statistics, 1990. CA 1990; 40:9.

LYMPHADENOPATHY

Guillermo Gonzalez-Osete, M.D.
Manuel Modiano, M.D.

There are more than 500 lymph nodes in the human body that may become enlarged in response to numerous stimuli: (1) infection (bacterial, viral, parasitic, spirochetal, chlamydial, mycobacterial, or fungal), (2) drug reactions (phenytoin, serum sickness), (3) malignancy (head and neck, GI, breast, rectal, lymphoma), and (4) miscellaneous conditions (sarcoidosis, systemic lupus erythematosus).

A. New-onset lymphadenopathy of <7 days' duration is unlikely to be malignant.

B. Recurrent or long-term (>7–14 days) lymphadenopathy (unilateral or bilateral) requires a full work-up. Most experienced clinicians see the patient again in 2–4 weeks to determine whether the node is increasing before embarking on a full work-up. The associated symptoms of fever, weight loss, or night sweats suggest malignancy (lymphoma B symptoms) or infection. Regional symptoms such as chest tightness, dysphagia, shortness of breath, and/or facial swelling suggest mediastinal disease and require a CT scan of the chest. Complaints of fullness in the abdomen, early satiety, and pain radiating to the shoulders or back necessitate abdominal CT to rule out pancreatic, renal, or other intraperitoneal lesions. Unilateral leg swelling (after deep vein thrombosis is ruled out) may require pelvic CT to rule out regional lymphadenopathy causing extrinsic compression.

C. Serologic studies and blood cultures help differentiate among infections, collagen vascular disease, and malignancy. Among the most common infectious causes are infectious mononucleosis, toxoplasmosis, syphilis, Epstein-Barr virus, HIV, and cytomegalovirus. If the history is suspicious and the patient is or was living in an endemic area, these causes must be ruled out.

D. Lymph node enlargement in the head and neck area requires a careful ENT evaluation, including biopsy of suspicious lesions; if ENT findings are normal, the patient may need to undergo a triple endoscopy procedure with evaluation of nasal, bronchial, and esophageal passages. Only if endoscopic findings are normal should fine needle biopsy of the lymph node be considered.

E. The supraclavicular area is often affected by breast cancer, lymphomas (Hodgkin's and non-Hodgkin's), and metastases from the lung and GI tract (esophagus, stomach, pancreas). Supraclavicular nodes are easily biopsied and are highly diagnostic.

F. Enlarged axillary lymph nodes are often a sign of breast or lung cancer. They also are often affected by lymphoma and may be biopsied to obtain a diagnosis if the primary source cannot be found.

G. When inguinal nodes are enlarged, physical examination should focus on the anorectal region, perineum, vulva, penis, and scrotum. Perform sigmoidoscopy to rule out rectal or anal carcinoma, evaluate the genitourinary system by urinalysis. Pelvic CT may provide useful information. If CT findings are normal, proceed with biopsy. Tumor markers CEA, PSA, and OC125 may also provide guidance toward a diagnosis.

H. For a patient with generalized lymphadenopathy but no other signs or symptoms and no other organ involvement, consider biopsy of the most accessible region (not necessarily the largest). The diagnostic yield is better with supraclavicular, axillary, or inguinal nodes (in descending order). A key feature of these biopsies is the need for adequate amounts of tissue with the specimen sectioned to allow for light microscopy, fresh frozen tissue for markers, and a portion in glutaraldehyde for electron microscopy. Patients with nondiagnostic biopsies require close follow-up, especially those with atypical hyperplasia, since many may develop lymphoproliferative disorders. Also, consider angioimmunoblastic lymphadenopathy in patients with "hyperplasia." This can be done by an experienced immunopathologist.

References

Copeland EM, McBride C. Axillary metastases from unknown primary sites. Ann Surg 1973; 178:25.
Moore RD, Weisberger AS, Bowerfind ES. An evaluation of lymphadenopathy in systemic disease. Arch Intern Med 1957; 99:751.
Portlock C, Goffinet DR. Lymphadenopathy. In: Clinical problems in oncology. 2nd ed. Boston: Little, Brown, 1986:38.
Saltzstein S. The fate of patients with nondiagnostic lymph node biopsies. Surgery 58:659.
Schroeder K, Franssila KO. Atypical hyperplasia of lymph nodes: a follow-up study. Cancer 1979; 44:1155.
Sinclair S, Beckman E, Eliman L. Biopsy of enlarged superficial lymph nodes. JAMA 1974; 228:602.
Weksler BB, Moore A. The lymphomas. In: Andreoli TE, Carpenter CCJ, Plum F, Smith LH Jr, eds. Cecil essentials of medicine. 2nd ed. Philadelphia: WB Saunders, 1990:380.
Zuelzer W, Kaplan J. The child with lymphadenopathy. Semin Hematol 1975; 12:323.

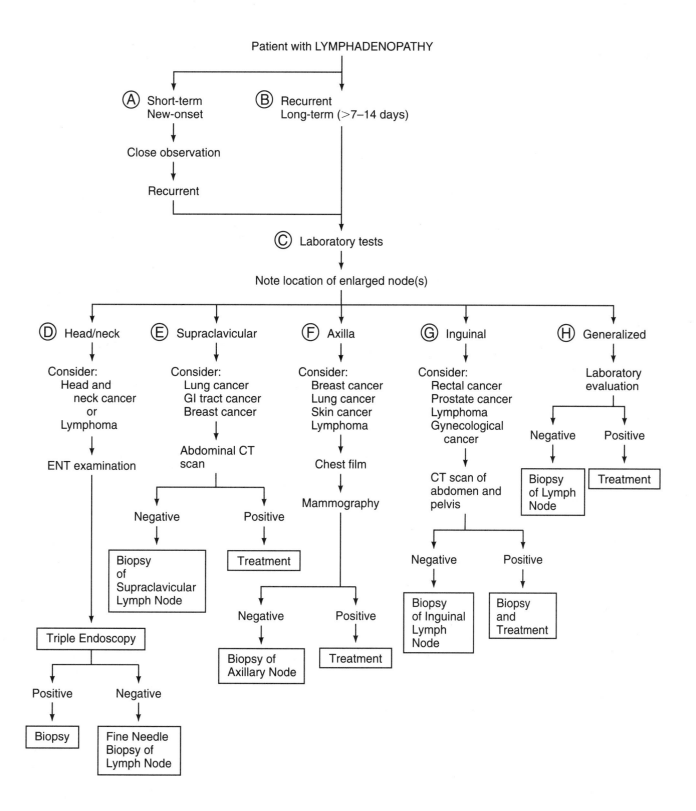

Patient with LYMPHADENOPATHY

Ⓐ Short-term
New-onset

Ⓑ Recurrent
Long-term (>7–14 days)

Close observation

Recurrent

Ⓒ Laboratory tests

Note location of enlarged node(s)

Ⓓ Head/neck

Consider:
Head and
neck cancer
or
Lymphoma

ENT examination

Triple Endoscopy

Positive   Negative

Biopsy   Fine Needle
Biopsy of
Lymph Node

Ⓔ Supraclavicular

Consider:
Lung cancer
GI tract cancer
Breast cancer

Abdominal CT
scan

Negative   Positive

Biopsy
of
Supraclavicular
Lymph Node

Treatment

Ⓕ Axilla

Consider:
Breast cancer
Lung cancer
Skin cancer
Lymphoma

Chest film

Mammography

Negative   Positive

Biopsy of
Axillary Node

Treatment

Ⓖ Inguinal

Consider:
Rectal cancer
Prostate cancer
Lymphoma
Gynecological
cancer

CT scan of
abdomen and
pelvis

Negative   Positive

Biopsy
of Inguinal
Lymph
Node

Biopsy
and
Treatment

Ⓗ Generalized

Laboratory
evaluation

Negative   Positive

Biopsy of Lymph
Node

Treatment

ADJUVANT THERAPY CHOICES IN BREAST CANCER

Ellen M. Chase, B.S.
Manuel Modiano, M.D.

Currently, 75–80% of newly diagnosed breast cancers are stage I or II; in approximately two-thirds no axillary lymph nodes are involved. Despite the apparent localized pattern at presentation, early systemic spread is common. The value of adjuvant systemic therapy after local definitive treatment has been established in both pre- and postmenopausal axillary node–positive (ANP) women, and (more recently) in axillary node–negative (ANN) women, a group thought to have a more favorable outcome. For ANP patients, medical oncology management issues relate primarily to choice of systemic treatment. For ANN women, issues relate to identification of the patients at highest risk for recurrence (who may benefit from aggressive treatment) and those at lowest risk (who may be spared the side effects of systemic therapy). Ideally, all patients should be managed by a multidisciplinary team. Although participation in a clinical trial may not be feasible for many patients, clinical research trials should be included as treatment options in discussions with individual patients.

A. The goal of initial definitive local treatment is local control of disease. Despite the potential for local failure in conserved breast tissue, numerous randomized studies (many with follow-up of 8–17 years) show no survival advantage for mastectomy over breast conservation. The 1990 NIH Early Breast Cancer Consensus Development Conference concluded that breast conservation treatment is appropriate primary therapy for most women with stage I or II breast cancer and is preferable because it provides survival equivalent to total mastectomy while preserving the breast. Women with tumors ≤5 cm may be candidates for limited resection if the breast is large enough to avoid distortion. Women with multicentric disease, those who would not achieve a cosmetic advantage by breast conservation, and those with certain collagen vascular diseases are not good candidates. The current recommended approach is local excision with clear margins, level I–II axillary node dissection, and breast irradiation to 4500–5000 rad with or without a radiation boost to the area of the primary tumor. The surgical approach for individual patients should be discussed in conjunction with radiation therapy and medical oncology so that all options, recurrence rates, and follow-up can be fully explained. Patients managed with breast conservation techniques should have close follow-up with regular mammography.

B. A number of patient variables and tumor characteristics relating to differentiation, rate of proliferation, and aggressiveness or invasiveness have been evaluated as prognostic factors in early-stage breast cancer. Data on very long follow-up of patients receiving only local-regional definitive treatment underscore the importance of axillary node involvement, tumor size, and nuclear grade in the natural history and prognosis of this disease. Although several newer variables such as flow cytometry, cathepsin D, and HER-2/neu oncogene expression appear promising, the clinical value of these remains to be defined.

C. The risk of recurrence after local therapy is directly related to the number of involved axillary nodes. This is a key factor in developing a management approach. Recurrence rates are lowest in women with no or few positive nodes. Prognosis is particularly poor in women with >10 positive nodes, and very aggressive approaches should be considered.

D. Tumor size is an important predictor of outcome and may be particularly helpful in ANN patients. The most favorable outcome is in women with tumors <1 cm. Infiltrating ductal or lobular carcinomas have a poorer prognosis than other types (tubular, colloid [mucinous], papillary). Nuclear grade also appears to be closely related to outcome (higher grade associated with higher rate of relapse), but this is not routinely reported and there are problems with reproducibility. Patients with T1N0 tumors >1 cm and other histologic criteria associated with aggressive disease may have improved disease-free survival (DFS) as a result of adjuvant systemic therapy.

E. Adjuvant systemic therapy has been clearly shown to reduce the rate of recurrence in ANN patients by approximately one-third. Reduced mortality rates are seen in nearly all trials, although this is not statistically significant in most. Benefit has been demonstrated in both pre- and postmenopausal patients and in both ER-negative and ER-positive patients. Of particular interest is the ability of tamoxifen to reduce ipsilateral breast tumor recurrences in ER-positive patients treated by breast conservation. Careful consideration of available risk factor information may identify patients who will benefit most from treatment.

F. Women with estrogen receptor (ER) negative tumors frequently have early relapse and a poor prognosis and may benefit from more aggressive treatment. Knowledge of ER status should be supplemented by information about other prognostic factors.

G. Adjuvant chemotherapy results in a highly significant improvement in both DFS and overall survival (OS) in premenopausal ANP women. According to the 1985 NIH Consensus Development Conference, combination chemotherapy should be the standard of care regardless of receptor status. Treatment given over 4–6 months seems to be as effective as longer therapy. For ER-positive, postmenopausal patients, tamoxifen is the standard of care, providing greater DFS and OS than no systemic treatment. Current trials

Patient with INVASIVE BREAST CARCINOMA

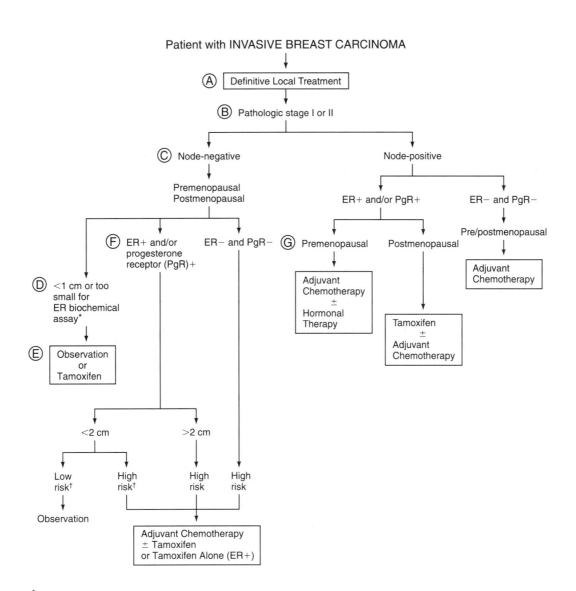

*Occult, small, or mammographically detected invasion tumor too small for bioochemical assay registered and observed on intergroup trial. Flow cytometry for prospective correlations.

†% S phase, ploidy determined by central laboratory using flow cytometry as part of intergroup trial.

are evaluating the benefit of adding cytotoxic drugs and optimal scheduling of the chemohormonal elements. For ER-negative, postmenopausal patients, maturing data from randomized studies show improved DFS and significantly improved OS with adjuvant chemotherapy. More intensive chemotherapy is under investigation.

References

Bonadonna G. Conceptual and practical advances in the management of breast cancer. Karnofsky Memorial Lecture. J Clin Oncol 1989; 7:1380.

Carter CL, Allen C, Henson DE. Relation of tumor size, lymph node status, and survival in 24,740 breast cancer cases. Cancer 1989; 63:181.

Fisher B, Costantino J, Redmond C, et al. A randomized clinical trial evaluating tamoxifen in the treatment of patients with node-negative breast cancer who have estrogen-receptor-positive tumors. N Engl J Med 1989; 320:479.

McGuire WL, Tandon AK, Allred DC, et al. How to use prognostic factors in axillary node-negative breast cancer patients. J Natl Cancer Inst 1990; 82:1006.

Osborne CK. Prognostic factors in breast cancer. Principles and Practice of Oncology Updates 1990; 4.

National Institutes of Health Consensus Development Conference on Treatment of Early Stage Breast Cancer, Bethesda, MD: National Cancer Institute, 1991.

Rosen PP, Groshen S, Saigo PE, et al. J Clin Oncol 1989; 7:355, 1239.

CARCINOMA OF UNKNOWN PRIMARY SITE

Antonio C. Buzaid, M.D.

Carcinoma of an unknown primary site constitutes up to 10% of referrals to cancer centers. One definition is no apparent primary site after complete history and physical examination, basic laboratory studies (including urinalysis and stool sample for occult blood), and chest film, with additional studies only as suggested by detectable abnormalities. The goal of additional studies is to identify the primary site, particularly in clinical situations in which potentially curative or effective therapy is available.

A. The history should focus on symptoms that could lead to the primary site (e.g., abdominal cramps, persistent cough, previous tobacco use). The physical examination should include a careful breast, pelvic, testicular, rectal, and skin evaluation. Examine lymph node–bearing areas for adenopathy.

B. The pathologic examination is the single most important step in determining the primary site. Adequate tissue samples should be provided to experienced pathologists who have access to electron microscopy and the most modern techniques in histochemical and immunohistochemical staining. At the time of surgery, the biopsy specimen should be divided into three portions: one portion snap frozen without fixation for immunohistochemical studies, one placed in glutaraldehyde for electron microscopy, and one into formalin for routine processing.

C. If the pathology evaluation does not suggest a primary site and labels the specimen as adenocarcinoma or poorly differentiated carcinoma, patients should undergo a baseline evaluation including beta-hCG; alpha-fetoprotein; CT scan of the chest (optional by some authors), abdomen, and pelvis; mammography (for women); and serum prostatic-specific antigen (PSA) and acid phosphatase (in men). Elevated beta-hCG and alpha-fetoprotein is suggestive of a germ cell tumor. Elevated acid phosphatase (prostatic fraction) and PSA is suggestive of metastatic prostate cancer. Elevation of PSA alone, however, may be secondary to benign prostatic hypertrophy. All other serum markers are not specific enough to be clinically helpful.

D. A special clinical subset includes males <50 years old with rapidly growing, poorly differentiated carcinomas involving predominantly midline structures (mediastinum, retroperitoneum) with or without bilateral pulmonary nodules. This clinical presentation is termed "extragonadal germ cell cancer syndrome." Approximately 10–15% of these patients may be cured with cisplatin-based chemotherapy. Therefore, they should be treated aggressively with chemotherapy regimens used for testicular cancer (e.g., VIP [VP-16, ifosfamide, cisplatin] or BEP [bleomycin, etoposide, cisplatin]).

E. Even in the absence of detectable ovarian disease, treat women who present with peritoneal carcinomatosis according to the guidelines established for therapy of advanced (stage III) ovarian carcinoma. Cytoreductive surgery followed by cisplatin-based combination chemotherapy produces long-term survival in approximately 10–20% of these patients.

F. The most common cause of adenocarcinoma or poorly differentiated carcinoma confined to the axillary nodes is occult breast cancer. Biopsy material should be analyzed for estrogen and progesterone receptors. The treatment of choice for these patients is modified radical mastectomy followed by adjuvant chemotherapy and, depending on receptor status, adjuvant hormonal therapy. The overall curability with surgery and adjuvant therapy appears to be similar to that for stage II breast cancer.

G. Inguinal node metastasis of unknown origin is a rare clinical presentation. Careful inspection of the skin, endoscopic evaluation of the anal canal and rectum, and gynecologic examination are of major importance. Patients in whom the primary tumor cannot be identified should undergo lymph node dissection of the affected area. After surgical resection, a 50% long-term survival was observed in one large series of 22 patients.

H. Squamous cell carcinoma is found in >70% of patients whose involved nodes are high in the neck or midneck. The most common occult primary sites include the nasopharynx, tonsil, base of tongue, and hypopharynx. It is often emphasized that a biopsy of high or midcervical nodes should not be performed until a search for the primary site has been completed because of an increased incidence of wound necrosis and an increased risk of local recurrence and even distant metastasis. However, other investigators have not observed such deleterious effects. An alternative approach is to perform a fine needle aspiration, which often has a high diagnostic yield. If the diagnosis is squamous cell carcinoma, patients should undergo MRI of the neck and a thorough ENT evaluation. This consists of direct laryngoscopy with random biopsies from the tonsil, nasopharynx, and base of the tongue of the affected side. Even if the primary cannot be identified, patients should undergo neck dissection followed by radiotherapy. The 5-year survival is 30–50%, depending on the extent of the disease at diagnosis.

I. Most patients do not fit into one of the subsets described here. Their work-up should be guided by symptoms or laboratory findings. An extensive "blind" work-up is not cost effective and therefore not

Patient with CARCINOMA OF UNKNOWN PRIMARY SITE

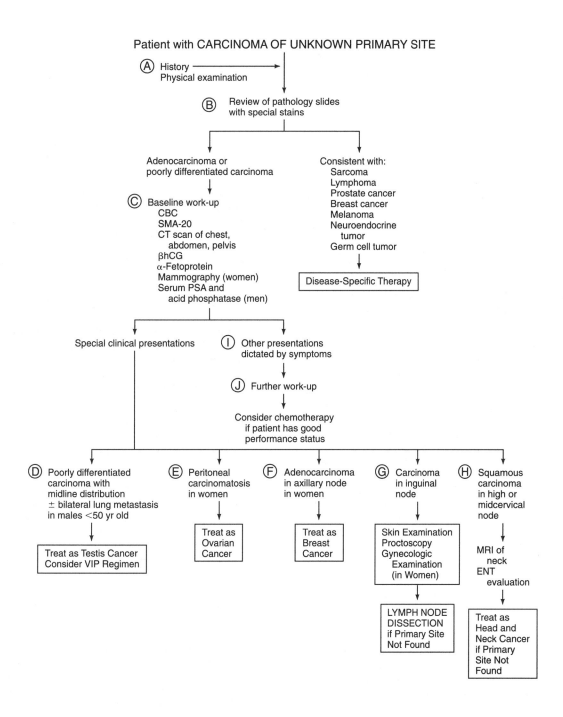

recommended. For instance, barium enema and upper GI series should be done only in patients who complain of abdominal discomfort or have iron-deficient anemia, and should not be part of a routine evaluation. Consider palliative chemotherapy, with either investigational or standard agents, in patients with good performance status.

J. If the pathology evaluation determines a specific diagnosis, patients should undergo disease-specific therapy. Even if the primary site is not found, patients can be treated according to the histology and not the primary site. For example, patients with widely metastatic neuroendocrine tumor should undergo regimens used in the treatment of small cell lung cancer.

References

Greco FA, Vaughn WK, Hainsworth JD. Advanced poorly differentiated carcinoma of unknown primary site: recognition of a treatable syndrome. Ann Intern Med 1986; 104:547.

Greenberg BR, Lawrence HJ. Metastatic cancer with unknown primary. Med Clin North Am 1988; 72:1055.

Sporn JR, Greenberg BR. Empiric chemotherapy in patients with carcinoma of unknown primary. Am J Med 1990; 88:49.

NEUTROPENIA AND FEVER

Antonio C. Buzaid, M.D.

Infection during episodes of chemotherapy-induced neutropenia is the most common cause of treatment-related mortality in oncology. Most infections originate in the alimentary tract, sinuses, lungs, and skin. The risk of a neutropenic patient developing infection is primarily dictated by the severity and duration of neutropenia. The lower the absolute granulocyte nadir and the more prolonged the neutropenia, the higher is the risk that serious infection will occur. Fever is a common symptom in cancer patients and may have many causes, including infection, the presence of the tumor itself, inflammation, transfusion of blood products, and chemotherapeutic and antimicrobial drugs. In neutropenic patients, however, fever is usually secondary to infection, especially if they have <500 granulocytes/μl.

A. In addition to a search for localizing symptoms, the medical history taking should identify any special circumstance or immunologic defect that may predispose the patient to certain opportunistic infections. For example, patients with Hodgkin's disease are at increased risk for herpes zoster and cryptococcal meningitis; those who have undergone bone marrow transplantation are at risk for severe interstitial pneumonia, especially with cytomegalovirus (CMV); and those on high-dose steroids are at increased risk for pneumocystis pneumonia and fungal infections. The use of steroids may further mask the signs and symptoms of infection and cloud the seriousness of the clinical picture.

B. Physical examination of neutropenic patients should be thorough and include meticulous evaluation of the oral cavity, genitalia, and perianal regions. Evaluate the entire integument, especially sites of vascular access and previous invasive procedures, as potential portals for infection. Recognize, however, that the characteristic signs and symptoms of infections are often absent in neutropenic patients because they are unable to mount an adequate inflammatory response. For instance, pyuria may be detectable in only 11% of patients with urinary infections, and purulent sputum in only 8% of patients with pneumonias.

C. The initial medical evaluation should be rapidly performed. In addition to the routine blood tests, patients should have blood cultured from two separate sites, urine culture, and a chest film. Other cultures and tests such as lumbar puncture, abdominal radiography, and bronchoscopy should be performed only if clinically indicated. Even with a comprehensive evaluation, a specific pathogen is initially identified in only 30–50% of patients. With profound neutropenia (<100 cell/μl), bacteremias can be documented in about 20–30% of febrile episodes.

D. Antimicrobial therapy should be directed against the pathogens responsible for most primary infections. Aerobic gram-negative bacilli, especially *Klebsiella*, *Escherichia coli*, and *Pseudomonas aeruginosa*, account for up to 50% of all culture-confirmed infections. The incidence of coagulase-negative staphylococci, and other gram-positive bacteria, however, has risen significantly in recent years and represents 30–50% of isolates in some hospitals. Most commonly, an aminoglycoside is combined with a beta-lactam with antipseudomonal activity (e.g., gentamicin plus mezlocillin or cefoperazone). In patients with marked renal impairment, consider the combination of a penicillin and a third-generation cephalosporin, both with antipseudomonal activity.

E. If the patient becomes rapidly afebrile, no organism is identified, all sites of infection resolve, and the absolute neutrophil count (ANC) is ≥500/μl, the antibiotic regimen can be discontinued after 7 days.

F. The management of patients who remain neutropenic but have been afebrile for >5 days and are doing clinically well remains controversial. If antibiotics are stopped, monitor these patients carefully. If they spike again, they should be immediately pancultured and restarted on broad-spectrum antibiotics. Neutropenic patients who are not doing well clinically should be continued on antibiotics until ANC is ≥500/μl.

G. Patients who remain neutropenic and febrile at day 4 but are doing well clinically may continue the same initial regimen for a few more days. However, if there is clinical deterioration, add vancomycin to the initial regimen if not included initially. If fever persists at day 7, start amphotericin to cover the possibility of fungal infections. During antibiotic treatment, conduct a thorough examination every day and include the skin, oral cavity, genitalia, perianal areas, and sites of venous access. Any medical complaint must be taken seriously and pursued without delay. For instance, mild discomfort in the maxillary region is often the first sign of a grave fungal infection, usually caused by *Aspergillus* or *Mucor*; tenderness in the perianal area may indicate a superimposed anaerobic infection; and diffuse abdominal pain may be the first clue to the diagnosis of typhlitis. In patients showing evidence of progressive disease, consider a change to different antibiotics.

Patient with FEVER ≥38° C AND ABSOLUTE NEUTROPHIL COUNT <1000/μl

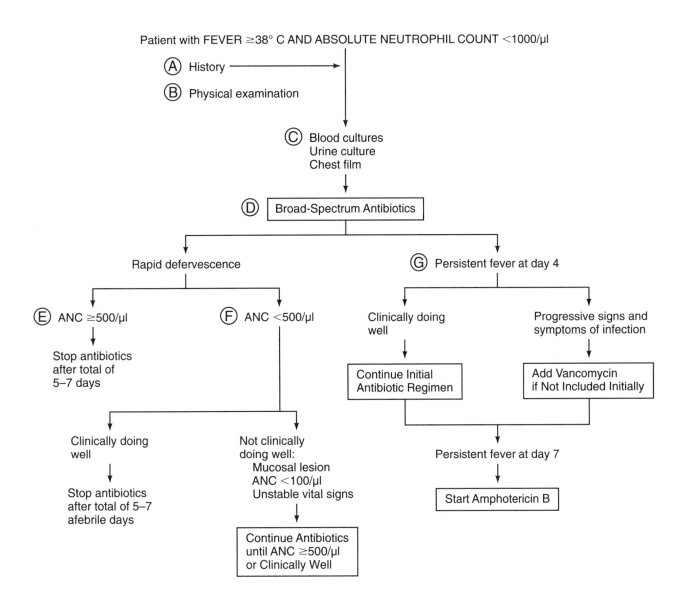

References

Hughes WT, Armstrong D, Bodey GP, et al. Guidelines for the use of antimicrobial agents in neutropenic patients with unexplained fever. J Infect Dis 1990; 161:381.

Lazarus HM, Creger RJ, Gerson SL. Infectious emergencies in oncology patients. Semin Oncol 1989; 16:543.
Pizzo PA. Evaluation of fever in the patient with cancer. Eur J Cancer Clin Oncol 1989; 25 (Suppl 2):S9.

PATHOLOGIC FRACTURES

Irwin E. Harris, M.D.

A. Plain radiography provides most of the information about the underlying lesion and directs future decision making. Technetium-labeled methylenediphosphonate bone scanning is a sensitive indicator of multiple skeletal involvement, except in myeloma, in which little reactive bone is formed. The skeleton is the third most common site of metastasis from adenocarcinoma; skeletal metastases are present in 70% of patients. Diffuse loss of mineral homogeneity throughout the skeleton suggests osteoporosis, osteomalacia, or marrow replacement by leukemia, lymphoma, or myeloma.

B. Nine percent of carcinomatous metastases are solitary, especially those of neuroblastoma and hypernephroma. A solitary bone lesion in a patient >40 years of age is most likely metastasis, whereas it may be a primary bone tumor in a patient <40 years of age.

C. The primary tumor is found in only one third of patients with skeletal metastases; most of those diagnosed have breast or prostate primaries. Undetected primaries are most likely lung or kidney. The recommended diagnostic strategy is history, physical examination, routine laboratory studies, chest radiography, urinalysis, intravenous pyelography (IVP) or abdominal CT, and mammography (in women). Additional tests detect primaries in only a few patients.

D. In most cases, tissue diagnosis does not alter the therapy, but it may if the lesion is a primary bone tumor or if the metastatic lesion can justifiably be resected, as in hypernephroma, thyroid carcinoma, or plasmacytoma. Resection of a solitary hypernephroma metastasis may result in a 30% 5-year survival rate.

E. Patients with metastatic disease have a short life expectancy. Internal fixation can be supplemented with methylmethacrylate for immediate stability, and prosthetic replacement can be used even in the young. Treat impending fractures with prophylactic fixation when the lesion is painful, with a lesion >2.5 cm in diameter, or when >50% of the diameter of the cortex is destroyed. Treat shafts of the femur, humerus, tibia, and subtrochanteric femur with intramedullary nail. Intertrochanteric and supracondylar fractures of the femur are treated with nail and side plate. Treat the distal tibia and distal humerus with flexible rods and bone cement. Use cemented prosthetic replacement for fractures of the femoral neck, acetabulum, and proximal tibia. Fracture stabilization is followed by radiotherapy.

(Continued on page 224)

Patient with FRACTURE

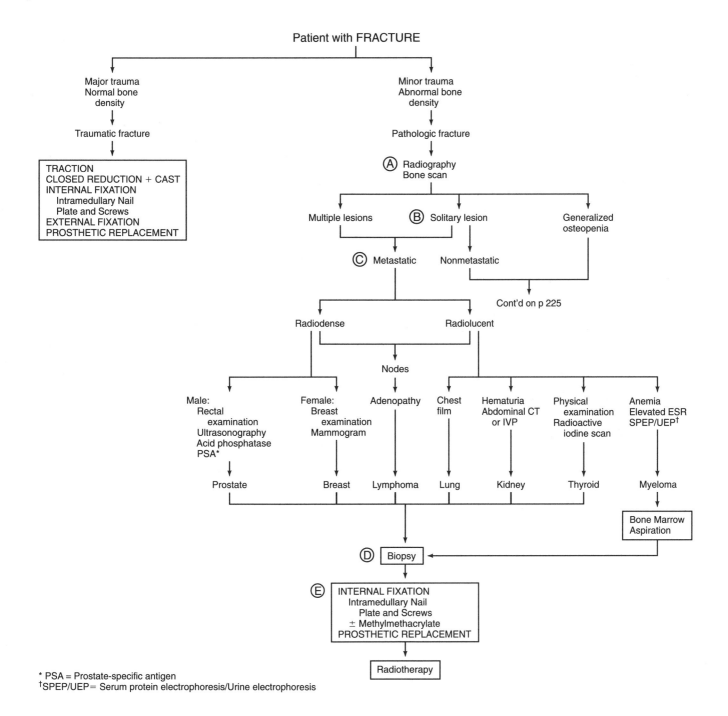

Major trauma
Normal bone density
↓
Traumatic fracture
↓

TRACTION
CLOSED REDUCTION + CAST
INTERNAL FIXATION
  Intramedullary Nail
  Plate and Screws
EXTERNAL FIXATION
PROSTHETIC REPLACEMENT

Minor trauma
Abnormal bone density
↓
Pathologic fracture
↓
Ⓐ Radiography
  Bone scan

Multiple lesions — Ⓑ Solitary lesion — Generalized osteopenia

Ⓒ Metastatic   Nonmetastatic

Cont'd on p 225

Radiodense — Radiolucent

Nodes

Male:
Rectal examination
Ultrasonography
Acid phosphatase
PSA*
↓
Prostate

Female:
Breast examination
Mammogram
↓
Breast

Adenopathy
↓
Lymphoma

Chest film
↓
Lung

Hematuria
Abdominal CT or IVP
↓
Kidney

Physical examination
Radioactive iodine scan
↓
Thyroid

Anemia
Elevated ESR
SPEP/UEP†
↓
Myeloma
↓
Bone Marrow Aspiration

Ⓓ Biopsy

Ⓔ INTERNAL FIXATION
Intramedullary Nail
Plate and Screws
± Methylmethacrylate
PROSTHETIC REPLACEMENT
↓
Radiotherapy

* PSA = Prostate-specific antigen
†SPEP/UEP= Serum protein electrophoresis/Urine electrophoresis

F. The differential diagnosis of a fractured solitary bone lesion is listed. Localized osteopenia due to failure to use a limb can occur with pain, reflex sympathetic dystrophy, previous cast immobilization, and paralytic conditions. Fractures are often seen in previously irradiated bone and in Paget's disease. The latter is distinguished from prostatic carcinoma by enlargement of the involved bone and coarsened, rather than destroyed, trabeculation.

G. Benign primary bone tumors often have intact cortex, distinct margins, and solid homogeneous periosteal reactions. Malignant tumors show destruction of cortex, indistinct margins, and lamellated or sunburst periosteal reactions.

H. Cast treatment without biopsy is justified for a benign bone tumor having a diagnostic radiographic appearance and self-healing behavior (e.g., unicameral bone cyst, metaphyseal fibrous cortical defect, eosinophilic granuloma, enchondroma, fibrous dysplasia). Biopsy is indicated when the diagnosis is uncertain or when the lesions are not likely to heal without resection or curettement and grafting (e.g., aneurysmal bone cysts, giant cell tumor, chondromyxoid fibroma, osteoblastoma, chondroblastoma). A cast may be used for healing of the cortex before definitive treatment. Steroid instillation is effective in obliterating unicameral bone cysts if cast immobilization of a fracture is unsuccessful.

I. Before biopsy, perform MRI to determine the extent of marrow and soft tissue involvement in primary malignant tumors of bone, although cortical destruction is better seen on CT. A fracture through a primary bone sarcoma most often necessitates amputation. However, if the cortical fracture is small and displacement is minimal, the patient may still be a candidate for resection and limb salvage, especially if preoperative adjuvant chemotherapy is administered. Treat chondrosarcomas by surgery alone.

J. Both metastatic and metabolic disease may involve the spine, proximal femurs, and ribs. Osteoporosis characteristically results in fractures of the distal radius and femoral neck. Osteomalacia more commonly affects the subtrochanteric femur and successive ribs at the same distance from the spine; 30% of patients with hip fracture have osteomalacia. Osteomalacia, marked by excess of unmineralized osteoid, can be of vitamin D deficiency, poor absorption of calcium or vitamin D enterically, vitamin D resistant form, or renal osteodystrophy. Osteoporosis can result from immobilization and disuse or from endocrinopathy (hyperthyroidism, hypercortisolism, or hyperparathyroidism), or it may be idiopathic (the type I postmenopausal variety is a loss of trabecular more than cortical bone; the type II senile variety is an equal loss of both).

References

Albright JA, Gillespie TE, Butard TR. Treatment of bone metastases. Semin Oncol 1980; 17:418.

Mankin HJ. Rickets, osteomalacia, and renal osteodystropy. An update. Orthop Clin North Am 1990; 21:81.

Simon MA, Bartucci EJ. The search for the primary tumor in patients with skeletal metastases of unknown origin. Cancer 1986; 58:1088.

Yazawa Y, Frassica FJ, Chao EY, et al. Metastatic bone disease; a study of the surgical treatment of 166 pathologic humeral and femoral fractures. Clin Orthop 1990; 251:213.

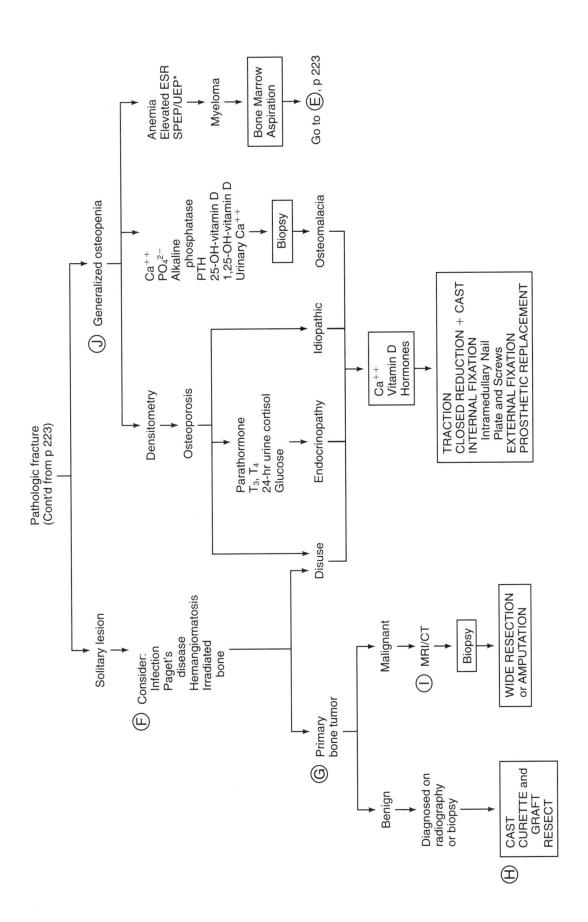

Pathologic fracture
(Cont'd from p 223)

Solitary lesion

F Consider:
Infection
Paget's disease
Hemangiomatosis
Irradiated bone

G Primary bone tumor

Benign

Diagnosed on radiography or biopsy

H CAST
CURETTE and GRAFT
RESECT

Malignant

I MRI/CT

Biopsy

WIDE RESECTION or AMPUTATION

Disuse

Generalized osteopenia

Densitometry

Osteoporosis

Parathormone
T₃, T₄
24-hr urine cortisol
Glucose

Endocrinopathy

Idiopathic

Ca⁺⁺
Vitamin D
Hormones

Ca⁺⁺
PO₄²⁻
Alkaline phosphatase
PTH
25-OH-vitamin D
1,25-OH-vitamin D
Urinary Ca⁺⁺

Biopsy

Osteomalacia

Anemia
Elevated ESR
SPEP/UEP*

Myeloma

Bone Marrow Aspiration

Go to E, p 223

TRACTION
CLOSED REDUCTION + CAST
INTERNAL FIXATION
Intramedullary Nail
Plate and Screws
EXTERNAL FIXATION
PROSTHETIC REPLACEMENT

*SPEP/UEP = Serum protein electrophoresis/Urine electrophoresis

225

CLINICAL CONSIDERATION FOR BONE MARROW TRANSPLANT CANDIDATES

Catherine Azar, M.D.
Mary Bordenave, Pharm.D., ITT (ASCP)

The efficacy of chemotherapeutic agents in the treatment of malignancy is limited by the life-threatening toxicities associated with escalations in the dosages of these drugs. Bone marrow toxicity is usually the dose-limiting factor for most agents. Furthermore, many cancers are or become resistant to standard dosages of chemotherapeutic agents. The goal of bone marrow transplantation (BMT) is to overcome disease resistance to treatment by using higher doses of these agents and to avoid excessive hematopoietic toxicity by "rescuing" the patient with infusions of bone marrow.

A. The most common nonmalignant diseases in which BMT is indicated are immunodeficiency disorders, severe aplastic anemia, genetic disorders of hematopoiesis, inborn errors of metabolism, and thalassemia. The most common malignant diseases are hematologic, including acute and chronic myelogenous leukemia, acute lymphoblastic leukemia, myelodysplasias, multiple myeloma, Hodgkin's disease, and non-Hodgkin's lymphoma. The solid tumors most often treated successfully with BMT are breast cancer, testicular carcinoma, and neuroblastoma. Not all tumors respond to high-dose chemotherapy with bone marrow rescue, even if they are chemotherapy sensitive. However, if a patient has a tumor that is amenable to BMT, chemosensitivity with standard-dose therapy is probably the most important prognostic factor for BMT success.

B. Timing is extremely important. BMT is not a procedure for an end-stage cancer patient. It is most successful in early stages of disease. Treating a patient in remission or one with minimal disease leads to a much more favorable outcome than treating one in full-blown relapse.

C. Evaluate performance status and organ function before committing a patient to BMT. Only patients in excellent physical condition can withstand BMT without severe toxicity. Increasing age contributes to morbidity and mortality.

D. Potential BMT patients should receive irradiated blood products before and after BMT. They must be screened for cytomegalovirus (CMV). Before their CMV status is known, they should receive only CMV-negative blood products. Avoid blood products from potential marrow donors because of the increased risk of graft rejection. In patients with aplastic anemia, avoid transfusing any blood products. The more transfusions these patients receive, the poorer is their outcome after BMT.

E. The first BMTs were done using monozygous twins (syngeneic graft) or HLA-identical siblings (allogeneic graft). Unfortunately, not every person requiring BMT has an HLA-matched sibling or a twin. Today, bone marrow or stem cell rescue can come from several other sources. A patient can be his or her own donor (autologous transplant). Bone marrow registry programs are available that enable patients to be matched with unrelated donors according to their specific HLA type.

F. Patients with hematologic malignancies often have more bone marrow involvement than those with solid tumors. Several options are available to find suitable donors for these patients if there are no related donors. Among these are the use of matched unrelated donors and the purging of autologous marrow using chemicals or monoclonal antibodies targeted at the tumor cells. Another option is the collection of peripheral stem cells; the patient undergoes cytophoresis with a cell separator and then progenitor cells are collected.

G. Autologous marrow reinfusion eliminates the issues of donor availability and graft-versus-host disease (GVHD). GVHD is also not an issue when the donor is an identical twin. However, the use of matched unrelated donors or slightly mismatched related donors increases the risk of GVHD. The possibility of GVHD influences the choice of types of BMT. Although GVHD can lead to many life-threatening complications, it can also cure some patients with leukemia ("graft-versus-leukemia effect"). Unfortunately this phenomenon is not seen in patients with lymphoma, multiple myeloma, or solid tumors, who should be treated with autologous marrow to avoid the complications of GVHD.

References

Buckner CD, Sanders JE, Storb R. Bone marrow transplantation. In: Advances and controversies in thalassemia therapy: bone marrow transplantation and other approaches. New York: Alan R. Liss, 1989.

Cheson BD, Lacerna L, Leyland-Jones B, et al. Autologous bone marrow transplantation: current status and future directions. Ann Intern Med 1989; 110:51.

Lasky LC. Hematopoietic reconstitution using progenitors recovered from blood. Transfusion 1989; 29:552.

Storb R. Bone marrow transplantation. In: DeVita VT, Hellman S, Rosenberg SA, eds. Cancer: principles and practice of oncology. 3rd ed. Philadelphia: JB Lippincott, 1989.

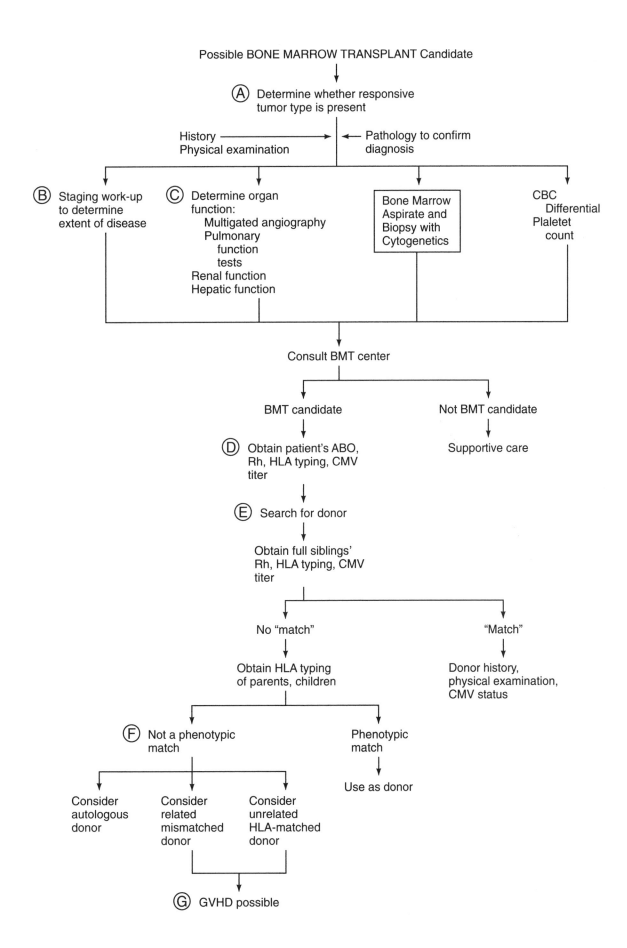

Possible BONE MARROW TRANSPLANT Candidate

Ⓐ Determine whether responsive
tumor type is present

History ⟶ ⟵ Pathology to confirm
Physical examination   diagnosis

Ⓑ Staging work-up
to determine
extent of disease

Ⓒ Determine organ
function:
    Multigated angiography
    Pulmonary
      function
      tests
  Renal function
  Hepatic function

Bone Marrow
Aspirate and
Biopsy with
Cytogenetics

CBC
Differential
Plaletet
count

Consult BMT center

BMT candidate

Not BMT candidate

Supportive care

Ⓓ Obtain patient's ABO,
Rh, HLA typing, CMV
titer

Ⓔ Search for donor

Obtain full siblings'
Rh, HLA typing, CMV
titer

No "match"

"Match"

Obtain HLA typing
of parents, children

Donor history,
physical examination,
CMV status

Ⓕ Not a phenotypic
match

Phenotypic
match

Use as donor

Consider
autologous
donor

Consider
related
mismatched
donor

Consider
unrelated
HLA-matched
donor

Ⓖ GVHD possible

SECONDARY MALIGNANCIES IN PATIENTS PREVIOUSLY TREATED FOR CANCER

Charles W. Taylor, M.D.

The use of combination chemotherapy and radiotherapy has met with great success in patients with certain types of cancer. There now exists a large population of patients who are long-term cancer survivors but who are at risk of developing secondary, treatment-related malignancies. Patients at highest risk are children or young adults previously treated for Hodgkin's disease, acute leukemia, retinoblastoma, Wilms' tumor, or soft tissue sarcoma. Such patients are commonly given a combination of chemotherapy and radiotherapy, and thus it is often difficult to accurately define the specific etiologic agent causing the second malignancy. However, drugs such as cyclophosphamide, procarbazine, BCNU, CCNU, and DTIC are known from animal studies to be carcinogens. In addition to direct carcinogenic effects, chemotherapy drugs may also have immunosuppressive effects that contribute to the development of secondary malignancies.

A. In taking the history of a patient previously treated for and presumably cured of malignancy, pay attention to the details of previous treatment (specific drugs, duration of treatment, total radiation dose) as well as current symptoms. Since the most common secondary malignancies are non-Hodgkin's lymphoma and acute leukemia, pay particular attention on physical examination to the presence of lymphadenopathy and/or organomegaly, and inspect closely the CBC.

B. Non-Hodgkin's lymphoma should be strongly considered in this group of patients if lymphadenopathy or organomegaly is detected on physical examination. However, solid tumors that may metastasize to lymph nodes must also be considered. Skin cancers observed include both epidermoid skin tumors and malignant melanoma.

C. The diagnostic tests are designed to establish a tissue diagnosis (lymph node or other accessible tumor site biopsy) and define the extent of disease. These issues must be addressed before treatment options can be discussed.

D. Cyclophosphamide may be acutely toxic to bladder mucosa, resulting in hemorrhagic cystitis, or may lead to a malignant change in bladder mucosal cells after long-term exposure. Patients presenting with bladder cancer are commonly asymptomatic except for irritative bladder symptoms and/or the presence of hematuria.

E. Urinary cytology may give a presumptive diagnosis of bladder cancer, but the definitive diagnosis must be made by cystoscopic examination and transurethral biopsy. Staging evaluations should cover sites of common metastatic spread, including lung and bone.

F. In patients with abnormal CBCs after previous cancer treatment, especially those with leukocytosis, leukopenia, or immature WBCs, there should be a high suspicion of malignant transformation to leukemia or myelodysplastic syndromes. Interestingly, the latent period for the development of secondary leukemias is shorter than that for the development of secondary solid tumors (4–6 years versus approximately 10 years).

G. Secondary leukemias are usually acute nonlymphocytic leukemias and constitute approximately 10% of all leukemias. Patients commonly develop a preleukemic phase characterized by cytopenias, macrocytosis, and/or circulating immature cells. Some patients may have a persistent myelodysplasia-type syndrome, but many progress to acute leukemia. Treatment of secondary acute leukemias or myelodysplastic syndromes is particularly difficult and, these patients have a much poorer response to combination chemotherapy than those with de novo disease. A bone marrow aspirate and biopsy should be performed to confirm the diagnosis.

H. Exposure to ionizing radiation has been associated with development of many different types of malignancies. After exposure to high doses of ionizing radiation after atomic bomb explosions, an increased incidence of leukemia, multiple myeloma, lung cancer, breast cancer, stomach cancer, and urinary tract cancer was observed. Cancers associated with therapeutic radiation can occur within the radiation field, and secondary sarcomas have been reported by many authors. Patients previously treated with radiotherapy to the neck area (especially those who received low doses of radiation) for Hodgkin's disease, other malignancies, or benign conditions are at risk for the development of both hypothyroidism and thyroid cancer.

References

Coleman CN, Tucker MA. Secondary cancers. In: DeVita VT, Hellman S, Rosenberg SA, eds. Cancer, principles and practices of oncology. Philadelphia: JB Lippincott, 1989:2181.

Greene MH, Wilson J. Second cancer following lymphatic and hematopoietic cancers in Connecticut, 1935–82. Natl Cancer Inst Monograph 1985; 68:191.

Penn I. Secondary neoplasms as a consequence of transplantation and cancer therapy. Cancer Detect Prev 1988; 12:39.

Patient with HISTORY OF CANCER PREVIOUSLY TREATED WITH
CHEMOTHERAPY AND/OR RADIOTHERAPY

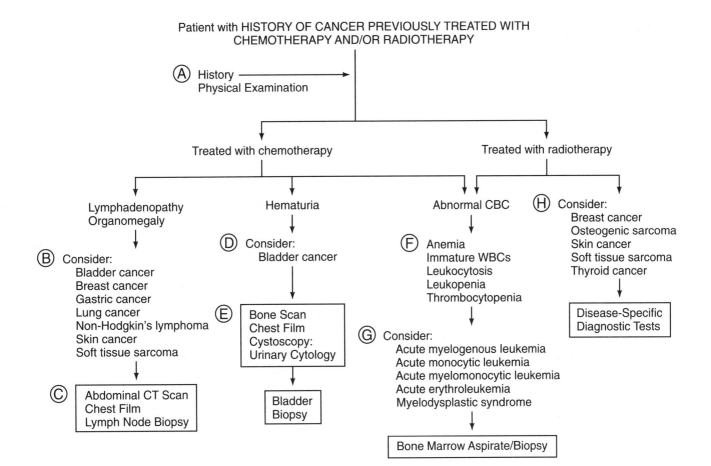

(A) History
Physical Examination

Treated with chemotherapy

Treated with radiotherapy

Lymphadenopathy
Organomegaly

Hematuria

Abnormal CBC

(H) Consider:
Breast cancer
Osteogenic sarcoma
Skin cancer
Soft tissue sarcoma
Thyroid cancer

(B) Consider:
Bladder cancer
Breast cancer
Gastric cancer
Lung cancer
Non-Hodgkin's lymphoma
Skin cancer
Soft tissue sarcoma

(D) Consider:
Bladder cancer

(F) Anemia
Immature WBCs
Leukocytosis
Leukopenia
Thrombocytopenia

Disease-Specific
Diagnostic Tests

(E) Bone Scan
Chest Film
Cystoscopy:
Urinary Cytology

(G) Consider:
Acute myelogenous leukemia
Acute monocytic leukemia
Acute myelomonocytic leukemia
Acute erythroleukemia
Myelodysplastic syndrome

(C) Abdominal CT Scan
Chest Film
Lymph Node Biopsy

Bladder
Biopsy

Bone Marrow Aspirate/Biopsy

SUPERIOR VENA CAVAL SYNDROME

Frederick R. Ahmann, M.D.

A. Obstruction of the superior vena cava (SVC) occurs when this thin-walled vessel is invaded, compressed, or thrombosed. Blockage of the blood flow frequently leads to development of the easily recognized superior vena caval syndrome (SVCS) with venous distention, facial edema, headache, tachypnea, cyanosis, and plethora. SVCS has commonly been characterized as an acute or subacute oncologic emergency, but recent reassessments of published experiences with this syndrome suggest that the establishment of a diagnosis is important and can be accomplished safely even if biopsies of tissue exposed to elevated venous pressures, and a brief delay in the initiation of therapy, are necessary.

B. In a patient with the above-noted signs and symptoms, confirmation that the SVC is obstructed is usually not required, as most patients have a mass visible on radiography. However, should confirmation be needed, this can be safely accomplished with either contrast or a nuclear venography. Nuclear venography is preferable in view of a lower injection volume of contrast, but both are associated with low complication rates.

C. Since the 1950s, bronchogenic carcinomas have been the leading cause of SVCS. Hence, for many years histologic confirmation of the diagnosis was thought to be unnecessary as palliative therapy was the only treatment possible. Recent advances in the treatment of small cell lung cancer and lymphoproliferative disorders, plus the low but present incidence of benign etiologies of this syndrome for which radiotherapy is not palliative and is potentially complicating, mandate accurate pretherapy assessment. There is minimal evidence to suggest that diagnostic procedures (including bronchoscopy, lymph node biopsies, mediastinoscopy, and thoracotomies) carry an excessive risk. Thus, the evaluation of these patients should be similar to that of any patient with a lung mass.

D. Standard palliative therapy for SVCS has been radiotherapy. Some debate persists as to the optimal dose, schedule, and fields of treatment, but in general approximately 50–70% of treated patients are reported to achieve symptomatic improvement within 2 weeks of initiation of radiotherapy. However, radiotherapy is no longer the sole or even the initial therapy for many patients. In a recent review, 40% of all cases of SVCS were due to small cell lung cancer; most of the remaining cases were secondary to lymphomas. Thus, up to 50% of all causes of SVCS are malignancies for which combination chemotherapy is needed to accomplish the therapeutic objectives of improved quality of life and prolonged survival. SVCS can cause distressing signs and symptoms that should be palliated in a timely fashion. However, because many such patients may have small cell lung cancer or lymphoma together with a definite incidence of benign etiologies, an accurate histologic diagnosis should be pursued in all patients with SVCS unless there are extenuating circumstances. Only with a definite histologic diagnosis can a rational therapeutic choice be made for both relieving SVCS and maximizing survival potential.

References

Ahmann FR. A reassessment of the clinical implications of the superior vena caval syndrome. J Clin Oncol 1984; 2:961.

Dombernowsky P, Hansen HH. Combination chemotherapy in the management of superior vena caval obstruction in small cell anaplastic carcinoma of the lung. Acta Med Scand 1978; 204:5123.

Perez CA, Presant CA, Van Amburg AL. Management of superior vena cava syndrome. Semin Oncol 1978; 5:123.

Patient with SUPERIOR VENA CAVAL SYNDROME

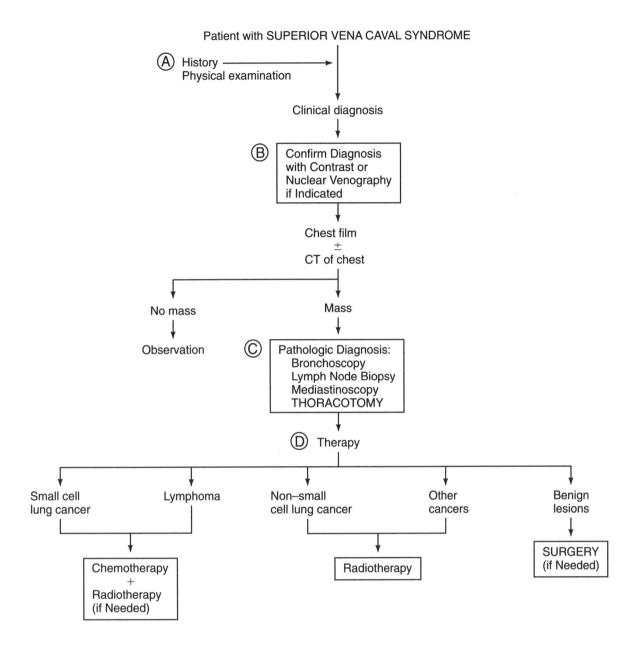

SPINAL CORD COMPRESSION

Guillermo Gonzalez-Osete, M.D.
Manuel Modiano, M.D.

Approximately 5% of systemic cancers involve the spinal cord. Spinal cord compression is a medical emergency in which a delay in treatment often causes irreversible loss of neurologic function.

A. Tumors that most commonly affect the spinal cord are of lung, breast, prostate, and lymphoma; less common are myeloma, melanoma, and genitourinary tract tumors. An important presenting sign is back pain, either of recent onset or old pain that has returned or increased. Pain is present in 97% of all cord compressions, followed in frequency by weakness (76%) and paresthesias (57%) along a bilateral or unilateral dermatomal distribution. There is associated bowel and bladder dysfunction in 51% of patients with more advanced disease. In a few patients there is no history of cancer, and pain is the initial presentation.

B. Even when the physical examination does not reveal signs of spinal cord compression, obtain plain radiographs of the painful region to rule out neoplastic involvement. If the plain films are negative, consider non-neoplastic causes (rheumatoid arthritis, aortic aneurysm, spondylosis, herniated disc, spinal tuberculosis, osteoarthritis, osteomyelitis). Proceed with a detailed work-up if any of the following are present: pain with tenderness to percussion over the affected vertebral body, bilateral muscle weakness in the extremities, sensory changes, loss of deep tendon reflexes, or bowel or bladder incontinence.

C. If plain films reveal a lesion in a painful area, follow with MRI or myelography, which have comparable sensitivity and specificity. Myelography is an invasive procedure that requires technical skill and the use of contrast. MRI is not invasive and helps in detecting intramedullary lesions, but patients may have difficulty lying still on the hard table or may have claustrophobia. Also, MRI is not always available. If these studies show a lesion, there is a 90% probability of cord compression.

D. If MRI is negative and clinical findings suggest cord involvement, proceed with myelography. Myelography will help determine the upper and lower extent of the lesion and ascertain if there is more than one lesion. If a complete block is found on lumbar myelography, cisternal myelography or MRI is required to identify the upper end of the block. If both studies are negative, there is no cord compression.

E. The choice of treatment depends on the type of tumor, the level of the block, the rapidity of onset and duration of symptoms, previous treatment, and the clinical experience available. This medical emergency is treated vigorously with radiation or surgery in addition to steroids. Our current recommendation is to immediately give 10 mg IV dexamethasone, follow with 4 mg every 6 hours daily for at least 72 hours, and then rapidly taper as tolerated. Begin radiotherapy immediately after the diagnosis is established. The earlier a lesion is detected and treated, the better the functional outcome will be. Response rates are 30–80%. The total dose of radiation is 3000–4000 rad, delivered over 2–4 weeks.

F. Consider surgery (laminectomy, stabilization) when there is (1) no histologic diagnosis and cord compression is the presenting sign of cancer, (2) history of radiation therapy to the affected area, (3) neurologic progression of disease despite steroids and radiotherapy, (4) instability requiring fixation, or (5) a high cervical lesion. After surgery, give radiotherapy to avoid recurrences. Initial response to combined surgery and radiation is 20–100%, depending on tumor type and timing of treatment. The best prognostic index for eventual recovery of function is pretreatment status: 60% of patients who are ambulatory at diagnosis remain so postoperatively, whereas only 7% of those who are paraplegic at diagnosis are ambulatory after treatment.

G. When plain films are negative and physical examination is not definitive, adjust pain medications and observe. If pain persists or worsens or if the history is highly suspicious, perform MRI and proceed accordingly.

References

Gilbert RW, Kim J-H, Posner JB. Epidural spinal cord compression from metastatic tumor: diagnosis and treatment. Ann Neurol 1978; 3:40.

Maranzano E, et al. Radiation therapy in metastatic spinal cord compression. Cancer 1991; 67:1333.

Rodichok L, et al. Early diagnosis of spinal epidural metastases. Am J Med 1981; 70:1181.

Wasserstrom W, Glass PJ, Posner JB. Diagnosis and treatment of leptomeningeal metastases from solid tumors: experience with 90 patients. Cancer 1982; 49:759.

Willson JKV, Masaryk T. Neurologic emergencies in the cancer patient. Semin Oncol 1989; 16:490.

Young RF, Post EM, King GA. Treatment of spinal epidural metastases. J Neurosurg 1980; 53:741.

SPINAL CORD COMPRESSION Suspected

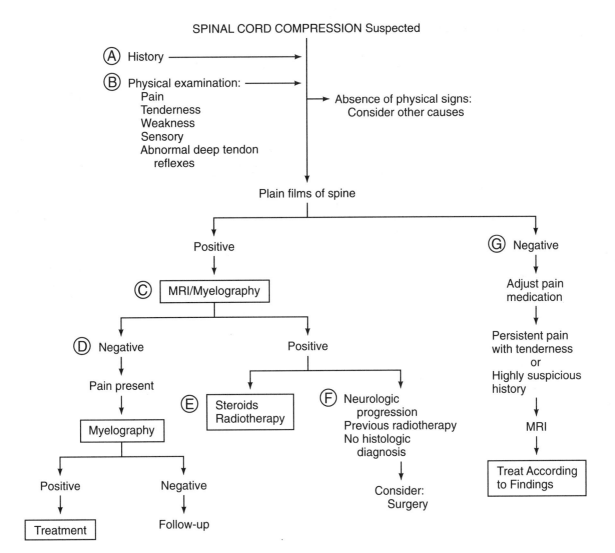

(A) History

(B) Physical examination:
   Pain
   Tenderness
   Weakness
   Sensory
   Abnormal deep tendon
      reflexes

Absence of physical signs:
Consider other causes

Plain films of spine

Positive

(G) Negative

(C) MRI/Myelography

(D) Negative

Positive

Adjust pain
medication

Pain present

(E) Steroids
Radiotherapy

(F) Neurologic
progression
Previous radiotherapy
No histologic
   diagnosis

Persistent pain
with tenderness
or
Highly suspicious
history

Myelography

Consider:
Surgery

MRI

Positive

Negative

Treat According
to Findings

Treatment

Follow-up

INFECTIOUS DISEASE

FOREIGN TRAVEL: IMMUNIZATIONS AND INFECTIONS

Rodney D. Adam, M.D.

A. Ascertain the patient's travel plans to determine the risk of exposure to various infections and the appropriate precautions. This includes countries of travel, whether city or rural, and purpose and duration of trip. Determine which illnesses are endemic or epidemic in the region to be visited and whether chloroquine-resistant *Plasmodium falciparum* is present. Malaria is not found in most cities outside equatorial Africa, but the water supply may be contaminated in urban or rural areas. In general, exposure to endemic infections is greater during longer trips and those to more rural areas.

B. Common means of acquiring infections include endogenous food and water and mosquitos; exposure to these sources should be limited as much as possible. HIV infection, endemic in many parts of the world, is spread sexually and by blood transfusion and reused needles. Other STDs, including gonorrhea and chancroid, are also common in many areas. Sexual abstinence, condom use, and avoidance of contaminated needles or transfusion of untested blood limit exposure to these agents.

C. Cholera vaccine has poor efficacy and high toxicity, and cholera is uncommon in most areas. Canine rabies is common in many areas, and human diploid vaccine for postexposure prophylaxis is not readily available. In highly endemic areas where exposure is a possibility, consider pre-exposure immunization. Hepatitis B is common in many areas; consider vaccination for travelers with potential occupational (e.g., medical workers) or sexual exposure.

D. Malaria is common in most tropical and subtropical regions. Most cases being caused by *P. falciparum* and *P. vivax*. Chloroquine is effective preventive therapy for *P. vivax* and chloroquine-sensitive *P. falciparum*. Mefloquine is the recommended preventive agent in 1992 for chloroquine-resistant *P. falciparum*, and doxycycline is a reasonable alternative, but recommendations are continually changing. Consult current CDC recommendations.

E. Febrile illnesses in returning travelers may be the result of routine viral infections. However, malaria is a common, treatable, and frequently fatal infection and is thus a primary consideration.

F. If the malaria smear is positive but does not definitively identify the species, the patient should be presumed to have *P. falciparum* infection, which should be assumed to be drug resistant if the person received preventive therapy. Patients with definite or probable *P. falciparum* malaria should be hospitalized for treatment. The recommended treatment changes frequently; consult current recommendations (e.g., CDC).

G. The infections in the algorithm are only a partial list and are geographically variable. For example, scrub typhus (rickettsial) is common in Malaysia, and several viral causes of hemorrhagic fever (e.g., Lassa fever) are found in equatorial Africa. If a hemorrhagic fever is suspected on the basis of thrombocytopenia, leukopenia, or coagulopathy, contact the CDC for proper isolation precautions.

H. Diarrhea occurring during travel or within a few days of return is most commonly caused by pathogenic *Escherichia coli* but may be caused by *Shigella*, *Salmonella*, *Campylobacter*, or other agents. Bloody diarrhea suggests shigellosis or amebiasis and stool WBCs are found with *Shigella*, invasive *E. coli*, *Campylobacter*, and some *Salmonella* infections. In the absence of specific findings, empiric therapy with TMP/SMX or a quinolone is appropriate. Further diagnostic steps or changes in therapy depend on initial findings and response to therapy.

I. Diarrhea with malabsorption but no blood or WBCs suggests giardiasis, cryptosporidiosis, isosporiasis, strongyloidiasis, or tropical sprue. *Entamoeba histolytica* causes a colitis (as do *Shigella*, *Campylobacter*, and sometimes *Salmonella*) characterized by rectal pain and bloody stools but an absence of WBCs. Initial studies include stools for ova and parasites (O&P), WBCs, and culture.

J. This partial list includes infections that are uncommon in short-term travelers but may be seen in long-term travelers or immigrants from endemic areas.

Person TRAVELS TO FOREIGN AREA

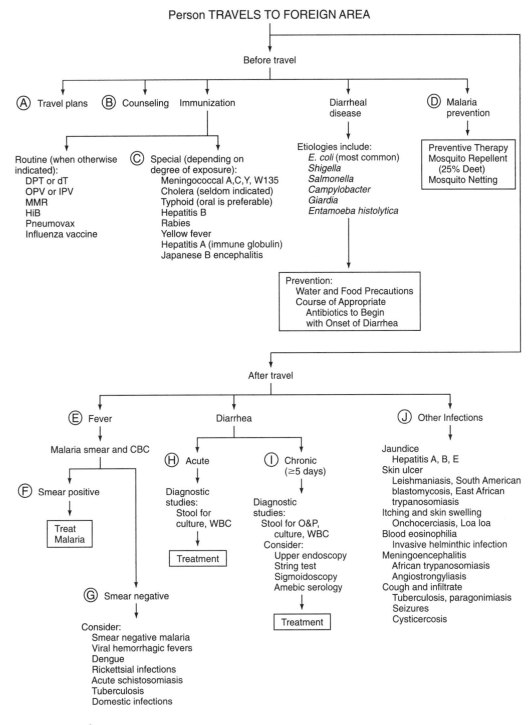

Before travel

Ⓐ Travel plans   Ⓑ Counseling   Immunization   Diarrheal   Ⓓ Malaria
                                                       disease   prevention

Routine (when otherwise   Ⓒ Special (depending on   Etiologies include: Preventive Therapy
indicated):   degree of exposure):   *E. coli* (most common)   Mosquito Repellent
    DPT or dT   Meningococcal A,C,Y, W135   *Shigella*   (25% Deet)
    OPV or IPV   Cholera (seldom indicated)   *Salmonella*   Mosquito Netting
    MMR   Typhoid (oral is preferable) *Campylobacter*
    HiB   Hepatitis B   *Giardia*
    Pneumovax   Rabies   *Entamoeba histolytica*
    Influenza vaccine   Yellow fever
                                 Hepatitis A (immune globulin)
                                 Japanese B encephalitis

                                                       Prevention:
                                                           Water and Food Precautions
                                                           Course of Appropriate
                                                               Antibiotics to Begin
                                                               with Onset of Diarrhea

After travel

Ⓔ Fever   Diarrhea   Ⓙ Other Infections

Malaria smear and CBC   Jaundice
                                                                       Hepatitis A, B, E
Ⓕ Smear positive   Ⓗ Acute   Ⓘ Chronic   Skin ulcer
                                    (≥5 days)   Leishmaniasis, South American
Treat   Diagnostic   blastomycosis, East African
Malaria   studies: Diagnostic   trypanosomiasis
                         Stool for   studies: Itching and skin swelling
                         culture, WBC   Stool for O&P,   Onchocerciasis, Loa loa
                                             culture, WBC   Blood eosinophilia
                     Treatment   Consider: Invasive helminthic infection
                                        Upper endoscopy   Meningoencephalitis
Ⓖ Smear negative   String test   African trypanosomiasis
                                        Sigmoidoscopy   Angiostrongyliasis
Consider: Amebic serology   Cough and infiltrate
    Smear negative malaria   Tuberculosis, paragonimiasis
    Viral hemorrhagic fevers   Treatment   Seizures
    Dengue   Cysticercosis
    Rickettsial infections
    Acute schistosomiasis
    Tuberculosis
    Domestic infections

References

Hill DR, Pearson RD. Health advice for international travel. Ann Intern Med 1988; 108:839.

Lobel HO, Bernard KW, Williams SL, et al. Effectiveness and tolerance of long-term malaria prophylaxis with mefloquine. JAMA 1991; 265:361.

Steffen R, Rickenbach M, Wilhelm U, et al. Health problems after travel to developing countries. J Infect Dis 1987; 156:84.

Studemeister MD. Travel medicine for the primary care physician. West J Med 1991; 154:418.

U.S. Department of Health and Human Services, Public Health Service, Centers for Disease Control. Health Information for International Travel, 1989.

Woodruff BA, Pavia AT, Blake PA. A new look at typhoid vaccination — information for the practicing physician. JAMA 1991; 265:756.

ACUTE AND SUBACUTE MENINGITIS

Steven D. Salas, M.D.
Richard M. Mandel, M.D.

A. Papilledema and/or focal neurologic deficits in a patient with meningeal symptoms suggests the possibility of a cerebral abscess. In this setting, lumbar puncture may disturb intracranial pressures and precipitate herniation.

B. Common underlying conditions in patients with brain abscess and other parameningeal foci include endocarditis, lung abscess, sinusitis, middle ear infection, and antecedent head trauma or neurosurgery. Therefore, blood cultures should be obtained and empiric therapy designed according to likely pathogens (see below).

C. If the CNS imaging procedure reveals a mass lesion, a neurologic and/or neurosurgical evaluation may be indicated. In patients with focal neurologic findings, altered sensorium, and temporal horn cerebritis, herpes simplex encephalitis should be considered and empiric therapy instituted pending diagnostic confirmation. Brain biopsy may be indicated, depending on the clinical circumstances.

D. In patients with signs and symptoms of acute meningitis, initiation of emergent antibiotic therapy within 30 minutes is critical in treating the potentially lethal progression of this disease. Waiting for CT scan or CSF Gram's stain may waste valuable therapeutic time. Start patients on empiric antibiotics on the basis of minimal data; further revision of the antimicrobial regimen may be undertaken after evaluation of the complete history, physical examination, and CSF analysis.

E. In normal immunocompetent hosts the most likely organisms include *Streptococcus pneumoniae, Neisseria meningitidis,* and (less likely), *Haemophilus influenzae.* Elderly patients may present in a more subtle fashion, encountering the usual organisms and others such as *Staphylococcus aureus, Listeria monocytogenes,* and gram-negative bacilli.

F. Common etiologic agents in compromised hosts include: (1) in diabetic and oncology patients, *S. pneumoniae, Staphylococcus aureus,* gram-negative bacilli, *Cryptococcus neoformans;* (2) in alcoholic patients, *S. pneumoniae;* (3) in steroid-treated and AIDS patients, *C. neoformans, Mycobacterium tuberculosis;* and (4) in AIDS patients, acute HIV meningitis.

G. Patients with closed head trauma encounter *S. pneumoniae* as well as gram-negative bacilli.

H. After open head trauma or neurosurgery, be concerned about *Staphylococcus* species and gram-negative bacilli. In procedures that traverse sinuses, upper respiratory flora are common.

I. Intraventricular shunt devices are associated with organisms such as *Staphylococcus epidermidis, Propionibacterium acnes,* diphtheroids, and gram-negative bacilli.

(Continued on page 238)

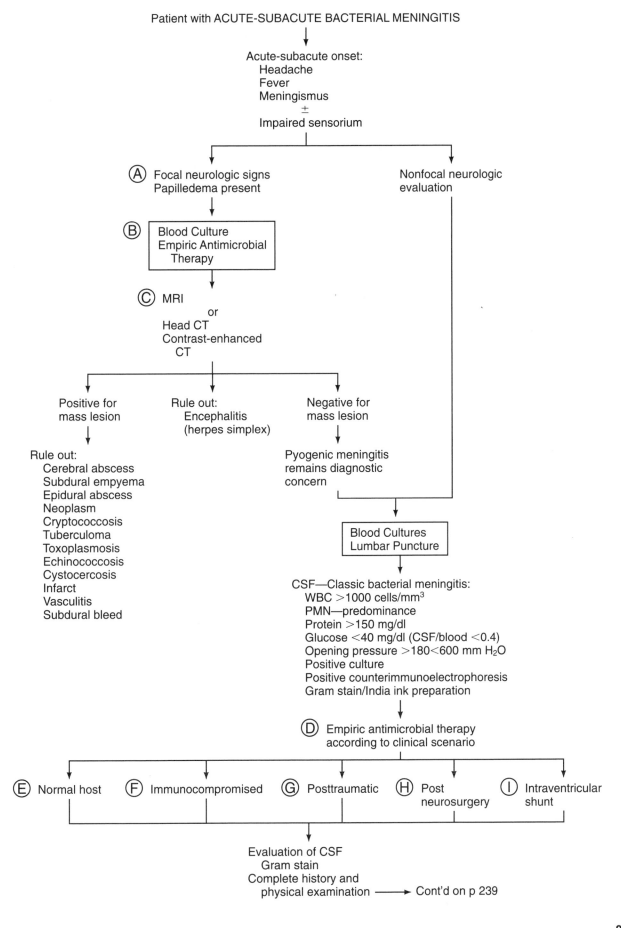

Patient with ACUTE-SUBACUTE BACTERIAL MENINGITIS

Acute-subacute onset:
　　Headache
　　Fever
　　Meningismus
　　±
　　Impaired sensorium

(A) Focal neurologic signs
　　Papilledema present

Nonfocal neurologic
evaluation

(B) | Blood Culture
Empiric Antimicrobial
　Therapy |

(C) MRI
　　or
　　Head CT
　　Contrast-enhanced
　　　CT

Positive for
mass lesion

Rule out:
Encephalitis
(herpes simplex)

Negative for
mass lesion

Rule out:
　　Cerebral abscess
　　Subdural empyema
　　Epidural abscess
　　Neoplasm
　　Cryptococcosis
　　Tuberculoma
　　Toxoplasmosis
　　Echinococcosis
　　Cystocercosis
　　Infarct
　　Vasculitis
　　Subdural bleed

Pyogenic meningitis
remains diagnostic
concern

| Blood Cultures
Lumbar Puncture |

CSF—Classic bacterial meningitis:
　　WBC >1000 cells/mm^3
　　PMN—predominance
　　Protein >150 mg/dl
　　Glucose <40 mg/dl (CSF/blood <0.4)
　　Opening pressure >180<600 mm H$_2$O
　　Positive culture
　　Positive counterimmunoelectrophoresis
　　Gram stain/India ink preparation

(D) Empiric antimicrobial therapy
　　according to clinical scenario

(E) Normal host　(F) Immunocompromised　(G) Posttraumatic　(H) Post
neurosurgery　(I) Intraventricular
shunt

Evaluation of CSF
　Gram stain
　Complete history and
　　physical examination ⟶ Cont'd on p 239

J. At this juncture, re-evaluate empiric therapy and start appropriate antimicrobial therapy based on Gram's stain evaluation. Centrifuged CSF is positive in 60–90% of cases of culture-positive meningitis. Positive cultures further guide therapy.

K. If no bacteria are seen on Gram's stain, the differential diagnosis expands. Cryptococcal meningitis can be ruled out by India ink preparation, cryptococcal antigen determination, and fungal culture.

L. In the absence of cryptococcal disease and if the CSF demonstrates a normal sugar level and absent or minimal cells, investigate a parameningeal focus (p 242).

M. Polymorphonuclear leukocytes in the CSF may be reflective of partially treated bacterial disease, early TB, or viral meningitis.

N. If the CSF demonstrates leukocytes with a mononuclear cell response, the glucose can be used to discriminate between viral meningitis versus partially treated bacterial, fungal, or tuberculous meningitis (p 240). If partially treated bacterial meningitis is a diagnostic consideration, antimicrobial therapy should be continued.

O. Treatment for tuberculous meningitis is indicated if there is strong ancillary evidence for this infection. Note that an appropriate CSF-AFB smear results from the spun sediment of 10 ml of CSF. The AFB cultures may take 6 weeks to turn positive; therefore, consider empiric therapy when clinical suspicion is high. Note that many of these presentations may not be classic and it is important to call in consultants to help with the subtle nuances of this extensive differential diagnosis.

References

Kaufman BA. Meningitis in the neurosurgical patient. Infect Dis Clin North Am 1990; 4:677.

McGee ZA, Baringer JR. Acute meningitis. In: Mandell GL, et al, eds. Principles and practice of infectious diseases. 3rd ed. New York: Churchill Livingstone, 1990:741.

Wispelwey B, et al. Bacterial meningitis in adults. Infect Dis Clin North Am 1990; 4:645.

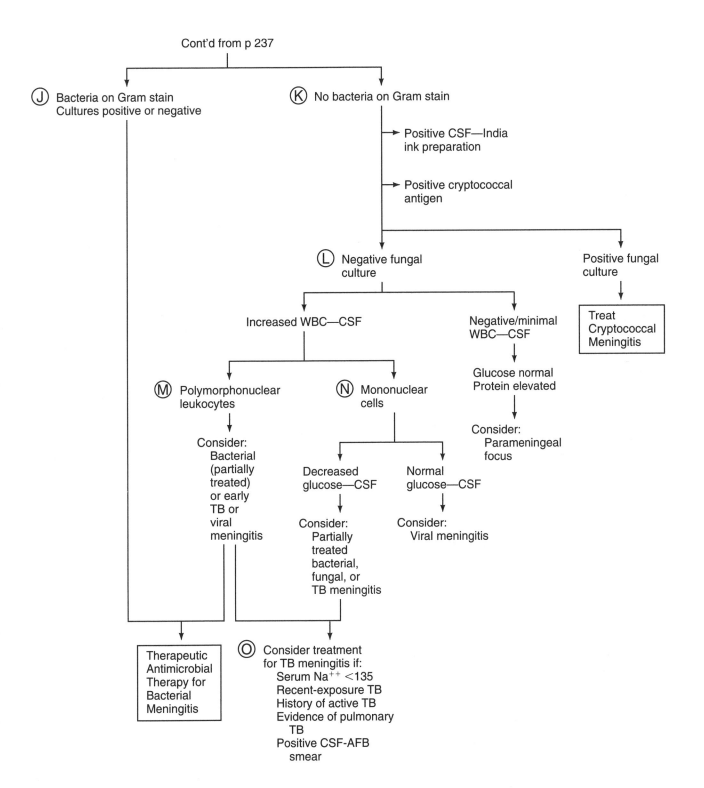

Cont'd from p 237

Ⓙ Bacteria on Gram stain
Cultures positive or negative

Ⓚ No bacteria on Gram stain

→ Positive CSF—India ink preparation

→ Positive cryptococcal antigen

Ⓛ Negative fungal culture

Positive fungal culture

Treat Cryptococcal Meningitis

Increased WBC—CSF

Negative/minimal WBC—CSF

Glucose normal Protein elevated

Consider: Parameningeal focus

Ⓜ Polymorphonuclear leukocytes

Consider: Bacterial (partially treated) or early TB or viral meningitis

Ⓝ Mononuclear cells

Decreased glucose—CSF

Consider: Partially treated bacterial, fungal, or TB meningitis

Normal glucose—CSF

Consider: Viral meningitis

Therapeutic Antimicrobial Therapy for Bacterial Meningitis

Ⓞ Consider treatment for TB meningitis if:
Serum Na^{++} <135
Recent-exposure TB
History of active TB
Evidence of pulmonary TB
Positive CSF-AFB smear

CHRONIC MENINGITIS

Jeffrey L. Silber, M.D.
Mark J. DiNubile, M.D.

A. In patients with chronic meningitis there is the insidious onset of headache, often accompanied by fever, nausea, vomiting, lethargy, and confusion. By convention, symptoms and CSF abnormalities must be present for at least 4 weeks. Differentiate chronic or persistent meningitis from the syndrome of recurrent meningitis.

B. Perform CT scan or MRI of the brain in all patients with chronic meningitis. The scan may identify a mass lesion, hydrocephalus, and/or contrast enhancement of the basilar meninges. If not contraindicated, perform a lumbar puncture. The CSF profile characteristically shows elevated protein and lymphocytic pleocytosis. The formula is never in itself diagnostic, but certain findings may suggest particular etiologies (e.g., hypoglycorrhachia is commonly found in tuberculous and fungal meningitis).

C. In most cases the history is nonspecific. Travel, outdoor activity, sexual habits, or other exposures occasionally help to focus the evaluation. Previous antimicrobial therapy may obscure the detection of bacterial infections such as endocarditis.

D. The physical examination sometimes reveals signs of associated systemic illness. Focality in the neurologic examination may reflect an unrecognized mass lesion. Cranial nerve abnormalities suggest a basilar meningitis, usually caused by infection, sarcoid, or malignancy. If accessible lesions outside the CNS are found, they should be biopsied and cultured.

E. Tuberculosis (TB), sarcoid, or tumor may be found by chest radiography. Cytologic, microbiologic, or histopathologic examination of tissue, sputum, or fluid obtained from other body sites may confirm a diagnosis of a mycobacterial, fungal, or malignant process. Skin tests have minimal utility and should be limited to a PPD and anergy panel. Serologic tests for certain infections and connective tissue diseases can be helpful in the appropriate clinical context. Blood cultures should be obtained and incubated for 2 weeks to exclude bacterial endocarditis. Additional studies, such as mammography and endoscopy, may be indicated in selected cases.

F. Stains and cultures of CSF for bacteria, mycobacteria, and fungi are mandatory and often must be repeated. Large volumes (>10 cc) should be processed to maximize detection of fungal, mycobacterial, and tumor cells. Fungi can sometimes be demonstrated in ventricular CSF, even when lumbar fluid is negative. Additional studies of the CSF may be diagnostic, such as serologic tests for syphilis, Lyme disease, and certain fungi; cytology for malignancies; and India ink and antigen detection for cryptococcal organisms.

G. If all attempts at diagnosis prove futile, consider a directed biopsy of brain and meninges. The yield of blind meningeal biopsy is low, and this invasive procedure is usually reserved for undiagnosed patients who have a focal lesion or suffer a progressive decline in neurologic function.

H. If empiric therapy is undertaken, certain principles guide the strategy of therapeutic trials: (1) diagnostic efforts must continue during therapy; (2) therapeutic response is difficult to interpret because recovery is always protracted, even with the use of appropriate drugs; (3) trials should be made sequentially, not concurrently; (4) amphotericin B should be used last; and (5) corticosteroids should be avoided because of their potentially devastating effects in patients with fungal meningitis. A trial of antituberculous therapy is indicated in most undiagnosed cases. Despite all diagnostic and therapeutic efforts, sometimes no cause can be determined. Some cases can be categorized retrospectively as "chronic benign lymphocytic meningitis," a self-limited illness in which spontaneous clinical remission usually ensues within 6 months. Other patients have persistent neurologic symptoms and CSF abnormalities. Certain patients with "idiopathic" chronic meningitis have a poor prognosis; the etiology often remains undefined, despite postmortem examination.

References

Katzman M, Ellner JJ. Chronic meningitis. In: Mandell GL, Douglas RG Jr, Bennett JE, eds. Principles and practice of infectious diseases. New York: Churchill Livingstone, 1990:755.

Peacock JE Jr. Persistent neutrophilic meningitis. Infect Dis Clin North Am 1990; 4:747.

Wilhelm C, Ellner JJ. Chronic meningitis. Neurol Clin 1986; 4:115.

Patient with HEADACHE ± FEVER ± CHANGE IN MENTAL STATUS

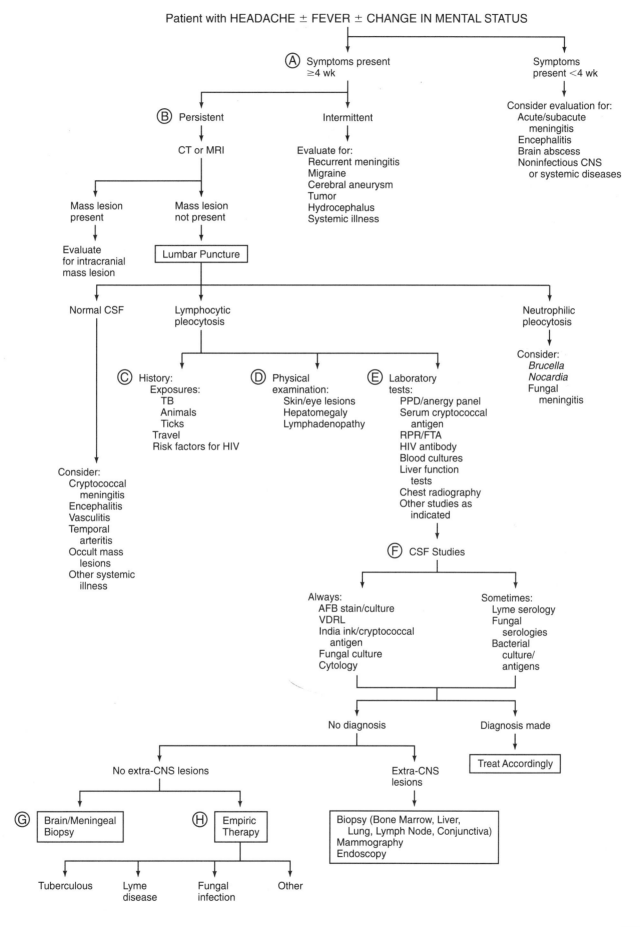

241

ASEPTIC MENINGITIS SYNDROME

Douglas Fish, M.D.
Richard M. Mandel, M.D.

A. A thorough history and physical examination is paramount. Note the season; medical history; degree of immunosuppression; previous exposure to tuberculosis and fungal disease; exposure to insects, animal excreta, and fresh water; travel; sexual history; HIV risk factors; medications, including recent antibiotics; immunization history; and contacts with family members or others who have also been ill. Look for evidence of rash, conjunctivitis, herpangina, otitis, and genital infection. Approach elderly and immunosuppressed individuals with a high index of suspicion for pyogenic meningitis. (Immunosuppression can be the result of steroid therapy, chemotherapy, transplants, alcoholism, asplenia, complement deficiency, and HIV infection.) If papilledema or focal neurologic signs are present, start empiric antimicrobial therapy and obtain CNS imaging studies before considering lumbar puncture (LP). A neurosurgical consultation may be indicated.

B. LP should be performed when meningitis is a considered diagnosis. "Aseptic meningitis syndrome" may be used to describe any acute-onset meningitis with a mononuclear cell pleocytosis and no other apparent cause after initial evaluation of routine stains and basic cultures. The benignity of the course of viral aseptic meningitis is easily defined retrospectively but may be difficult to ascertain in acutely ill patients. If available, counterimmunoelectrophoresis for bacterial antigens for *Streptococcus pneumoniae*, *Haemophilus influenzae*, and *Neisseria meningitidis* should be performed on CSF and urine. If one of these is positive, treat for the detected pathogen. A CSF WBC count <500 cells/mm^3 with a mononuclear predominance, a negative Gram's stain, a protein level <80–100 mg/dl, and a normal glucose level in a normal host suggests a viral meningitis, especially in summer or fall. A choice between antibiotic therapy and a course of observation must be made. If the above conditions are met, observation is appropriate; if not, antibacterial therapy pending the 48- to 72-hour culture results is prudent. These guidelines depend greatly on the patient's clinical appearance and the knowledge that the aforementioned criteria are not absolute. There may be some overlap during the early course between the CSF parameters of aseptic meningitis and acute pyogenic meningitis. CSF can be sent for enteroviral culture, and this may well be cost effective in some instances by reducing hospital stays and antibiotic usage. It is not uncommon to find a polymorphonuclear predominance early in viral meningitis. Repeating LP in 8–36 hours to seek a mononuclear shift is recommended. If the patient is in a high-risk group for pyogenic (treatable) meningitis (e.g., immunocompromised or elderly people) or has recently received antibiotics, raising the question of partially treated meningitis, give antibiotics pending 48- to 72-hour blood and CSF culture results, and postpone the decision regarding continuation of therapy until that time. Given the grave consequences of stopping therapy, it may be prudent in these instances to complete a course of therapy. An HIV evaluation may be indicated under appropriate clinical circumstances.

C. If a parameningeal focus (subdural empyema, epidural abscess, brain abscess) is suspected, perform a head CT scan with contrast or MRI, especially if the patient has sinusitis or otitis. If results are abnormal, start treatment with appropriate antibiotics to cover for the identified infection and obtain a neurosurgical consultation. Examination of the spine for tenderness and appropriate imaging procedures may be indicated to rule out an epidural abscess or vertebral osteomyelitis. With loss of higher integrative function, consider herpes simplex encephalitis and perform MRI.

D. Infectious etiologies such as fungal or tuberculous meningitis, Lyme disease, rickettsial disease, leptospirosis, brucellosis, syphilis, and amebae may present as aseptic meningitis. In addition, endocarditis and bacterial toxins such as those from *Staphylococcus aureus* may cause a CSF pleocytosis. Consider potential noninfectious causes of aseptic meningitis. The following may all cause this syndrome: drugs such as trimethoprim, trimethoprim-sulfamethoxazole, and nonsteroidal anti-inflammatory agents; heavy metals; spinal and neurosurgical procedures; tumors; hematologic malignancies; sarcoidosis; collagen vascular diseases such as systemic lupus erythematosus, vasculitis, and Behçet's disease; postseizure effect; and Mollaret's meningitis. There may be considerable overlap between aseptic and chronic meningitides.

References

Connoly KJ, Hammer SM. The acute aseptic meningitis syndrome. Infect Dis Clin North Am 1990; 4:599.

Gordon MF, Allen M, Coyle PK. Drug induced meningitis. Neurology 1990; 40:163.

McGee ZA, Boringer Jr. Acute meningitis. In: Mandell GL, Douglas RG Jr, Bennett JE, eds. Principles and practice of infectious diseases. 3rd ed. New York: Churchill Livingstone, 1990:741.

Meyer NM Jr, Johnson RT, Crawford IP, et al. Nervous system syndromes of "viral" etiology. Am J Med 1960; 27:334.

Patient with ASEPTIC MENINGITIS SYNDROME

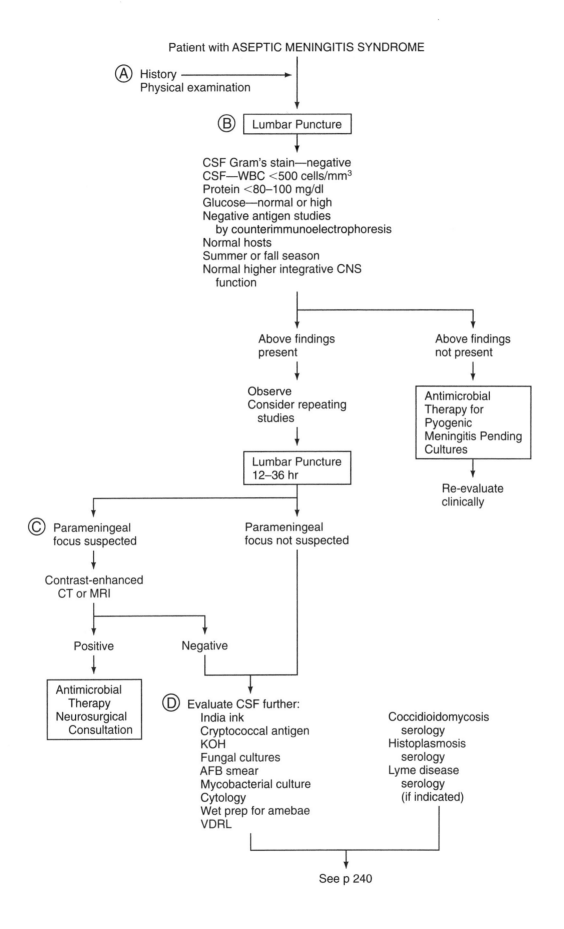

Ⓐ History
Physical examination

Ⓑ Lumbar Puncture

CSF Gram's stain—negative
CSF—WBC <500 cells/mm³
Protein <80–100 mg/dl
Glucose—normal or high
Negative antigen studies
    by counterimmunoelectrophoresis
Normal hosts
Summer or fall season
Normal higher integrative CNS
    function

Above findings
present

Above findings
not present

Observe
Consider repeating
    studies

Antimicrobial
Therapy for
Pyogenic
Meningitis Pending
Cultures

Lumbar Puncture
12–36 hr

Re-evaluate
clinically

Ⓒ Parameningeal
focus suspected

Parameningeal
focus not suspected

Contrast-enhanced
CT or MRI

Positive   Negative

Antimicrobial
Therapy
Neurosurgical
Consultation

Ⓓ Evaluate CSF further:
India ink
Cryptococcal antigen
KOH
Fungal cultures
AFB smear
Mycobacterial culture
Cytology
Wet prep for amebae
VDRL

Coccidioidomycosis
    serology
Histoplasmosis
    serology
Lyme disease
    serology
    (if indicated)

See p 240

SEXUALLY TRANSMITTED DISEASES

George William Estes, M.D.
Richard M. Mandel, M.D.

A. Obtain the history in as factual and nonjudgmental a manner as possible. Specifically seek risk factors known to correlate with sexually transmitted diseases (STDs): sexual activity; age <25 years; multiple sexual partners; history of STDs, prostitution, or contact with a prostitute; illicit drug use; and residence in a detention center. Other useful history includes sexual practices, duration of symptoms and signs, recent related medical treatment of a partner, travel, immunosuppression, and self-treatment (especially with topical or systemic antibiotics). The physical examination should include not only the genitalia but the lower abdomen, pubic and inguinal areas, inner thighs, anus, and rectum plus a thorough pelvic examination in females. Look for extragenital sites of infection as well.

B. Perhaps because of the psychological importance of the sexual organs, a patient may suspect an STD but have a history and physical findings inconsistent with any STD.

C. STDs should be viewed as sentinel events identifying patients participating in unsafe sexual practices. Seek co-existing STDs in patients who present for evaluation. Counseling should be offered and consist of a minimum of discussion of safe sex techniques and an offer of HIV testing (with appropriate consent and before-and-after test counseling).

D. Given the increasing incidence of syphilis, its consequences, and the favorable cost-benefit status of testing, all patients with an STD should receive a serum nontreponemal test (SNT).

E. Regardless of sexual practices, women should have rectal swabs cultured; the history will dictate whether pharyngeal cultures are necessary. Homosexual men should routinely undergo urethral, rectal, and pharyngeal cultures. Gram staining of extraurethral sites is not recommended.

F. Many cases of nongonococcal urethritis (NGU) are caused by *Chlamydia trachomatis;* some of the remainder are caused by *Ureaplasma urealyticum*. *C. trachomatis* can cause urethritis or epididymitis (including asymptomatic forms). In women it can cause symptomatic or asymptomatic urethritis, endocervicitis, endometritis, pelvic inflammatory disease, and the Fitz-Hugh–Curtis perihepatitis syndrome. Obstructive infertility, ectopic pregnancy, and neonatal infections may be serious sequelae of this infection. As optimal treatment regimens change, consult current CDC recommendations.

G. *N. gonorrhoeae* is a fastidious organism that requires the use of selective media and a CO_2-enriched atmosphere for growth.

H. As a function of its dynamic resistance patterns, optimal treatment regimens for *N. gonorrhoeae* change; consult current CDC recommendations. NGU frequently coexists with gonococcal disease and should be treated concurrently.

I. A Gram-stained smear of urethral discharge or a swab containing four or more neutrophils per oil (1000×) field is abnormal and indicates acute urethritis. Lesser numbers do not exclude this diagnosis.

J. Optimal control of STDs requires notification of partners. If the presenting patient is unable or unwilling to do so, local health departments can facilitate this process. It is less than desirable to "blindly" treat a partner; a thorough evaluation is required. However, it is often necessary to treat contacts empirically owing to sufficiently high rates of infectivity of the STDs.

K. Examine the first 10 cc of a voided urine specimen; 15 or more neutrophils in 5 high-day (400×) fields strongly suggests urethritis.

L. Vaginitis due to *Trichomonas vaginalis* can be asymptomatic, but women typically complain of vaginal discharge, pruritus, and dyspareunia. Men infected with *T. vaginalis* are typically asymptomatic but need to be treated.

M. Patients with small amounts of discharge (minimal inflammatory response) are best re-evaluated in the morning before voiding.

(Continued on page 246)

SEXUALLY TRANSMITTED DISEASE Suspected

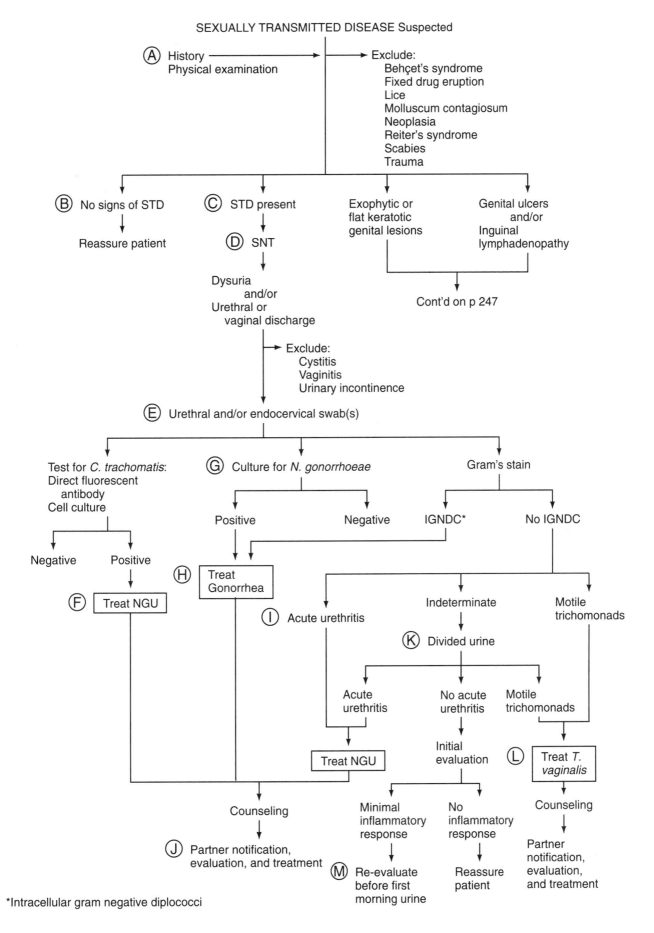

Ⓐ History
Physical examination

Exclude:
Behçet's syndrome
Fixed drug eruption
Lice
Molluscum contagiosum
Neoplasia
Reiter's syndrome
Scabies
Trauma

Ⓑ No signs of STD

Reassure patient

Ⓒ STD present

Ⓓ SNT

Dysuria
and/or
Urethral or
vaginal discharge

Exophytic or
flat keratotic
genital lesions

Genital ulcers
and/or
Inguinal
lymphadenopathy

Cont'd on p 247

Exclude:
Cystitis
Vaginitis
Urinary incontinence

Ⓔ Urethral and/or endocervical swab(s)

Test for *C. trachomatis*:
Direct fluorescent
antibody
Cell culture

Ⓖ Culture for *N. gonorrhoeae*

Gram's stain

Negative   Positive

Positive   Negative

IGNDC*   No IGNDC

Ⓕ Treat NGU

Ⓗ Treat
Gonorrhea

Ⓘ Acute urethritis

Indeterminate

Motile
trichomonads

Ⓚ Divided urine

Acute
urethritis

No acute
urethritis

Motile
trichomonads

Treat NGU

Initial
evaluation

Ⓛ Treat *T.
vaginalis*

Counseling

Counseling

Ⓙ Partner notification,
evaluation, and treatment

Minimal
inflammatory
response

No
inflammatory
response

Partner
notification,
evaluation,
and treatment

Ⓜ Re-evaluate
before first
morning urine

Reassure
patient

*Intracellular gram negative diplococci

245

N. The true incidence of human papillomavirus (HPV) infection is unknown, but reasonable estimates place it at 10–20% of sexually active adults. Infected patients may have overt warts, minimally symptomatic lesions, subclinical infections, or latent infections. In an effort to detect subclinical lesions, examination aided by magnification and acetic acid (aceto-whitening) is becoming commonplace; cervical Pap smears are already standard care. Certain strains of HPV have been strongly associated with cervical neoplasia, and are now also implicated in neoplasias of the vulva, penis, and anus. It is suggested that partners of patients with HPV also undergo evaluation.

O. Recent studies have identified genital ulcer disease as an independent risk factor for HIV infection.

P. The easiest and most common methods of examination are dark-field and phase-contrast direct microscopy.

Q. A lesion is considered negative for treponemes only after three sequential negative examinations have been performed. However, further evaluation and appropriate therapy should not be delayed while data are being collected.

R. Treatment failure or reinfection must be assumed before the sero-fast state is considered.

S. Treatment regimens vary according to the stage of disease or the presence of concomitant HIV infection. Consult current CDC recommendations before initiating therapy.

T. Biological false-positive SNTs are well known, and multiple noninfectious etiologies may be implicated.

U. The best predictor of the cause of genital ulcers is local prevalence patterns. Differentiation is not reliably possible on clinical grounds alone; laboratory studies are essential.

V. Both lymphogranuloma venereum and donovanosis are rare (<100 cases reported per annum and 11 cases reported in 1988, respectively) in the United States.

W. For identification of herpes simplex virus (HSV) as a cause of genital ulcer, Tzanck and Pap smears of lesions are quick and inexpensive. However, they are insensitive, do not allow for differentiation of HSV I or II when positive, and do not exclude HSV when negative. Tissue culture methods are the "gold standard" but are time consuming and expensive.

X. First episodes of HSV should be treated. This results in decreased viral shedding and severity and duration of symptoms. The decision regarding when, and for how long, to institute prophylaxis is less clear and must be made with the patient's input on a case-by-case basis. Therapy has no impact on subsequent recurrence.

Y. A positive Gram-stained smear classically shows gram-negative coccobacilli in a "school of fish" or "fingerprint" configuration. The laboratory should be notified that *Haemophilus ducreyi* is a possibility when submitting specimens.

Z. Chancroid was once uncommon in the general U.S. population but has become more common since 1985. Currently, >3000 cases per annum are reported. For treatment regimens, refer to current CDC recommendations.

References

Centers for Disease Control. Sexually transmitted diseases treatment guidelines. MMWR 1989; 38:S–8.

Handsfield HH. Sexually transmitted diseases. Infect Dis Clin North Am 1987; 1:1.

Holmes King K, Mardh Per-Anders, Sparling PF, Wiesner PJ, eds. Sexually transmitted diseases. 2nd ed. New York: McGraw-Hill, 1990.

Mandell GL, Douglas RG, Bennett JE, eds. Principles and practices of infectious diseases. 3rd ed. New York: Churchill Livingstone, 1990.

Martin DH. Sexually transmitted diseases. Med Clin North Am 76:6.

Zenilman JM. Sexually transmitted diseases treatment guidelines. Rev Infect Dis 1990; 12:S–6.

Cont'd from p 245

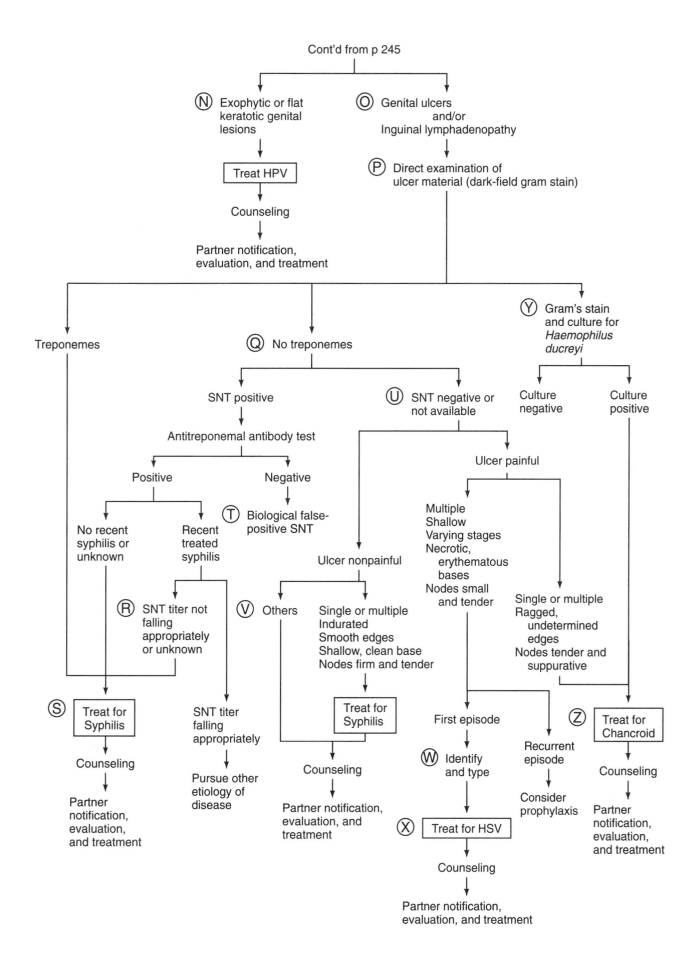

247

APPROACH TO THE NEWLY DIAGNOSED HIV-POSITIVE PATIENT

J. Kevin Carmichael, M.D.

HIV infection is most commonly diagnosed by detection of serum antibodies. The most commonly used test is the enzyme-*l*inked *i*mmuno*s*orbent *a*ssay (ELISA), which has both a sensitivity and specificity >98%. The predictive power of a positive ELISA varies with the prevalence of HIV in the population tested. A positive test in a person with a history of high-risk behaviors is probably a true positive, and a positive test in a person without such a history is likely a false positive. Consequently a person should not be definitively diagnosed as HIV-infected until a confirmatory test such as a Western blot or an HIV immunofluorescence assay is also positive.

A. Counseling the HIV-infected person is a continuous process beginning with pretest counseling and lasting throughout the infection. There are certain "imperatives" as follows: (1) the distinction between HIV infection and AIDS, (2) the natural history of HIV infection and available intervention/treatment measures, (3) methods of transmission and the prevention of transmission, and (4) referral to community resources. The burden of counseling rests with the physician, but many other resources are often available and should be used to complement physician counseling.

B. Obtain a general history. Pay special attention to any history of and treatment of sexually transmitted diseases, mycobacterial infections, and AIDS-defining illnesses.

C. Baseline laboratory testing should be performed. Specific complaints may require additional testing for evaluation. An immunization review should also be obtained (Table 1).

D. An HIV-focused review of systems is critical in HIV management. Review of systems should include fatigue, weight loss, anorexia, anxiety, depression, fever, chills, night sweats, adenopathy, skin rash or bruising, headache, sinus or ear pain, visual changes, oral sores, odynophagia, dysphagia, shortness of breath, dyspnea on exertion, cough, abdominal pain, diarrhea, genital-rectal sores/pain, arthritis, muscle weakness, forgetfulness, and discoordination.

E. Patients may be divided into three groups based on CD4 count: (1) CD4 >500. These patients are at low risk for opportunistic infection. They may be at increased risk for bacterial infections (especially *Streptococcus pneumoniae* and *Haemophilus influenzae*), tuberculosis (TB), and herpes zoster. No *Pneumocystis carinii* pneumonia (PCP) prophylaxis is indicated. Antiretroviral therapy is controversial because of the lack of research-proven benefits. (2) CD4 between 500 and 200. Risk of opportunistic infection increases as the CD4 count approaches 200. Patients often have symptoms of HIV infection such as lymphadenopathy, fever, fatigue, weight loss, and diarrhea. Dermatologic problems, TB, herpes zoster, and Kaposi's sarcoma are more common than in those with CD4 >500. No PCP prophylaxis is indicated. Antiretroviral therapy with zidovudine appears to delay progression to AIDS in persons with CD4 <500. (3) CD4 <200: These patients are at risk for opportunistic infection. PCP prophylaxis is indicated. Antiretroviral therapy with zidovudine appears to delay disease progression.

F. At this time antiretroviral therapy with zidovudine is recommended for all HIV-infected persons with CD4 <500. It is recommended that two CD4 counts <500, 1 month apart, be obtained before initiation of zidovudine. The recommended dose is 500 to 600 mg daily in divided doses. Didanosine and Zalcitchine have been approved by the FDA for use as alternative antiretroviral agents.

G. Patients with CD4 <200 *or* with previous PCP should receive PCP prophylaxis. Three drugs are commonly used for this: trimethoprim-sulfamethoxazole, dapsone, and pentamidine aerosol. There is comparative research in progress evaluating the optimal dosage, relative efficacy, and risks of these three measures. Many clinicians prefer oral therapy for as long as it is tolerated.

H. CD4 count is currently the best indicator of immune status in HIV-infected persons and has the greatest clinical utility. Remember, there is considerable short-term variability of CD4 count and thus patterns and trends are more significant than isolated numbers. The recommended time interval between repeat CD4 counts is every three months.

TABLE 1 Immunization of HIV Infected Adults

	Asymptomatic	Symptomatic
Pneumococcal	Yes	Yes
Influenza	No	Yes
Td	Yes	Yes
Hepatitis B	Consider on an individual basis	

From MMWR 1989; 38:205.

Patient with POSITIVE HIV ANTIBODY TEST RESULT

(A) Counseling

(B) History
Physical examination

(C) Baseline laboratory testing:
    CBC with differential, platelets
    CD4 count
    SMAC (least expensive assessment
        of renal, hepatic, and
        nutritional status)
    RPR
    HBsAg, HBsAb
    PPD with control (in HIV-infected
        patients >5 mm of induration
        is considered positive)
    Coccidioidomycosis serology
        (if in or from an endemic area)
    Chest film (PA and lateral)
    Immunization review

(D) Review of systems

(E) Stage based on CD4 count

CD4 >500

CD4 >200 but <500

(F) Initiate Antiretroviral
    Therapy

CD4 <200

Initiate Antiretroviral
Therapy

(G) Initiate Pneumocystis
    Prophylaxis

(H) Repeat CD4
    every 3 mo

Repeat CD4
every 3 mo

Repeat CD4
every 3 mo

References

Carmichael JK, Carmichael CG. Guidelines for the ambulatory care of HIV infected persons. Miami, Fla: Dade County Area Health Education Center Program, 1992.

Cohen PT, Sande MA, Volberding PA. The AIDS knowledge base. Waltham, Mass: Medical Publishing Group, 1990.

Guidelines for prophylaxis Against *Pneumocystis carinii* pneumonia for persons with human immunodeficiency virus. MMWR 1989; 38:S-5.

State-of-the-Art Conference on azidothymidine therapy for early HIV infection. Am J Med 1990; 89:335.

THE ACUTELY ILL HIV-POSITIVE PATIENT

Douglas Fish, M.D.
Richard M. Mandel, M.D.

A. A careful history and physical examination can give valuable clues to the chief complaint and point the work-up in the right direction. Specific questions about dietary habits, travel, and social habits may be particularly helpful.

B. Fever is very common in HIV-positive individuals and should be of particular concern when it is new or increased from patient's baseline. If neutropenic, the patient should be hospitalized and begun on empiric antibiotic therapy while a source is sought. If the absolute neutrophil count (ANC) is >750 cells/mm³, disposition must be based on clinical appearance, suspected source of fever, ability to treat as an outpatient, and degree of supportive care at home. Infection may stem from systemic, pulmonary, CNS, urinary tract, GI tract, cutaneous, reticuloendothelial, ocular, or ENT sources. Malignancy (especially non-Hodgkin's lymphoma), collagen vascular disease, and drug fever must also be included in the differential diagnosis.

C. An acute visual change as manifested by scotomata, flashes, floaters, or decreased acuity demands immediate funduscopic examination. Maintain a very low threshold for ophthalmologic referral.

D. If retinal hemorrhages are seen, urgent ophthalmologic confirmation is indicated and treatment for presumed CMV retinitis should be initiated, especially if the ophthalmologist considers the lesion sight threatening. *Toxoplasma gondii* and *Pneumocystis carinii* can infect the eye and should be considered, as should noninfectious causes of retinopathy. Cotton wool spots (white lesions on the retina) may be followed and require no therapy. If the fundoscopic examination is normal but visual acuity (V/A) or visual field testing abnormal, an initial ophthalmologic referral is indicated.

E. Diarrhea may range in severity from mild to life threatening. The need for hospitalization depends on the degree of dehydration.

F. Initial evaluation of diarrhea includes fecal leukocytes; culture for *Salmonella, Shigella,* and *Campylobacter;* ova and parasites ×3; AFB; and *Cryptosporidium* staining. If the patient is or has recently been on antibiotics, *Clostridium difficile* toxin should also be obtained. Obtain blood cultures if the patient is febrile, since bacteremia from the GI tract is not uncommon in the HIV-seropositive patient.

G. If diarrhea persists and the above studies are unrevealing, perform proctosigmoidoscopy with biopsy for culture and histopathology with special stains, looking for bacterial, chlamydial, viral, fungal, and mycobacterial infection as well as malignancy and inflammatory bowel disease. Small bowel biopsy is indicated when lower GI endoscopy and stool studies fail to reveal a diagnosis and diarrhea is persistent.

H. Rash is common in HIV-positive people. Xerosis, seborrheic dermatitis, dermatophyte infection, and scabies typically respond to standard therapies. Oral, perioral, anal, and perianal herpes simplex infections occur frequently, as does varicella zoster. These infections can disseminate, and hospitalization for therapy is required if they do. HIV-positive individuals seem more prone to drug eruptions. If there is doubt as to the cause of a rash, early referral to a dermatologist is suggested. Suspicious lesions should be biopsied for routine, fungal, viral, and mycobacterial culture and sent for histopathology.

I. A good oral examination may provide valuable clues to a painful mouth and swallowing difficulties. Gingivitis, dental abscesses, thrush, and herpes simplex are common and readily treatable. Severe oropharyngeal involvement is frequently associated with esophageal disease. If initial therapy fails or no oropharyngeal pathology is noted, upper GI endoscopy with biopsy is necessary, looking for yeast, infection with herpes virus or Cytomegalovirus, aphthous ulcers, Kaposi's sarcoma or other malignancies, and oral or other GI problems.

References

Chaisson RE, Volberding PA. Clinical manifestations of HIV infection. In: Mandell GL, Douglas RC Jr, Bennett JE, eds. Principles and practices of infectious diseases. 3rd ed. New York: Churchill Livingston, 1990:1059.

Gerberding JL. Diagnosis and management of HIV-infected patients with diarrhea. J Antimicrob Chemother 1989; 23(Suppl. A):83.

Henderly DE, Jampol LM. Diagnosis and treatment of cytomegalovirus retinitis. J Acquir Immune Defic Syndr 1991; 4(Suppl. 1):6.

Hollander H. The acutely ill HIV-positive patient. In: Callaham ML, Barton CW, Schumaker HM, eds. Decision making in emergency medicine. Philadelphia: BC Decker, 1990:202.

Johanson JF, Sonnenberg A. Efficient management of diarrhea in the acquired immunodeficiency syndrome (AIDS). Ann Intern Med 1990; 112:942.

ACUTELY ILL HIV-POSITIVE PATIENT

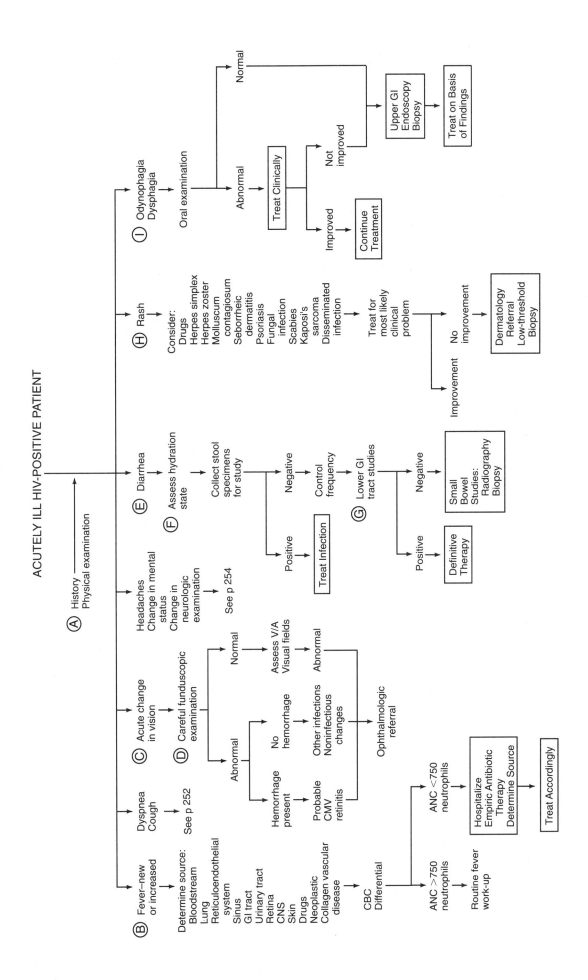

Ⓐ History
Physical examination

Ⓑ Fever—new or increased
Determine source:
Bloodstream
Lung
Reticuloendothelial system
Sinus
GI tract
Urinary tract
Retina
CNS
Skin
Drugs
Neoplastic
Collagen vascular disease

CBC Differential

ANC >750 neutrophils → Routine fever work-up

ANC <750 neutrophils → Hospitalize / Empiric Antibiotic Therapy / Determine Source → Treat Accordingly

Dyspnea Cough → See p 252

Ⓒ Acute change in vision
Ⓓ Careful funduscopic examination
Abnormal
  Hemorrhage present → Probable CMV retinitis
  No hemorrhage → Other infections / Noninfectious changes → Ophthalmologic referral
Normal → Assess V/A Visual fields → Abnormal

Headaches
Change in mental status
Change in neurologic examination → See p 254

Ⓔ Diarrhea
Ⓕ Assess hydration state → Collect stool specimens for study
  Positive → Treat Infection
  Negative → Control frequency
Ⓖ Lower GI tract studies
  Positive → Definitive Therapy
  Negative → Small Bowel Studies: Radiography Biopsy

Ⓗ Rash
Consider:
Drugs
Herpes simplex
Herpes zoster
Molluscum contagiosum
Seborrheic dermatitis
Psoriasis
Fungal infection
Scabies
Kaposi's sarcoma
Disseminated infection
→ Treat for most likely clinical problem
  Improvement
  No improvement → Dermatology Referral / Low-threshold Biopsy

Ⓘ Odynophagia Dysphagia → Oral examination
  Abnormal → Treat Clinically
    Improved → Continue Treatment
    Not improved → Upper GI Endoscopy Biopsy → Treat on Basis of Findings
  Normal → Upper GI Endoscopy Biopsy

251

PULMONARY INFECTIONS IN THE HIV-INFECTED PATIENT

Neil M. Ampel, M.D.

A. A critical issue in the evaluation of HIV-infected patients with pulmonary disease is the number of circulating CD4 or T-helper lymphocytes. Opportunistic pulmonary infections are less likely to occur if the CD4 count is >200/μl (or >20% of total lymphocytes), and they become increasingly frequent as the CD4 count drops below these levels. *Pneumocystis carinii* pneumonia (PCP) is by far the most common opportunistic infection in HIV-infected patients, ultimately occurring in >80% of all such individuals. Dyspnea, an abnormal chest radiograph, and a CD4 count <200/μl all make an HIV-related opportunistic pulmonary infection likely.

B. The chest radiographic pattern plays an important role in management. A diffuse pattern strongly suggests PCP. Fungal infections such as coccidioidomycosis or histoplasmosis occasionally also present this way and sometimes occur with *P. carinii* as the cause of the pneumonic process. In 10% of cases of PCP, the chest radiograph is normal.

C. In patients with diffuse chest radiographic patterns, obtain an arterial blood gas. To determine if the patient has a mild arteriolar-alveolar block despite normal arterial P_{O_2}, perform either exercise oximetry or a gallium scan of the lung. The former consists of walking the patient on a treadmill and measuring O_2 saturation; a drop in O_2 saturation during exercise indicates an arteriolar-alveolar block. The gallium scan takes several days. An increased uptake in the lungs suggests PCP. If either test is positive, initiate a diagnostic work-up and start empiric therapy for PCP. If these tests are negative and the patient is clinically stable, observation is appropriate.

D. If the arterial P_{O_2} on room air is <90 mm Hg, the patient has a significant arteriolar-alveolar block. Initiate an aggressive work-up to determine the cause of the pulmonary process and begin empiric therapy for PCP, since this is the most common cause of this presentation.

E. Focal chest radiographic abnormalities are distinctly uncommon in PCP unless the patient has been receiving aerosolized pentamidine prophylaxis. In this case, PCP often presents with a focal upper lobe infiltrate, sometimes with cavitation and sometimes with a nodular appearance. If such a chest radiographic pattern is seen in a patient on aerosolized pentamidine, further diagnostic tests to exclude PCP are needed. Since diagnostic yields with noninvasive methods are much lower in patients on this form of prophylaxis, consider bronchoscopy with transbronchial biopsy to establish the cause of the chest radiograph abnormality.

F. The work-up for PCP should include obtaining pulmonary secretions, either through saline induction of a sputum sample or by bronchoalveolar lavage (BAL). Examination of such specimens for an etiologic organism should include stains that at the least detect *P. carinii*. Stains for fungi and mycobacteria should also be performed and examined on such specimens. If the induced-sputum specimen is nondiagnostic or if there is a possibility of more than one pathogen, BAL should be performed. A transbronchial biopsy is not necessary in most cases unless the patient has been on aerosolized pentamidine prophylaxis. Empiric therapy for PCP includes trimethoprim-sulfamethoxazole or IV pentamidine.

G. If a focal pulmonary infiltrate is encountered and the patient is not on aerosolized pentamidine, initiate a work-up for pneumonias other than PCP. Besides acute bacterial pneumonias, consider fungal pneumonias, such as coccidioidomycosis, histoplasmosis, and cryptococcosis, and rule out tuberculosis. Evaluation of expectorated sputum may be enough to establish the diagnosis, but some cases require a more invasive method to obtain pulmonary secretions.

References

CDC. Guidelines for prophylaxis against *Pneumocystis carinii* pneumonia for persons infected with human immunodeficiency virus. MMWR 1989; 38 (S-5):1.

Jules-Elysee KM, Stover DE, Zaman MB, et al. Aerosolized pentamidine: effect on diagnosis and presentation of *Pneumocystis carinii* pneumonia. Ann Intern Med 1990; 750.

Kovacs JA, Masur H. Opportunistic infections. In: DeVita VT Jr, Hellman S, Rosenberg SA, eds. AIDS. Etiology, diagnosis, treatment, and prevention. 2nd ed. Philadelphia: JB Lippincott, 1988:199.

Mills J. *Pneumocystis carinii* and *Toxoplasma gondii* infections in patients with AIDS. J Infect Dis 1986; Rev Infect Dis 8:1001.

Phair J, Muñoz A, Detels R, Kaslow R, Rinaldo C, Saah A, and the Multicenter AIDS Cohort Study Group. The risk of *Pneumocystis carinii* pneumonia among men infected with human immunodeficiency virus type 1. N Engl J Med 1990; 322:161.

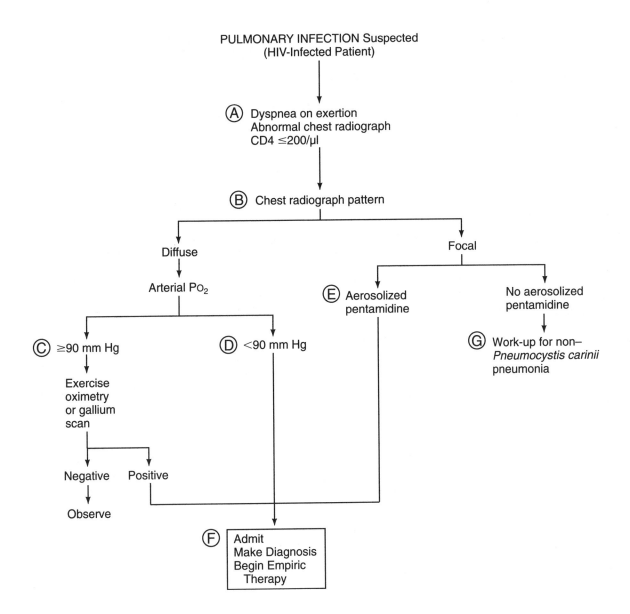

PULMONARY INFECTION Suspected
(HIV-Infected Patient)

Ⓐ Dyspnea on exertion
Abnormal chest radiograph
CD4 ≤200/µl

Ⓑ Chest radiograph pattern

Diffuse

Focal

Arterial PO₂

Ⓔ Aerosolized
pentamidine

No aerosolized
pentamidine

Ⓒ ≥90 mm Hg

Ⓓ <90 mm Hg

Ⓖ Work-up for non–
Pneumocystis carinii
pneumonia

Exercise
oximetry
or gallium
scan

Negative   Positive

Observe

Ⓕ Admit
Make Diagnosis
Begin Empiric
   Therapy

CENTRAL NERVOUS SYSTEM INFECTIONS IN THE HIV-INFECTED PATIENT

Neil M. Ampel, M.D.

A. Many infections can occur in the CNS of HIV-infected patients. A useful approach is to determine whether they present as a mass lesion producing a focal deficit on neurologic examination, or without such a deficit. By far the most common lesions producing focal neurologic deficits in HIV-infected patients are cerebral toxoplasmosis and CNS lymphoma. Other possibilities include progressive multifocal leukoencephalopathy (PML), bacterial brain abscesses, tuberculomas, and fungal brain abscesses. If a patient with HIV infection presents with a focal neurologic deficit, a CT scan of the head should be performed before a lumbar puncture to rule out a space-occupying CNS lesion.

B. If a mass lesion is detected, the key differential point is whether more than one is present. If so, the diagnosis of cerebral toxoplasmosis is more likely and CNS lymphoma less likely. *Toxoplasma* brain abscesses tend to be at the junction of the gray and white matter and usually demonstrate surrounding edema and ring enhancement with contrast. The presence of serum antibodies to *Toxoplasma gondii* does not establish the diagnosis, but their absence strongly suggests another diagnosis. In the case of multiple ring-enhancing lesions with positive serum *Toxoplasma* antibodies, it is not unreasonable to treat empirically for cerebral toxoplasmosis, although some clinicians may still perform a brain biopsy at this point. PML also presents with multiple lesions on CT, but it differs from cerebral toxoplasmosis in that the lesions are in the white matter only, are usually hypodense, and are nonenhancing with contrast.

C. If a single lesion is found on CT, CNS lymphoma is most likely. One approach before brain biopsy is to perform an MRI scan of the head, since this is more sensitive than CT. The presence of multiple lesions on MRI and positive serum *T. gondii* antibodies again suggests cerebral toxoplasmosis. Under these conditions, empiric treatment for toxoplasmosis may also be started. If a single lesion is found, perform a brain biopsy to establish the diagnosis of CNS lymphoma.

D. If there is no response to therapy for toxoplasmosis within 2 weeks or if the patient develops toxicities

from the therapy, making continued treatment difficult, perform a brain biopsy to establish the nature of the lesion.

E. If no mass lesion is detected on CT, a lumbar puncture may be safely performed and the work-up continued as described for nonfocal neurologic disorders. Alternatively, MRI may be done to further exclude any space-occupying CNS lesion before performing the lumbar puncture, provided that the patient is clinically stable and the MRI can be obtained without significant delay.

F. The most common treatable cause of nonfocal CNS infection during HIV infection is cryptococcal meningitis. CSF values in this condition may be disarmingly normal. Most commonly, there is a CSF pleocytosis of ≤20 cells/μl, predominantly of lymphocytes, with low CSF glucose and elevated protein. CSF cryptococcal antigen titers are usually positive and often markedly elevated (>1:1000). Culture of the CSF for *Cryptococcus neoformans* is invariably positive but usually takes several days. The India ink test is insensitive and should not be used. A positive CSF cryptococcal antigen test should lead to empiric therapy for cryptococcosis.

G. CNS syphilis is being recognized as increasingly common among HIV-infected patients. The presence of any CSF abnormality in association with a positive VDRL test in the CSF should lead to a presumptive diagnosis of CNS syphilis, and treatment with high-dose IV penicillin.

H. Several entities not infrequently cause an abnormal CSF profile in HIV-infected patients other than cryptococcosis and CNS syphilis. The most common is HIV infection itself. Early infection is usually manifested as acute aseptic meningitis. Later in the course of the disease, patients may develop dementia with cognitive slowing and diffuse cortical atrophy on CT. Herpes virus infections due to herpes simplex, herpes varicella-zoster, and cytomegalovirus may also cause a CSF pleocytosis. Bacterial meningitis is not more common among HIV-infected patients than in other hosts, but occasionally occurs.

CENTRAL NERVOUS SYSTEM INFECTION Suspected
(HIV-Infected Patient)

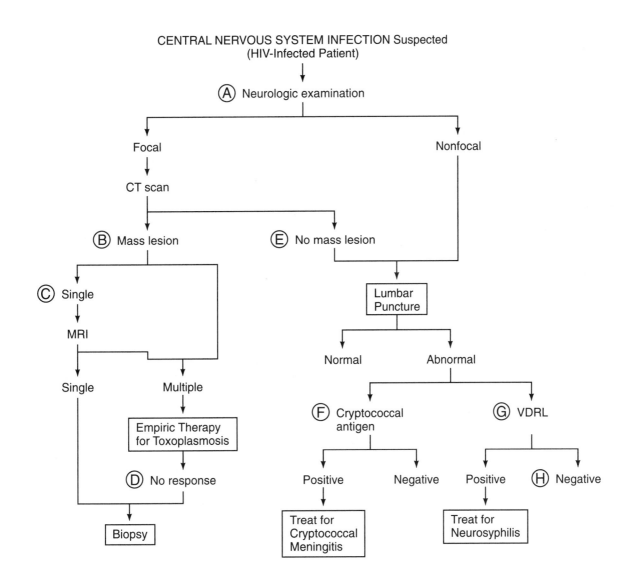

References

Brew B, Rosenblum M, Price RW. Central and peripheral nervous system complications of HIV infection and AIDS. In: DeVita VT Jr, Hellman S, Rosenberg SA, eds. AIDS. Etiology, diagnosis, treatment, and prevention. 2nd ed. Philadelphia: JB Lippincott, 1988:185.

Chuck SL, Sande MA. Infections with *Cryptococcus neoformans* in the acquired immunodeficiency syndrome. N Engl J Med 1989; 321:794.

Elder GA, Sever JL. Neurologic disorders associated with AIDS retroviral infection. Rev Infect Dis 1988; 10:286.

Luft BJ, Remington JS. Toxoplasmic encephalitis. J Infect Dis 1988; 157:1.

Musher DM, Hamill RJ, Baughn RE. Effect of human immunodeficiency virus (HIV) infection on the course of syphilis and on the response to treatment. Ann Intern Med 1990; 113:872.

SEPSIS

Neil M. Ampel, M.D.

A. There are no standardized definitions embracing the concepts of sepsis and septic shock. Bone recently defined *sepsis* as the clinical evidence of infection, with fever or hypothermia, tachypnea, and tachycardia. The *sepsis syndrome* represents a more severe manifestation, encompassing sepsis with evidence of inadequate organ perfusion, such as the inability to maintain adequate oxygenation, oliguria, or elevated serum lactate. Finally, *septic shock* is defined as the sepsis syndrome with hypotension. Although gram-negative aerobic bacilli are the most common causes of these syndromes, any number of pathogenic organisms, including gram-positive bacteria and fungi, may produce the same physiologic responses. Blood cultures may or may not be positive.

B. The basic approach to managing a patient with presumed sepsis involves three steps. First, attempt to restore the patient to physiologic normalcy. Intravascular volume should be repleted to maintain an adequate blood pressure. In less severe cases, this is done by administration of crystalloid fluids. In patients with evidence or a history of congestive heart failure, a pulmonary artery catheter may be needed. With severe hypotension, it may be necessary to add pressor agents, particularly dopamine, to IV fluids to maintain adequate blood pressure and renal function. In addition, supplemental oxygen should be administered. In severe cases, intubation and mechanical ventilation may be required. Pulmonary expiratory end-diastolic pressure (PEEP) may be needed to maintain adequate arterial oxygenation, but should be used in amounts that do not affect blood pressure. Finally, metabolic abnormalities should be corrected. Many clinicians administer sodium bicarbonate if the serum pH falls to ≤7.2, but others believe this may be deleterious. Hyperglycemia, hypoglycemia, and serum electrolyte disorders should be monitored and corrected as necessary.

C. Once basic support has been achieved, seek the cause of the infection. A thorough history and physical examination will elucidate the source of the infection in most patients. The most common causes of sepsis include urinary tract infection (UTI) with extension to the renal parenchyma, pneumonia, and intravascular line infection. Occasionally a GI catastrophe, such as perforation, ischemic colitis, or abscess, is the cause. Appropriate radiologic tests based on the history and physical examination should be ordered. In general, a chest radiograph is always needed. Other radiographs, including CT scan of the abdomen, are necessary only if the history and physical examination suggest an abdominal or retroperitoneal process. Standard laboratory tests should include a CBC, an arterial blood gas, and measurement of serum electrolytes and creatinine. A urinalysis should be obtained.

D. In all cases, blood cultures should be drawn: at least three, all from separate venipunctures. This ensures that a contaminating microorganism is not mistaken for a pathogen, and increases the likelihood of detecting a true bacteremia. Although some clinicians advocate waiting at least 20 min between each blood culture, it is appropriate to obtain them one after another. Other cultures should be obtained based on the history, physical examination, and radiographic findings. If there is evidence of pneumonia, a Gram's stain of a sputum specimen should be examined and the specimen plated for culture. If the urinalysis demonstrates pyuria, obtain a urine culture. If possible, examine a Gram's stain of the urinary sediment.

E. Once basic support has been provided, the source of infection assessed, and appropriate cultures obtained, begin empiric antibiotic therapy. Ideally, in the critically ill patient, the time between initial contact and initiation of antimicrobial therapy should not be >30 mins. The choice of antimicrobial therapy depends on the presumed source of infection, the most common microorganisms involved, and any complicating factors, such as renal failure. For presumed UTI with sepsis, antibiotics should be directed against gram-negative aerobic bacilli and the enterococcus. Penicillin or ampicillin plus either an aminoglycoside or an extended-spectrum third-generation cephalosporin are reasonable choices. If the GI tract is the presumed source, add an agent active against anaerobic gram-negative bacilli to the above regimen. Metronidazole, clindamycin, or chloramphenicol are appropriate choices. For pneumonia, base empiric antibiotic therapy on the results of Gram's stain of the sputum. If gram-positive cocci in clusters are seen, an antistaphylococcal agent, such as nafcillin or a first-generation cephalosporin, is reasonable. If gram-positive diplococci are the predominant organisms present, penicillin is a good empiric agent. If gram-negative bacilli are detected, a broad-spectrum cephalosporin, such as cefuroxime, ceftriaxone, or ceftazidime, is appropriate. Finally, if an intravascular line infection is suspected, treat both gram-positive cocci and gram-negative aerobic bacilli. Administer nafcillin or vancomycin plus an aminoglycoside or an extended-spectrum third-generation cephalosporin. In all cases, therapy may have to be subsequently modified in relation to the patient's response to treatment and the results of the microbiologic cultures. Future treatment for gram-negative aerobic bacillary shock may include monoclonal antibody therapy, but this approach is still experimental. To date, high-dose corticosteroids have not proved beneficial and are not recommended for sepsis or septic shock.

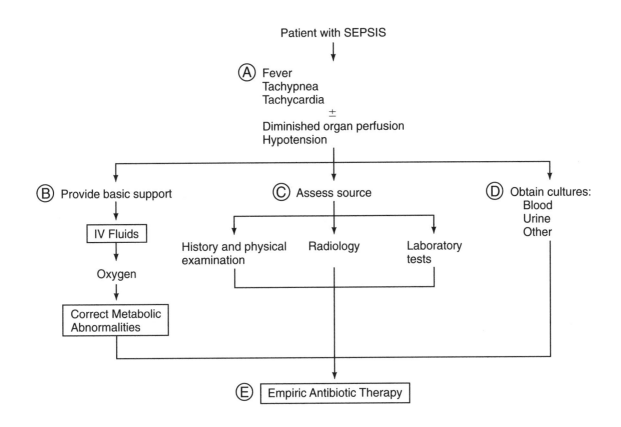

References

Bone RC. Sepsis, the sepsis syndrome, multi-organ failure: a plea for comparable definitions. Ann Intern Med 1991; 114:332.

Luce JM. Pathogenesis and management of septic shock. Chest 1987; 91:883.

Parker MM. Current management of septic shock. Infect Med 1989; March/April:47.

The Veterans Administration Systemic Sepsis Cooperative Study Group. Effect of high-dose glucocorticoid therapy on mortality in patients with clinical signs of systemic sepsis. N Engl J Med 1987; 317:659.

Wolff SM. Monoclonal antibodies and the treatment of gram-negative bacteremia and shock. N Engl J Med 1991; 324:486.

TOXIC SHOCK SYNDROME

Simone A. Ince, M.D.
Richard M. Mandel, M.D.

Toxic shock syndrome (TSS) is the name given to the myriad of clinical findings caused by infection with an exotoxin-producing species of *Staphylococcus aureus,* first described in 1978 in children. Afflicted adults had similar clinical features of high fever, erythroderma, and hypotension along with variable organ system dysfunction, including nausea, vomiting, diarrhea, mental confusion, renal failure, hepatic failure, and thrombocytopenia. In 1980 it was noted that this syndrome occurred with increasing frequency in young menstruating females, particularly those who used superabsorbent tampons. Surgical and nonsurgical wounds, postpartum infection, abscesses, osteomyelitis, pneumonia, and sinusitis have been reported to cause nonmenstrual TSS. Contraceptive sponge and diaphragm use has also been implicated in a few cases of TSS. Nonmenstrual TSS is considerably less common than the menstrual form: at most 15% of reported cases.

A. It is essential to determine the presence or absence of hypotension, with implications not only for treatment, but for early exclusion of some of the exanthems of various other diseases that may masquerade as the erythroderma of TSS (Table 1). Measles is most prominent in children and young adults but can occur in any age group. Prodromal symptoms of high fever, malaise, irritability, conjunctivitis, photophobia, hacking cough, nasal discharge, and (variably) Koplik's spots are followed in 3 to 4 days by a red maculopapular rash. Within 3 days the rash spreads from the face to the trunk and extremities; it may coalesce in areas, giving the appearance of erythroderma. The rash typically persists for 6 days and disappears in the order in which it appeared. Measles can be differentiated from TSS by the absence of hypotension. Rocky Mountain spotted fever (RMSF), an acute febrile illness caused by infection with *Rickettsia rickettsiae,* is transmitted via tick bite and is characterized by the abrupt onset of fever, headache, chills, and a pink macular rash on the extremities. This progresses over 2 to 3 weeks to a deep red maculopapular rash on the trunk and extremities. Again, the history and the rare presence of hypovolemic hypotension differentiate RMSF from TSS. Leptospirosis is an acute febrile illness caused by infection with the spirochete *Leptospira,* usually via contact with infected animal urine or tissue. Farmers, trappers, and abattoir workers are at increased risk. The onset is sudden with fever and chills, headache, myalgia, pharyngeal and conjunctival injection, and a macular/maculopapular/urticarial rash on the trunk. Hypotension is absent.

B. If hypotension is present with a fever >38.9° C, consider an infectious process leading to sepsis.

Perform a thorough work-up with blood cultures, chest film, urinalysis, and lumbar puncture if there are signs of CNS involvement. The presence of classical erythroderma narrows the possible diagnoses to TSS and "toxic streptococcus" syndrome. The erythroderma may be delayed, localized, or evanescent; therefore, continue to suspect TSS.

C. A different entity, re-described in the mid-1980s and associated with many of the signs and symptoms of TSS, is the "toxic streptococcus" syndrome. Caused by an exotoxin-producing species of group A beta-hemolytic streptococcus (*S. pyogenes*), it too is characterized by fever, hypotension, rash, and multiple organ failure. This syndrome, however, is often secondary to an obvious source of infection; search for cellulitis, fasciitis/myositis, or a pulmonary source leading to the systemic illness.

D. The CDC definition of TSS is given in Table 1. Fever, hypotension, and rash consisting of a diffuse erythroderma, often described as sunburn, are major characteristics, along with multiple organ involvement: GI, muscular, renal, liver, blood, CNS, and mucous membrane abnormalities. In most cases of TSS, desquamation of rash-afflicted areas occurs about 1 week after the onset. In the absence of desquamation, all three major criteria plus more than five organ systems involved must be present to comply with the CDC definition. If desquamation is present, all three major criteria plus more than three organ systems involved are sufficient for diagnosis.

TABLE 1   CDC Criteria for Diagnosis of TSS

Temperature >38.9° C
Systolic BP <90 mm Hg
Rash with subsequent desquamation, especially on palms and soles
Involvement of ≥3 of the following organ systems:
　　Gastrointestinal: vomiting, profuse diarrhea
　　Muscular: severe myalgias or >fivefold increase in creatine kinase
　　Mucous membranes (vagina, conjunctivae, or pharynx): frank hyperemia
　　Renal insufficiency: BUN or creatinine at least twice upper limit of normal, with pyuria in absence of urinary tract infection
　　Liver: hepatitis; bilirubin, SGOT, SGPT at least twice upper limit of normal
　　Blood: thrombocytopenia <100,000/mm^3
　　CNS: disorientation without focal neurologic signs
Negative results of serologic tests for Rocky Mountain spotted fever, leptospirosis, and measles

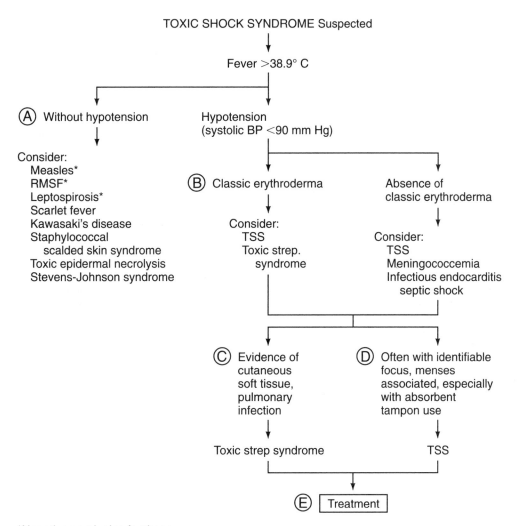

TOXIC SHOCK SYNDROME Suspected

Fever >38.9° C

Ⓐ Without hypotension

Hypotension
(systolic BP <90 mm Hg)

Consider:
  Measles*
  RMSF*
  Leptospirosis*
  Scarlet fever
  Kawasaki's disease
  Staphylococcal
    scalded skin syndrome
  Toxic epidermal necrolysis
  Stevens-Johnson syndrome

Ⓑ Classic erythroderma

Absence of
classic erythroderma

Consider:
TSS
Toxic strep.
  syndrome

Consider:
TSS
Meningococcemia
Infectious endocarditis
  septic shock

Ⓒ Evidence of
cutaneous
soft tissue,
pulmonary
infection

Ⓓ Often with identifiable
focus, menses
associated, especially
with absorbent
tampon use

Toxic strep syndrome

TSS

Ⓔ Treatment

*Negative serologies for these
diseases are required to make the
diagnosis of TSS by CDC definition.

References

E.   TSS carried a mortality rate of approximately 5.0% in 1980 and 0% in 1989. Cases of nonmenstrual TSS carry a slightly increased mortality. The diagnosis is made on the basis of clinical findings and associated tampon use. An obvious infectious source is present only in a minority of patients, although a thorough search for such a source should be made. Blood cultures are rarely positive. Treatment hinges on early diagnosis, vigorous fluid replacement, pressor and ventilatory support if needed, tampon removal, vaginal douche, drainage of abscesses, and antibiotic therapy with a penicillinase-resistant penicillin.

Barter T, Dascal A, Carrol K, Curley FJ. Toxic strep syndrome—a manifestation of group A streptococcal infection. Arch Intern Med 1988; 148:1421.
Broome CV. Epidemiology of TSS in the US: overview. Rev Infect Dis 1989; 11(Suppl 1):S14.
Centers for Disease Control. Reduced incidence of menstrual toxic shock syndrome. MMWR 1991; 39:421.
Chesney PJ. Clinical aspects and spectrum of Illness of TSS: overview. Rev Infect Dis. 1989; 11(Suppl 1):S1.
Waldvogel F, Mandell, et al. Staphylococcus aureus—including toxic shock syndrome. In: Mandel, et al, eds. Principles and practice of infectious diseases. New York: Churchill Livingstone, 1990:1480.

STAPHYLOCOCCUS AUREUS BACTEREMIA

Jeffrey L. Silber
Mark J. DiNubile

Staphylococcus aureus is one of the most common causes of both community-acquired and nosocomial bacteremia. In most cases, *S. aureus* bacteremia is a consequence of a local infection that enters the bloodstream after an insult to normally protective skin structures. Serious complications and poor outcome are common despite the availability of potent antistaphylococcal antibiotics.

Once in the bloodstream, *S. aureus* has the propensity to infect both normal and damaged organs, including heart valves, viscera, bones, and joints, in addition to shunts and orthopedic hardware. Patients with *S. aureus* bacteremia who have no overt evidence of endocarditis or metastatic infection may still harbor occult infection of vital structures. It was commonly recommended that all patients with *S. aureus* bacteremia be treated for at least 4 weeks. Although the diagnosis of endocarditis can never be totally excluded, the clinical settings in which patients are at low risk of endocarditis can be defined. The challenge is to identify patients unlikely to have endocarditis or other hidden foci of infection after *S. aureus* bacteremia and who are therefore candidates for shorter courses (usually 2 weeks) of antibiotic therapy.

A. The approach to patients with *S. aureus* bacteremia should emphasize the primary site of infection. The absence of a demonstrable initial focus of infection suggests endocarditis. If the bacteremia was clearly related to a removable focus (e.g., an intravascular line), the patient is relatively unlikely to have or develop endocarditis.

B. When blood cultures remain persistently positive for >48 hours or, in presumed line-related bacteremia, 24 hours after the line has been removed, the patient should be assumed to have endovascular infection.

C. Patients with a prosthetic device should usually be treated as if that prosthesis has been seeded. Patients with a visceral abscess, pneumonia, osteomyelitis, or septic arthritis should be assumed to have endocarditis, as should all IV drug users. Some patients with skin infections may be candidates for short-course therapy.

D. Echocardiography is occasionally helpful but not routinely indicated. The presence of a vegetation mandates at least 4 weeks of treatment.

E. Patients considered for short-course therapy should show no evidence of active infection on repeated evaluations, including a careful examination at the end of 2 weeks of treatment. Patients with a removable primary focus of infection, short-lived bacteremia, no prosthetic devices, and a "negative" echocardiogram (if done) who have responded promptly to antibiotic therapy and show no evidence of ongoing infection may be treated with appropriate antistaphylococcal antibiotics for 2 weeks. Most other patients require longer courses of therapy, usually 4–6 weeks. In some, surgical intervention (e.g., incision and drainage, valve replacement) may also be needed. On completion of therapy, all patients (especially those receiving short-course therapy) need close clinical follow-up for several weeks. Those who relapse should be retreated with longer courses of antibiotics and evaluated for endovascular or other foci of infection.

References

Bayer AS, Lam K, Gintzon L, et al. *Staphylococcus aureus* bacteremia: clinical, serologic, and echocardiographic findings in patients with and without endocarditis. Arch Intern Med 1987; 147:457.

Dajani AS, Bisno AL, Chung KJ, et al. Prevention of bacterial endocarditis. Recommendations by the American Heart Association. JAMA 1990; 264:2919.

Mylotte JM, McDermott C, Spooner JA. Prospective study of 114 consecutive episodes of *Staphylococcus aureus* bacteremia. Rev Infect Dis 1987; 9:891.

Sheagren JN. *Staphylococcus aureus:* the persistent pathogen. N Engl J Med 1984; 310:1368, 1437.

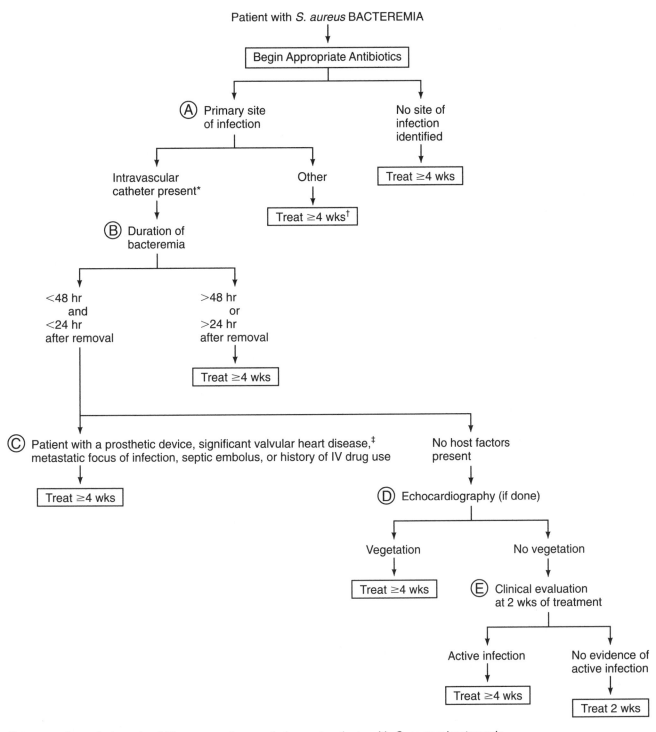

Patient with *S. aureus* BACTEREMIA

Begin Appropriate Antibiotics

(A) Primary site of infection

No site of infection identified
Treat ≥4 wks

Intravascular catheter present*

Other
Treat ≥4 wks†

(B) Duration of bacteremia

<48 hr and <24 hr after removal

>48 hr or >24 hr after removal
Treat ≥4 wks

(C) Patient with a prosthetic device, significant valvular heart disease,‡ metastatic focus of infection, septic embolus, or history of IV drug use
Treat ≥4 wks

No host factors present

(D) Echocardiography (if done)

Vegetation
Treat ≥4 wks

No vegetation
(E) Clinical evaluation at 2 wks of treatment

Active infection
Treat ≥4 wks

No evidence of active infection
Treat 2 wks

*Intravascular catheters should be removed promptly in most patients with *S. aureus* bacteremia.

†Patients with a skin or soft tissue source of infection may be candidates for short-course therapy. For these selected patients, management should proceed as for intravascular catheter–derived infection.

‡Previous bacterial endocarditis, most congenital cardiac malformations, hypertrophic cardiomyopathy, rheumatic and other acquired valvular dysfunction, and mitral valve prolapse with regurgitation, as per American Heart Association indications for endocarditis prophylaxis before surgical, dental, and endoscopic procedures (Dajani AS, Bisno AL, Chung KJ, et al. JAMA 1990; 264:2919).

HEPATITIS EXPOSURE

Stephen J. Gluckman, M.D.
Mark J. DiNubile, M.D.

Hepatitis is inflammation of the liver that can result from infections or other causes. Some infections are contagious, and a subset of these are potentially preventable after a significant exposure. It is impossible to advise a patient after exposure to hepatitis without ascertaining the relevant historical information. Three particularly important questions must be addressed: (1) *Type of hepatitis* — e.g., A, B, C, Epstein-Barr virus, cytomegalovirus, alcohol, or drug. Each type has its own specific risks for transmission and strategies for prevention. (2) *Any history of hepatitis*— If a person has already had the type of viral hepatitis to which he or she has been exposed, there is no risk of acquiring it again. (3) *Type of exposure*— Each type of infectious hepatitis has particular modes of transmission. Not only does a person have to be "exposed," but the contact must be sufficient for transmission of infection to occur.

A. If a person exposed to hepatitis A has already had it, only reassurance is required.

B. If the exposed person is not known to have had hepatitis A, the type of exposure becomes important. Hepatitis A is spread via the fecal-oral route. Persons at increased risk for the disease are close personal, household, or day-care contacts. In addition, this virus has been responsible for epidemics related to contaminated food or water. If the exposure has not occurred in one of these settings, no intervention is necessary. If the exposure has been of one of these types and has occurred within the previous 2 weeks, immune globulin (IG), 0.02 ml/kg, is indicated.

C. If a person exposed to hepatitis B has already had it, there is no further risk.

D. If the exposed person is not known to have had hepatitis B, the type of exposure becomes critical. If the exposure was via a contaminated blood transfusion, there is no effective prevention. If the situation involves a newborn of a mother with hepatitis B, the child should receive 0.5 ml of hepatitis B immune globulin (HBIG) within 12 hours of birth, and active immunization should be started.

E. If the exposure was via a contaminated needlestick or permucosal exposure to infectious blood within the past week or through sexual contact in the previous 2 weeks, and if the patient has never received hepatitis B vaccine, prophylaxis is indicated. The proper approach is to obtain a tube of blood to test for hepatitis B core antibody (HBcAb) and administer a dose of HBIG (0.06 ml/kg). If the antibody test is positive, the patient has already had hepatitis B and no further prophylaxis is indicated. If negative, active immunization against hepatitis B should usually be initiated within 1 week of exposure. If the patient has already received hepatitis B vaccine, ascertain the response to the vaccine. In a known responder, the level of hepatitis B surface antibody (HBsAb) should be determined. If the levels are adequate (≥10 sample ratio units [SRU]), no further prophylaxis is needed. If the levels are <10 SRU, a booster dose of vaccine is indicated. A known nonresponder should usually receive HBIG (0.06 ml/kg) on two occasions 1 month apart. When patients do not know their response status to the vaccine, check the level of HBsAb: If ≥10 SRU, nothing further is required; if <10 SRU, give HBIG (0.06 ml/kg) and a single booster dose of the vaccine.

F. If a person exposed to hepatitis C has already had it, there is no further risk.

G. There are no proved interventions after exposure to hepatitis C. Hepatitis C is a major cause of post-transfusion hepatitis, but intervention after transfusion is unlikely to be effective. The virus also appears to be contagious via sticks from contaminated needles, permucosal contact with blood, and sexual relations. Since IG contains some antibody against this virus, it is reasonable to give IG (0.06 ml/kg) for prophylaxis after these types of exposure.

H. When a person has had exposure to hepatitis but the type is unknown, it may be prudent to administer a single dose of IG (0.06 ml/kg) if the exposure is of the type that could transmit type A, B, or C hepatitis.

Reference

Recommendations of the Immunization Practices Advisory Committee (ACIP). Protection against viral hepatitis. MMWR 1990; 39:1.

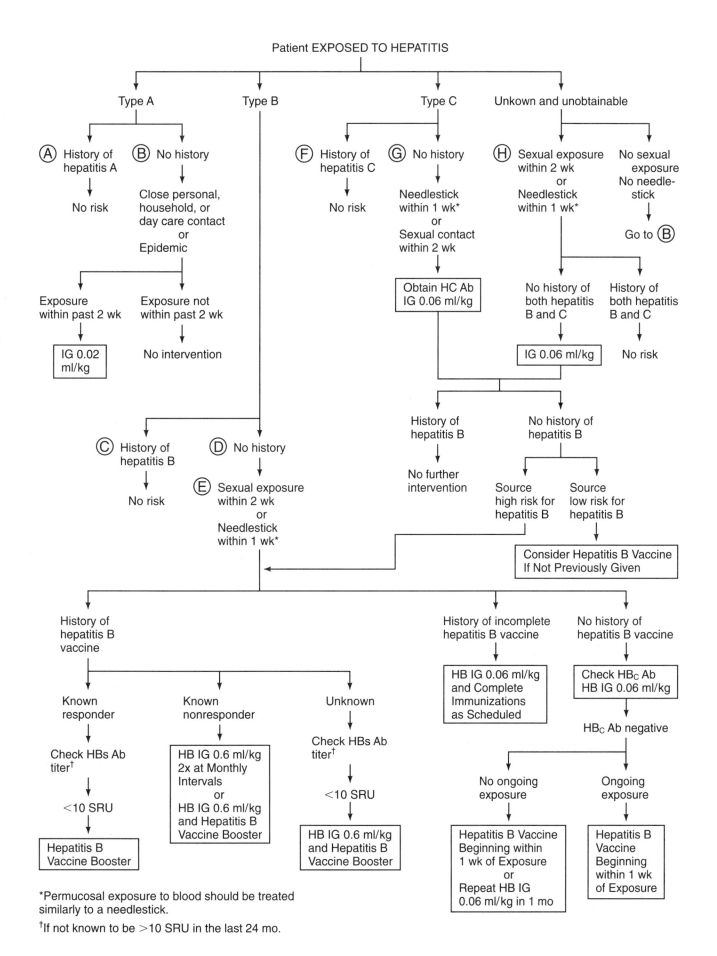

Patient EXPOSED TO HEPATITIS

Type A   Type B   Type C   Unknown and unobtainable

(A) History of hepatitis A

No risk

(B) No history

Close personal, household, or day care contact or Epidemic

Exposure within past 2 wk

Exposure not within past 2 wk

IG 0.02 ml/kg

No intervention

(F) History of hepatitis C

No risk

(G) No history

Needlestick within 1 wk* or Sexual contact within 2 wk

Obtain HC Ab IG 0.06 ml/kg

(H) Sexual exposure within 2 wk or Needlestick within 1 wk*

No sexual exposure No needle-stick

Go to (B)

No history of both hepatitis B and C

History of both hepatitis B and C

IG 0.06 ml/kg

No risk

History of hepatitis B

No further intervention

No history of hepatitis B

Source high risk for hepatitis B

Source low risk for hepatitis B

Consider Hepatitis B Vaccine If Not Previously Given

(C) History of hepatitis B

No risk

(D) No history

(E) Sexual exposure within 2 wk or Needlestick within 1 wk*

History of hepatitis B vaccine

History of incomplete hepatitis B vaccine

No history of hepatitis B vaccine

HB IG 0.06 ml/kg and Complete Immunizations as Scheduled

Check HB$_C$ Ab HB IG 0.06 ml/kg

HB$_C$ Ab negative

Known responder

Known nonresponder

Unknown

Check HBs Ab titer[†]

Check HBs Ab titer[†]

<10 SRU

HB IG 0.6 ml/kg 2x at Monthly Intervals or HB IG 0.6 ml/kg and Hepatitis B Vaccine Booster

<10 SRU

Hepatitis B Vaccine Booster

HB IG 0.6 ml/kg and Hepatitis B Vaccine Booster

No ongoing exposure

Ongoing exposure

Hepatitis B Vaccine Beginning within 1 wk of Exposure or Repeat HB IG 0.06 ml/kg in 1 mo

Hepatitis B Vaccine Beginning within 1 wk of Exposure

*Permucosal exposure to blood should be treated similarly to a needlestick.

[†]If not known to be >10 SRU in the last 24 mo.

263

FEVER OF UNKNOWN ORIGIN

Seth Weissman, M.D.
Richard M. Mandel, M.D.

The strict definition of fever of unknown origin (FUO) is (1) duration of at least 3 weeks, (2) temperature >38.3° C on several occasions, and (3) unknown cause after routine work-up. These criteria tend to eliminate protracted viral illness or other self-limited etiologies from being classified as FUO. Instruct patients to check their temperature at least twice daily. Sustained fever is seen with typhoid fever or miliary tuberculosis (TB). Intermittent fever is most often seen with abscesses and other pyogenic infections. In the absence of other symptoms (chills, sweats, and tachycardia) or abnormal results on initial work-up, consider diagnoses such as exaggerated circadian temperature rhythm and factitious fever. Although the pattern of fever generally is not helpful in determining the cause of FUO, it may aid in diagnosing cases of tertian or quartan malaria, cyclic neutropenia, or Hodgkin's disease (with the Pel-Ebstein fever characterized by 5–10 days of fever alternating with 5–10 days of afebrility). Fever lasting >6 months suggests granulomatous disease or adult Still's disease.

A. Most associated symptoms are nonspecific (e.g., malaise, sweats, weight loss, myalgias). Obtain a thorough history of travel (especially to regions where malaria, tuberculosis, or certain mycoses are endemic), animal exposure (zoonotic infections), insect bites (rickettsial infections), previous surgery, and occupational exposures (berylliosis).

B. Physical examination must be painstakingly thorough and often repeated. Pay particular attention to skin, eyes, teeth, sinuses, lymph nodes, heart, abdomen, pelvis, rectum, and extremities.

C. Resist the urge to "shotgun" the work-up. Reasonable routine testing includes CBC with differential, hepatic and muscle enzymes, multiple (up to six) blood cultures, and urine for analysis and culture (including three morning specimens for AFB analysis). Stool examination for ova and parasites may be indicated. The choice of serologic tests is guided by the history and physical examination. Consider VDRL and HIV antibody tests in patients with appropriate risk factors. Other serologies may include a streptozyme panel, antibody titers to mycoses, agents responsible for many zoonotic infections, amebiasis, as well as to cytomegalovirus (CMV) and the hepatitis viruses. Do not order these tests for every patient. If there is a low pretest probability of the specific disease, expect more false than true positives. Serum should be frozen and saved for potential use in comparing acute and convalescent titers. In the absence of clinical suspicion of disease, ANA, rheumatoid factor, and serum protein electrophoresis are seldom diagnostic. ESR is nonspecific. Although ESR >100 mm/hr suggests vasculitis, it can also be seen with neoplasm, TB, or pyogenic infection. Skin testing may reveal a positive PPD, exposure to fungal pathogens, or anergy, which suggests sarcoidosis, miliary tuberculosis, Whipple's disease, Hodgkin's disease, or some other malignancy. Chest films are routine. Examination of CSF in the absence of specific CNS signs or symptoms is usually not indicated, initially.

D. Infection is the most common cause of FUO in adults. However, as the duration of FUO increases, the probability of an infectious etiology decreases. Two important systemic infections to consider are TB and infectious endocarditis (IE). When TB presents as FUO, extrapulmonary involvement predominates. Patients with miliary TB may have a negative PPD and a normal chest film. Bone marrow and liver biopsies may be necessary for diagnosis. IE is rare in the absence of a murmur, and only 5% are truly culture negative. Four to six negative blood cultures (obtained at least 5–10 days after the patient is off antibiotics) should eliminate this possibility. Peripheral stigmata of IE may suggest the diagnosis. Echocardiography is helpful if vegetations are seen.

E. Intra-abdominal abscesses are the most common type of localized infection to cause FUO. Use abdominal and pelvic CT and ultrasonography to investigate this possibility. Osteomyelitis is commonly encountered as FUO. Radionuclide bone scan reveals abnormalities earlier than plain radiographs. Also consider odontogenic abscess and infections of the biliary tree, urinary tract, and sinuses.

F. Innumerable other infectious agents may be responsible for FUO. Except for CMV or HIV, viruses rarely cause FUO. The search for other infectious agents must be tailored to the patient.

G. Neoplasm is the second most common cause of FUO in adults, and lymphoma is the most common neoplasm. Fever also occurs with leukemia, myelodysplasia, and solid tumors, including renal cell carcinoma, hepatoma, adenocarcinoma of the colon, carcinomatosis, and atrial myxoma.

H. Among the collagen vascular or autoimmune etiologies are systemic lupus erythematosus (fever as the only presenting symptom in <5%), Still's disease, vasculitis, and drug hypersensitivity reactions. Strongly consider temporal arteritis in elderly patients, even in the absence of classical physical findings. Patients often have ESR >100 mm/hr. Erythema multiforme, rheumatic fever, and polymyalgia rheumatica may uncommonly present with fever as the chief complaint.

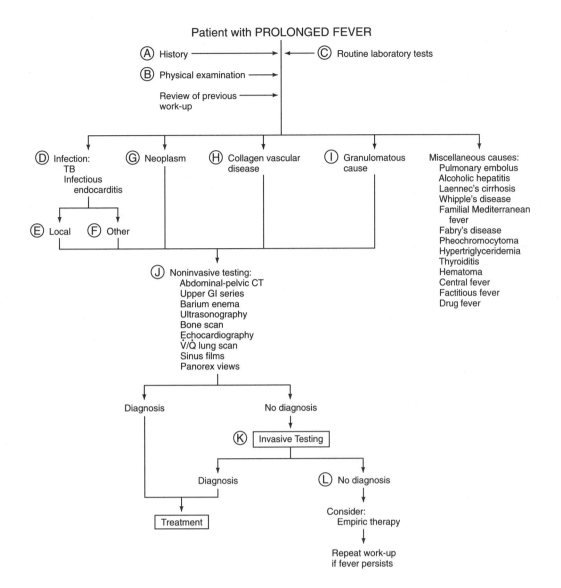

Patient with PROLONGED FEVER

Ⓐ History
Ⓑ Physical examination
Review of previous work-up
Ⓒ Routine laboratory tests

Ⓓ Infection:
TB
Infectious endocarditis

Ⓖ Neoplasm

Ⓗ Collagen vascular disease

Ⓘ Granulomatous cause

Miscellaneous causes:
Pulmonary embolus
Alcoholic hepatitis
Laennec's cirrhosis
Whipple's disease
Familial Mediterranean
   fever
Fabry's disease
Pheochromocytoma
Hypertriglyceridemia
Thyroiditis
Hematoma
Central fever
Factitious fever
Drug fever

Ⓔ Local   Ⓕ Other

Ⓙ Noninvasive testing:
Abdominal-pelvic CT
Upper GI series
Barium enema
Ultrasonography
Bone scan
Echocardiography
V̇/Q̇ lung scan
Sinus films
Panorex views

Diagnosis

No diagnosis

Ⓚ Invasive Testing

Diagnosis

Ⓛ No diagnosis

Treatment

Consider:
Empiric therapy

Repeat work-up
if fever persists

I. In one study of patients with FUO lasting >1 year, granulomatous causes were more common than neoplastic or autoimmune ones. Entities include granulomatous hepatitis of unknown etiology, sarcoidosis, and Crohn's disease. When granulomas are found on liver biopsy rule out other potential infectious and noninfectious causes before diagnosing granulomatous hepatitis of unknown etiology.

J. The noninvasive work-up should be thorough but tempered by one's best judgment of clinical probabilities.

K. If the work-up to this point is still unrevealing, proceed with biopsies of bone marrow and liver. Samples should be cultured for bacteria, mycobacteria, viruses, and fungi and sent for histologic study. Other biopsy sites may include skin, lymph nodes, muscle, temporal artery, or any organ or bodily fluid found to be suspicious on work-up. Reserve laparotomy for patients with fever and abdominal pain whose etiology remains unknown after noninvasive study.

L. The cause may remain unknown in 5–15% of patients even after thorough evaluation. These patients tend to have a low mortality rate and good prognosis, and fever often resolves spontaneously. Therapeutic trials tend to obscure the picture and there probably is no role for empiric antibiotics in FUO. Trials of antipyretics, nonsteroidal anti-inflammatory drugs, and even corticosteroids (if a noninfectious etiology is certain) may bring symptomatic improvement. The work-up may need to be repeated in several weeks to months if fevers persist.

References

Dinarello CA, Wolff SM. Fever of unknown origin. In: Mandel GL, et al, eds. Principles and practice of infectious diseases. 3rd ed. New York: Churchill Livingstone, 1990:468.

Larson EB, Featherstone HJ, Petersdorf RG. Fever of undetermined origin: diagnosis and follow-up of 105 cases, 1970–80. Medicine. 1982; 61:269.

Swartz MN, Simon HB. Fever of undetermined origin. Sci Am 1990; 7:5.

NEPHROLOGY

CHRONIC RENAL FAILURE

Anwar Al-Haidary, M.B., M.R.C.P., M.Sc.
Joy L. Logan, M.D.

A. Renal ultrasonography is a sensitive, noninvasive test that will define kidney size and rule out chronic obstruction. Small kidneys (<10 cm in length) indicate chronic renal failure, but normal to large kidneys may be present in chronic renal failure as a result of diabetes, amyloid, or light-chain disease. Polycystic kidney disease also causes chronic renal failure and renomegaly, but the renal cysts are clearly discernible by ultrasonography after the age of 18. Cysts may also be found by ultrasound examination of the liver, pancreas, and ovaries of patients with polycystic kidney disease.

B. Pertinent historical data in chronic renal failure include symptoms or signs of extrarenal manifestations of connective tissue diseases or vasculitities (e.g., skin rashes, joint pains, neurologic complaints). Respiratory symptoms prompt consideration of Wegener's granulomatosis or Goodpasture's syndrome. A history of high-risk behaviors heightens consideration of chronic glomerulopathies resulting from hepatitis B or HIV. These diagnoses are supported by serologic studies (antinuclear antibody, C3/C4, antineutrophil cytoplasmic antibody, anti–glomerular basement membrane antibodies, cryoglobulins, HIV, and hepatitis B antibodies). Other historical factors pertinent to the differential diagnosis of chronic renal failure include a family history of renal disease, long-standing hypertension, or recurrent urinary tract infection (UTI). A drug history is also important, since analgesics (phenacetin), amphotericin B, cyclosporin A, and other agents may lead to chronic renal injury.

C. A lack of historical clues in a patient with small kidneys suggests a subclinical glomerulopathy as the cause of chronic renal failure, whether primary or secondary. Consider also chronic interstitial nephritis resulting from disorders of calcium or urate metabolism, as well as occult small vessel occlusion from cholesterol emboli.

D. Identification of light chains by urine protein electrophoresis suggests myeloma, amyloidosis, or light-chain disease. The urinary protein in amyloidosis is usually in the nephrotic range and the diagnosis is confirmed by peritoneal fat pad aspiration or rectal biopsy. Light-chain disease and myeloma can be confirmed by bone marrow examination and skeletal radiographs. Diabetic nephropathy usually presents with nephrotic-range proteinuria and hypertension, and the diagnosis is strongly supported by the finding of associated diabetic retinopathy.

E. After the initial evaluation of renal function and the exclusion of reversible factors (fluid overload/contraction, hypertension, UTI, obstruction), evaluate the patient periodically for signs or symptoms of uremia or fluid imbalance. Make regular assessment of renal function by determination of creatinine clearances and/or serum creatinine, BUN, electrolytes, calcium, phosphate, albumin, full blood counts, ferritin, PTH, and bone radiographs.

F. Stable patients with slow deterioration of renal function and minor uremic symptoms (pruritus, anemia, volume and/or electrolyte abnormalities responsive to conservative treatment, renal osteodystrophy) may be managed conservatively with appropriate pharmacologic and dietary therapy. Erythropoietin may be administered to correct the anemia.

G. Unanticipated deterioration in renal function prompts additional searches for reversible factors. Appearance of major uremic symptoms (e.g., nonresponsive volume overload, pericarditis, progressive neuropathy) in a patient without reversible factors requires consideration of renal replacement therapy via dialysis or transplantation.

References

Baldwin DS. Chronic glomerulonephritis: nonimmunologic mechanisms of progressive glomerular damage. Kidney Int 1982; 21:109.

Eschbach JW, Adamson JW. Recombinant human erythropoietin: implications for nephrology. Am J Kid Dis 1988; 11:203.

Hostetter TH, Olson JL, Rennke HG, et al. Hyperfiltration in remnant nephrons: a potentially adverse response to renal ablation. Am J Physiol 1981; 241:F85.

Krowlewski AS, Canessa M, Warren JH, et al. Predisposition to hypertension and susceptibility to renal disease in insulin-dependent diabetes mellitus. N Engl J Med 1988; 318:140.

Meyer TW, Anderson SA, Rennke HG, Brenner BM. Reversing glomerular hypertension stabilizes established glomerular injury. Kidney Int 1987; 31:752.

Morris PJ. Renal transplantation: indications, outcome, complications, and results. In: Schrier RW, Gottschalk CW, eds. Diseases of the kidney. 4th ed. Boston: Little, Brown, 1988:3229.

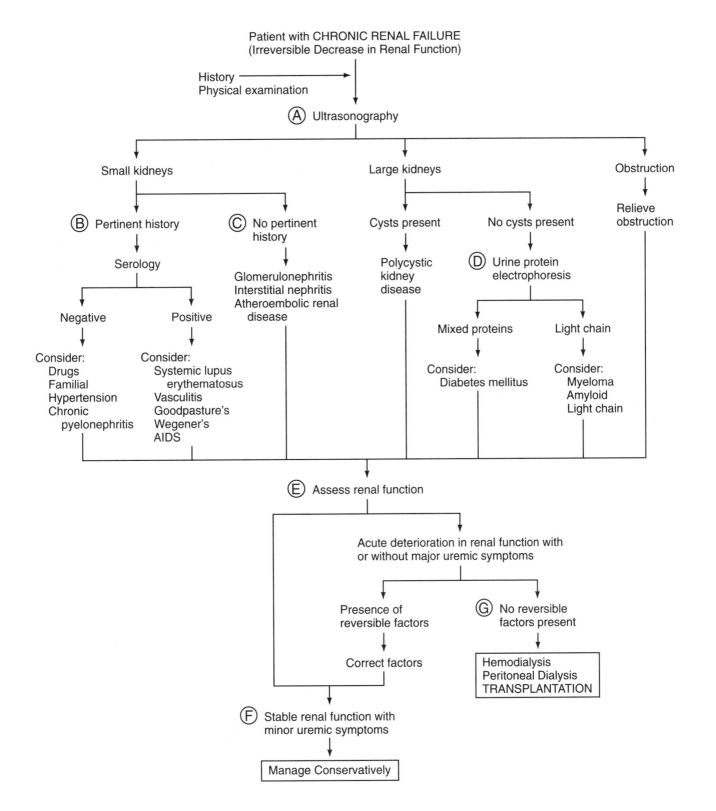

Patient with CHRONIC RENAL FAILURE
(Irreversible Decrease in Renal Function)

History
Physical examination

Ⓐ Ultrasonography

Small kidneys

Ⓑ Pertinent history

Serology

Negative

Consider:
Drugs
Familial
Hypertension
Chronic
pyelonephritis

Positive

Consider:
Systemic lupus
erythematosus
Vasculitis
Goodpasture's
Wegener's
AIDS

Ⓒ No pertinent history

Glomerulonephritis
Interstitial nephritis
Atheroembolic renal
disease

Large kidneys

Cysts present

Polycystic
kidney
disease

No cysts present

Ⓓ Urine protein electrophoresis

Mixed proteins

Consider:
Diabetes mellitus

Light chain

Consider:
Myeloma
Amyloid
Light chain

Obstruction

Relieve obstruction

Ⓔ Assess renal function

Acute deterioration in renal function with
or without major uremic symptoms

Presence of reversible factors

Correct factors

Ⓖ No reversible factors present

Hemodialysis
Peritoneal Dialysis
TRANSPLANTATION

Ⓕ Stable renal function with minor uremic symptoms

Manage Conservatively

ACUTE RENAL FAILURE

Anwar Al-Haidary, M.B., M.R.C.P., M.Sc.
David B. Van Wyck, M.D.

Acute renal failure (ARF) in hospitalized patients frequently involves multiple potential etiologies. The challenge is therefore to identify and correct dominant reversible factors and to prevent the complications anticipated after sudden loss of renal function. The history and physical examination should aim to identify or exclude evidence of systemic inflammatory disease, infection, volume and hemodynamic disturbances, medications, and allergies. Renal ultrasonography should be undertaken if historical or physical evidence suggests malignancy, urinary stone disease, solitary kidney (including transplanted), neurogenic bladder, or bladder outlet obstruction. Careful examination of a fresh urine specimen is essential.

A. In the patient with ARF, muddy brown casts and epithelial cell casts suggest acute tubular necrosis (ATN), WBC casts acute interstitial nephritis (AIN), and RBC casts rapidly progressive glomerulonephritis (RPGN). Obtain a random urine sample for analysis of sodium (U_{Na}, P_{Na}) and creatinine (U_{cr}, P_{cr}) concentration, and calculation of fractional excretion of sodium (Fe_{Na}):

$$Fe_{Na}(\%) = \frac{U_{Na} \times P_{cr}}{U_{cr} \times P_{Na}} \times 100$$

B. ATN results from ischemic or toxic damage to renal tubular epithelium. Ischemia can usually be identified by inspection of the patient and recent blood pressure recordings. The most common causes of nephrotoxic ATN include drugs (especially aminoglycosides, amphotericin B, cisplatin), radiocontrast material, heavy metals (mercury, lead), hemoglobin, myoglobin (see A), and multiple myeloma (with light-chain deposition). Since the BUN and P_{cr} rise proportionately in ATN, a normal ratio of 10–20:1 is often seen. U_{Na} >20 mEq/L or Fe_{Na} >1.0% supports the diagnosis of ATN, but lower values for either test may be seen, particularly early in the course of ischemic ATN.

C. Although myoglobin is not directly nephrotoxic, luminal obstruction of the renal tubules with myoglobin casts and intense myoglobin-mediated intrarenal vasoconstriction frequently combine to produce ARF after breakdown of muscle tissue (rhabdomyolysis). The diagnosis of rhabdomyolysis is suggested by high serum concentrations of other intracellular constituents, including potassium, phosphate, and urate, and is confirmed by elevated plasma creatine kinase levels, a positive urine dipstick test for heme without urinary RBCs by microscopy, and a positive test for myoglobinuria. The low BUN/P_{cr} ratio accompanying renal failure in this disorder reflects the high load of creatine released from damaged muscle. The risk of ARF after rhabdomyolysis is increased by hypotension or dehydration; vigorous efforts to maintain brisk urinary output are accordingly indicated. Common causes of rhabdomyolysis include trauma, drug overdose (alcohol and cocaine), and heat stroke. Although decreased protein intake, drugs (including sulfamethoxazole and cimetidine), and acidosis can also lower the BUN/P_{cr} ratio, these laboratory abnormalities are not usually associated with ARF.

D. Inflammation of the tubulointerstitial region of the kidney may be associated with acute or chronic renal failure. If the etiology is bacterial, as in pyelonephritis, treatment requires appropriate antibiotics. The most common noninfectious cause of interstitial nephritis is a drug-induced allergic reaction. Methicillin, penicillin, cephalothin, nonsteroidal anti-inflammatory drugs (NSAIDs), and cimetidine are strongly associated with AIN. Other penicillins and cephalosporins, as well as the sulfonamides, thiazides, and furosemides, are also likely offenders. In most patients, partial to full recovery is expected after withdrawal of the responsible agent. Since the role of steroid therapy in AIN is uncertain, prednisone (60 mg/day with rapid taper) should be administered only to patients with severe disease (P_{cr} >2.5–3.0 mg/dl).

E. Consider rapidly progressing glomerulonephritis (RPGN) whenever rapid deterioration in renal function is accompanied by RBC casts and proteinuria. Serologic examination is the key to differential diagnosis. In particular, low plasma complement levels are frequently found in immune complex–mediated diseases, including postinfectious glomerulonephritis, membranoproliferative glomerulonephritis, cryoglobulinemia, and (in the presence of antinuclear antibodies) systemic lupus erythematosus; a positive test for antineutrophil cytoplasmic antibody strongly suggests either Wegener's granulomatosis or a necrotizing systemic vasculitis. Definitive diagnosis is established by renal biopsy, in which RPGN is histologically defined as crescent formation involving >50% of glomeruli.

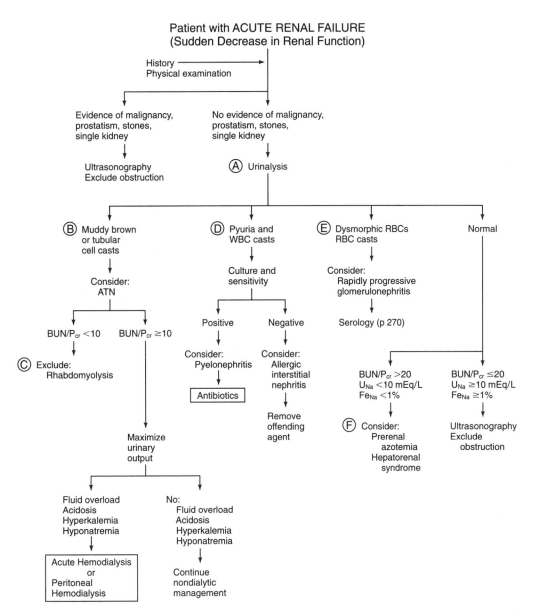

Patient with ACUTE RENAL FAILURE
(Sudden Decrease in Renal Function)

History ——————
Physical examination

Evidence of malignancy, prostatism, stones, single kidney

No evidence of malignancy, prostatism, stones, single kidney

Ultrasonography
Exclude obstruction

Ⓐ Urinalysis

Ⓑ Muddy brown or tubular cell casts

Consider:
ATN

BUN/P$_{cr}$ <10   BUN/P$_{cr}$ ≥10

Ⓒ Exclude:
Rhabdomyolysis

Maximize urinary output

Fluid overload
Acidosis
Hyperkalemia
Hyponatremia

Acute Hemodialysis
or
Peritoneal Hemodialysis

No:
Fluid overload
Acidosis
Hyperkalemia
Hyponatremia

Continue nondialytic management

Ⓓ Pyuria and WBC casts

Culture and sensitivity

Positive   Negative

Consider:
Pyelonephritis

Antibiotics

Consider:
Allergic interstitial nephritis

Remove offending agent

Ⓔ Dysmorphic RBCs RBC casts

Consider:
Rapidly progressive glomerulonephritis

Serology (p 270)

BUN/P$_{cr}$ >20
U$_{Na}$ <10 mEq/L
Fe$_{Na}$ <1%

Ⓕ Consider:
Prerenal azotemia
Hepatorenal syndrome

Normal

BUN/P$_{cr}$ ≤20
U$_{Na}$ ≥10 mEq/L
Fe$_{Na}$ ≥1%

Ultrasonography
Exclude obstruction

F. In prerenal disease, enhanced tubular reabsorption of solutes and water predominates over the rather modest fall in glomerular filtration rate. Since urea and creatinine are both filtered, but urea is avidly reabsorbed and creatinine is not, an elevated BUN/P$_{cr}$ ratio results. U$_{Na}$ <10 mEq/L or Fe$_{Na}$ <1% provides further evidence that intrinsic renal function is intact and that prerenal causes for azotemia should be sought, including volume depletion, hypotension, congestive heart failure, cirrhosis, NSAID administration, and severe bilateral renal artery stenosis. In hepatorenal syndrome, ARF in association with cirrhosis and ascites is characterized by low U$_{Na}$ (often <10 mEq/L) and Fe$_{Na}$ (<1%). The interpretation of BUN/P$_{cr}$ ratios may be rendered unreliable by disorders of protein metabolism. For example, hepatic cirrhosis and protein malnutrition are associated with low BUN levels, whereas GI bleeding, hypercatabolism, high protein intake (often from parenteral nutrition), and corticosteroid administration are all associated with elevated BUN levels.

References

Ebert TH. Hematuria. In: Greene HL, Glassock RJ, Kelley MA, eds. Introduction to clinical medicine. Philadelphia: BC Decker, 1991.

Espinal CH, Gregory AW. Differential diagnosis of acute renal failure. Clin Nephrol 1980; 13:73.

Falk RJ, Hogan S, Carey TS, Jennette C. Clinical course of anti-neutrophil cytoplasmic antibody-associated glomerulonephritis and systemic vasculitis. Ann Intern Med 1990; 113:656.

Galpin JE, Shinaberger JH, Stanley TM, et al. Acute interstitial nephritis due to methicillin. Am J Med 1978; 65:756.

Rose BD. In: Pathophysiology of renal disease. 2nd ed. New York: McGraw-Hill, 1987:65.

PROTEINURIA

Anwar Al-Haidary, M.B., M.R.C.P., M.Sc.
David B. Van Wyck, M.D.

A. Proteinuria is the presence of >150 mg/day of protein in the urine. Perform protein electrophoresis of a 24-hour urine specimen in any patient with proteinuria identified by dipstick urine examination, because quantification and characterization of the protein excreted are essential to differential diagnosis and treatment.

B. The presence of nephrotic range proteinuria (>3.5 g/day) implies glomerular disease or glomerulonephritis (GN). Characteristically, the main component of glomerular proteinuria is albumin, and there is no monoclonal protein component. Diabetes is one of the most frequent causes of nephrotic syndrome in adults. It can be readily excluded by history, physical examination (with particular attention to retinal changes), and normal fasting blood glucose. Rarely, diabetic retinopathy can be excluded only by fluorescein angiography.

C. In the absence of diabetes, the most common causes of nephrotic syndrome in adults include focal sclerosing GN, membranous GN, and amyloidosis, which can be distinguished only by tissue examination (renal biopsy). Serologic investigation may be rewarding, nevertheless. Systemic lupus erythematosus (SLE) is characterized by elevated antinuclear antibody (ANA). Complement components C3 and C4 may be low in SLE, postinfectious GN, cryoglobulinemia, and membranoproliferative GN. Positive antinuclear neutrophil cytoplasmic antibody (ANCA), formerly thought to be specific for Wegener's granulomatosis, is known to be associated also with the GN of systemic vasculitis. Hepatitis B virus or HIV antigenemia are well described etiologies of nephrotic syndrome, and the presence of either renders further diagnostic studies unnecessary. A number of drugs, including gold, penicillamine, phenytoin, captopril, and nonsteroidal anti-inflammatory agents, have been shown to cause nephrotic syndrome; withdrawal of the offending agents generally prompts resolution of proteinuria.

D. Renal biopsy remains the best means of establishing the definitive diagnosis of most causes of nephrotic syndrome. Treatment is aimed at the underlying condition, control of excessive protein losses, and managing the expected complications of nephrotic syndrome (edema, ascites, and increased risk of infections and deep venous thrombosis). A low-protein diet, angiotensin II converting enzyme (ACE) inhibitors, and calcium channel blockers have proved effective in decreasing proteinuria in patients with nephrotic syndrome from a wide range of causes.

E. Although patients showing proteinuria of <3.5 g/day may suffer from the same disorders of glomerular function seen in nephrotic syndrome, low-grade proteinuria is also frequently seen in patients with primarily extrarenal disorders such as congestive cardiac failure or uncontrolled hypertension. Similarly, significant proteinuria that arises during a febrile illness or after heavy exercise does not suggest a pathologic condition. Orthostatic proteinuria is a benign condition that usually remits spontaneously and is characterized by significant proteinuria only when the patient is active and in the upright position. Like transient and benign persistent forms, orthostatic proteinuria has a typically benign course.

F. The presence of monoclonal protein in the urine and in plasma suggests plasma cell dyscrasia. Further examination by immunoelectrophoresis, bone marrow aspiration, and skeletal radiography is needed to exclude multiple myeloma. In the absence of evidence for myeloma, consider secondary amyloidosis, light-chain disease, and B-cell lymphoproliferative disorders. Definitive diagnosis of amyloidosis may require tissue biopsy. Management consists of treating the underlying disorder.

References

Clive DM. Proteinuria. In: Greene HL, Glassock RJ, Kelley MA, eds. Introduction to clinical medicine. Philadelphia: BC Decker, 1991:508.

Rose BD. Pathophysiology of renal disease. 2nd ed. New York: McGraw-Hill, 1987.

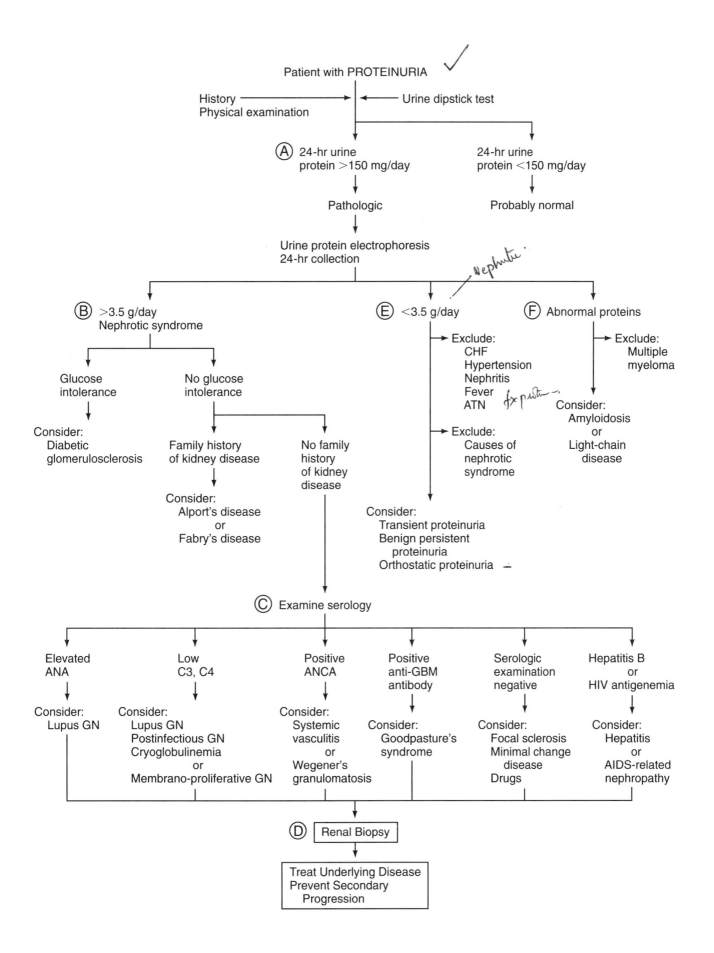

Patient with PROTEINURIA

History — Physical examination → ← Urine dipstick test

(A) 24-hr urine protein >150 mg/day — 24-hr urine protein <150 mg/day

Pathologic — Probably normal

Urine protein electrophoresis
24-hr collection

Nephritic.

(B) >3.5 g/day
Nephrotic syndrome

(E) <3.5 g/day

(F) Abnormal proteins

Glucose intolerance — No glucose intolerance

Consider:
Diabetic glomerulosclerosis

Family history of kidney disease — No family history of kidney disease

Consider:
Alport's disease
or
Fabry's disease

→ Exclude:
CHF
Hypertension
Nephritis
Fever
ATN   *fx prostra –*

→ Exclude:
Causes of nephrotic syndrome

Consider:
Transient proteinuria
Benign persistent proteinuria
Orthostatic proteinuria –

→ Exclude:
Multiple myeloma

Consider:
Amyloidosis
or
Light-chain disease

(C) Examine serology

Elevated ANA

Low C3, C4

Positive ANCA

Positive anti-GBM antibody

Serologic examination negative

Hepatitis B or HIV antigenemia

Consider:
Lupus GN

Consider:
Lupus GN
Postinfectious GN
Cryoglobulinemia
or
Membrano-proliferative GN

Consider:
Systemic vasculitis
or
Wegener's granulomatosis

Consider:
Goodpasture's syndrome

Consider:
Focal sclerosis
Minimal change disease
Drugs

Consider:
Hepatitis
or
AIDS-related nephropathy

(D) Renal Biopsy

Treat Underlying Disease
Prevent Secondary Progression

HEMATURIA

Anwar Al-Haidary, M.B., M.R.C.P., M.Sc.
David B. Van Wyck, M.D.

A. Since the presence or absence of cellular urinary casts is pivotal to the evaluation of patients with hematuria, several freshly voided urine sediments should be closely examined by the physician. The presence of RBC casts virtually establishes the diagnosis of glomerulonephritis (GN) or vasculitis. Dysmorphic changes in urinary RBCs, best observed under interference phase-contrast microscopy, likewise suggest glomerular origin.

B. Perform serologic tests (antinuclear antibody for systemic lupus erythematosus [SLE], cryoglobulins for essential mixed cryoglobulinemia, antineutrophil cytoplasmic antibody for Wegener's and vasculitis, and anti–glomerular basement membrane antibodies for Goodpasture's syndrome) as soon as glomerular disease is detected. Also, examine the plasma C3 and C4 components of complement, since low levels are a hallmark of GN associated with SLE, infections, cryoglobulinemia, and membranoproliferative GN.

C. If the above serologic examination is unrewarding and the patient has normal renal function, normal blood pressure, and proteinuria <300 mg/day, consider the diagnosis of IgA nephropathy (Berger's disease). This relatively common presentation of GN shows a typically benign course. Hypertension, renal insufficiency, or high-grade proteinuria, regardless of the pathologic diagnosis, suggests a less favorable prognosis, and in the opinion of many nephrologists requires tissue evaluation.

D. Normal-shaped RBCs and the absence of cellular casts, acellular casts, or significant proteinuria (>300 mg/day) suggest extraglomerular bleeding. The common causes of extraglomerular hematuria in adults include prostatic disease, kidney and urinary stones, malignancy, and trauma. In children, urinary stones and trauma are main causes of nonglomerular hematuria.

E. Pyuria, defined as >4 WBCs per high-power field, is commonly associated with bacteriuria. Pyuria without evidence of infection suggests the diagnosis of interstitial nephritis. Acute interstitial nephritis is characterized by fever, skin rash, eosinophilia, and eosinophiluria, most commonly in association with antibiotic administration. Chronic interstitial nephritis is found in association with a wide variety of drugs, heavy metal intoxication, metabolic abnormalities, and therapeutic radiation.

References

Ebert TH. Hematuria. In: Greene HL, Glassock RJ, Kelley MA, eds. Introduction to clinical medicine. Philadelphia: BC Decker, 1991.

Falk RJ, Hogan S, Carey TS, Jennette C. Clinical course of antineutrophil cytoplasmic antibody–associated glomerulonephritis and systemic vasculitis. Ann Intern Med 1990; 113:656.

Rodicio JL. Idiopathic IgA nephropathy. Kidney Int 1984; 25:717.

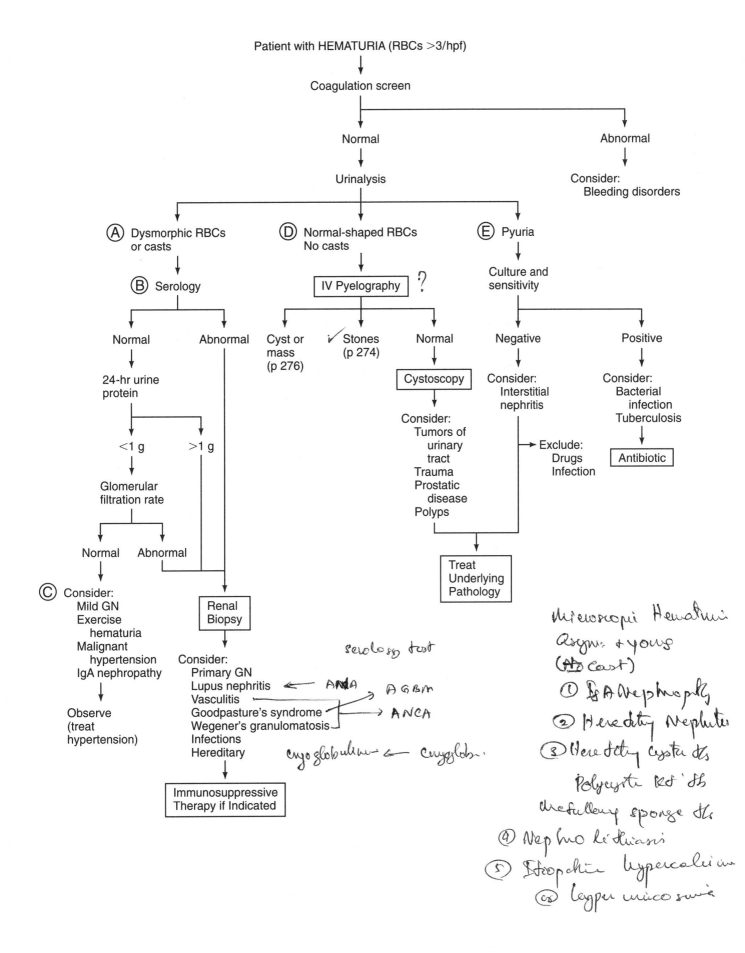

Patient with HEMATURIA (RBCs >3/hpf)

Coagulation screen

Normal → Urinalysis

Abnormal → Consider: Bleeding disorders

(A) Dysmorphic RBCs or casts

(D) Normal-shaped RBCs No casts

(E) Pyuria

(B) Serology

Normal → 24-hr urine protein

Abnormal

<1 g → Glomerular filtration rate

>1 g

Normal

Abnormal

(C) Consider:
Mild GN
Exercise hematuria
Malignant hypertension
IgA nephropathy

Observe (treat hypertension)

Renal Biopsy

Consider:
Primary GN
Lupus nephritis
Vasculitis
Goodpasture's syndrome
Wegener's granulomatosis
Infections
Hereditary

Immunosuppressive Therapy if Indicated

IV Pyelography ?

Cyst or mass (p 276)

✓ Stones (p 274)

Normal → Cystoscopy

Consider:
Tumors of urinary tract
Trauma
Prostatic disease
Polyps

Culture and sensitivity

Negative → Consider: Interstitial nephritis

Positive → Consider: Bacterial infection Tuberculosis → Antibiotic

Exclude: Drugs Infection

Treat Underlying Pathology

Handwritten notes:

serology test

Lupus nephritis ← ANA

A GBM

→ ANCA

cryoglobulin ← cryoglob.

Microscopic Hematuria
Asymp. + young
(No cast)
① IgA Nephropathy
② Hereditary Nephritis
③ Hereditary cystic dis
Polycystic kd dis
Medullary sponge dis
④ Nephrolithiasis
⑤ Idiopathic hypercalciuria
⑥ Hyper uricosuria

KIDNEY STONES

James L. McGuire, M.D.
David B. Van Wyck, M.D.

Kidney stones are frequently manifested by sharp colicky pain radiating to the groin, testicle, or tip of the urethra, often accompanied by gross hematuria. Common clinical presentations also include nephrocalcinosis, renal damage, and staghorn calculi. Although urinary stone disease is common, approximately 40% of patients suffer only a single episode of stone passage. Thus, intensive investigation and treatment is directed toward patients with special risk factors, including family history of stone disease, history of major stone complication, solitary kidney, age at onset <20 years, and associated predisposing conditions such as renal tubular acidosis, urinary infection with urea-splitting organisms, and malabsorption syndromes. Chemical analysis is extremely useful in distinguishing the four main stone types. Struvite or infection stones account for 20% of all stones and are found in urine infected with urea-splitting organisms. Urate stones account for 5% and commonly arise in the setting of hyperuricemia and gout. Cystine stones comprise 3% of the total and result from a renal tubular defect promoting urinary cystine loss. Clinical setting and chemical analysis render the diagnosis of these disorders readily apparent. The pathogenesis and treatment of calcium and uric acid containing stones is detailed in the decision tree.

A. A detailed history is useful in identifying high calcium intake, usually from dairy products; high salt intake, which promotes calcium excretion; fluid intake inadequate to match losses; malabsorption syndromes, which are associated with calcium oxalate stones; previous urinary tract infections or procedures; or use of medications such as vitamin D or calcium-containing antacids.

B. A 24-hour urine collection for calcium, urate, creatinine, and pH may be the single most important test in patients with calcium kidney stones. The demonstration of hypercalciuria is pivotal. In the absence of major reversible causes of hypercalciuria, consider the diagnosis of idiopathic hypercalciuria from hyperabsorption of calcium. A low urinary volume <1 L per day may aggravate the degree of urinary supersaturation in patients with stones. High urate excretion predisposes to stone formation, whether pure urate or mixed. Most patients with calcium oxalate nephrolithiasis show urine pH values >6.5. In approximately 50% of patients, no obvious abnormality is apparent on routine urine collection. In some of these remaining patients, urinary levels of the stone inhibitor citrate may be low.

C. Treatment strategies for patients with calcium-containing stones should begin with generous fluid intake (over 2 L per day) and, in the presence of hypercalciuria, dietary restriction of calcium and sodium. Thiazide (e.g., hydrochlorothiazide, 25–50 mg/day) lowers both calcium and oxalate excretion. Cellulose sodium phosphate (Calcibind) has been suggested for idiopathic calcium hyperabsorption, but its cost and the high level of GI intolerance has limited its use. Give allopurinol (300 mg/day, adjusted downward for renal insufficiency) for hyperuricosuria.

References

Coe FI, Parks JH. Pathophysiology of kidney stones and strategies for treatment. Hosp Pract 1988; 23:185.

McGuire JL. Kidney stones. In: Greene HL, Glassock RJ, Kelley MA, eds. Introduction to clinical medicine. Philadelphia: BC Decker, 1991:519.

Pak CYC, Fuller C. Idiopathic hypocitrauric calcium-oxalate nephrolithiasis successfully treated with potassium citrate. Ann Intern Med 1986; 104:33.

Preminger GM, Pak CYC. The practical evaluation and selective medical management of nephrolithiasis. Semin Urol 1985; 3:170.

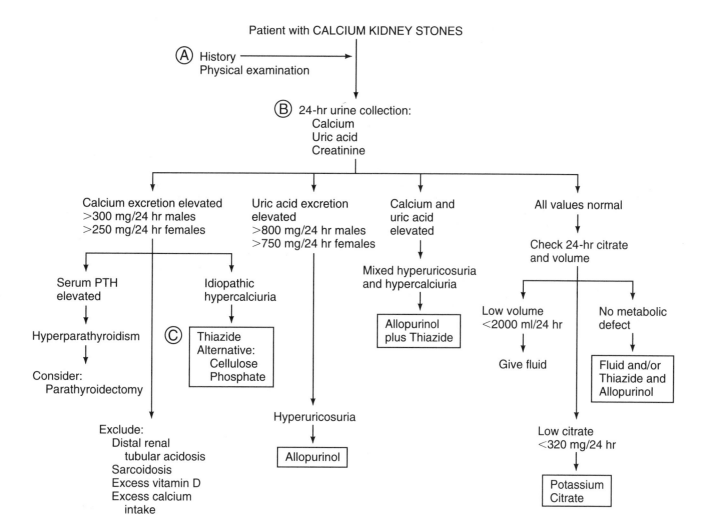

Patient with CALCIUM KIDNEY STONES

Ⓐ History
Physical examination

Ⓑ 24-hr urine collection:
Calcium
Uric acid
Creatinine

Calcium excretion elevated
>300 mg/24 hr males
>250 mg/24 hr females

Uric acid excretion
elevated
>800 mg/24 hr males
>750 mg/24 hr females

Calcium and
uric acid
elevated

All values normal

Serum PTH
elevated

Idiopathic
hypercalciuria

Hyperparathyroidism

Consider:
Parathyroidectomy

Ⓒ Thiazide
Alternative:
Cellulose
Phosphate

Exclude:
Distal renal
tubular acidosis
Sarcoidosis
Excess vitamin D
Excess calcium
intake

Hyperuricosuria

Allopurinol

Mixed hyperuricosuria
and hypercalciuria

Allopurinol
plus Thiazide

Check 24-hr citrate
and volume

Low volume
<2000 ml/24 hr

Give fluid

No metabolic
defect

Fluid and/or
Thiazide and
Allopurinol

Low citrate
<320 mg/24 hr

Potassium
Citrate

275

RENAL CYSTS AND MASSES

David B. Van Wyck, M.D.

A. Flank pain, palpable abdominal mass, or hematuria frequently heralds a renal mass or cystic disease. Begin evaluation of patients with these findings with a CT scan or ultrasonography (US). In general, superior sensitivity renders CT sufficient for the definitive diagnosis of most lesions, and necessary when US evidence is equivocal. When CT is inconclusive, arteriography or needle aspiration may be required.

B. Simple renal cysts are the most common renal masses, occurring in 50% of patients >50 years of age. Although usually asymptomatic and discovered incidentally on a plain film of the abdomen, intravenous pyelography (IVP), or renal US, simple cysts occasionally cause flank or abdominal pain. There may be a single cyst or multiple cysts involving both kidneys. Distinguishing simple cysts from two more serious conditions, polycystic kidney disease (PKD) and solid masses, such as renal cell carcinoma or a renal abscess, is the most important task in the differential diagnosis, and is aided by criteria established for the use of US and CT. The criteria favoring a simple cyst on US are (1) sharp margins with smooth walls, (2) no echoes (anechoic) within the cyst, and (3) a strong posterior wall echo, indicating good transmission through the water-filled cyst. When all three criteria are fulfilled, the likelihood of a malignancy is extremely small and no further evaluation is required. When there is incomplete renal visualization, evidence of calcifications or septa, or multiple cysts that may obscure a potential carcinoma, CT is required. A simple cyst is considered to be present on CT if (1) the cyst is sharply demarcated from the surrounding parenchyma and has smooth, thin walls; (2) the fluid within the cyst is homogeneous (like water) with a density of 0 to 20 Hounsfield units; and (3) there is no enhancement of the cyst fluid after administration of radiocontrast media. The need for cyst puncture is virtually eliminated by the use of US and CT, and should be considered only if the initial, noninvasive procedures cannot confirm a benign cyst.

C. Single or multiple cysts may arise in the course of chronic renal failure. Although acquired cystic disease is occasionally found in patients before dialysis, its incidence may exceed 50% among patients who have undergone dialysis for >3 years. The relatively high incidence of neoplasia associated with acquired cystic disease has prompted recommendations to regularly monitor end-stage renal disease (ESRD) patients sonographically. The diagnostic approach to simple cysts should also be used in patients with acquired renal cystic disease.

D. Adult PKD is responsible for 10–12% of cases of ESRD. Inherited as an autosomal dominant disorder and progressing uniformly to chronic renal failure, adult PKD occurs in approximately 1 of every 1250 live births. Penetrance is complete if the patient lives to 80 years of age. Symptoms of flank pain, abdominal discomfort, and hematuria frequently do not become apparent until the age of 40–50, when they may be associated with hypertension and renal insufficiency. Diagnosis by US is straightforward in advanced disease but may be less reliable in the early stages: a negative US cannot with complete certainty rule out PKD in patients <40. However, CT can detect smaller cysts, lowering the age at which a negative study virtually excludes disease to about 20–25.

E. Medullary cystic disease, unlike the previously mentioned disorders, is rare. Occurring in children, it progresses inevitably to ESRD by the age of 20–40. Since the course of disease is slow and largely asymptomatic, patients frequently present with evidence of advanced renal disease. The diagnosis of medullary cystic disease is often made by inference from the clinical presentation and the common feature of a positive family history. Multiple small and occasional large cysts at the corticomedullary junction are distinctive features on US.

F. Since patients with medullary sponge kidney are frequently asymptomatic, the diagnosis may never be made unless urinary tract infection or passage of a stone prompt IVP. With the exception of stone formation, medullary sponge kidney is a benign disorder with an excellent long-term prognosis, and no specific therapy is needed. Recurrent stone formers may benefit from a thiazide diuretic for hypercalciuria, allopurinol for hyperuricosuria, or potassium citrate for hypocitraturia (p 274).

G. Renal cell carcinoma may arise as a mass lesion, cystic degeneration of a mass, or malignant conversion of a cyst. Symptoms are frequently absent or not specific to the kidney, so that most tumors are discovered during evaluation of hematuria; the full triad of flank pain, palpable mass, and hematuria is seen in <10% of patients. Associated findings include fever, either anemia or erythrocytosis, hepatic dysfunction, and hypercalcemia. CT is pivotal in the diagnosis and staging of renal cell carcinoma and has largely replaced arteriography as the definitive diagnostic study. Small lesions <2 cm may be detected before distortion of the renal outline by abnormal heterogeneous enhancement after injection of contrast.

Patient with RENAL MASS OR CYSTIC DISEASE

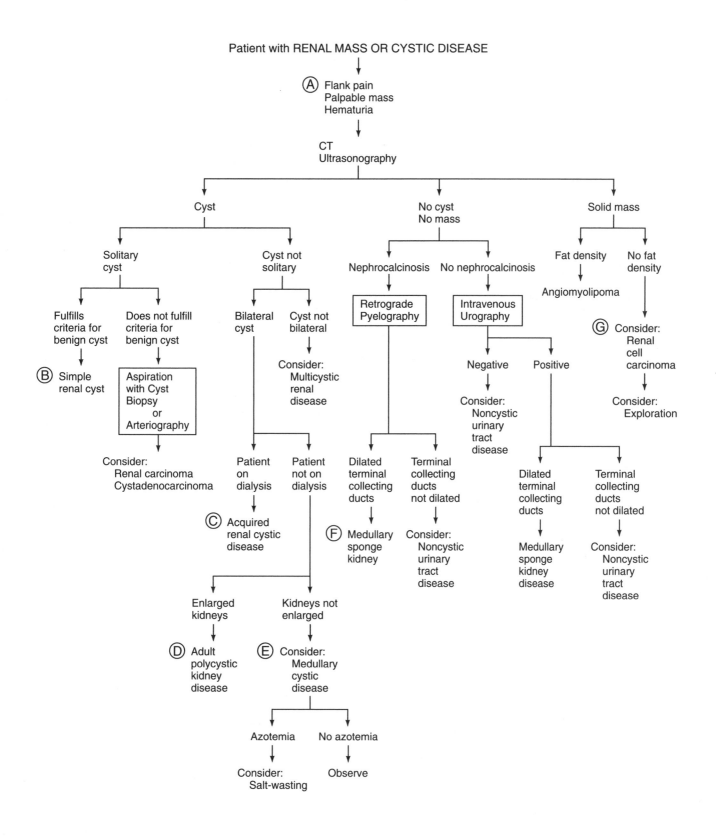

References

Gardner KD. Cystic kidneys. Kidney Int 1988; 33:610.

Grantham JJ. Polycystic kidney disease—an old problem in a new context. N Engl J Med 1988; 319:944.

Rose BD, Black RM. Manual of clinical problems in nephrology. Boston: Little, Brown, 1988:314.

Warshauer DM, McCarthy SM, Street L, et al. Detection of renal masses: sensitivities and specificities of excretory urography/linear tomography, US and CT. Radiology 1988; 169:363.

METABOLIC ACIDOSIS

Hillary Don, M.D.

A. Metabolic acidosis is defined as a decrease in measured blood bicarbonate accompanied by the appearance of a base deficit. It does not include the small, immediate, mandatory physiologic response to *acute respiratory alkalosis* (change $HCO_3^- = 0.2 \times$ change $PaCO_2$), which is not associated with a base deficit. At normal $PaCO_2$, the CO_2 combining power measured with plasma electrolytes should be 1.0–1.5 mEq greater than the HCO_3^- calculated with the blood gas determination: greater differences suggest discrepant sampling times, or excess heparin or processing time for the blood gas sample. When serum HCO_3^- is low but the blood pH >7.43, the metabolic acidosis is likely to be in partial compensation for a respiratory alkalosis (change in $HCO_3^- = 0.5 \times$ change $PaCO_2$). On the other hand, when serum HCO_3^- is low and pH is <7.39, assume metabolic acidosis to be the primary disorder and expect a secondary respiratory alkalosis (change $PaCO_2 = 1.1 \times$ change HCO_3^-). When pH is between these two values, mixed defects are present and the primary lesion must be distinguished by the clinical setting.

B. The physiologic anion gap $[AG = Na^+ - (Cl^- + HCO_3^-)]$ is 12 mEq/L. An increase in circulating organic acid anions such as lactate or acetoacetate produces a rise in serum antiglobulin that matches the fall in serum HCO_3^- milliequivalent for milliequivalent. If the fall in HCO_3^- exceeds the increase in antiglobulin, a mixed anion gap and non–anion gap acidosis is present; this may arise when there are renal and extrarenal disorders or, more commonly, during early or resolving phases of ketoacidosis when the ketoacid clearance rate exceeds the rate at which depleted HCO_3^- buffers are regenerated. Metabolic acidoses showing an elevated anion gap are limited to (1) a short list of drug and poison ingestions, including methanol, salicylates, ethylene glycol, paraldehyde, paracetamol, and butanone; and (2) in the absence of suspicious ingestions, the diabetic and alcoholic ketoacidoses.

C. The use of $NaHCO_3$ to correct metabolic acidosis is controversial, because it may transiently increase $PaCO_2$, increase cerebral acidosis, decrease serum K^+, increase Na^+, shift the oxyhemoglobin curve to the left, and contribute to a postrecovery overshoot metabolic alkalosis. However, in certain instances the correction of acidemia may improve cardiac function and potentiate the action of vasoactive drugs. Some authors therefore advise cautious administration of $NaHCO_3$ (base deficit $\times$ 0.1 $\times$ kg body weight), when pH is <7.2 and volume replacement with saline has failed. The pH should not be corrected above 7.25 with $NaHCO_3$.

D. Predisposing factors for lactic acidosis are tissue hypoxia (shock, hypotension, congestive heart failure, hypoxemia), systemic disorders (sepsis, liver failure, leukemia, convulsions, strychnine poisoning, abnormal gut flora), drugs or toxins (butanone, paracetamol, ritodrine), and inborn errors of metabolism (glucose-6 phosphatase deficiency). D-Lactate is not detected by the usual enzymatic methods for lactate and requires special analysis. Treatment is of the underlying cause, but a pH <7.2 may need to be partially corrected with $NaHCO_3$ (see C). Dichloroacetate stimulates pyruvate dehydrogenase and has been successfully used to treat lactic acidosis. D-Lactate is treated by a nonabsorbable antibiotic such as vancomycin.

E. Non–anion gap acidosis (hyperchloremic metabolic acidosis) results from either increased loss of HCO_3^- or insufficient acid excretion and HCO_3^- production by the kidney. Non–anion gap acidosis can be caused by administration of acid (NH_4Cl, $CaCl_2$, arginine HCl), by loss of HCO_3^- through the GI tract (diarrhea, small bowel fistula, ileostomy), or by loss through the kidney (renal tubular acidosis, mineralocorticoid deficiency states such as Addison's disease, carbonic anhydrase inhibition). Aldosterone deficiency is suspected by the clinical picture (weight loss, increased skin pigmentation, hypotension) or previous administration of steroids. Treatment of the underlying condition whenever possible is the key. Unlike the situation in elevated anion gap acidoses, $NaHCO_3$ therapy is mandatory in most non–anion gap acidoses.

References

Androgue H, Wilson H, Boyd AE III, et al. Plasma acid-base patterns in diabetic ketoacidosis. N Engl J Med 1982; 307:1603.

Don H. Metabolic Acidosis. In: Don H, ed. Decision making in critical care. Toronto: BC Decker, 1985:164.

DuBose TD Jr. Clinical approach to patients with acid-base disorders. Med Clin North Am 1983; 67:799.

Lever E, Jaspan JB. Sodium bicarbonate therapy in severe diabetic ketoacidosis. Am J Med 1983; 75:263.

Stacpoole PW, Harman EM, Curry SH, et al. Treatment of lactic acidosis with dichloroacetate. N Engl J Med 1983; 309:390.

Stolberg L, Rolfe R, Gitlin N, et al. D-Lactic acidosis due to abnormal gut flora. Diagnosis and treatment of two cases. N Engl J Med 1982; 306:1344.

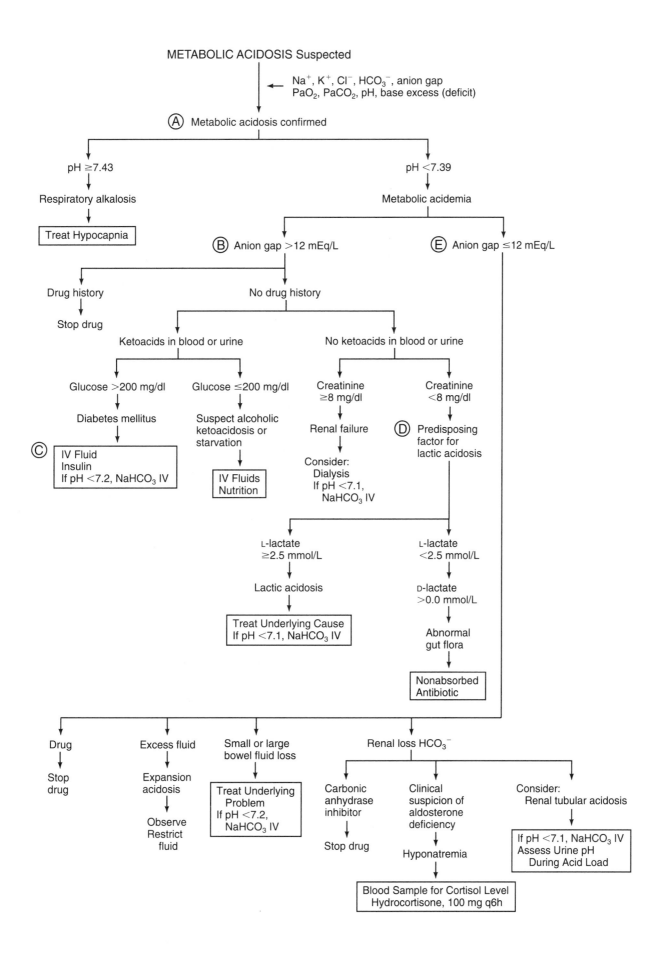

METABOLIC ACIDOSIS Suspected

← Na⁺, K⁺, Cl⁻, HCO₃⁻, anion gap
PaO₂, PaCO₂, pH, base excess (deficit)

Ⓐ Metabolic acidosis confirmed

pH ≥7.43

Respiratory alkalosis

Treat Hypocapnia

pH <7.39

Metabolic acidemia

Ⓑ Anion gap >12 mEq/L

Drug history

Stop drug

No drug history

Ketoacids in blood or urine

Glucose >200 mg/dl

Diabetes mellitus

Ⓒ IV Fluid
Insulin
If pH <7.2, NaHCO₃ IV

Glucose ≤200 mg/dl

Suspect alcoholic
ketoacidosis or
starvation

IV Fluids
Nutrition

No ketoacids in blood or urine

Creatinine
≥8 mg/dl

Renal failure

Consider:
Dialysis
If pH <7.1,
NaHCO₃ IV

Creatinine
<8 mg/dl

Ⓓ Predisposing
factor for
lactic acidosis

L-lactate
≥2.5 mmol/L

Lactic acidosis

Treat Underlying Cause
If pH <7.1, NaHCO₃ IV

L-lactate
<2.5 mmol/L

D-lactate
>0.0 mmol/L

Abnormal
gut flora

Nonabsorbed
Antibiotic

Ⓔ Anion gap ≤12 mEq/L

Drug

Stop
drug

Excess fluid

Expansion
acidosis

Observe
Restrict
fluid

Small or large
bowel fluid loss

Treat Underlying
Problem
If pH <7.2,
NaHCO₃ IV

Renal loss HCO₃⁻

Carbonic
anhydrase
inhibitor

Stop drug

Clinical
suspicion of
aldosterone
deficiency

Hyponatremia

Blood Sample for Cortisol Level
Hydrocortisone, 100 mg q6h

Consider:
Renal tubular acidosis

If pH <7.1, NaHCO₃ IV
Assess Urine pH
During Acid Load

279

METABOLIC ALKALOSIS

Hillary Don, M.D.

When alkalemia is severe, metabolic alkalosis produces paresthesias, obtundation, tetany, and convulsions. Cardiac arrhythmias may be precipitated, particularly in the presence of digitalis, and volume depletion is common. The O_2-hemoglobin dissociation curve is shifted to the left, impeding tissue oxygen uptake.

A. Metabolic alkalosis is confirmed by an increase in measured blood bicarbonate, a reciprocal decrease in Cl^-, and an increase in base excess. It does not include the small, immediate, mandatory physiologic increase in HCO_3^- in response to *acute respiratory acidosis* (change $HCO_3^- = 0.1 \times$ change $PaCO_2$). At normal $PaCO_2$, the CO_2 combining power measured with plasma electrolytes should be 1.0–1.5 mEq greater than the HCO_3^- calculated with the blood gas determination; greater differences suggest discrepant sampling times, or excess heparin or processing time for the blood gas sample. Elevated plasma HCO_3^- with a blood pH <7.39 suggests that the metabolic alkalosis is secondary, compensating for a primary chronic respiratory acidosis. Since compensation is slow in onset and slow to resolve, metabolic alkalosis may persist after rapid correction of respiratory acidosis. A pH >7.43 suggests a primary metabolic alkalosis with alkalemia. When pH lies between these two levels, a mixed lesion is present and the primary deficit must be distinguished by information gained from the clinical setting. A modest compensatory respiratory acidosis with reduction in tidal volume and maintained respiratory rate (change in $PaCO_2 = 0.7 \times$ change in HCO_3^-) usually accompanies the metabolic alkalemia. However, the $PaCO_2$ rarely exceeds 60 mm Hg, and total absence of compensation is not abnormal for moderate degrees of metabolic alkalosis. Hypoxemia may be present, requiring titration of F_IO_2 to maintain adequate O_2 saturation. Mechanical ventilation is not necessary; if it is already in use for some other reason, take care to restrict minute ventilation to prevent a compounding respiratory alkalosis.

B. Metabolic alkalosis may occur from exogenous sources of alkali, including administration of oral citrate (Shohl's) solutions, citrated blood, acetate in IV hyperalimentation, excessive $NaHCO_3$ during treatment of metabolic acidosis, and absorbable antacids. Cation exchange resins (Kayexalate) and possibly neutral phosphate (Neutra-Phos) potentiate absorption of otherwise nonabsorbable antacids. Alkalosis caused by administered alkali, loss of acid from the stomach, or diuretics (thiazides, ethacrynic acid, furosemide) is usually associated with hypovolemia, which prevents renal bicarbonate excretion. Selective dehydration (water loss) causes a rise in HCO_3^- concentration, a condition referred to as contraction alkalosis. Treatment with IV normal saline, coupled with cautious KCl replacement, restores effective renal perfusion, permits renal excretion of bicarbonate, and thereby corrects alkalemia (saline responsive).

C. High urine Cl^-, in the absence of diuretics, provides evidence that volume depletion is not present and that alkalosis therefore will not be corrected by saline infusion (so-called saline unresponsive). A high urine Cl^- therefore turns attention to the possibility of hypermineralocorticolism (primary or secondary to corticosteroid ingestion). Renal failure plus alkali administration, and severe K^+ deficiency, may also be suspected. If renal function is intact, an aldosterone antagonist (aldactone) may be effective. Rarely, correction of severe alkalemia requires intravenous HCl (0.2 mol/L). Other forms of titratable H^+ are available, but may precipitate hepatic coma (NH_4Cl) and may increase intracellular alkalosis (NH_4Cl, arginine HCl). Alternatively, hemodialysis and peritoneal dialysis readily correct metabolic alkalosis and may be the safest and most expeditious treatment when hypervolemia is present, particularly in the presence of renal failure.

References

Cogan MG, Liu F, Berger BE, et al. Metabolic alkalosis. Med Clin North Am 1983; 67:903.

Don H. Metabolic Alkalosis. In: Don H, ed. Decision making in critical care. Toronto: BC Decker, 1985:166.

Javaheri S, Shore NS, Rose B, Kazemi H. Compensatory hypoventilation in metabolic alkalosis. Chest 1982; 81:296.

Madias NE, Levey AS. Metabolic alkalosis due to absorption of "nonabsorbable" antacids. Am J Med 1983; 74:155.

Rothe KF. Hydrochloric acid for metabolic alkalosis. Lancet 1983; 1:1332.

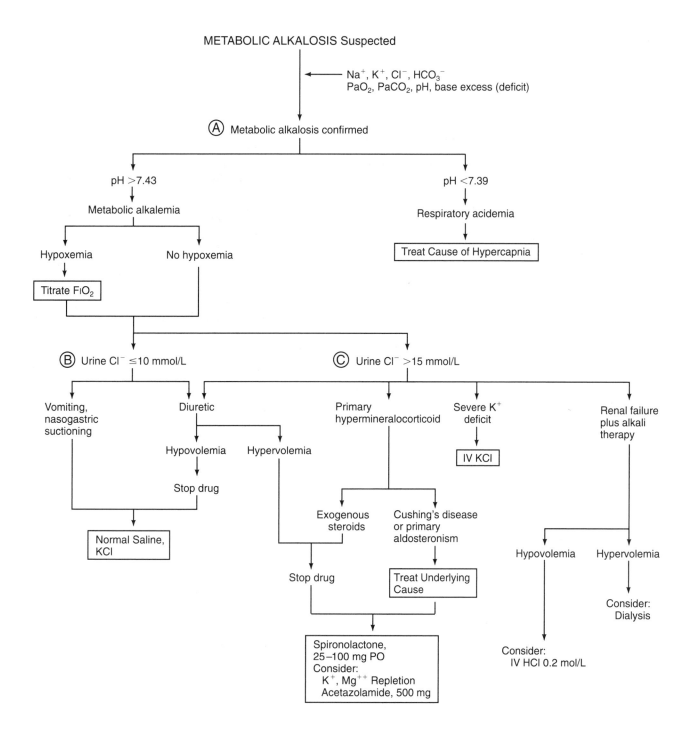

METABOLIC ALKALOSIS Suspected

Na⁺, K⁺, Cl⁻, HCO₃⁻
PaO₂, PaCO₂, pH, base excess (deficit)

Ⓐ Metabolic alkalosis confirmed

pH >7.43
Metabolic alkalemia

pH <7.39
Respiratory acidemia

Treat Cause of Hypercapnia

Hypoxemia
Titrate FiO₂

No hypoxemia

Ⓑ Urine Cl⁻ ≤10 mmol/L

Ⓒ Urine Cl⁻ >15 mmol/L

Vomiting, nasogastric suctioning

Diuretic
Hypovolemia   Hypervolemia
Stop drug

Primary hypermineralocorticoid

Severe K⁺ deficit
IV KCl

Renal failure plus alkali therapy

Normal Saline, KCl

Exogenous steroids

Cushing's disease or primary aldosteronism

Stop drug

Treat Underlying Cause

Hypovolemia   Hypervolemia

Spironolactone,
25–100 mg PO
Consider:
  K⁺, Mg⁺⁺ Repletion
  Acetazolamide, 500 mg

Consider:
IV HCl 0.2 mol/L

Consider:
Dialysis

HYPONATREMIA

Anwar Al-Haidary, M.B., M.R.C.P., M.Sc.

A. Sodium concentrations may be spuriously low when excess lipid or protein displaces sodium and water from plasma (so-called pseudohyponatremia). Simple inspection of plasma samples reveals the lactescence of hyperlipidemia and increased viscosity of hyperproteinemic states. Plasma osmolality remains normal.

B. When both plasma sodium and plasma osmolality are low, true hypotonic hyponatremia exists. The important diagnostic task is to determine whether the apparent free water excess is absolute or relative; despite hyponatremia, total body sodium may be low (hypovolemia), normal (euvolemic), or high (hypervolemia).

C. In hypovolemic states, the renal imperative to maintain effective circulating blood volume overrides its role in regulating plasma osmolality. Despite decreased plasma osmolality, hypovolemic hyponatremia is characterized by nonosmotic secretion of antidiuretic hormone (ADH) secretion and avid salt and water retention. Management should be directed at correcting the underlying disorder and re-establishing normal effective circulating volume.

D. Euvolemic hyponatremia is caused by persistent nonosmotic secretion of ADH in the absence of evidence of either volume depletion or salt retention. Total body sodium is normal and the U_{Na} reflects daily intake of sodium. Water restriction with treatment of the underlying disorder is the cornerstone of treatment. If hyponatremia is accompanied by seizures or mental status changes, initial therapy should include infusion of 3% saline, with diuretics if volume overload is threatened, sufficient to raise the plasma sodium $0.75-1.0$ mEq/L per hour until the plasma sodium rises above 120 mEq/L, followed by water restriction. The syndrome, which has been termed "reset osmostat," is generally not severe and does not require specific therapy.

E. Hypo-osmolar states associated with excess total body sodium and extracellular fluid expansion are easily recognized by evidence of pulmonary or peripheral edema. When renal function is intact, the pathophysiology resembles that in hypovolemic hyponatremia: decreased effective circulating volume brought on by heart failure, liver disease, or nephrotic syndrome causes avid retention of both salt and water; if the resultant total body increase in water is greater than that of salt, hyponatremia develops. Low U_{Na} excretion is the key finding. When acute or chronic renal failure is present, salt and water excretion are both limited and the low plasma sodium concentration reflects greater intake of water than of salt. Treatment entails water restriction, diuretics, and therapy for the underlying condition. Severe hyponatremia with mental status changes, hypervolemia, and renal failure may require emergency dialysis.

F. Hyponatremia associated with hypertonic states reflects the presence of impermeant nonsodium solutes circulating in high concentrations in plasma. These substances draw fluid from the intracellular into the extracellular space to maintain osmotic equilibrium across cell membranes, thereby diluting plasma sodium: e.g., it is calculated that for every 100 mg/dl in blood sugar the S_{Na} decreases by 1.6 mEq/L.

References

Anderson RJ. Hospital associated hyponatremia. Kidney Int 1986; 29:1237.

Arieff AI. Hyponatremia, convulsions, respiratory arrest, and permanent brain damage after elective surgery in healthy women. N Engl J Med 1986; 314:1529.

Ayus JC, Krothapalli RK, Arieff AI. Changing concepts in treatment of severe symptomatic hyponatremia. Am J Med 1985; 78:897.

Buckalew VM Jr. Hyponatremia: pathogenesis and management. Hosp Pract 1986; 21:49.

Humes HD. Disorders of sodium and water balance. In: Humes HD, ed. Pathophysiology of electrolyte and renal disorders. New York: Churchill Livingstone, 1986.

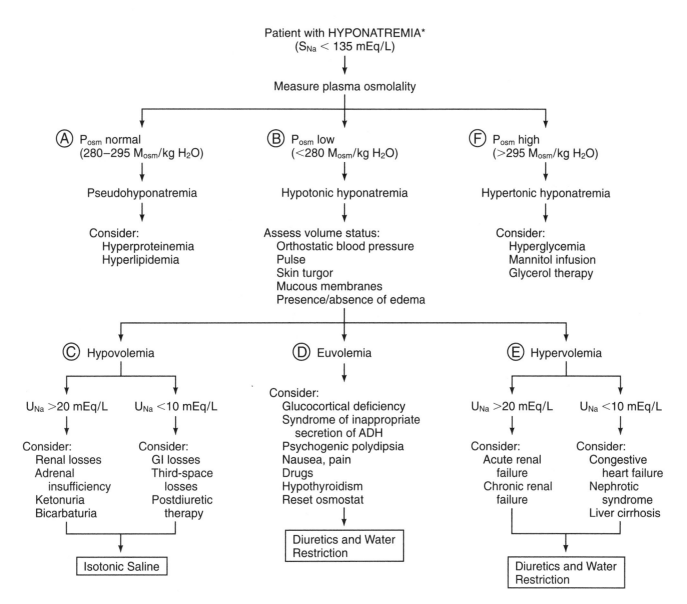

Patient with HYPONATREMIA*
($S_{Na} < 135$ mEq/L)

↓

Measure plasma osmolality

(A) P_{osm} normal
(280–295 M_{osm}/kg H_2O)

↓

Pseudohyponatremia

↓

Consider:
  Hyperproteinemia
  Hyperlipidemia

(B) P_{osm} low
(<280 M_{osm}/kg H_2O)

↓

Hypotonic hyponatremia

↓

Assess volume status:
  Orthostatic blood pressure
  Pulse
  Skin turgor
  Mucous membranes
  Presence/absence of edema

(F) P_{osm} high
(>295 M_{osm}/kg H_2O)

↓

Hypertonic hyponatremia

↓

Consider:
  Hyperglycemia
  Mannitol infusion
  Glycerol therapy

(C) Hypovolemia

U_{Na} >20 mEq/L

Consider:
  Renal losses
  Adrenal
    insufficiency
  Ketonuria
  Bicarbaturia

U_{Na} <10 mEq/L

Consider:
  GI losses
  Third-space
    losses
  Postdiuretic
    therapy

Isotonic Saline

(D) Euvolemia

Consider:
  Glucocortical deficiency
  Syndrome of inappropriate
    secretion of ADH
  Psychogenic polydipsia
  Nausea, pain
  Drugs
  Hypothyroidism
  Reset osmostat

Diuretics and Water Restriction

(E) Hypervolemia

U_{Na} >20 mEq/L

Consider:
  Acute renal
    failure
  Chronic renal
    failure

U_{Na} <10 mEq/L

Consider:
  Congestive
    heart failure
  Nephrotic
    syndrome
  Liver cirrhosis

Diuretics and Water Restriction

*Adapted from Humes HD, ed. Pathophysiology of electrolyte disorders. Melbourne: Churchill Livingstone, 1986:55; with permission.

HYPERNATREMIA

Anwar Al-Haidary, M.B., M.R.C.P., M.Sc.

Disorders of plasma sodium concentration frequently reflect either a net gain or loss of body water, or an imbalance between the change in body water and the change in total body sodium. Since hypernatremia, regardless of fluid status, is a potent stimulus for thirst, it must be assumed that the patient presenting with hypernatremia has either a diminished thirst reflex (as in organic brain disease) or limited access to water (severe debilitation). The diagnostic approach centers on careful assessment of body fluid status, using both the physical examination and laboratory information. Treatment is guided by the etiology of the disorder. Because compensatory mechanisms to prevent brain shrinkage are slow to reverse, correction of chronic hypernatremia should be timed accordingly to be completed over 1–3 days.

A. In hypovolemic hypernatremia, substantial loss of hypotonic fluids without water replacement has occurred. Water loss therefore exceeds sodium loss, but both water and sodium deficits exist. The hypotonic fluid loss could be of renal origin, as suggested by high U_{Na} (>20 mEq/L) and low U_{osm} (<300 mOsm/L), or extrarenal origin as evidenced by low U_{Na} (<10 mEq/L) and high U_{osm}. Isotonic saline should be administered until volume depletion has been reversed, followed by hypotonic saline infusion until the electrolyte disorder has been corrected. Approximate water deficit can be calculated by the following formula:

Water deficit = 0.5 × body weight (kg) × ([P_{Na}/140] −1),

assuming that total body water in a volume-depleted patient is approximately 50% of body weight.

B. When there is pure water loss and total body sodium remains normal, isovolemic hypernatremia results. Excessive water loss can occur when there is a defect in the production or release of antidiuretic hormone (ADH) (e.g., in central diabetes insipidus [DI]) or in renal response to ADH (nephrogenic DI). The hallmark of this disorder is polyuria with low U_{osm}. On the other hand, normal renal function ensures that when the water loss is due to extrarenal factors such as respiratory or skin losses, the U_{osm} will be elevated. Appropriate management entails gradual rehydration with 5% dextrose in water and treatment of the underlying disorder.

C. When sodium salts are added abruptly and in massive amounts to extracellular fluid (ECF), hypernatremia results. Administration of hypertonic $NaHCO_3$ during cardiac resuscitation, excessive infusion of hypertonic saline, and enteric tube feeding each has been implicated in iatrogenic hypernatremia. The rapid ECF volume expansion and intracellular fluid volume contraction that follows hypertonic sodium infusion may lead to pulmonary edema. Diuretics should therefore be given promptly and the resultant sodium and water losses replaced with equal volumes of dextrose in water. Patients with poor renal function who remain oliguric in response to diuretics require dialysis.

References

Humes HD. Disorders of sodium and water balance. In: Humes HD, ed. Pathophysiology of electrolyte and renal disorders. New York: Churchill Livingstone, 1986.

Marsden PA, Halperin ML. Pathophysiological approach to patients presenting with hypernatremia. Am J Nephrol 1985; 5:229.

Narins RG, Jones ER, Stom MC, et al. Diagnostic strategies in disorders of fluid, electrolyte and acid-base homeostasis. Am J Med 1982; 72:496.

Synder NA, Feigal EW, Arieff AI. Hypernatremia in elderly patients. Ann Intern Med 1987; 107:309.

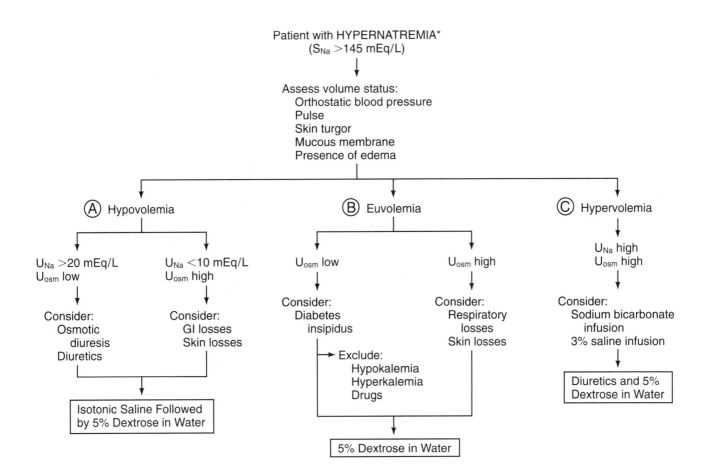

Patient with HYPERNATREMIA*
(S_{Na} >145 mEq/L)

Assess volume status:
  Orthostatic blood pressure
  Pulse
  Skin turgor
  Mucous membrane
  Presence of edema

(A) Hypovolemia

U_{Na} >20 mEq/L
U_{osm} low

Consider:
  Osmotic
    diuresis
  Diuretics

U_{Na} <10 mEq/L
U_{osm} high

Consider:
  GI losses
  Skin losses

Isotonic Saline Followed
by 5% Dextrose in Water

(B) Euvolemia

U_{osm} low

Consider:
  Diabetes
    insipidus

Exclude:
  Hypokalemia
  Hyperkalemia
  Drugs

U_{osm} high

Consider:
  Respiratory
    losses
  Skin losses

5% Dextrose in Water

(C) Hypervolemia

U_{Na} high
U_{osm} high

Consider:
  Sodium bicarbonate
    infusion
  3% saline infusion

Diuretics and 5%
Dextrose in Water

*Adapted from Humes HD, ed. Pathophysiology of electrolyte
disorders. Melbourne: Churchill Livingstone, 1986:68; with permission.

HYPOKALEMIA

Catherine S. Thompson, M.D.
David M. Clive, M.D.

Hypokalemia usually arises through some disorder in the external potassium balance. Of the 70 mEq of potassium per day ingested by the average American, virtually all is absorbed, and 80% is excreted through the kidneys; the rest is lost in the feces, largely through intestinal secretion. Dietary deficiency of potassium is uncommon in American society. Generally, it is seen only in chronically ill and malnourished people or in alcoholics. Any state characterized by metabolic alkalosis leads to hypokalemia. The shift of potassium from the extracellular space into the intracellular space during alkalosis not only lowers the plasma potassium level but also enhances the gradient for potassium excretion in the distal tubule of the kidney. The major effects of hypokalemia are on electrically excitable cells, particularly skeletal and cardiac muscle cells. Muscle weakness is common in severe hypokalemia, and rhabdomyolysis may actually occur. Marked hypokalemia produces characteristic ECG changes. Cardiac arrhythmias are the most dangerous complication of hypokalemia. Hypokalemia has effects on the kidney itself. In potassium deficiency states, the kidneys lose the ability to concentrate urine, which leads to polyuria (e.g., nephrogenic diabetes insipidus).

A. Patients with hypokalemia should be questioned about dietary ingestion of potassium and the use of medications, including diuretics or laxatives, that can cause potassium depletion. Symptoms such as vomiting or diarrhea or a family history of hypokalemia are additional important features. The physical examination provides clues if the patient has signs of volume depletion (hypotension or tachycardia) or if it detects the presence of GI fistulas, a nasogastric drainage tube, or ureterosigmoidostomy.

B. Initial laboratory assessment of hypokalemic patients includes an electrolyte profile, blood pH, and urine electrolytes (urine sodium, potassium, chloride). Serum aldosterone and renin level tests are occasionally helpful.

C. Hypokalemia is caused by one of two mechanisms (Table 1). The first mechanism is extrarenal in origin (increased extrarenal losses or reduced potassium intake); the second is increased renal losses. The two mechanisms are differentiated on the basis of urine potassium content: a urine potassium level >20 mEq/L in the presence of hypokalemia indicates excess renal loss.

D. Extrarenal potassium losses may occur as a result of diarrhea, vomiting, continuous nasogastric suction, or profuse sweating.

E. Hypokalemia is not uncommon among patients being treated with diuretics. The potassium losses are attributable to the increased distal delivery of sodium, which occurs as a result of the renal tubular actions of the diuretic. The metabolic "contraction" alkalosis, which these medications engender, also contributes to potassium wasting. Disorders characterized by glucocorticoid or mineralocorticoid excess (e.g., Cushing's syndrome, Conn's syndrome, and Bartter's syndrome) are also causes of potassium loss. In these patients, kaliuresis is driven by the mineralocorticoid effects of the hormones on the tubular cells and by the metabolic alkalosis that occurs in these physiologic states.

F. Adequate treatment of hypokalemia caused by true body potassium depletion requires identification of the underlying cause of the disorder and then specific interventions to replete potassium stores (Table 2). Volume depletion should be corrected in hypokalemic individuals with excessive GI fluid losses; medications that aggravate hypokalemia, specifically diuretics, should be discontinued. In most cases, potassium repletion can be accomplished with oral potassium supplements. In patients with severe hypokalemia (potassium <2.5 mEq/L) or with cardiac arrhythmias referable to hypokalemia, IV repletion is indicated. In these patients, administer potassium salts no faster than 10–20 mEq/hr; pay close attention to cardiac rhythm and serum potassium concentration.

TABLE 1 Causes of Hypokalemia

Reduced potassium intake
Renal losses
  Tubular defects (renal tubular acidosis)
  Metabolic alkalosis
  Diuretics
  Mineralocorticoid excess
  Edematous disorders
  Bartter's syndrome
  Magnesium deficiency
  Filtered, nonreabsorbable anions
  Leukemia
Extrarenal losses
  Vomiting, nasogastric suction
  Losses from large intestine
  Biliary drainage
  Profuse sweating

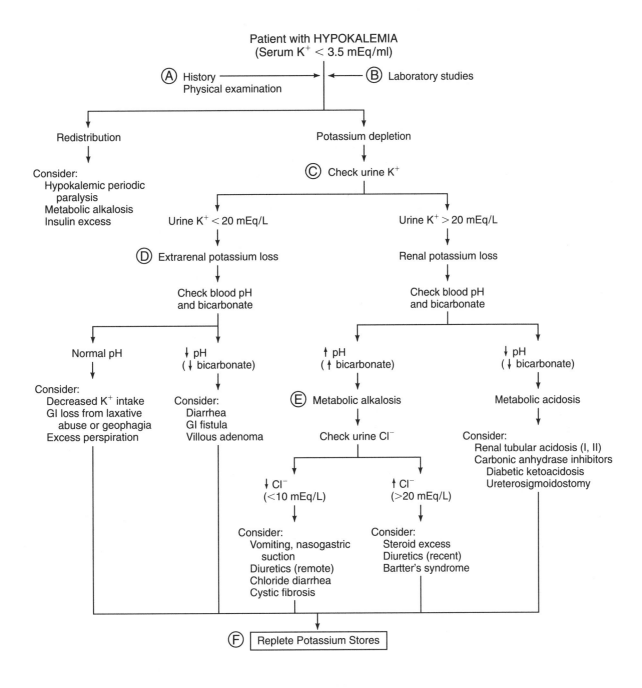

Patient with HYPOKALEMIA
(Serum K$^+$ < 3.5 mEq/ml)

(A) History — (B) Laboratory studies
Physical examination

Redistribution

Consider:
  Hypokalemic periodic
    paralysis
  Metabolic alkalosis
  Insulin excess

Potassium depletion

(C) Check urine K$^+$

Urine K$^+$ < 20 mEq/L

(D) Extrarenal potassium loss

Check blood pH
and bicarbonate

Normal pH

Consider:
  Decreased K$^+$ intake
  GI loss from laxative
    abuse or geophagia
  Excess perspiration

↓ pH
(↓ bicarbonate)

Consider:
  Diarrhea
  GI fistula
  Villous adenoma

Urine K$^+$ > 20 mEq/L

Renal potassium loss

Check blood pH
and bicarbonate

↑ pH
(↑ bicarbonate)

(E) Metabolic alkalosis

Check urine Cl$^-$

↓ Cl$^-$
(<10 mEq/L)

Consider:
  Vomiting, nasogastric
    suction
  Diuretics (remote)
  Chloride diarrhea
  Cystic fibrosis

↑ Cl$^-$
(>20 mEq/L)

Consider:
  Steroid excess
  Diuretics (recent)
  Bartter's syndrome

↓ pH
(↓ bicarbonate)

Metabolic acidosis

Consider:
  Renal tubular acidosis (I, II)
  Carbonic anhydrase inhibitors
  Diabetic ketoacidosis
  Ureterosigmoidostomy

(F) Replete Potassium Stores

TABLE 2 Treatment of Hypokalemia

Acute
  IV replacement (potassium chloride or potassium phosphate)
    ≤ 20 mEq/hr or 200 mEq/day
Chronic
  Increased dietary supply (citrus fruits, etc.)
  Oral solutions (potassium chloride, potassium citrate)
  Oral tablets (avoid enteric-coated preparations)
  Potassium-sparing agents (spironolactone, triamterene)

References

Brown RS. Extrarenal potassium homeostasis. Kidney Int 1986;
    30:116.
DeFronzo R. Hyperkalemia and hyporeninemic hypoaldoster-
    onism. Kidney Int 1980; 17:118.
Gabow PA, Peterson LN. Disorders of potassium metabolism.
    In: Schrier RW, ed. Renal and electrolyte disorders. 3rd
    ed. Boston: Little, Brown, 1986:207.
Stein JH. Hypokalemia: common and uncommon causes.
    Hosp Pract 1988; 23:55.
Tannen RL. Potassium disorders. In: Kokko JP, Tannen RL,
    eds. Fluids and electrolytes. Philadelphia: WB Saunders,
    1986.
Valtin H. Renal dysfunction: mechanisms involved in fluid and
    solute imbalance. Boston: Little, Brown, 1979:89.

HYPERKALEMIA

Catherine S. Thompson, M.D.
David M. Clive, M.D.

Hyperkalemia is potentially the most rapidly lethal of all electrolyte disturbances. ECG changes may be seen when the potassium concentration in the plasma rises to ≥ 5 mEq/L. With further increases in serum potassium concentrations, cellular irritability and eventually lethal arrhythmias develop.

A. Patients with hyperkalemia should be questioned closely about dietary intake of potassium, including the use of salt substitutes (KCl). Some drugs, including potassium-sparing diuretics, beta-adrenergic blockers, nonsteroidal anti-inflammatory drugs (NSAIDs), and angiotensin-converting enzyme inhibitors, can aggravate a hyperkalemia tendency in certain patients. A history of renal disease or recent reduction in urinary output is also important.

B. Laboratory assessment of hyperkalemic patients should include serum electrolytes, creatinine, BUN, and acid-base status. Additional tests such as aldosterone and renin levels may provide information regarding renal tubular disorders that lead to hyperkalemia. "Spurious" hyperkalemia can be excluded by obtaining a plasma potassium level, which will be normal if the hyperkalemia is the result of cell lysis after the blood specimen is obtained.

C. An elevated plasma potassium level confirms hyperkalemia. The three chief mechanisms of hyperkalemia are increased excretory load, decreased excretory capacity, and transcellular potassium movement (Table 1).

D. Eating a potassium-rich diet is unlikely to provoke hyperkalemia because of the extraordinary capacity of the kidney to dispose of excess potassium. However, the combination of renal insufficiency plus a normal or high potassium intake may lead to hyperkalemia, a constant concern in patients with kidney disease. Diets must be modified accordingly.

E. Disorders leading to decreased urinary excretion of potassium include glucocorticoid and mineralocorticoid deficiency, renal tubule secretory defects, and acute renal failure.

F. Hyperkalemia arises not infrequently as a result of perturbations in the internal mechanism of potassium balance. Metabolic acidosis can provoke hyperkalemia through transcellular shifting of potassium stores. Tissue necrosis or toxic injury to cells can also cause leakage of potassium into the extracellular space. Potassium deficiency, with or without hyperglycemia, can lead to impaired cellular potassium intake.

G. The treatment of hyperkalemia exploits both the internal and external pathways of potassium disposition (Table 2). Internal mechanisms are the fastest acting (i.e., one can engender shifts of potassium into cells more quickly than one can remove potassium

TABLE 1 Causes of Hyperkalemia

Increased excretory load
  Dietary excess
  Iatrogenic
  Tissue breakdown
Decreased excretory ability
  Acute and chronic renal failure
  Mineralocorticoid insufficiency
  Hyporeninemic hypoaldosteronism
  Potassium-sparing diuretics
  Renal tubular defects (acute interstitial
    nephritis, transplant kidney)
Transcellular potassium movement
  (Metabolic) acidosis
  Exercise
  Endocrine abnormalities (diabetes mellitus)
  Periodic paralyses
  Drugs (e.g., succinylcholine, digitalis)
  Osmolar load

from the body). Thus, rapidly administer insulin and alkalinizing agents (sodium bicarbonate) to patients with life-threatening degrees of hyperkalemia. Calcium salts may also be administered because these have a membrane-stabilizing effect, although they do not engender potassium movement in and of themselves. To reduce total body potassium stores, ion-exchange resins like sodium polystyrene sulfate (e.g., Kayexalate) are introduced into the GI tract. These absorb potassium from the gut and release, in exchange, a sodium molecule. For hyperkalemic patients with renal insufficiency, emergent dialysis may be required.

References

Brown RS. Extrarenal potassium homeostasis. Kidney Int 1986; 30:116.

Cox M, Sterns R, Singer I. The defense against hyperkalemia: the roles of insulin and aldosterone. New Engl J Med 1978; 299:525.

DeFronzo R. Hyperkalemia and hyporeninemic hypoaldosteronism. Kidney Int 1980; 17:118.

Gabow PA, Peterson LN. Disorders of potassium metabolism. In: Schrier RW, ed. Renal and electrolyte disorders. 3rd ed. Boston: Little, Brown, 1986:207.

Goldfarb S, et al. Acute hyperkalemia induced by hyperglycemia: hormonal mechanisms. Ann Intern Med 1976; 84:426.

Rose BD. Clinical physiology of acid-base and electrolyte disorders. 3rd ed. New York: McGraw-Hill, 1989.

Stein JH. Hypokalemia: common and uncommon causes. Hosp Pract 1988; 23:55.

Tannen RL. Potassium disorders. In: Kokko JP, Tannen RL, eds. Fluids and electrolytes. Philadelphia: WB Saunders, 1986.

Valtin H. Renal dysfunction: mechanisms involved in fluid and solute imbalance. Boston: Little, Brown, 1979:89.

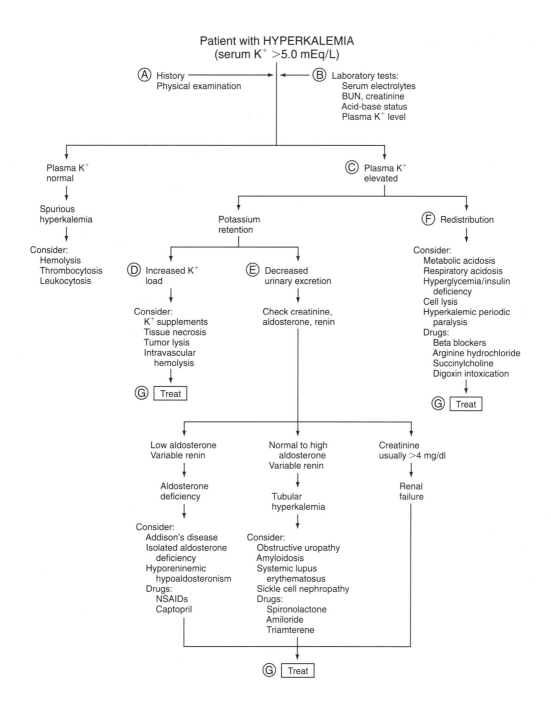

Patient with HYPERKALEMIA
(serum K$^+$ >5.0 mEq/L)

Ⓐ History
Physical examination

Ⓑ Laboratory tests:
Serum electrolytes
BUN, creatinine
Acid-base status
Plasma K$^+$ level

Plasma K$^+$ normal

Ⓒ Plasma K$^+$ elevated

Spurious hyperkalemia

Consider:
Hemolysis
Thrombocytosis
Leukocytosis

Potassium retention

Ⓕ Redistribution

Ⓓ Increased K$^+$ load

Ⓔ Decreased urinary excretion

Consider:
K$^+$ supplements
Tissue necrosis
Tumor lysis
Intravascular hemolysis

Check creatinine, aldosterone, renin

Consider:
Metabolic acidosis
Respiratory acidosis
Hyperglycemia/insulin deficiency
Cell lysis
Hyperkalemic periodic paralysis
Drugs:
Beta blockers
Arginine hydrochloride
Succinylcholine
Digoxin intoxication

Ⓖ Treat

Ⓖ Treat

Low aldosterone
Variable renin

Normal to high aldosterone
Variable renin

Creatinine usually >4 mg/dl

Aldosterone deficiency

Tubular hyperkalemia

Renal failure

Consider:
Addison's disease
Isolated aldosterone deficiency
Hyporeninemic hypoaldosteronism
Drugs:
NSAIDs
Captopril

Consider:
Obstructive uropathy
Amyloidosis
Systemic lupus erythematosus
Sickle cell nephropathy
Drugs:
Spironolactone
Amiloride
Triamterene

Ⓖ Treat

TABLE 2   Treatment of Hyperkalemia

Drug	Dose	Time of Onset	Duration of Action	Mechanism
Calcium gluconate	1 amp, 10% solution	1–5 min	30–120 min	Membrane stabilization
NaHCO$_3$	1–2 amp (bolus)	5–10 min	2 hr	Redistribution
Glucose/insulin	50 g dextrose, 10 units regular insulin	Rapid	Variable	Redistribution
Sodium polystyrene sulfonate resin (Kayexalate)	15–30 g PO or rectally	10–60 min	As long as continued	Increased excretion
Mineralocorticoid replacement	For specific indications	—	—	Increased excretion
Dialysis	For severe hypokalemia	—	—	—

HYPOMAGNESEMIA

Anwar Al-Haidary, M.B., M.R.C.P., M.Sc.
David B. Van Wyck, M.D.

Hypomagnesemia is a common finding in patients hospitalized with severe disease. Because several factors, including hyperaldosteronism and cisplatin therapy, enhance renal excretion of both magnesium and potassium, and because hypomagnesemia may provoke both potassium and calcium depletion, hypomagnesemia should be suspected whenever hypokalemia or hypocalcemia are resistant to supplementation. Increased renal loss of magnesium is the most common pathogenesis of hypomagnesemia, but excessive extrarenal losses or transcellular redistribution are also seen.

A. Redistribution of magnesium from the extracellular space to the bone may be responsible for acute hypomagnesemia after parathyroidectomy (so-called hungry bone syndrome). Similarly, saponification of magnesium has been thought responsible for hypomagnesemia in acute pancreatitis.

B. Hypomagnesemia frequently complicates management of chronic alcoholics. Although acutely rising alcohol levels may increase renal magnesium excretion, the pathogenesis of hypomagnesemia among most alcoholics is most likely due to poor dietary intake, coupled with increased stool losses with diarrhea and increased renal losses with hypophosphatemia, if present. Increased intestinal losses are responsible for hypomagnesemia associated with intestinal malabsorption, chronic diarrhea, laxative abuse, short bowel syndrome, inflammatory bowel syndromes, and biliary fistulas.

C. Defective tubular reabsorption of magnesium has been identified in patients developing hypomagnesemia after cisplatin therapy, and may contribute to magnesium wasting during recovery from acute tubular necrosis, urinary obstruction, and renal transplant rejection. Since renal tubular reabsorption of magnesium is impaired by natriuresis or calciuresis, magnesium depletion may complicate the course of diuretic therapy (particularly with loop diuretics), high-volume saline infusion, hyperaldosteronism, hypercalcemia and hypervitaminosis D.

D. Initiate treatment of chronic hypomagnesemia due to malabsorption and renal magnesium wasting with oral magnesium replacement (magnesium oxide, 250–500 mg four times daily). Acute hypomagnesemia, or chronic hypomagnesemia unresponsive to oral supplements, is appropriately managed with a 3-day replacement plan requiring IV therapy as follows: *Day 1.* Dilute 12 ml of a 50% solution of $MgSO_4$ in 1000 ml of a glucose-containing solution, and infuse over 3 hours; follow with 10 ml in each of two 1000-ml solutions, and infuse through the remainder of the first day. *Day 2.* Dilute 10 ml of $MgSO_4$ in the daily IV fluid volume and infuse over the second day. *Day 3.* Same as day 2.

References

Brautbar N, Gruber HE. Magnesium and bone disease. Nephron 1986; 44:1.

Flink EB. Therapy of magnesium deficiency. Ann NY Acad Sci 1969; 162:901.

Goldfarb S, Kelepouris E. Disorders of serum phosphate, magnesium and calcium. In: Humes HD, ed. Pathophysiology of electrolyte and renal disorders. New York: Churchill Livingstone, 1986.

Lim P, Jacob E. Magnesium deficiency in patients on long-term diuretic therapy for heart failure. Br Med J 1972; 3:620.

Whang R. Magnesium deficiency: pathogenesis, prevalence and clinical implications. Am J Med 1987; 82(Suppl. 3A):25.

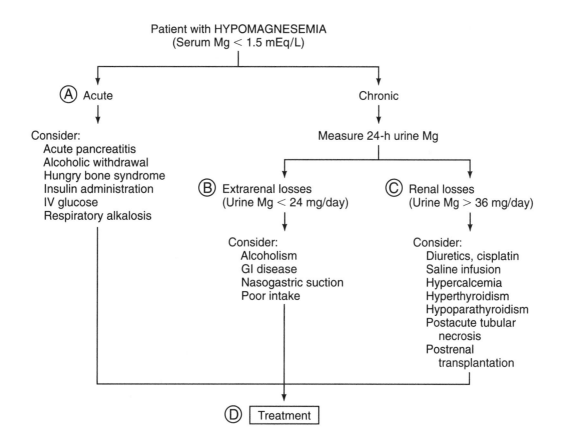

Patient with HYPOMAGNESEMIA
(Serum Mg < 1.5 mEq/L)

Ⓐ Acute

Consider:
    Acute pancreatitis
    Alcoholic withdrawal
    Hungry bone syndrome
    Insulin administration
    IV glucose
    Respiratory alkalosis

Chronic

Measure 24-h urine Mg

Ⓑ Extrarenal losses
(Urine Mg < 24 mg/day)

Consider:
    Alcoholism
    GI disease
    Nasogastric suction
    Poor intake

Ⓒ Renal losses
(Urine Mg > 36 mg/day)

Consider:
    Diuretics, cisplatin
    Saline infusion
    Hypercalcemia
    Hyperthyroidism
    Hypoparathyroidism
    Postacute tubular
        necrosis
    Postrenal
        transplantation

Ⓓ Treatment

HYPOPHOSPHATEMIA

Mark S. Siskind, M.D.
Robert F. Klein, M.D.
Steven T. Harris, M.D.

Although phosphate is predominantly an intracellular anion, cell function and integrity are determined by both its intracellular and extracellular concentrations. Serum phosphate concentrations >1.5 mg/dl rarely produce symptoms. When phosphate levels fall below this threshold, widespread evidence of cell dysfunction may be seen, manifested by muscle weakness (including heart failure and respiratory insufficiency), rhabdomyolysis, hemolytic anemia, impaired leukocytic chemotaxis and phagocytosis, and diminished platelet aggregation. CNS findings may range from anorexia and malaise to ataxia, delirium ("hypophosphatemic madness"), seizures, and coma.

A. Asymptomatic hypophosphatemia can be treated orally with skim milk (0.9 mg phosphate/ml), Neutra-Phos (3.33 mg/ml), or Phospho-Soda (129 mg/ml) (Table 1). Unfortunately, diarrhea often complicates oral phosphate repletion. Phosphate should be replaced parenterally when hypophosphatemia is symptomatic or complicated, or when the patient is asymptomatic but oral therapy has failed or is not a practical option. An appropriate regimen for uncomplicated hypophosphatemia is 2.5 mg phosphorus/kg IV over 6 hours, with a dosage increase to 5 mg phosphorus/kg IV over 6 hours in symptomatic patients. Parenteral administration should be stopped when the serum phosphate level reaches 2.0 mg/dl. Monitoring blood levels should be particularly painstaking during phosphate repletion in patients with renal failure, as fatal hyperphosphatemia may occur. Calcium and (if hypomagnesemia is also present) magnesium supplementation may be required during phosphate repletion to prevent hypocalcemic tetany. The calcium must not be added to phosphate-containing solutions, or precipitation of calcium salts will occur. Other potential hazards of parenteral phosphate administration include hypotension, as well as hyperkalemia and hypernatremia, which may result from the particular phosphate preparation used.

B. The cause of hypophosphatemia is usually readily apparent from inspection of the patient and the clinical setting. Hypophosphatemia arises from either total body phosphate depletion or movement of phosphate from the extracellular to the intracellular space. Phosphate depletion may occur after reduced dietary intake (starvation, chronic alcoholism), increased renal losses (renal "leak," hypomagnesemia, hyperparathyroidism), or increased nonrenal losses (secretory diarrhea, vomiting, laxative abuse). Diabetic ketoacidosis is associated with both low intake of dietary phosphate and high urinary losses. Iatrogenic causes are common, however. Phosphate absorption is blocked by phosphate-binding antacids, diuretic therapy enhances renal phosphate excretion, and profound transcellular shifts of phosphate frequently occur during nutritional refeeding with IV glucose solutions or hyperalimentation. The hypophosphatemia accompanying respiratory alkalosis is due to a shift of phosphate into the intracellular compartment, is associated with neither phosphate depletion nor symptoms, and requires no phosphate replacement. Because only a small fraction of total body phosphate resides in the extracellular fluid space, the degree of body phosphate deficit cannot be reliably assessed by serum level alone. Therefore, patients at greatest risk for hypophosphatemia require careful monitoring of serum phosphate, especially during inception of nutritional therapy. Hyperalimentation fluids should contain a phosphate concentration of 12–15 mmol/L to provide an adequate amount of phosphate.

TABLE 1 Therapeutic Phosphorus Preparations

Preparation	Phosphate (mmol/ml)	Phosphorus (mg/ml)	Sodium (mEq/ml)	Potassium (mEq/ml)
Oral				
Whole cow's milk	0.029	0.9	0.025	0.035
Neutra-Phos	0.107	3.33	0.095	0.095
Phospho-Soda	4.15	128.65	4.822	0
Acid Na phosphate	1.018	35.54	1.015	0
Neutral Na phosphate	0.673	20.86	1.214	0
Parenteral				
Neutral Na phosphate	0.09	2.8	0.161	0
Neutral Na, K phosphate	0.1	3.1	0.162	0.019
Na phosphate	3.0	93.0	4.0	0
K phosphate	3.003	93.11	0	4.36

From Klein RF, Harris ST. Hypophosphatemia. In: Don H, ed. Decision making in critical care. Philadelphia: BC Decker, 1985:170.

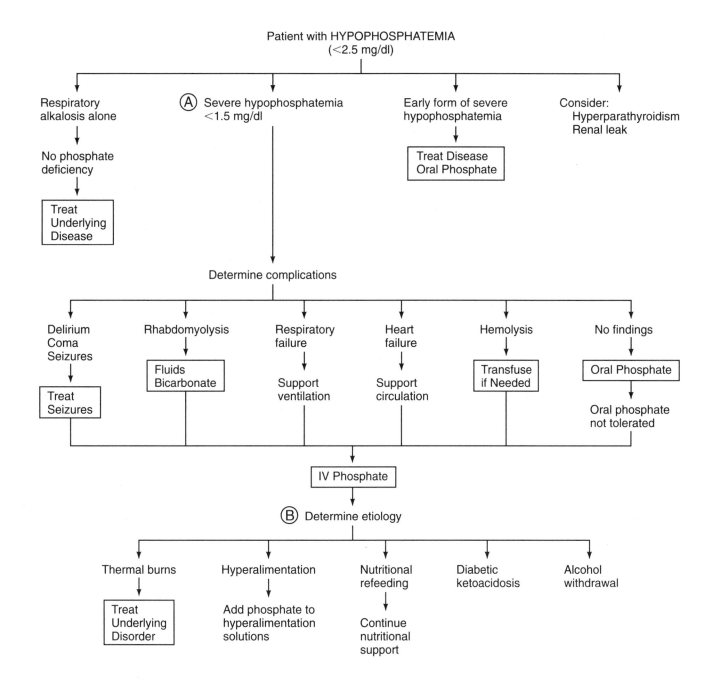

Patient with HYPOPHOSPHATEMIA
(<2.5 mg/dl)

Respiratory
alkalosis alone

No phosphate
deficiency

Treat
Underlying
Disease

Ⓐ Severe hypophosphatemia
<1.5 mg/dl

Early form of severe
hypophosphatemia

Treat Disease
Oral Phosphate

Consider:
Hyperparathyroidism
Renal leak

Determine complications

Delirium
Coma
Seizures

Treat
Seizures

Rhabdomyolysis

Fluids
Bicarbonate

Respiratory
failure

Support
ventilation

Heart
failure

Support
circulation

Hemolysis

Transfuse
if Needed

No findings

Oral Phosphate

Oral phosphate
not tolerated

IV Phosphate

Ⓑ Determine etiology

Thermal burns

Treat
Underlying
Disorder

Hyperalimentation

Add phosphate to
hyperalimentation
solutions

Nutritional
refeeding

Continue
nutritional
support

Diabetic
ketoacidosis

Alcohol
withdrawal

References

Fitzgerald FT. Clinical hypophosphatemia. Annu Rev Med 1978; 29:177.

Klein RF, Harris ST. Hypophosphatemia. In: Don H, ed. Decision making in critical care. Toronto: BC Decker, 1985:170.

Knochel JP. The pathophysiology and clinical characteristics of severe hypophosphatemia. Arch Intern Med 1977; 137:203.

Knochel JP. Hypophosphatemia and phosphorus depletion. In: Brenner BM, Rector FC, eds. The kidney. 4th ed. Philadelphia: WB Saunders, 1991:888.

Lentz RD, Brown DM, Kjelistrand CM. Treatment of severe hypophosphatemia. Ann Intern Med 1978; 89:941.

CHOOSING A CHRONIC DIALYSIS MODALITY

Joseph I. Shapiro, M.D.

Patients who present with end-stage renal disease (ESRD) may be successfully treated with renal transplantation (p 296), hemodialysis, or peritoneal dialysis modalities.

A. Both peritoneal dialysis and hemodialysis may safely be performed at home in some patients at less expense than in-center therapy. Moreover, although peritoneal dialysis may be performed in-center, it is not economically feasible for extended periods and is not truly a therapeutic option.

B. Next, it must be decided whether hemodialysis or peritoneal dialysis is superior. Both of the basic dialysis modalities have several advantages and disadvantages. Hemodialysis requires adequate vascular access, which is preferably an arteriovenous fistula and less desirably a Gore-Tex graft. Semipermanent venous catheters ("permacaths") may also be used, although they do not function as well or remain patent as long as arteriovenous fistulas. Hemodialysis also requires a relatively stable blood pressure during the therapy. In-center facilities are generally expert in optimizing hemodynamics of patients during hemodialysis and still report a considerable incidence of symptomatic hypotension with dialysis treatments. Candidates for home hemodialysis should have exceptionally stable hemodynamics. Peritoneal dialysis patients must have a suitable peritoneal membrane for dialysis therapy to be effective. Although patients who have had considerable abdominal surgery or a number of peritoneal infections may have an unsuitable peritoneal membrane, it is probably wrong to exclude most of these patients without a therapeutic trial.

C. Peritoneal dialysis may be prescribed as chronic ambulatory peritoneal dialysis that involves very long dwell times spaced throughout the day, or chronic cycling peritoneal dialysis in which the patient has relatively rapid exchanges performed with the aid of a mechanical cycler, usually at night during sleep. The former has the advantage of better middle molecule clearance and less total expense (as no cycler is necessary), with the negative features of more connections and disconnections (which increase the risk of infection) and greater protein losses across the membrane. Depending on the permeability characteristics of the peritoneal membrane as well as the efficiency of abdominal lymphatic absorption of dialysate, one may be preferable to the other.

D. In deciding between home and in-center hemodialysis and peritoneal dialysis, psychological and social considerations are as important as the medical factors. Home dialysis requires increased motivation of the patient, and often the patient's family, especially for home hemodialysis in which a hemodialysis partner is essential. Home dialysis also requires a suitable dwelling place with adequate space for peritoneal dialysis or hemodialysis supplies and a water supply suitable for hemodialysis. Patient compliance with prescribed therapy, as well as communication with dialysis physicians and staff, must be good for home dialysis to be a reasonable alternative. Because of these constraints and other issues, home dialysis appears to be gradually losing popularity in the United States.

E. The choice of one modality does not necessarily exclude a subsequent switch to another. Frequently, patients develop frustration with in-center hemodialysis over time and may desire a home-based alternative, although at the onset of their need for dialytic therapy, involvement with home hemodialysis or peritoneal dialysis seemed overwhelming. Conversely, other patients may develop complications or find difficulties, both medical and social, with home dialysis and subsequently choose to dialyze in center. Therefore, a certain empiricism may be justified in choosing dialysis modalities in the knowledge that it is relatively easy to switch to an alternative.

References

Henderson LW. Symptomatic hypotension during hemodialysis. Kidney Int 1980; 17:571.

Henderson LW, Cheung AK, Chenoweth DE. Choosing a membrane. Am J Kidney Dis 1983; 3:5.

Maher JF. Physiology of the peritoneum. Implications for peritoneal dialysis. Med Clin North Am 1990; 74:985.

Mattern WD, McGaghie WC, Rigby RJ, et al. Selection of ESRD treatment: an international study. Am J Kidney Dis 1989; 13:457.

Merrill JP. Dialysis versus transplantation in the treatment of end-stage renal disease. Annu Rev Med 1978; 29:343.

Patient needs CHRONIC DIALYSIS THERAPY

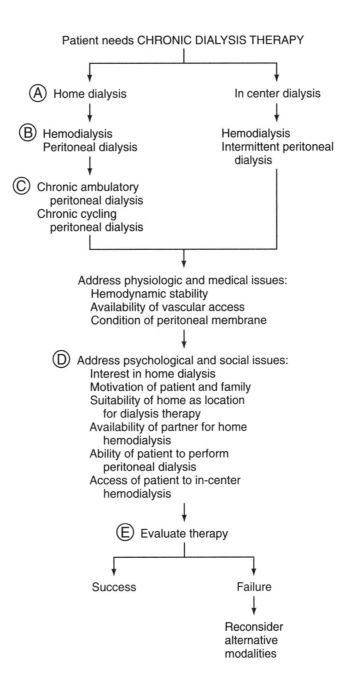

Ⓐ Home dialysis

In center dialysis

Ⓑ Hemodialysis
Peritoneal dialysis

Hemodialysis
Intermittent peritoneal
dialysis

Ⓒ Chronic ambulatory
peritoneal dialysis
Chronic cycling
peritoneal dialysis

Address physiologic and medical issues:
Hemodynamic stability
Availability of vascular access
Condition of peritoneal membrane

Ⓓ Address psychological and social issues:
Interest in home dialysis
Motivation of patient and family
Suitability of home as location
for dialysis therapy
Availability of partner for home
hemodialysis
Ability of patient to perform
peritoneal dialysis
Access of patient to in-center
hemodialysis

Ⓔ Evaluate therapy

Success

Failure

Reconsider
alternative
modalities

SELECTION OF PATIENTS FOR TRANSPLANTATION

Joseph I. Shapiro, M.D.

Most transplant nephrologists believe it is the right of every end-stage renal disease (ESRD) patient to be considered for renal transplantation, a procedure that in the long run is less expensive than chronic hemodialysis therapy. Moreover, although a definite survival advantage of renal transplantation over chronic hemodialysis or peritoneal dialysis has been difficult to demonstrate, most patients enjoy a considerably better quality of life with a renal transplant than with alternative ESRD therapy. A relative shortage of organs still exists, but with improvements in organ harvesting and storage and improved awareness of potential organ donors, it is possible that most patients with ESRD may ultimately receive a renal transplant.

A. To determine whether the patient is interested in a renal transplant, education of the patient as to the risks and benefits of renal transplantation is required. If a patient is willing to consider renal transplantation, the transplant team must address the risks and benefits for that patient, and first determine the safety of the procedure for him or her.

B. Perform a detailed history and physical examination as well as baseline laboratory (CBC, prothrombin time, partial thromboplastin time, chemistry panel, HIV Ab, HBsAg, CMV Ab, urine culture, urinalysis) and other screening tests (chest film, ECG) in all potential kidney transplant recipients. Pay careful attention to the nature of the underlying renal disease as well as the presence of extrarenal disease that would be relevant to either the transplant procedure itself or the chronic immunosuppression required. Diseases that recur in high incidence in the transplant kidney (e.g., focal glomerulosclerosis, Goodpasture's syndrome, oxalosis) are relative but not absolute contraindications to renal transplantation. Diseases of relevance to the procedure include diabetes mellitus (which increases the likelihood of coronary artery disease or neurogenic bladder) and abnormalities of the urinary tract architecture. Diseases of relevance to the chronic immunosuppression required include infection with HIV-1, currently an absolute contraindication to renal transplantation; the presence of noncutaneous cancer, a very strong contraindication to a transplant; infection or lack of infection with cytomegalovirus (CMV), which could influence management of the recipient if given a CMV-positive kidney; or a history of psychosocial difficulties, which might suggest potential difficulties for the patient in complying with a transplantation medical regimen.

C. In selected patients, further evaluation of potential problems is indicated before transplantation. Diabetic patients should receive a detailed cardiac evaluation even if there is no history of chest discomfort, because of the high incidence of silent myocardial ischemia in these patients. Similarly, vesicoureterography is warranted in diabetics because of the high incidence of neurogenic bladder and reflux in this population. A multidisciplinary approach is needed in patients with significant extrarenal diseases. Age itself is not a contraindication to renal transplantation, although the likelihood of significant extrarenal disease that could adversely affect the success and safety of transplantation does increase with age.

D. If it is determined that transplantation would be safe for the patient, the next step is to decide between a living related and a cadaveric transplant. In general, living related transplants have little survival advantage over cadaveric transplants unless the tissue match is excellent (e.g., a six-antigen or two-haplotype match). Other reasons to favor a living related transplant are high plasma renin activity, making it difficult to obtain a cadaveric transplant, or the patient's failure to thrive with alternative therapy. As waiting times (and waiting list lengths) vary considerably from center to center, the enthusiasm for living related transplants for this latter indication also vary. Potential living related kidney donors should not be considered if they have significant extrarenal disease or a significant possibility of developing renal disease. Hypertension is still considered a contraindication to donating a kidney. In addition, any reluctance of the potential donor to go through the organ donation procedure should dampen the enthusiasm for the transplant considerably. The choice of living nonrelated transplants is controversial at this time because of the considerable ethical issues surrounding this practice.

References

Fryd DS. The selection of cadaver kidney recipients (letter). JAMA 1988; 259:840.

Guttmann RD. Renal transplantation (second of two parts). N Engl J Med 1979; 301:1038.

Merrill JP. Dialysis versus transplantation in the treatment of end-stage renal disease. Annu Rev Med 1978; 29:343.

Riehle RA Jr, Steckler R, Naslund EB, et al. Selection criteria for the evaluation of living related renal donors. J Urol 1990; 144:845.

Yoshimura N, Oka T. Medical and surgical complications of renal transplantation: diagnosis and management. Med Clin North Am 1990; 74:1025.

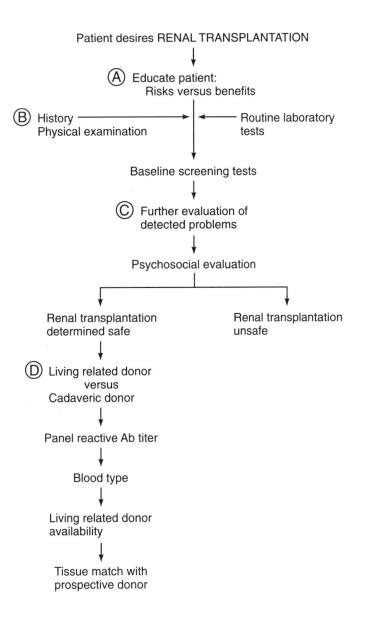

Patient desires RENAL TRANSPLANTATION

(A) Educate patient:
Risks versus benefits

(B) History ———————→ ←——— Routine laboratory
Physical examination tests

Baseline screening tests

(C) Further evaluation of
detected problems

Psychosocial evaluation

Renal transplantation   Renal transplantation
determined safe   unsafe

(D) Living related donor
versus
Cadaveric donor

Panel reactive Ab titer

Blood type

Living related donor
availability

Tissue match with
prospective donor

FEVER IN A TRANSPLANT PATIENT

Joseph I. Shapiro, M.D.

A. Fever in a transplant patient offers a considerable differential diagnosis, including virtually all the conventional causes of fever as well as special considerations related to the immunosuppressive agents used to prevent or treat allograft rejection, plus allograft rejection itself. This can be simplified somewhat by examining the clinical situation in which the fever occurred. Fevers may be related to rejection, infection, drug reactions, malignancies, or collagen vascular diseases.

B. Infections must be considered first, and because of the impaired ability of immunosuppressed transplant recipients to combat infection, must be addressed with expediency and aggressiveness. Infections can be categorized as conventional and opportunistic, i.e., related primarily to the immunosuppression used. The likelihood of a given infectious agent causing fever is related to duration of time since the transplant. In the early post-transplant period, the most likely infectious causes of fever are bacterial, most commonly urinary tract infections and wound infections with the usual pathogens. Urinary infections may lead to pyelonephritis with a higher than usual incidence because of the high incidence of reflux into the transplant ureter and kidney as well as the immunosuppressive agents employed. Pyelonephritis in a transplant patient typically is associated with renal failure, in contrast to native kidney pyelonephritis in which the contralateral kidney usually maintains renal function at normal. Opportunistic infections in this period are not common, although herpes simplex may occur. When a cytomegalovirus (CMV)-negative recipient receives a CMV-positive kidney, primary CMV infection is likely. For this reason, CMV prophylaxis with immune globulin may be indicated in this setting. In the intermediate period, opportunistic infections are more likely than conventional bacterial infections. *Pneumocystis* infections were once extremely common during this period, but their incidence has become low with the common use of either trimethoprim-sulfamethoxasole or inhaled pentamidine prophylaxis. CMV reactivations remain a common infectious cause of fever during this time. The likelihood of this infection becoming symptomatic is directly related to the amount of immunosuppression the patient has received. *Nocardia* and fungal infections such as cryptococcosis and aspergillosis may also complicate over-immunosuppression. Conventional infections in this time period. Later after transplant, infections in general are considerably less common, and opportunistic and conventional infections occur with comparable frequency. *Pneumocystis* infections are unlikely >6 months after transplant whether or not prophylaxis has been employed.

C. Acute rejection is another cause of fever in transplant recipients. This may be seen with hyperacute rejection (extremely uncommon) or with acute rejection. Even patients with severe chronic rejection leading to reinstitution of dialysis therapy may develop fever when immunosuppression is tapered off. With cyclosporine immunosuppression, fever does not accompany rejection with as high a frequency as was seen before the availability of this agent.

D. Drug reactions may cause fever in transplant patients, although this is not common, possibly because of the immunosuppressive agents (which are also anti-inflammatory) used.

E. Similarly, collagen vascular disorders such as systemic lupus erythematosus or polyarteritis nodosa may cause fever in transplant patients, but this is less likely because of the immunosuppressive agents.

F. Malignancies may complicate renal transplant care, especially when excessive amounts of immunosuppression are employed. Although skin tumors represent a considerable percentage of these malignancies, lymphoproliferative disorders occur with considerably increased incidence compared with age-matched controls. These are particularly likely to occur in the late post-transplant period and appear to be related to the net amount of immunosuppression received. Polyclonal B-cell lymphomas related to Epstein-Barr virus infection have recently been described in renal transplant recipients. These infections may show a response to lower doses of immunosuppression and antiviral therapy initially, but are extremely difficult to treat in later stages, especially when they become monoclonal.

References

Masur H, Cheigh JS, and Stubenbord WT. Infection following renal transplantation: a changing pattern. Rev Infect Dis 1982; 4:1208.

Penn I. Malignancies associated with immunosuppressive or cytotoxic therapy. Surgery 1978; 83:492.

Peterson PK, Balfour HH Jr, Fryd DS, et al. Fever in renal transplant recipients: causes, prognostic significance and changing patterns at the University of Minnesota Hospital. Am J Med 1981; 71:345.

Rubin RH, Wolfson JS, Cosimi AB, Tolkoff-Rubin NE. Infection in the renal transplant recipient. Am J Med 1981; 70:405.

Tolkoff-Rubin NE, Cosimi AB, Russell PS, Rubin RH. A controlled study of trimethoprim-sulfamethoxazole prophylaxis of urinary tract infection in renal transplant recipients. Rev Infect Dis 1982; 4:614.

Tolkoff-Rubin NA, Rubin RH, Keller EE, et al. Cytomegalovirus infection in dialysis patients and personnel. Ann Intern Med 1978; 89:625.

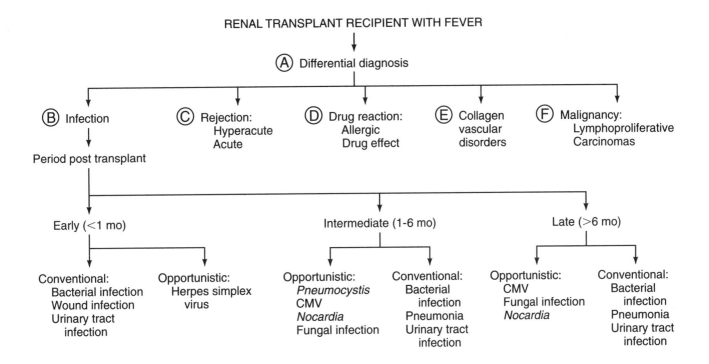

RENAL TRANSPLANT RECIPIENT WITH FEVER

Ⓐ Differential diagnosis

Ⓑ Infection

Ⓒ Rejection:
   Hyperacute
   Acute

Ⓓ Drug reaction:
   Allergic
   Drug effect

Ⓔ Collagen
   vascular
   disorders

Ⓕ Malignancy:
   Lymphoproliferative
   Carcinomas

Period post transplant

Early (<1 mo)

Conventional:
   Bacterial infection
   Wound infection
   Urinary tract
      infection

Opportunistic:
   Herpes simplex
   virus

Intermediate (1-6 mo)

Opportunistic:
   Pneumocystis
   CMV
   Nocardia
   Fungal infection

Conventional:
   Bacterial
      infection
   Pneumonia
   Urinary tract
      infection

Late (>6 mo)

Opportunistic:
   CMV
   Fungal infection
   Nocardia

Conventional:
   Bacterial
      infection
   Pneumonia
   Urinary tract
      infection

NEUROLOGY

ACUTE HEADACHE

Jeanette K. Wendt, M.D.

Headache is a common complaint in Western society, but fortunately most patients who present with acute headache have benign conditions.

A. Patients with sudden onset of headache and no history of head trauma require a full neurologic evaluation to exclude a subarachnoid hemorrhage. Perform a CT scan of the head first. This can be negative up to 15% of those with subarachnoid hemorrhage. Most neurologists perform a lumbar puncture in all patients with sudden onset of severe headache who have a negative CT scan, regardless of the presence or absence of nuchal rigidity. If subarachnoid hemorrhage is seen on CT, a lumbar puncture is not necessary.

B. Every patient with a recent history of head trauma who presents with focal neurologic complaints or findings or has altered mental status should undergo a head CT. Those patients with no focal complaints and a normal neurologic examination can be observed and treated symptomatically. However, if their condition deteriorates or if they fail to improve with conservative treatment, perform CT. Skull radiography has limited usefulness in the evaluation of head trauma.

C. Sinusitis is an overdiagnosed cause of headache. The diagnosis of sinus headache should be made only in the context of recent upper respiratory illness, purulent nasal discharge, fever, and localized tenderness over the sinus area. Sinus radiography can confirm the diagnosis but is seldom necessary for the initial evaluation and treatment.

D. The most common category of headache in patients presenting to emergency rooms is the nonmigrainous vascular headache secondary to systemic infection. These patients typically are febrile and have other symptoms of systemic illness. The neurologic examination is normal and there is no nuchal rigidity.

E. In patients with no history of headache, a new headache may represent their first migraine or tension headache. For the initial migraine headache it is often necessary to perform a complete neurologic evaluation, including CT. The role of hypertension in headache is not clearly understood and it is probably overdiagnosed as a cause of headache. When diastolic blood pressures are >120 mm Hg, this may be the source of headache. Patients in pain from any cause may have elevation of blood pressure. Therefore, exclude other causes in patients who present with headache and blood pressure.

F. In individuals >50 years of age who present with headache, temporal arteritis should be excluded as an etiology. The headache may be unilateral or bilateral and the temporal arteries are often thickened and tender. It is important to make an early diagnosis to prevent the visual loss that can occur from thrombosis of the ophthalmic artery. The ESR is usually elevated but a temporal artery biopsy is diagnostic. Treatment consists of high-dose prednisone.

References

Edmeads J. Emergency management of headache. Headache 1988; 28:675.

Little N. Acute head pain. Emerg Med Clin North Am 1987; 5:687.

Raskin NH. Headache. New York: Churchill Livingstone, 1988.

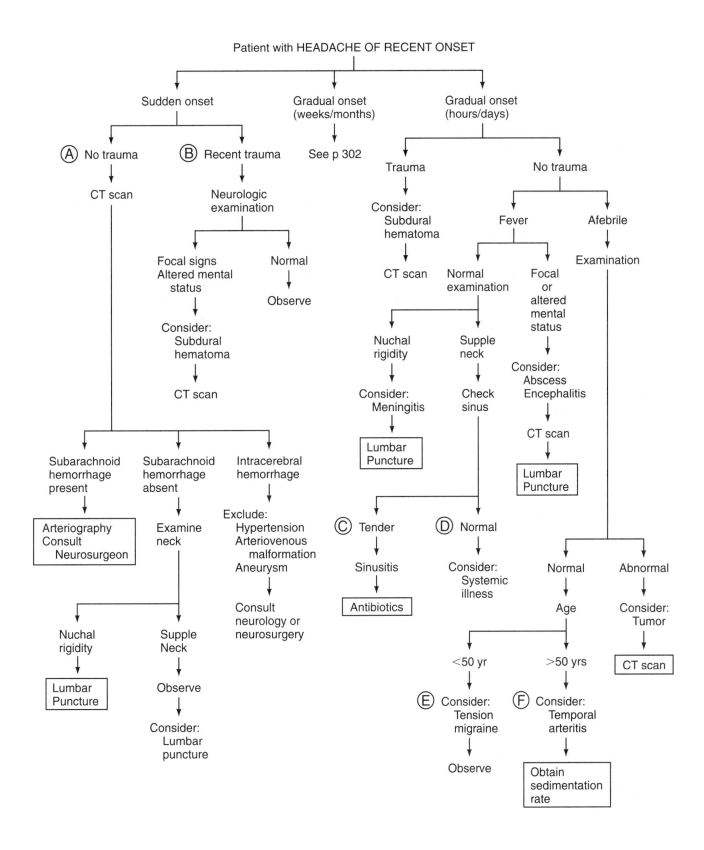

Patient with HEADACHE OF RECENT ONSET

Sudden onset

Ⓐ No trauma

CT scan

Ⓑ Recent trauma

Neurologic examination

Focal signs Altered mental status

Normal

Observe

Consider: Subdural hematoma

CT scan

Gradual onset (weeks/months)

See p 302

Gradual onset (hours/days)

Trauma

Consider: Subdural hematoma

CT scan

No trauma

Fever

Normal examination

Focal or altered mental status

Afebrile

Examination

Nuchal rigidity

Supple neck

Consider: Meningitis

Check sinus

Consider: Abscess Encephalitis

Lumbar Puncture

CT scan

Lumbar Puncture

Subarachnoid hemorrhage present

Subarachnoid hemorrhage absent

Intracerebral hemorrhage

Arteriography Consult Neurosurgeon

Examine neck

Exclude: Hypertension Arteriovenous malformation Aneurysm

Consult neurology or neurosurgery

Nuchal rigidity

Supple Neck

Lumbar Puncture

Observe

Consider: Lumbar puncture

Ⓒ Tender

Sinusitis

Antibiotics

Ⓓ Normal

Consider: Systemic illness

Normal

Age

Abnormal

Consider: Tumor

CT scan

<50 yr

>50 yrs

Ⓔ Consider: Tension migraine

Observe

Ⓕ Consider: Temporal arteritis

Obtain sedimentation rate

301

CHRONIC HEADACHE

Jeanette K. Wendt, M.D.

Most patients with chronic headache have benign conditions. Those with more serious neurologic disorders can usually be diagnosed on the basis of a careful history and examination.

A. A careful history is the most important aspect in the evaluation of headache patients, because there are no diagnostic tests for most headache disorders. Important aspects of the history include rapidity of onset, location, age, constancy of the pain, symptoms of systemic illness, and focal neurologic complaints.

B. Migraine headaches are more common in women, with the age of onset before age 50. Classic migraine is a headache preceded by a focal neurologic deficit, usually lasting 15–30 minutes. The most common auras are visual, but sensory, motor, speech, or brain-stem symptoms may occur. The headache is usually but not always unilateral; is throbbing and accompanied by nausea and/or vomiting, photophobia, and phonophobia; is typically aggravated by physical activity; and last hours to a few days.

C. Individuals who have ≤1 migraines per month can usually be treated with abortive and symptomatic medications only. The most effective abortive agents are ergotamine; isometheptene, usually in combination with dichloralphenazone; high doses of nonsteroidal anti-inflammatory drugs (NSAIDs); or dihydroergotamine. Symptomatic medications include antiemetics, NSAIDs, mild tranquilizers, and narcotic analgesics.

D. Patients with >1 migraine headache per month should be given prophylactic medications, including tricyclic antidepressants, beta blockers, and calcium channel blockers. Methysergide is usually reserved for patients who do not respond to or cannot take the other prophylactic medications. Each prophylactic agent should be given in adequate doses and for 3–4 weeks before its effectiveness is determined.

E. Cluster headaches are severe, unilateral, usually periorbital, dull, boring pain that is relatively short in duration (usually 45 minutes to 1 hour) but may recur many times during a day and often wakes the patient from sleep. Cluster headaches are more common in men, may be precipitated by alcohol, and must be associated with at least one associated symptom such as lacrimation, rhinorrhea, conjunctival injection, nasal congestion, forehead and facial sweating, ptosis, or miosis. The attacks occur in clusters, each lasting

an average of 2–3 months. Acute headaches can be treated with ergotamine and high-flow oxygen. Cluster headaches should be treated prophylactically in all patients because of their severity.

F. Patients with analgesic rebound headaches take daily or almost daily analgesics. These may be the simple analgesics such as acetaminophen or aspirin, or these combined with caffeine and minor tranquilizers. It is the overuse of these medications that perpetuates and escalates the headache cycle. Only by discontinuing the offending medications can effective prophylactic treatment be found. Some patients require hospitalization during the withdrawal period for symptomatic treatment of the often severe withdrawal headache and the associated nausea, vomiting, and dehydration. An aggressive prophylactic treatment program is necessary after withdrawal of the analgesics.

G. Patients with ergotamine dependency have daily or almost daily headaches alleviated only by ergotamine. When attempts to discontinue the ergotamine are made, a severe and protracted withdrawal headache occurs. Prophylactic medications are usually not effective while the excessive ergotamine use continues. These patients usually require hospitalization. An effective treatment of the withdrawal headache consists of IV phenothiazines or metoclopramide and IV dihydroergotamine. Once the patient has been withdrawn from the ergotamine, institute an aggressive prophylactic regimen.

H. Tension headache is a common complaint. The typical description is of a bilateral-pressure, dull, bandlike pain associated with neck muscle tightness and often precipitated by emotional stress. There is often associated scalp tenderness but not nausea, vomiting, photophobia, or phonophobia. Make a careful search for aggravating or precipitating factors. Relaxation and biofeedback can lessen the severity and frequency of the headaches. Some patients may require prophylactic medications such as tricyclic antidepressants or beta blockers.

References

Rapoport AM. Analgesic rebound headache. Headache 1988; 28:662.
Saper JR. Ergotamine dependency—a review. Headache 1987; 27:435.

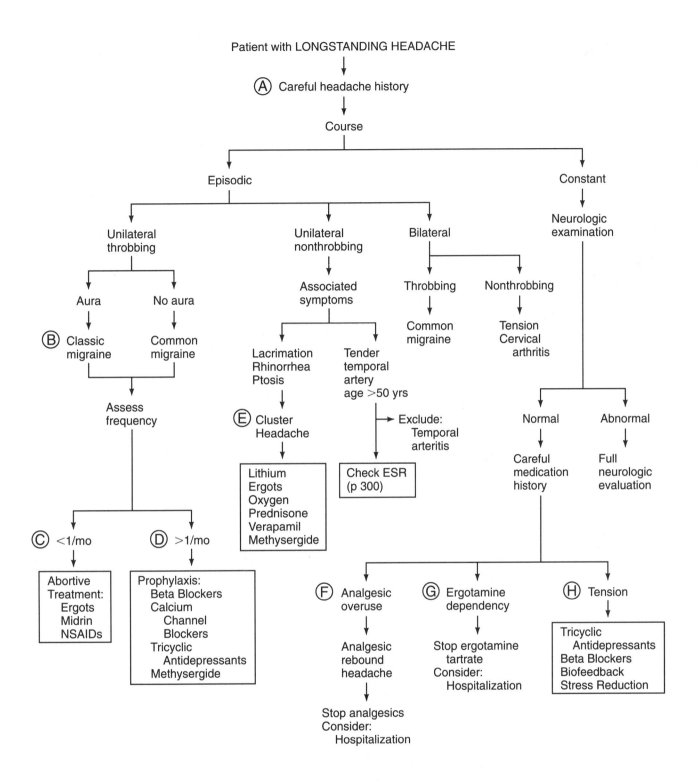

Patient with LONGSTANDING HEADACHE

Ⓐ Careful headache history

Course

Episodic — Constant

Episodic:

Unilateral throbbing
- Aura → Ⓑ Classic migraine
- No aura → Common migraine

→ Assess frequency
- Ⓒ <1/mo → Abortive Treatment: Ergots, Midrin, NSAIDs
- Ⓓ >1/mo → Prophylaxis: Beta Blockers, Calcium Channel Blockers, Tricyclic Antidepressants, Methysergide

Unilateral nonthrobbing → Associated symptoms
- Lacrimation, Rhinorrhea, Ptosis → Ⓔ Cluster Headache → Lithium, Ergots, Oxygen, Prednisone, Verapamil, Methysergide
- Tender temporal artery age >50 yrs → Exclude: Temporal arteritis → Check ESR (p 300)

Bilateral
- Throbbing → Common migraine
- Nonthrobbing → Tension, Cervical arthritis

Constant:

Neurologic examination
- Normal → Careful medication history
  - Ⓕ Analgesic overuse → Analgesic rebound headache → Stop analgesics Consider: Hospitalization
  - Ⓖ Ergotamine dependency → Stop ergotamine tartrate Consider: Hospitalization
  - Ⓗ Tension → Tricyclic Antidepressants, Beta Blockers, Biofeedback, Stress Reduction
- Abnormal → Full neurologic evaluation

TRANSIENT ISCHEMIC ATTACKS

Merrill C. Kanter, M.D.

Transient ischemic attacks (TIAs) are brief episodes of focal neurologic deficits caused by interruption of blood flow to the brain that does not last long enough to cause permanent infarction. The deficit must resolve within 24 hours to be classified as a TIA and usually lasts <1 hour. TIAs are an important indicator of cerebrovascular and cardiovascular disease. The risk of cerebral infarction is highest in the first few months after a TIA; thus, early intervention and treatment are crucial. Myocardial infarction (MI) is the most common cause of death in patients with TIA; therefore, a thorough cardiac history and evaluation is indicated.

A. Focal neurologic deficits occur in a number of conditions other than vascular ischemic events. Vascular events have an abrupt onset; the maximal effect is usually seen within minutes. Conditions such as subdural hematoma, metabolic abnormalities, demyelinating disorders, brain abscesses, and brain tumors often have a more insidious onset. Occasionally they present with transient deficits, but more commonly persistent abnormalities remain. A focal seizure or migraine may present with transient focal neurologic deficits but is usually accompanied by other symptoms. Involuntary movements, loss of consciousness, incontinence, or confusion suggest a seizure. Visual scintillations or severe headache occur in transient episodes in migraine patients.

B. The pattern of neurologic deficits indicates the vascular territory involved. Carotid artery ischemia causes weakness or sensory loss that may involve the contralateral face, arm, and leg. If the speech center is affected, aphasia may be present. Blindness in one eye (amaurosis fugax) is seen with carotid artery disease (p 306). Vertebrobasilar TIAs usually involve a combination of ataxia, diplopia, dysarthria, complete blindness, dysphagia, and varying patterns of limb weakness.

C. When a TIA is in the vertebrobasilar distribution, evaluation includes imaging of the brain to exclude nonvascular causes (e.g., hemorrhage, arteriovenous malformation, tumor). This can be done with a CT scan; however, MRI gives a more detailed view of the cerebellum and brain stem and is the procedure of choice if available. Hematologic evaluation includes CBC (differential, platelet count), prothrombin and activated partial thromboplastin times, VDRL (FTA) test, ESR, fasting glucose, electrolytes, liver and kidney function, lipid profile, and urinalysis. Cardiac evaluation includes chest film and ECG. If these are abnormal or if there is clinical evidence of cardiac disease, transthoracic echocardiography and/or a Holter monitor may identify thrombi or arrhythmias.

In patients <45 years old, those with left atrial abnormalities, and those with suspected embolic disease, transesophageal echocardiography can identify left atrial thrombi.

D. The same hematologic and risk factor evaluation is performed for carotid artery TIAs. CT of the head will rule out nonvascular causes. Noninvasive neurovascular testing is important in these patients. Carotid duplex ultrasonography, including B-mode and Doppler evaluation of the extracranial carotid system, is the procedure of choice for initial evaluation; it assesses the degree of stenosis present and plaque characteristics. Ultrasonography can be used as a screening procedure to determine the need for surgical evaluation; it is also a noninvasive method for follow-up evaluation. If surgery is considered, perform cerebral arteriography. This visualizes the intracranial and extracranial vessels, providing an accurate assessment of the degree of extracranial stenosis and amount of intracranial vascular disease.

E. Management includes modification of risk factors such as hypertension, diabetes mellitus, hypercholesterolemia, smoking, and obesity. Treat vertebrobasilar TIAs with aspirin, 325 mg/day. If TIAs persist, consider low-intensity anticoagulation with heparin and then low-dose warfarin for 3–6 months. Ticlopidine hydrochloride, 250 mg twice a day, is also useful in patients whose symptoms persist on aspirin or those who are aspirin allergic. Because of the risk of neutropenia, complete blood counts must be checked every 2 weeks for the first 3 months.

Management of carotid artery TIAs involves determining the degree of carotid stenosis. If there is an ipsilateral stenosis of ≥70%, carotid endarterectomy along with best medical treatment is more beneficial than medical therapy alone. Best medical treatment is usually aspirin, 325–1300 mg/day; lower dosages cause fewer GI side effects. Anticoagulant therapy is beneficial when a cardiac source is identified. Consider anticoagulation for patients with a thrombus, prosthetic valve, recent MI, or chronic arrhythmia. Less well established indications are crescendo TIAs and persistent TIAs on aspirin therapy. Use low-dose anticoagulation for 3–6 months and then re-evaluate the need for it. Because long-term anticoagulation may increase the risk of hemorrhagic complications, a retrial of antiplatelet therapy is often used. Ticlopidine hydrochloride, 250 mg twice a day, may be useful in patients who are aspirin allergic or whose TIAs persist on aspirin therapy. Check CBCs every 2 weeks for the first 3 months.

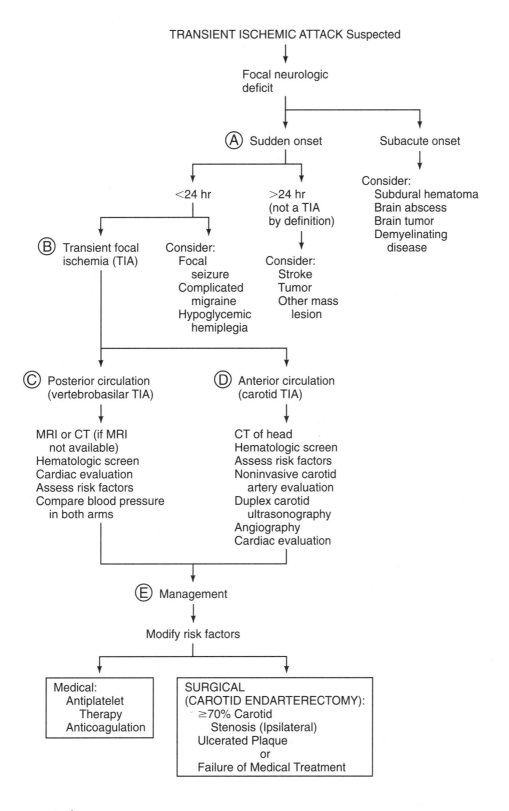

TRANSIENT ISCHEMIC ATTACK Suspected

Focal neurologic deficit

Ⓐ Sudden onset

Subacute onset

Consider:
   Subdural hematoma
   Brain abscess
   Brain tumor
   Demyelinating
     disease

<24 hr

>24 hr
(not a TIA
by definition)

Ⓑ Transient focal
   ischemia (TIA)

Consider:
   Focal
     seizure
   Complicated
     migraine
   Hypoglycemic
     hemiplegia

Consider:
   Stroke
   Tumor
   Other mass
     lesion

Ⓒ Posterior circulation
   (vertebrobasilar TIA)

Ⓓ Anterior circulation
   (carotid TIA)

MRI or CT (if MRI
   not available)
Hematologic screen
Cardiac evaluation
Assess risk factors
Compare blood pressure
   in both arms

CT of head
Hematologic screen
Assess risk factors
Noninvasive carotid
   artery evaluation
Duplex carotid
   ultrasonography
Angiography
Cardiac evaluation

Ⓔ Management

Modify risk factors

Medical:
   Antiplatelet
     Therapy
   Anticoagulation

SURGICAL
(CAROTID ENDARTERECTOMY):
   ≥70% Carotid
     Stenosis (Ipsilateral)
   Ulcerated Plaque
     or
Failure of Medical Treatment

References

Hass WK, Easton JD, Adams HP, et al. A randomized trial comparing ticlopidine hydrochloride with aspirin for the prevention of stroke in high-risk patients. Ticlopidine Aspirin Stroke Study Group. N Engl J Med 1989; 321(8):501–507.

Mohr JP, Pessin MS. Stroke: pathophysiology, diagnosis, and management. New York: Churchill Livingstone, 1986: 293–336.

North American Symptomatic Carotid Endarterectomy Trial (NASCET) Investigators. Benefit of carotid endarterectomy for patients with high-grade stenosis of the internal carotid artery. Stroke 1991; 22:816–817.

TRANSIENT MONOCULAR VISUAL LOSS

Merrill C. Kanter, M.D.

Patients with transient monocular visual loss require urgent evaluation. The risk of permanent visual loss from temporal arteritis is high (~35%) and timely evaluation and treatment can prevent further visual loss. If the temporary visual loss is due to vascular ischemia, it is commonly referred to as amaurosis fugax (AF). An episode of AF is an indicator of increased risk of stroke similar to that of a hemispheric transient ischemic attack (TIA). In the presence of carotid artery disease, AF is a marker of increased risk of cardiac death.

A. Temporal arteritis may cause blindness due to thrombosis of the central retinal artery secondary to giant cell arteritis. Presentation usually includes headache, visual loss or changes, and symptoms of fever, anorexia, and weight loss. Leukocytosis, anemia, and elevated ESR are commonly seen. The disease process is self-limited over a period of months. Therapy with high-dose steroids can prevent further visual impairment, although restoration of vision is variable. Other disorders that can present with unilateral visual changes and headache include migraine and occipital seizures. These often have a homonymous hemianopsia that has been misinterpreted by the patient as a monocular loss of vision. A positive visual phenomenon such as scintillating scotoma may be seen in migraine or seizure patients.

B. AF is typically described as impairment of vision that begins in the upper field of vision of one eye and progresses to involve the entire visual field of that eye. It usually lasts seconds to minutes. AF occasionally can stop with a hemifield loss, ascend, or rarely progress across the visual field laterally. Repeat episodes of AF tend to follow a stereotyped pattern for each patient.

C. Vascular ocular diseases causing anterior ischemic optic neuropathy, occlusion of the central retinal vein, and malignant arterial hypertension can sometimes begin with attacks of AF. Nonvascular causes of AF include hemorrhage, increased intraorbital pressure, and congenital anomalies. Optic neuritis and glaucoma can present with transient visual loss. Papilledema from any cause can present with visual obscurations. These disorders can be identified with the aid of a careful opthalmologic examination showing abnormal ocular findings with a normal retina.

D. Laboratory evaluation of patients with a history of transient monocular visual loss includes the following: CBC differential and platelet count (polycythemia, leukemia, thrombocytosis); Westergren sedimentation rate (evidence of arteritis; giant cell or Takayasu's); fasting glucose (diabetes mellitus); prothrombin and partial thromboplastin times (if prolonged, check antiphospholipid antibodies); and lipid profile (hyperlipidemia).

E. Noninvasive carotid artery studies include duplex (B mode and Doppler) ultrasonography, transcranial Doppler, pneumoplethysmography, and ophthalmodynamometry. Identification of the percent stenosis and plaque characteristics helps assess the need for further, more invasive, evaluation. Carotid artery stenosis ≥70% is an indication for surgical intervention (ipsilateral carotid endarterectomy). Surgical intervention was recently shown to be far superior to medical treatment in a multicenter randomized trial. The trial is continuing to assess the risks/benefits of surgical versus medical treatment in patients with ipsilateral carotid stenoses of 30–69% who have had an ischemic event (stroke, TIA, AF). Total occlusion seen by duplex ultrasonography is not as accurate as arteriography; therefore, arteriography should be performed in all patients who show no flow on Doppler ultrasound, to evaluate the possibility of a very-high-grade stenosis. The treatment is very different for patients with total occlusion (best medical therapy) and those with tight stenosis (surgical therapy). The other noninvasive studies mentioned can provide further information about intracranial stenosis in patients in whom arteriography is not performed. CT or MRI scans can reveal clinically silent cerebral infarctions and nonvascular lesions.

F. If the ipsilateral carotid artery is normal, further evaluation to identify a source may include cardiac evaluation. Cardiac emboli may cause unilateral visual loss, although they are usually larger emboli and do not occlude the ophthalmic vessels. Hypoperfusion due to low cardiac output can occasionally cause AF, particularly with severe ipsilateral carotid disease.

References

Amaurosis Fugax Study Group. Current management of amaurosis fugax. Stroke 1990; 21:201.

Miller NR. Walsh and Hoyt's clinical neuro-ophthalmology. 4th ed. Baltimore: Williams & Wilkins, 1991:2300.

Patient with TRANSIENT MONOCULAR VISUAL LOSS

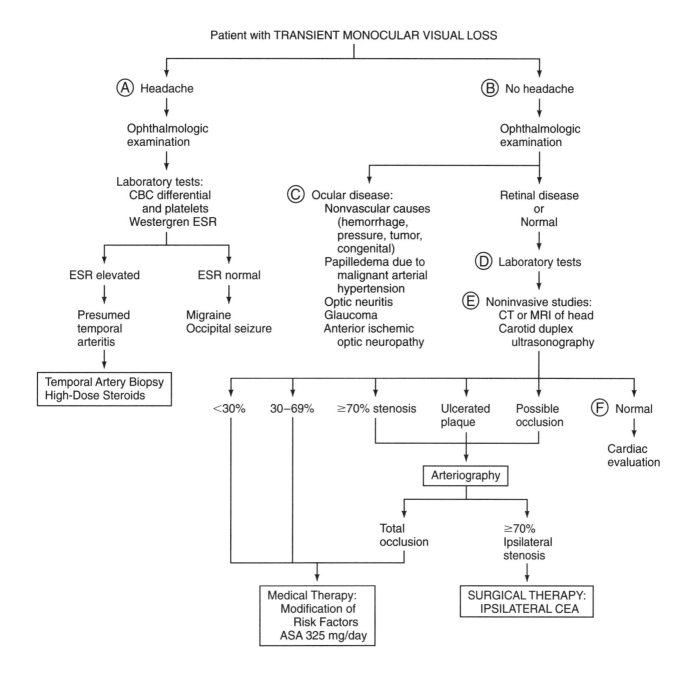

COMPLETED STROKE

Merrill C. Kanter, M.D.

A. Ischemia of a complete vascular region at the onset of symptoms causes a completed stroke. This may occur in the anterior circulation, where most commonly the middle cerebral artery is occluded and causes a hemiparesis and sensory loss contralateral to the lesion. In the posterior circulation, infarctions involving the lower brain stem are most common and cause a constellation of symptoms, including ataxia, dysarthria, diplopia, and facial weakness. It is important to differentiate among other focal neurologic deficits by using the history, physical examination, and neuroimaging (p 304). Seizures with Todd's paralysis or complicated migraine may present with sudden onset of focal neurologic deficits.

B. In completed stroke patients who are candidates for anticoagulation, it is important to evaluate any evidence of cerebral hemorrhage. Patients considered for anticoagulation are those at high risk for embolic strokes (i.e., cardiac source or recurrent strokes). Repeat a CT scan approximately 48 hours after the event. If there is no hemorrhagic transformation and the infarct is small to moderate in size, acute anticoagulation (heparin) followed by warfarin therapy is indicated. If hemorrhagic transformation has occurred, postpone anticoagulation for 8–10 days.

Re-evaluate the patient after the hemorrhage has resolved. This includes repeat CT of the head and reassessment of the medical, neurologic, and social risk factors for anticoagulation.

C. In the future there may be an opportunity to use thrombolytic agents. It appears that this will carry the caveat of early detection and intervention. This approach is similar to the early use of fibrinolytic agents in acute coronary artery thrombosis. If therapy can be started within a therapeutic window (probably within 6 hours after the stroke), there is great promise for such intervention. Controlled investigations are needed before there can be widespread use of this therapy.

References

Report of the WHO Task Force on Stroke and Other Cerebrovascular Disorders. Stroke: Recommendations on stroke prevention, diagnosis, and therapy. Stroke 1989; 20:1407–1431.

Wolf PA, D'Agostino RB, Belanger AJ, Kannel WB. Probability of stroke: a risk profile from the Framingham study. Stroke 1991; 22:312–318.

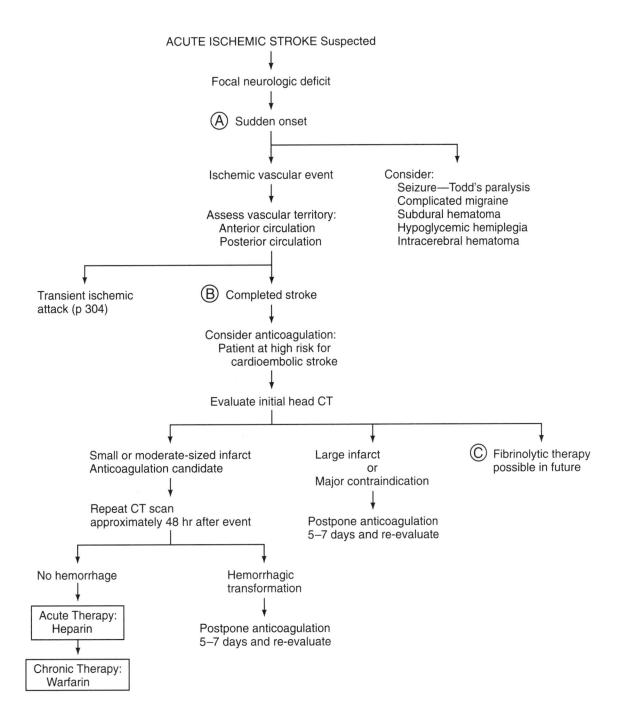

ACUTE ISCHEMIC STROKE Suspected

Focal neurologic deficit

(A) Sudden onset

Ischemic vascular event

Consider:
    Seizure—Todd's paralysis
    Complicated migraine
    Subdural hematoma
    Hypoglycemic hemiplegia
    Intracerebral hematoma

Assess vascular territory:
    Anterior circulation
    Posterior circulation

Transient ischemic attack (p 304)

(B) Completed stroke

Consider anticoagulation:
Patient at high risk for cardioembolic stroke

Evaluate initial head CT

Small or moderate-sized infarct
Anticoagulation candidate

Large infarct
or
Major contraindication

(C) Fibrinolytic therapy possible in future

Repeat CT scan approximately 48 hr after event

Postpone anticoagulation 5–7 days and re-evaluate

No hemorrhage

Hemorrhagic transformation

Acute Therapy:
Heparin

Postpone anticoagulation 5–7 days and re-evaluate

Chronic Therapy:
Warfarin

PROGRESSING STROKE

Merrill C. Kanter, M.D.

An ischemic stroke is a focal neurologic deficit that persists >24 hours. If only a portion of the vascular territory is involved (partial stroke), the stroke may worsen after its initial onset. Deterioration may occur over hours to days after the initial event. There are a variety of causes of worsening or progressing stroke, including both cerebral and systemic factors.

A. Patients who show neurologic deterioration after a partial stroke require re-examination, including a thorough neurologic, cardiac, and pulmonary evaluation. Clinical or laboratory evidence of infection, renal or hepatic failure, congestive heart failure, arrhythmias, or pulmonary embolism may cause significant worsening of neurologic symptoms. In addition, overzealous lowering of blood pressure can cause early neurologic deterioration in a patient who is usually hypertensive and now has compromised cerebral autoregulation because of ischemia. A repeat head CT scan is important in assessing the size of the infarction, recurrent strokes, edema, and secondary hemorrhage.

B. Cerebral causes of a progressive stroke include progressing thrombosis or recurrent emboli. If there are no contraindications to anticoagulation (systemic or cerebral hemorrhage, uncontrolled hypertension, large infarction) in the presence of progressing thrombosis or recurrent emboli, use IV heparin. Worsening neurologic deficits in patients with partial strokes in the posterior circulation are more often due to progressing thrombosis than in the anterior circulation.

Approximately 30–40% of patients with partial posterior circulation ischemia go on to progression of the thrombosis. Use acute therapy with heparin anticoagulation to prevent further ischemia. However, a thorough evaluation to exclude other causes of deterioration is important before considering anticoagulation.

C. If there is early CT evidence of hemorrhage or edema, intensive supportive care is needed. If the edema compromises brain-stem function or causes alteration of consciousness (i.e., a herniation syndrome), use hyperventilation and osmotic diuresis to control raised intracranial pressure.

D. Acute hydrocephalus or early seizure activity can occur, particularly in association with hemorrhage. Hydrocephalus can be treated and monitored with a ventriculoperitoneal shunt. Clinical deterioration due to a rapid increase in intracranial pressure because of an intracerebral hemorrhage warrants consideration of surgical evacuation of the hematoma.

References

Allen CMC, Harrison MJG, Wade DT. The management of acute stroke. Baltimore: The Johns Hopkins University Press, 1989:85.

Buchan A, Hachinski V. Atherothrombotic cerebrovascular disease. In: Johnson RT, ed. Current therapy in neurologic disease. 3rd ed. Philadelphia: BC Decker, 1990:177.

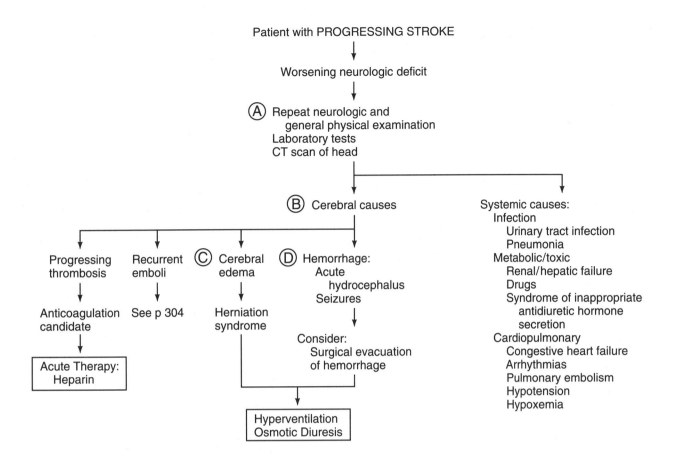

Patient with PROGRESSING STROKE

↓

Worsening neurologic deficit

↓

Ⓐ Repeat neurologic and
general physical examination
Laboratory tests
CT scan of head

Ⓑ Cerebral causes

Systemic causes:
  Infection
    Urinary tract infection
    Pneumonia
  Metabolic/toxic
    Renal/hepatic failure
    Drugs
    Syndrome of inappropriate
      antidiuretic hormone
      secretion
  Cardiopulmonary
    Congestive heart failure
    Arrhythmias
    Pulmonary embolism
    Hypotension
    Hypoxemia

Progressing
thrombosis

Recurrent
emboli

Ⓒ Cerebral
edema

Ⓓ Hemorrhage:
Acute
  hydrocephalus
Seizures

Anticoagulation
candidate

See p 304

Herniation
syndrome

Consider:
Surgical evacuation
of hemorrhage

Acute Therapy:
Heparin

Hyperventilation
Osmotic Diuresis

MEMORY LOSS

Geoffrey L. Ahern, M.D., Ph.D.

The pure amnestic syndrome is a disturbance of memory function with four characteristics: (1) the patient is alert, attentive, and motivated (i.e., not confused or depressed) and cognitive functions other than memory (e.g., language, visuospatial functions) are intact; (2) there is an anterograde amnesia (moving forward in time from the ictal event) in which there is impairment of new learning; (3) there is a retrograde amnesia in which information acquired before the ictus is not accessible—this accessibility is variable, with older memories more easily retrieved than more recently formed ones (Ribot's law); (4) confabulation (the production of implausible answers to questions regarding unretrievable information) may be present. The foregoing description is useful as a reference point, but keep in mind that memory disturbance can be seen in conjunction with a number of other neuropsychological abnormalities, particularly disorders of higher-order attention and concentration.

The amnestic syndrome appears to depend on damage to the limbic system, especially the temporal lobe (including the hippocampus and amygdala), dorsomedial nucleus of the thalamus, hypothalamus (particularly the mamillary bodies), and mesial portions of the frontal lobes and basal forebrain. The responsible lesions are usually (although not necessarily) bilateral and may result from a number of different insults.

A. Exogenous substance abuse (intentional or otherwise) may compromise memory functions. If a toxic screen results in a positive test for alcohol, consider a number of entities. First, the patient may be experiencing an alcoholic blackout. Second, alcoholics are subject to trauma; consider the entities discussed under **B.** Finally, the Wernicke-Korsakoff syndrome is usually encountered in alcoholics who suffer from poor nutrition (thiamine deficiency). Wernicke's encephalopathy (confusion, ataxia, ophthalmoplegia, and nystagmus) may progress to Korsakoff's syndrome, in which a chronic amnestic state is present (often accompanied by confabulation, particularly in the early stages). Thiamine replacement may be useful if given early; glucose may precipitate a deficiency state and therefore should not be given until thiamine is administered. In other populations, consider different substances (particularly prescription and over-the-counter medications). The elderly are particularly susceptible to cognitive side effects of common medications. Perhaps the best examples of this are anticholinergic compounds, which have been shown to interfere with memory processes.

B. A frequent cause of amnesia seen in clinical practice is head trauma. The damage done to the temporal lobe and orbitofrontal areas frequently affects memory processes. Concussion/contusion of the brain is the most likely etiologic agent in these cases, but also keep in mind the possibility of more severe injury, including subdural, epidural, and intracerebral hematoma. Accompanying alterations in attention and concentration are possible and perhaps even likely.

C. The tissues of the CNS are very sensitive to metabolic derangements. This is particularly true for those structures subserving higher-order attention/concentration and memory. Therefore, any insult, whether anoxic (e.g., cardiorespiratory arrest, carbon monoxide poisoning), hypoglycemia, or ischemic, may result in an amnestic state, with or without accompanying changes in attention and concentration. Herpes simplex encephalitis demonstrates a preference for attacking the temporal lobes. The resulting hemorrhagic encephalitis may lead to an amnestic state. Mass lesions should also be considered in the differential diagnosis of the amnestic syndrome. Entities in this group include aneurysms of the anterior communicating artery, pituitary lesions, and colloid cysts of the third ventricle.

D. Psychogenic amnesia does not resemble the organic amnesias. There is no anterograde amnestic gradient and the retrograde memory loss does not obey Ribot's law. Rather, the patient may forget only selective events from the past, usually of an unpleasant or traumatic nature. Selective biographical information may be lost, including personal identity (which is almost always preserved in organic amnesias). A remarkable indifference to the patient's own deficits may be observed. While psychogenic amnesia is generally thought to be a form of hysterical conversion, temporolimbic epilepsy or even frank malingering may produce a similar picture. Psychotherapy, hypnosis, or amobarbital (Amytal) interview may be useful in these cases; if epilepsy is suspected, EEG and appropriate anticonvulsant treatment may be indicated. Finally, a memory impairment may be seen after a course of electroconvulsive therapy (ECT).

E. Transient global amnesia (TGA) is usually seen in middle-aged individuals. It may occur after a period of physical exertion. The onset is abrupt and the patient often appears very confused and anxious, sometimes repeating the same questions over and over. The anterograde component can last several hours; the retrograde component may span a period of hours to years. The total episode may last 12–72 hours and generally does not recur. Vascular insufficiency has been suggested as the usual cause, but migraine, epilepsy, tumors, and diazepam overdose have also been implicated. Should a case of what appears to be classic TGA last longer than 3 days, consider the possibility of an irreversible cerebrovascular event involving the posterior cerebral circulation.

(Continued on page 314)

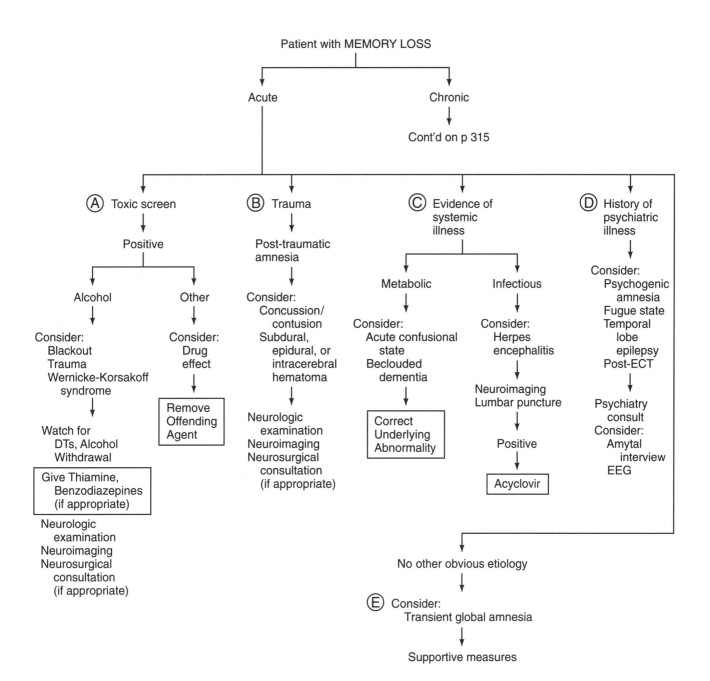

Patient with MEMORY LOSS

Acute

Chronic

Cont'd on p 315

Ⓐ Toxic screen

Positive

Alcohol

Consider:
  Blackout
  Trauma
  Wernicke-Korsakoff
    syndrome

Watch for
  DTs, Alcohol
  Withdrawal

Give Thiamine,
Benzodiazepines
(if appropriate)

Neurologic
  examination
Neuroimaging
Neurosurgical
  consultation
  (if appropriate)

Other

Consider:
  Drug
  effect

Remove
Offending
Agent

Ⓑ Trauma

Post-traumatic
amnesia

Consider:
  Concussion/
    contusion
  Subdural,
    epidural, or
    intracerebral
    hematoma

Neurologic
  examination
Neuroimaging
Neurosurgical
  consultation
  (if appropriate)

Ⓒ Evidence of
  systemic
  illness

Metabolic

Consider:
  Acute confusional
    state
  Beclouded
    dementia

Correct
Underlying
Abnormality

Infectious

Consider:
  Herpes
  encephalitis

Neuroimaging
Lumbar puncture

Positive

Acyclovir

Ⓓ History of
  psychiatric
  illness

Consider:
  Psychogenic
    amnesia
  Fugue state
  Temporal
    lobe
    epilepsy
  Post-ECT

Psychiatry
  consult
Consider:
  Amytal
    interview
  EEG

No other obvious etiology

Ⓔ Consider:
  Transient global amnesia

Supportive measures

F. Chronic memory loss is most likely to result from a degenerative dementing process. The best known of these entities is senile dementia of the Alzheimer type (SDAT). While it is true that the syndrome usually begins with an amnestic disorder, other higher-cortical functions (e.g., language, constructional abilities) are eventually compromised as well. SDAT is sometimes characterized as one of the "cortical" dementias, in contrast to the "frontal-subcortical" dementias that occasionally accompany extrapyramidal disorders such as Parkinson's disease or progressive supranuclear palsy (PSP). The amnestic problem seen in the "frontal-subcortical" dementias is often less of a true amnesia, per se, than "forgetting to remember"; in other words, the memory traces are there, but the patient has great difficulty retrieving them. Depression can look much the same as a "frontal-subcortical" dementia and should be considered in the differential diagnosis. It is important not to miss the diagnosis of depression, as it is one of the few causes of memory loss that can be treated (as opposed to the degenerative dementias discussed above). Multi-infarct dementia (MID) may show elements characteristic of either the "cortical" or "frontal-subcortical" dementias, depending on the areas in-volved. Stepwise progression, a pseudobulbar syndrome, and focal neurologic deficits are sometimes found. Finally, the same entities that can cause an acute confusional state may go on to produce a chronic confusional state, if they are not alleviated. Here too, it is important not to miss the diagnosis, because some amelioration of the impaired cognitive status may be possible if the offending condition is treated.

References

Ahern GL, Daffner KR, Duffy JD, Mesulam MM. Selected topics in behavioral neurology. In: Hyman SE, Jenike MA, eds. Manual of clinical problems in psychiatry. Boston: Little, Brown, 1990:111.

Butters N, Miliotis P. Amnesic disorders. In: Heilman KM, Valenstein E, eds. Clinical neuropsychology. 2nd ed. New York: Oxford, 1985:403.

Kapur N. Memory disorders in clinical practice. London: Butterworths, 1988.

Signoret JL. Memory and amnesias. In: Mesulam MM, ed. Principles of behavioral neurology. Philadelphia: FA Davis, 1985:169.

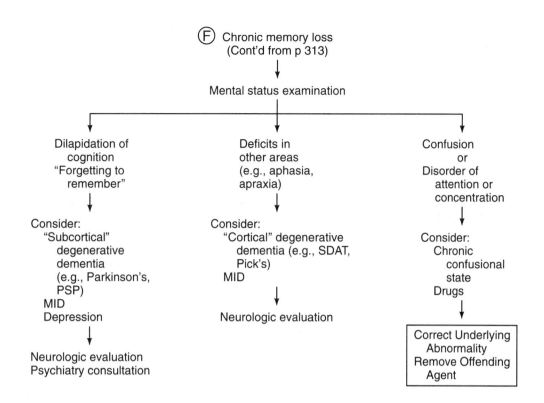

F Chronic memory loss
(Cont'd from p 313)

↓

Mental status examination

Dilapidation of
cognition
"Forgetting to
remember"

↓

Consider:
"Subcortical"
degenerative
dementia
(e.g., Parkinson's,
PSP)
MID
Depression

↓

Neurologic evaluation
Psychiatry consultation

Deficits in
other areas
(e.g., aphasia,
apraxia)

↓

Consider:
"Cortical" degenerative
dementia (e.g., SDAT,
Pick's)
MID

↓

Neurologic evaluation

Confusion
or
Disorder of
attention or
concentration

↓

Consider:
Chronic
confusional
state
Drugs

↓

Correct Underlying
Abnormality
Remove Offending
Agent

DIZZINESS

William A. Sibley, M.D.

Complaints of "dizziness" from a patient may mean near-syncope, including hyperventilation/anxiety attacks (p 492); a peripheral vestibular disorder (such as vestibular neuronitis, labyrinthitis, Meniere's disease, internal auditory artery thrombosis, nonspecific vascular disturbances in the inner ear, or benign paroxysmal positional vertigo); a central vestibular disturbance (brain-stem disorders: multiple sclerosis, lateral medullary infarction; temporal lobe disturbance: e.g., vertigo as the aura of a complex partial seizure); or ataxia (p 326).

A. The sensation of dizziness due to near-syncope or hyperventilation/anxiety is commonly referred to also as "giddiness."

B. When there is a false sense of motion, the sensation is called "vertigo," and this symptom usually implies dysfunction of the vestibular system. The most common type of vertigo is rotary. When vertigo is severe, it is often associated with nausea and vomiting.

C. In Meniere's disease, there is distention of the membranous labyrinth in one or both ears that fluctuates in severity. During a period of increased pressure in the labyrinth, patients typically have a feeling of fullness in the affected ear, an increase in the chronic tinnitus and deafness in that ear, and acute vertigo. The severity of each attack varies greatly; at the onset of very severe vertigo, some patients lose consciousness briefly. The duration is typically hours to a few days. With repeated attacks, there is increased deafness. In most patients with Meniere's disease, deafness precedes the episodic vertigo, but in some, episodes of vertigo precede the deafness. Acoustic neuromas and other posterior fossa tumors seldom produce episodic vertigo of this kind.

D. Acute labyrinthitis, due to either bacterial or viral infection, is much less common, and there is hearing loss associated with the vertigo.

E. Benign paroxysmal positional vertigo is a fairly common disorder, thought to be due to a loose or dislodged otolith in one ear. Vertigo occurs only in certain positions of the head (e.g., looking up, lying on the right side) and usually starts after a brief latent interval (a few seconds) after the head assumes the offending position. Changing position usually relieves symptoms rapidly. Most cases begin suddenly, without apparent cause; others follow head trauma. In older persons the syndrome may be due to vascular insults in the inner ear. Symptoms commonly subside in a few months but may recur.

F. Vestibular neuronitis is an acute illness lasting 6–8 weeks. There is usually rapid onset of rotary vertigo, which is almost always worse on the first day of the illness. There is no hearing loss. After the first day the severity of vertigo rapidly subsides, and in the later weeks of the illness it occurs only with rapid head movement. Vestibular neuronitis is a syndrome rather than a disease and probably has a variety of causes.

G. Multiple sclerosis may produce an attack of vertigo lasting several days, seldom longer, and caused by a new plaque in the floor of the fourth ventricle. In addition to nystagmus, patients usually have other typical symptoms or signs of the illness: e.g., double vision, extraocular muscle palsies, Babinski's sign. In older individuals a lateral medullary infarct (Wallenberg's syndrome) is often heralded by vertigo; examination also shows Horner's syndrome, unilateral palatal weakness, and ipsilateral loss of pain in the face and opposite side of the body.

H. To distinguish when a complaint of "dizziness" is really due to ataxia, always question whether it is present only when walking. When the sensation is also present while sitting, recumbent, or standing, it cannot be explained as ataxia.

References

Baloh RW, Honrubia V. Clinical neurophysiology of the vestibular system. 2nd ed. Philadelphia: FA Davis, 1990.
Drachman DA, Hart CW. An approach to the dizzy patient. Neurology 1972; 22:323.

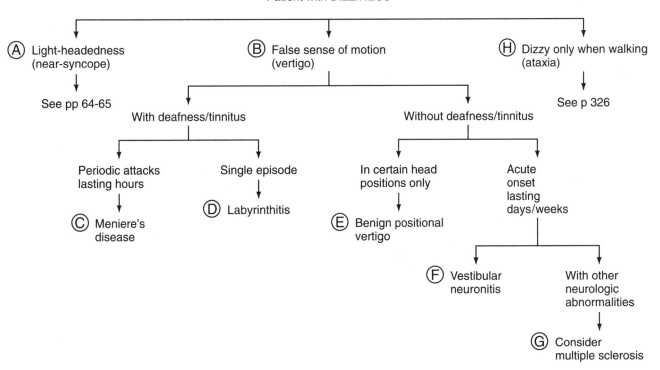

Patient with DIZZINESS

A) Light-headedness (near-syncope)

See pp 64-65

B) False sense of motion (vertigo)

With deafness/tinnitus

Periodic attacks lasting hours

C) Meniere's disease

Single episode

D) Labyrinthitis

Without deafness/tinnitus

In certain head positions only

E) Benign positional vertigo

Acute onset lasting days/weeks

F) Vestibular neuronitis

With other neurologic abnormalities

G) Consider multiple sclerosis

H) Dizzy only when walking (ataxia)

See p 326

SEIZURES

K.J. Oommen, M.D.

A seizure is the subjective or objective behavioral manifestation of an abnormal, excessive, neural discharge within the CNS. The focus of origin and nature of this discharge determines the clinical presentation. The advent of closed circuit television monitoring and simultaneous EEG led to the classification of seizures by the International League Against Epilepsy (ILAE) in 1981 and of Epilepsies and Epileptic Syndromes in 1985.

A. After an initial seizure, take a careful history. If there is evidence of previous undiagnosed episodes of seizures, this should be considered a recurrent seizure or epilepsy. Search for precipitating factors such as sleep deprivation and use of alcohol or stimulant drugs, including over-the-counter preparations. Look for underlying diseases that by themselves or because of their treatment would cause seizures. Thus, a patient with a history of diabetes may develop hyperglycemia resulting in seizures, or may suffer from hypoglycemia as a result of overdose of insulin or hypoglycemic agents. Treatment for hypertension with diuretics may cause hyponatremia, and patients with hypoparathyroidism may develop hypocalcemic tetani and seizures. Treatment should be directed toward the underlying cause of the problem. In addition to neurologic evaluation, perform EEG, MRI, and a complete metabolic screen.

B. With seizures of focal onset, the first question is whether consciousness is preserved or impaired during the seizure. When consciousness is impaired, it is a complex partial seizure; if not, it is called a simple partial seizure. Simple partial sensory seizures consist of paresthesias, special sensory symptoms (smell or taste), affective symptoms (fear or anxiety), psychic symptoms (derealization or depersonalization), dysmnesic symptoms (deja vu or jamais vu), and visual symptoms as well as auditory phenomena. Motor symptoms may include a focal motor jerk that either remains localized or progresses to involve other parts of the body in sequence (jacksonian march). A seizure of partial onset that eventually becomes convulsive is referred to as a secondary generalized seizure.

C. Generalized seizures may be convulsive or nonconvulsive. The latter can be diagnosed with EEG. In typical absence, the EEG shows three/sec spike and wave discharges. In atypical absence, the EEG may show four to six cycles/sec spike and wave discharges. Behaviorally, myoclonic jerks or automatisms may be seen. In atonic or astatic seizures, patients lose tone and "crumble" to the ground. Violent rhythmic clonic and tonic movements of the extremities occur in generalized clonic-tonic-clonic seizures.

D. Frequently, one may see seizures in which the clinical phenomena are atypical. Patients may present with unusual or bizarre behavior akin to seizures. This type consists of an extremely wide range of events in which the EEG may be normal or unchanged from the preictal EEG during and after the episode. The patient may not respond to medical treatment and should be referred to an epilepsy center for video/EEG monitoring.

E. An unprovoked seizure may occur in 10% of the population. Isolated seizures in which the neurologic examination, EEG, and imaging studies are normal may not require antiepileptic treatment. However, even under these circumstances, recurrence is possible. Patients should be warned of the potential risks of future seizures. Laws regarding driving, employability, and reporting requirements to traffic authorities vary from state to state, and patients should be advised accordingly.

F. The decision to use antiepileptics is based on high risk. In a study of children from Halifax, Nova Scotia, three predictive factors were identified. With an abnormal neurologic examination, 73% had recurrence, as opposed to 47% of those with a normal neurologic examination. With complex partial seizures, 79% had recurrence, as opposed to 44% in tonic-clonic seizures. When EEG showed focal spikes, 68% had recurrence, as opposed to 60% of those with generalized spikes. In those with complex partial seizures and a focal EEG associated with an abnormal neurologic examination, the estimated recurrence was 96%.

References

Camfield PR, Camfield CS, Dooley JM, et al. Epilepsy after a first unprovoked seizure in childhood. Neurology 1985; 35:1657.

Proposal for the classification of the epilepsies and the epileptic syndromes. Commission on Classification and Terminology of the International League Against Epilepsy. Epilepsia 1985; 26:268.

Proposal for revised clinical and EEG classification of epileptic seizures. Commission on Classification and Terminology of the International League Against Epilepsy. Epilepsia, 1981; 22:489.

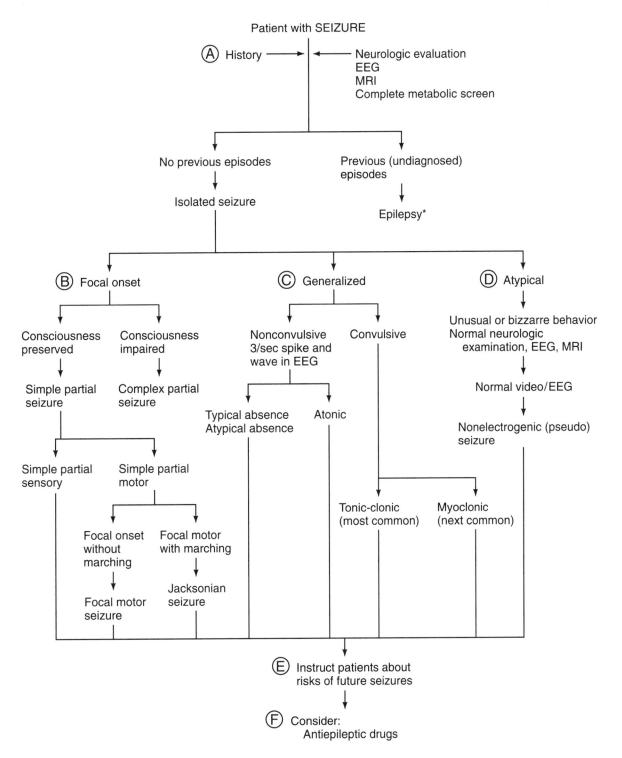

Patient with SEIZURE

Ⓐ History → | ← Neurologic evaluation
EEG
MRI
Complete metabolic screen

No previous episodes — Previous (undiagnosed) episodes

Isolated seizure — Epilepsy*

Ⓑ Focal onset

Consciousness preserved — Consciousness impaired

Simple partial seizure — Complex partial seizure

Simple partial sensory — Simple partial motor

Focal onset without marching — Focal motor with marching

Focal motor seizure — Jacksonian seizure

Ⓒ Generalized

Nonconvulsive 3/sec spike and wave in EEG — Convulsive

Typical absence Atypical absence — Atonic

Tonic-clonic (most common) — Myoclonic (next common)

Ⓓ Atypical

Unusual or bizzarre behavior
Normal neurologic examination, EEG, MRI

Normal video/EEG

Nonelectrogenic (pseudo) seizure

Ⓔ Instruct patients about risks of future seizures

Ⓕ Consider:
Antiepileptic drugs

*See second reference.

319

STATUS EPILEPTICUS

K.J. Oommen, M.D.

Status epilepticus (SE) is defined as continued seizures lasting at least 30 minutes without regaining of consciousness (except in simple partial status) between individual attacks. Convulsive SE is an acute neurologic emergency that carries a high mortality risk if untreated. A duration of 30 minutes of uninterrupted seizures is required for diagnosis, but in view of the high mortality rate and possibility of complications, institute treatment in any patient with the potential for SE.

A. Consciousness is preserved in cases of simple partial status; awareness of surroundings is impaired in the complex partial type.

B. Generalized SE may be convulsive or nonconvulsive. The convulsive type includes both tonic-clonic and myoclonic status. The tonic-clonic form carries the gravest prognosis; in the myoclonic form, there is continuous myoclonic activity, and consciousness may not be completely lost.

C. Assess cardiorespiratory function in the first 5 minutes and monitor the ECG and blood gases (ABGs). Administer oxygen and suction oral secretions if necessary.

D. In both partial and generalized seizures, blood should be drawn for CBC, electrolytes, renal and liver functions, antiepilepsy drug (AED) levels, and drug screen at 5–10 minutes. In those with a history of chronic alcoholism, give IV 5% dextrose in normal saline (D_5NS) with B complex and 100 mg of thiamine. Also, 2 ml magnesium sulfate may be given IM. Perform as thorough a neurologic evaluation as possible.

E. If a metabolic abnormality is present, it should be corrected. If there is no obvious metabolic derangement, start IV normal saline. In those with a history of diabetes and possible overdose, a Dextrostix test may provide quick determination of serum glucose levels. Unless the patient is hyperglycemic, give an IV bolus of 25 g glucose with B vitamins. If the seizures continue, start IV phenytoin at a concentration of no greater than 5 mg ml at a rate <50 mg min. During administration of phenytoin, monitor the ECG and blood pressure. If the seizures do not stop within 10 minutes of phenytoin infusion, acute CNS injury is very likely. Consider IV lorazepam or diazepam. However, the possibility of respiratory depression warrants caution in the use of benzodiazepines in such patients.

F. If the seizures stop, perform a CT scan of the head to rule out the presence of any structural lesion. If this is negative, MRI and EEG should also be performed electively.

G. If the seizures persist after phenytoin infusion, intubate the patient. Give phenobarbital, 10 mg/kg, at a rate of 100 mg/min. Additional doses at 10 mg/kg may be given as needed with monitoring of blood levels. A dose of 1 mg/kg should give approximately 1 μg/ml of phenobarbital serum concentration.

H. Alternatively, the patient may be placed in pentobarbital coma. Give a 5 mg/kg bolus of pentobarbital IV after intubation and artificial ventilation; 25–50 mg may be given every 2–5 minutes until the EEG shows burst suppression. Compressed spectral analysis (CSA), if available, may be used to monitor the electrical activity of the brain during pentobarbital coma.

I. Other choices include a 4% solution of paraldehyde, 0.12–0.3 ml/kg IV, over 15–30 minutes. The availability of paraldehyde may be limited in the United States. Glass syringes and rubber tubing may be necessary for administration. Other choices include lidocaine, 50–100 mg IV bolus followed by 1–2 mg/min IV. However, high doses of lidocaine itself can cause seizures; because of this and the variability in its CNS distribution, it is best avoided.

J. If the status is broken, CT of the head may be performed at this time. If this is abnormal (hemorrhage, abscess, or mass affect due to tumor or traumatic lesions such as epidural or subdural hematomas), consult a neurosurgeon for appropriate management. If the CT is negative, a spinal tap may be performed to rule out an infectious process or, in some cases, subarachnoid hemorrhage. These conditions should be appropriately managed if present.

K. If seizures continue despite these measures, general anesthesia should be instituted by a competent anesthesiologist. Neuromuscular blockade may be required to avoid musculoskeletal injuries.

L. The nonconvulsive generalized seizure of the absence variety may be indistinguishable from a complex partial status or a psychological fugue state except when myoclonic activity is present. EEG will help the diagnosis by showing the presence of three/sec spike and wave discharges as in classic absence, or four to six Hz discharges in atypical absence.

References

Leppik IE, Status Epilepticus. Neurol Clin 1986; 4:633.
Rashkin MC, Youngs C, Penovich P, Pentobarbital treatment of refractory status epilepticus. Neurology 1987; 37:500.
Status epilepticus in perspective. Neurology 1990; 40: Suppl 2.

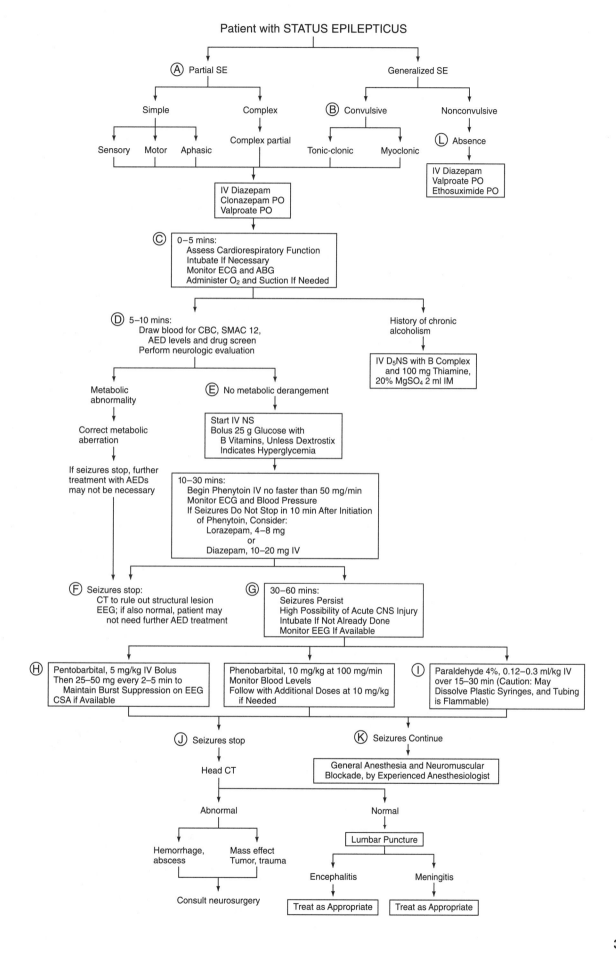

Patient with STATUS EPILEPTICUS

(A) Partial SE

Simple

Sensory   Motor   Aphasic

Complex

Complex partial

Generalized SE

(B) Convulsive

Tonic-clonic   Myoclonic

Nonconvulsive

(L) Absence

IV Diazepam
Valproate PO
Ethosuximide PO

IV Diazepam
Clonazepam PO
Valproate PO

(C) 0–5 mins:
Assess Cardiorespiratory Function
Intubate If Necessary
Monitor ECG and ABG
Administer O_2 and Suction If Needed

(D) 5–10 mins:
Draw blood for CBC, SMAC 12,
AED levels and drug screen
Perform neurologic evaluation

History of chronic
alcoholism

IV D_5NS with B Complex
and 100 mg Thiamine,
20% $MgSO_4$ 2 ml IM

Metabolic
abnormality

Correct metabolic
aberration

If seizures stop, further
treatment with AEDs
may not be necessary

(E) No metabolic derangement

Start IV NS
Bolus 25 g Glucose with
   B Vitamins, Unless Dextrostix
   Indicates Hyperglycemia

10–30 mins:
Begin Phenytoin IV no faster than 50 mg/min
Monitor ECG and Blood Pressure
If Seizures Do Not Stop in 10 min After Initiation
   of Phenytoin, Consider:
      Lorazepam, 4–8 mg
         or
      Diazepam, 10–20 mg IV

(F) Seizures stop:
CT to rule out structural lesion
EEG; if also normal, patient may
   not need further AED treatment

(G) 30–60 mins:
Seizures Persist
High Possibility of Acute CNS Injury
Intubate If Not Already Done
Monitor EEG If Available

(H) Pentobarbital, 5 mg/kg IV Bolus
Then 25–50 mg every 2–5 min to
   Maintain Burst Suppression on EEG
CSA if Available

Phenobarbital, 10 mg/kg at 100 mg/min
Monitor Blood Levels
Follow with Additional Doses at 10 mg/kg
   if Needed

(I) Paraldehyde 4%, 0.12–0.3 ml/kg IV
over 15–30 min (Caution: May
Dissolve Plastic Syringes, and Tubing
is Flammable)

(J) Seizures stop

Head CT

(K) Seizures Continue

General Anesthesia and Neuromuscular
Blockade, by Experienced Anesthesiologist

Abnormal

Hemorrhage,
abscess

Mass effect
Tumor, trauma

Consult neurosurgery

Normal

Lumbar Puncture

Encephalitis

Treat as Appropriate

Meningitis

Treat as Appropriate

WEAKNESS

Lynn M. Tolander, M.D.

Weakness is a term used loosely by patients and physicians alike, ranging in meaning from stiffness to numbness to fatigue to true lack of strength. This discussion refers only to the last-named meaning.

A. Important historical facts include type of onset and time course, fluctuations, relation to exercise, distribution (e.g., hemiparesis, paraparesis, quadriparesis, proximal, distal, bulbar), involvement of facial musculature, family history, medical history, and exposure to drugs or toxins. Also ask about associated symptoms such as cramps, pain, sensory loss, and myoglobinuria. The first step in the neuromuscular examination is to try to localize the lesion responsible for the weakness to the upper motor neuron (UMN), lower motor neuron (LMN), both, or neither. UMN signs include spasticity, hyperreflexia, clonus, and Babinski's sign; LMN signs include diminished muscle tone, atrophy, fasciculations, and hyporeflexia or areflexia.

B. UMN signs can generally be easily localized to above or below the foramen magnum, i.e., intracranial or spinal cord. Intracranial lesions typically cause a contralateral hemiparesis, often with associated signs such as aphasia, neglect, hemianopia, or hemisensory loss. An abrupt onset suggests a vascular event (stroke or hemorrhage), but occasionally tumors, abscesses, and multiple sclerosis (MS) present acutely. Investigation should include a brain CT or MRI scan and further tests, such as angiography, as indicated. In the acute setting when hemorrhage is suspected, a noncontrasted CT is the preferred test. When MS is suspected, MRI is superior.

C. In evaluating patients with potential spinal cord lesions, remember that with acute presentations, clear UMN signs may be initially lacking owing to spinal shock. However, a clear sensory and motor level is often present. Lesions at the lower cervical level may be accompanied by LMN signs at the level of the lesion, with UMN signs below the level. Another unique spinal cord presentation is the Brown-Séquard hemisection, which causes ipsilateral weakness and loss of position and vibratory sense, with contralateral loss of pain and temperature sense. Spinal cord lesions can be further divided into compressive (extramedullary) and intramedullary lesions. Pain tends to be a more prominent feature of compressive cord lesions. Herniated disc, epidural hematoma, epidural abscess, and epidural metastasis usually present acutely; osteophytic ridges and dural-based tumors (meningioma, neurofibroma) have a slower onset. Intramedullary lesions tend to be painless but cause early urinary dysfunction. Transverse myelitis has a quick onset and may be of viral, demyelinating, or vasculitic origin. Myelopathies can result from vitamin deficiencies (B_{12}, E), radiation, or HIV infection. Tumors of the spinal cord include astrocytomas and ependymomas. Traumatic lesions include contusion, severed cord, and delayed syrinx. Examples of vascular cord lesions are anterior spinal artery infarct and ruptured arteriovenous malformation. Congenital malformations of the cord and vertebral column may not produce symptoms until adolescence or adulthood. Hereditary spastic paraparesis is the name given to a slow degeneration of the cord; it affects older family members. Spinal cord lesions should be investigated with MRI or CT-myelography, and further tests such as lumbar puncture as indicated. Rapid intervention is often necessary to preserve remaining neurologic function.

D. Although variable in presentation, some conditions can be associated with both UMN and LMN findings on examination. Classically, this is seen in amyotrophic lateral sclerosis (ALS) owing to degeneration of the anterior horns and corticospinal tracts. ALS begins insidiously in middle or late life with bulbar or limb weakness, and progresses to death within 2–10 years. Helpful clues on examination include diffuse muscle wasting, bulbar weakness, fasciculations, Babinski's sign, and preserved sensation. Nerve conduction studies (NCS) are normal, while EMG demonstrates widespread denervation. Because of the dismal prognosis, a diagnosis of ALS should be made only after serial examinations and exclusion of potentially treatable disorders such as syringomyelia, brain stem or high spinal cord tumor, myasthenia gravis, lead toxicity, and neuropathy. Subacute combined degeneration (vitamin B_{12} deficiency), Friedreich's ataxia, and tabes dorsalis involve the corticospinal tracts as well as the dorsal columns and peripheral nerves, thereby causing weakness and sensory loss. Lesions of the termination of the spinal cord, or conus, cause paraparesis and (classically) saddle anesthesia and early urinary retention.

E. By far the largest group of disorders with LMN signs falls under the category of peripheral neuropathy (p 332). Lesions restricted to the anterior horn of the spinal cord produce LMN weakness, atrophy, and fasciculations. Spinal muscular atrophy, aside from the severe infantile form, tends to cause slowly progressive weakness beginning in childhood or adolescence. It has an autosomal recessive inheritance pattern. Poliovirus infection is rarely seen acutely any more. However, a postpolio syndrome has emerged as the cause of renewed weakness, atrophy, and cramps 30–40 years after the original illness. Cauda equina lesions, although often difficult to distinguish from conus lesions, are usually associated with pain and asymmetric paraparesis and sensory loss. Radiculopathies are characterized by loss of strength, sensation, and reflex in a dermatomal/myotomal pattern. Plexopathies tend to cause widespread sensorimotor loss

(Continued on page 324)

Patient with WEAKNESS

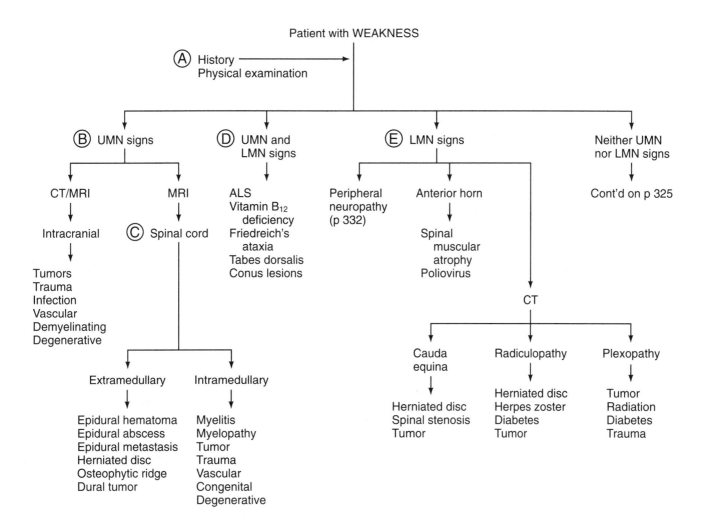

Ⓐ History ——————→
Physical examination

Ⓑ UMN signs

Ⓓ UMN and
LMN signs

Ⓔ LMN signs

Neither UMN
nor LMN signs

CT/MRI

MRI

ALS
Vitamin B₁₂
deficiency
Friedreich's
ataxia
Tabes dorsalis
Conus lesions

Peripheral
neuropathy
(p 332)

Anterior horn

Cont'd on p 325

Intracranial

Ⓒ Spinal cord

Spinal
muscular
atrophy
Poliovirus

Tumors
Trauma
Infection
Vascular
Demyelinating
Degenerative

CT

Cauda
equina

Radiculopathy

Plexopathy

Extramedullary

Intramedullary

Herniated disc
Spinal stenosis
Tumor

Herniated disc
Herpes zoster
Diabetes
Tumor

Tumor
Radiation
Diabetes
Trauma

Epidural hematoma
Epidural abscess
Epidural metastasis
Herniated disc
Osteophytic ridge
Dural tumor

Myelitis
Myelopathy
Tumor
Trauma
Vascular
Congenital
Degenerative

in one limb owing to involvement of the brachial or lumbosacral plexus. Pain is common when tumor is the cause of the plexopathy. Cauda equina lesions, radiculopathies, and plexopathies should be evaluated with CT or MRI. NCS/EMG can help differentiate a radiculopathy from a peripheral nerve lesion.

F. When weak patients lack clear UMN or LMN signs, have no sensory loss, and have normal to reduced tone and reflexes, the neuromuscular junction (NMJ) and muscle are possible sites of pathology.

G. By far the most common disease affecting the NMJ is myasthenia gravis (MG), in which autoantibodies attack the acetylcholine (ACh) receptor. A typical history is one of intermittent ptosis and diplopia. The muscles most often involved, in order, are the levator palpebrae; extraocular muscles; orbicularis oculi; facial muscles; muscles of mastication, swallowing, and phonation; and neck, shoulder and hip muscles. The symptoms worsen with exercise and improve with rest. Ptosis can often be elicited by having the patient look up at the ceiling for 1–2 minutes. There is a female predominance in young-onset cases and a male-predominance in older-onset cases. The purely ocular form is more common in older-onset males. The course is progressive or fluctuating; spontaneous remissions occasionally occur. The risk of myasthenic crisis is highest in the first year after onset. Diagnosis can be confirmed with electrophysiologic testing (specifically, repetitive nerve stimulation), the Tensilon test, and an ACh receptor antibody assay. Seek associated conditions such as hyperthyroidism and thymoma. The Eaton-Lambert, or myasthenic, syndrome is a paraneoplastic condition most commonly seen in patients with small cell lung cancer. It can be differentiated from MG by an increase rather than decrease in strength with muscle activity, and by electrophysiologic testing. Drugs that reduce neuromuscular transmission include penicillamine, aminoglycoside antibiotics such as gentamicin and kanamycin, and antiarrhythmics such as quinidine and lidocaine. Botulism is characterized by GI upset followed by weakness, ophthalmoplegia, and pupillary abnormalities.

H. Diseases of muscle are generally termed dystrophies or myopathies. The dystrophies are inherited; the myopathies are generally acquired. However, the naming of some inherited disorders such as the mitochondrial myopathies and congenital myopathies fails to follow the general rule.

I. Acquired myopathies fall into three main groups: endocrine, infectious/inflammatory, and drugs and toxins. The hyperthyroid state can produce the following forms of weakness: chronic thyrotoxic myopathy, thyroid ophthalmopathy, and thyrotoxic periodic paralysis. Diagnosis can be tricky. Chronic thyrotoxic myopathy is most often due to a nodular goiter. The degree of atrophy may be striking, and classic signs of hyperthyroidism are sometimes absent. Thyroid ophthalmopathy typically causes limitation of upward gaze, with or without exophthalmos. Diagnosis is made by orbital CT or MRI rather than thyroid function tests. Thyrotoxic periodic paralysis is a sporadic, not familial, disorder. It is associated with hypokalemia during attacks. Asian males are particularly predisposed. Hypothyroid myopathy is associated with increased muscle mass and slowed reflexes. It is often overlooked as a cause of elevated creatine kinase (CK). Hyperaldosteronism, acromegaly, Cushing's syndrome, hypophosphatemia, and hyperparathyroidism are other endocrinologic causes of myopathic weakness. Polymyositis (PM) and dermatomyositis (DM) are the prototype inflammatory myopathies. PM/DM typically begins in middle-aged individuals and has an acute to subacute onset. Early symptoms may be fatigue and difficulty in rising from a chair, climbing stairs, or combing hair. Myalgias are present in <50% of cases. The cervical and pharyngeal muscles may be involved, but, unlike MG, the extraocular muscles are spared. In dermatomyositis, there is a characteristic violaceous rash involving the eyelids and knuckles. Diagnostic evaluation should include thyroid function tests and a Tensilon test in uncertain cases, plus ESR, ANA, RF, CK, EMG, and muscle biopsy. Look for malignancy in older-onset individuals. Other infectious and inflammatory causes of myopathy are inclusion body myositis, bacteria and viruses, sarcoidosis, toxoplasmosis, trichinosis, and cysticercosis. A CBC with differential, CK, ESR, and muscle biopsy are necessary for diagnosis. Of drugs and toxins, steroids and ethanol are the most important causes of proximal myopathy. Steroid myopathy appears to be more common in women, in patients receiving treatment for >1 month, and in those taking fluorinated steroids such as dexamethasone. Muscle toxicity from ethanol includes an acute, painful necrotizing myopathy; chronic myopathy; and cardiomyopathy. Other drugs to consider include guanethidine, chloroquine, hydroxychloroquine, clofibrate, lovastatin, gemfibrozil, colchicine, zidovudine, doxorubicin, emetine (in ipecac), pentazocine, potassium-lowering diuretics, and heroin. Of note, the risk of myopathy in patients taking lovastatin increases with simultaneous administration of gemfibrozil or cyclosporine. Similarly, the risk of myopathy with clofibrate and with colchicine increases in patients with chronic renal insufficiency. Many drug-induced myopathies coexist with neuropathy or cardiomyopathy.

J. The inherited muscle disorders can usually be diagnosed clinically and then confirmed by CK, EMG, and muscle biopsy. The Duchenne and Becker forms of muscular dystrophy (MD) are X-linked and therefore primarily affect males. They are characterized by young age of onset, pseudohypertrophied muscles, cardiac involvement, severe proximal muscle weakness, and very high CK levels. The lifespan in Duchenne MD averages just two to three decades; in Becker MD the average is five decades. Definitive diagnosis can now be made by muscle biopsy showing deficiency of the protein dystrophin. Myotonic dystrophy is inherited in an autosomal dominant pattern and is the most common form of MD. It is unique in its characteristic myotonia, "hatchet facies," distal predominance of weakness, and multi-

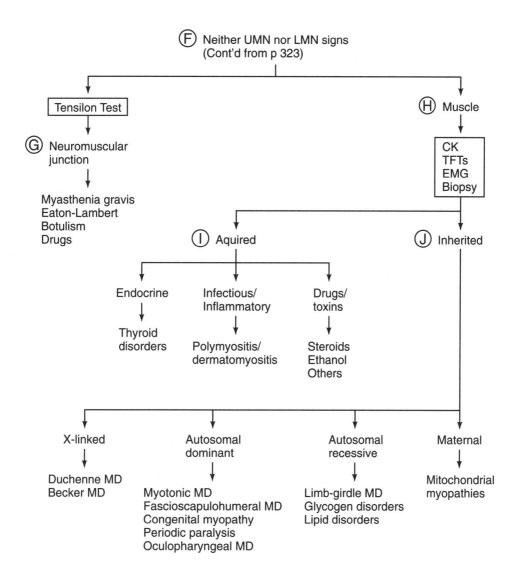

F Neither UMN nor LMN signs
(Cont'd from p 323)

Tensilon Test

G Neuromuscular
junction

Myasthenia gravis
Eaton-Lambert
Botulism
Drugs

H Muscle

CK
TFTs
EMG
Biopsy

I Aquired

Endocrine

Thyroid
disorders

Infectious/
Inflammatory

Polymyositis/
dermatomyositis

Drugs/
toxins

Steroids
Ethanol
Others

J Inherited

X-linked

Duchenne MD
Becker MD

Autosomal
dominant

Myotonic MD
Fascioscapulohumeral MD
Congenital myopathy
Periodic paralysis
Oculopharyngeal MD

Autosomal
recessive

Limb-girdle MD
Glycogen disorders
Lipid disorders

Maternal

Mitochondrial
myopathies

system involvement. Facioscapulohumeral (and sometimes peroneal) MD has an adolescent onset and an unmistakeable pattern of weakness. The congenital myopathies (central core, nemaline, myotubular) are generally mildly progressive and show distinct pathology on muscle biopsy. Familial hyper-/hypo-/normokalemic periodic paralysis is episodic in nature, as the name suggests. Onset is usually in early adulthood. Lastly, oculopharyngeal dystrophy is a late-onset, focal form of MD. Autosomal recessive muscle disorders include limb-girdle MD and disorders of glycogen and lipid metabolism. With improved classification of muscle disease, the category of limb-girdle MD has dwindled and consists of a heterogeneous group of patients. The juvenile form of spinal muscular atrophy must be considered in the differential diagnosis. McArdle's disease, phosphofructokinase deficiency, and carnitine palmitoyl transferase deficiency typically present with exercise-induced cramps and myoglobinuria. Measurement of low serum lactate in the ischemic lactate test suggests the diagnosis of McArdle's. Muscle biopsy with histochemical studies is necessary for definitive diagnosis of metabolic muscle disorders. The mitochondrial myopathies are a growing group of disorders characterized by weakness, fatigability, and multisystem involvement. Diagnosis must be confirmed by muscle biopsy.

References

Brooke MH. A clinician's view of neuromuscular disorders. 2nd ed. Baltimore: Williams & Wilkins, 1986.

Muscle disease. Neurol Clin 1988; 6:1.

Amyotrophic lateral sclerosis. Neurol Clin 1987; 5:1.

Targoff IN. Diagnosis and treatment of polymyositis and dermatomyositis. Comp Ther 1990; 16:16.

GAIT DISTURBANCES

William A. Sibley, M.D.

This chapter emphasizes those gait problems due to neurologic or neuromuscular disease, rather than those due to orthopedic problems.

A. In very early gait disorders it is often difficult even for experienced observers to be sure of the cause simply from inspection of the gait. Associated findings on neurologic examination may be crucial.

B. Bilateral Babinski's signs and very active deep tendon reflexes (DTRs) in the legs suggest an early paraparesis due to spinal cord disease, even though reduced strength in the legs may not be evident on direct muscle testing. In more advanced stages the paraparetic gait is a slow, labored, stiff process, and muscle weakness (especially in hip flexors and foot dorsiflexors) is easier to detect on examination.

C. Bilateral grasp reflexes and dementia suggest an apractic gait. Gait apraxia when fully developed resembles the first efforts of a toddler just learning to walk. There is a loss of the "blueprint" for walking; often the base is slightly widened and only a few difficult steps are possible. It is seen in bifrontal brain dysfunction such as that produced by bifrontal infarcts, advanced hydrocephalus, frontal tumors, Pick's disease, and very advanced Alzheimer's disease.

D. A steppage gait (exaggerated lifting of the knee with each step) suggests distal weakness of the leg, as might be seen in generalized peripheral neuropathy or peroneal nerve mononeuropathy (if unilateral). With generalized peripheral neuropathy, DTRs are absent or reduced, and weakness and sensory changes are greatest distally. With peroneal mononeuropathy, commonly due to nerve trauma at the fibular head, DTRs are normal.

E. An absent or reduced arm swing on one side suggests parkinsonism or early hemiparesis. Micrographia, cogwheel rigidity and flexion of the limbs and trunk, difficulty in rolling over in bed, aching shoulders, facial seborrhea, reduced voice volume, and poor facial expression are other features of parkinsonism. In advanced parkinsonism there is a disturbance of postural reflexes; the standing patient, when pushed, cannot make appropriate corrective movements to avoid falling. The gait may also become propulsive or retropulsive in advanced cases. Circumduction of the leg, increased tendon reflexes, and Babinski's sign on one side suggest a hemiparetic gait, usually indicating some diseases of the contralateral cerebral hemisphere.

F. Any widening of the gait base or abnormality on heel-shin coordination testing suggests an ataxic gait. There are at least three types of gait ataxia: truncal, sensory, and gait-and-extremity ataxia.

G. Truncal ataxia is an unsteady gait with normal finger-to-nose and heel-shin coordination tests. Tandem walking is difficult, if not impossible. In severe cases patients cannot even stand with one foot directly in front of the other. Truncal ataxia is seen with vestibular disorders, and thus in anyone having vertigo (p 316); it is also seen in some patients with drug-induced vestibular damage who do not have vertigo. Truncal ataxia also occurs with disease of the cerebellar vermis (e.g., medulloblastoma, alcoholic cerebellar degeneration).

H. Sensory ataxia is an unsteady gait due to loss of position sense in the toes. Many diseases associated with absent DTRs can be associated with this type of gait disorder. Unilateral loss of position sense usually does not produce a gait disorder.

I. Gait-and-extremity ataxia can occur with various types of drug intoxication that affect cerebellar function (e.g., alcohol, phenytoin, various sedatives and tranquilizers); it may also be seen in hypothyroidism. Such ataxia is also seen with diseases of the cerebellum and brain stem, including various types of cerebellar degeneration, multiple sclerosis, strokes, and tumors.

References

Gilman S. Gait disorders. In: Rowland LP, ed. Merritt's textbook of neurology. 8th ed. Philadelphia: Lea & Febiger, 1989:54.

Gilroy J, Meyer JS. Medical neurology. 3rd ed. New York: Macmillan, 1979.

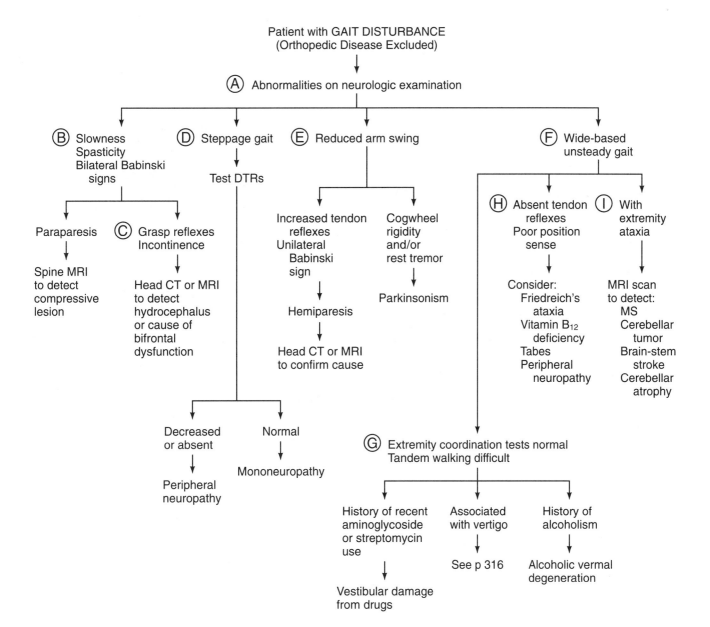

Patient with GAIT DISTURBANCE
(Orthopedic Disease Excluded)

Ⓐ Abnormalities on neurologic examination

Ⓑ Slowness
Spasticity
Bilateral Babinski
signs

Ⓓ Steppage gait

Test DTRs

Ⓔ Reduced arm swing

Ⓕ Wide-based
unsteady gait

Paraparesis

Ⓒ Grasp reflexes
Incontinence

Spine MRI
to detect
compressive
lesion

Head CT or MRI
to detect
hydrocephalus
or cause of
bifrontal
dysfunction

Increased tendon
reflexes
Unilateral
Babinski
sign

Cogwheel
rigidity
and/or
rest tremor

Ⓗ Absent tendon
reflexes
Poor position
sense

Ⓘ With
extremity
ataxia

Hemiparesis

Parkinsonism

Consider:
Friedreich's
ataxia
Vitamin B$_{12}$
deficiency
Tabes
Peripheral
neuropathy

MRI scan
to detect:
MS
Cerebellar
tumor
Brain-stem
stroke
Cerebellar
atrophy

Head CT or MRI
to confirm cause

Decreased
or absent

Normal

Peripheral
neuropathy

Mononeuropathy

Ⓖ Extremity coordination tests normal
Tandem walking difficult

History of recent
aminoglycoside
or streptomycin
use

Associated
with vertigo

History of
alcoholism

Vestibular damage
from drugs

See p 316

Alcoholic vermal
degeneration

TREMOR

Erwin B. Montgomery, Jr., M.D.

Tremor is defined as an involuntary movement that is regular in its rhythm. This distinguishes tremor from other involuntary movements such as myoclonus, chorea, atheotosis, and ballismus. Tremor is characterized by the situations in which it occurs, including resting, with movement (action) or when a posture is maintained. Some forms of tremor are present in more than one situation.

A. The signs of disdiadochokinesia (impaired rapidly alternating movements), ataxia, rebound (secondary to decreased muscle tone), and decomposition of movement (complex single movements broken down into sequence of simple movements) are often referred to as "cerebellar signs." This is a misnomer, because these signs can be associated with lesions elsewhere in the nervous system. Syndromes associated with "cerebellar signs" can be organized into precerebellar, cerebellar, and postcerebellar. Precerebellar refers to lesions of the sensory systems that ultimately project to the cerebellum. The cerebellum requires sensory information in order to adequately program movement. Postcerebellar refers to lesions that affect pathways from the cerebellum to motor cortex. These lesions prevent information regarding motor programming necessary for the normal execution of movement from reaching the motor cortex.

B. Flapping tremor is manifested by attempts to maintain a posture against resistance that is periodically interrupted by reduced muscular activity. This type of tremor is called "asterixis." Typically, when testing, the arms are held outstretched with the wrists bent back. Initially the subject is able to hold the position, but periodically the muscles relax and the posture is lost. Next the posture is regained. This cycle continues, producing a flapping tremor.

C. A coarse tremor is tested by having the patient hold their arms outstretched. A tremor appears and increases in amplitude as the patient attempts to maintain the posture. This is called a "wing-beating" tremor.

References

Findley LJ. The pharmacology of essential tremor. In: Marsden CD, Fahn S, eds. Movement disorders 2. London: Butterworths, 1987:359.

Gilman S, Bloedel JR, Lechtenberg R. Disorders of the cerebellum. Philadelphia: FA Davis, 1981.

Montgomery EB Jr. Signs and symptoms suggesting cerebellar dysfunction resulting from a cerebral lesion. Arch Neurol 1983; 40:422.

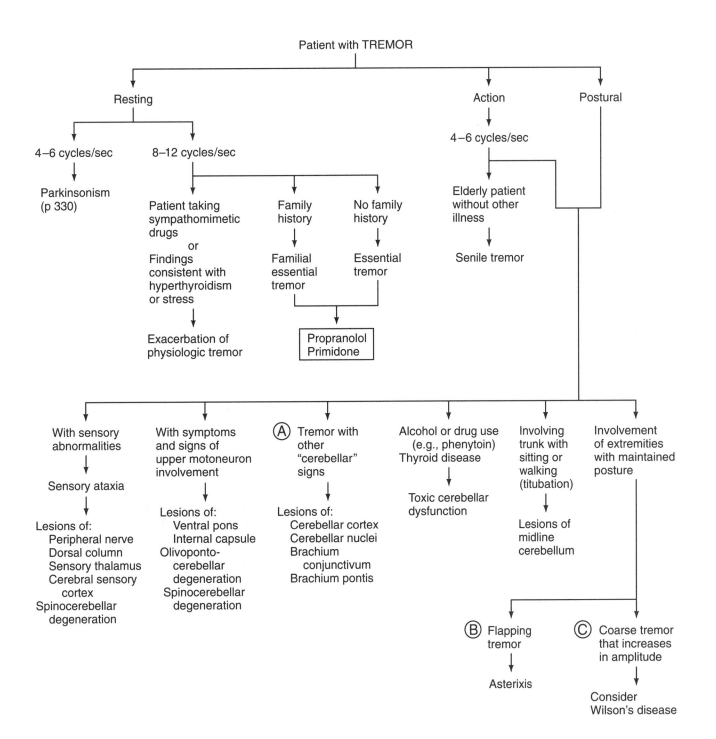

Patient with TREMOR

Resting

4–6 cycles/sec → Parkinsonism (p 330)

8–12 cycles/sec →

- Patient taking sympathomimetic drugs **or** Findings consistent with hyperthyroidism or stress → Exacerbation of physiologic tremor
- Family history → Familial essential tremor
- No family history → Essential tremor

Familial essential tremor / Essential tremor → Propranolol / Primidone

Action

4–6 cycles/sec → Elderly patient without other illness → Senile tremor

Postural

With sensory abnormalities → Sensory ataxia → Lesions of:
Peripheral nerve
Dorsal column
Sensory thalamus
Cerebral sensory cortex
Spinocerebellar degeneration

With symptoms and signs of upper motoneuron involvement → Lesions of:
Ventral pons
Internal capsule
Olivoponto-cerebellar degeneration
Spinocerebellar degeneration

Ⓐ Tremor with other "cerebellar" signs → Lesions of:
Cerebellar cortex
Cerebellar nuclei
Brachium conjunctivum
Brachium pontis

Alcohol or drug use (e.g., phenytoin) Thyroid disease → Toxic cerebellar dysfunction

Involving trunk with sitting or walking (titubation) → Lesions of midline cerebellum

Involvement of extremities with maintained posture

Ⓑ Flapping tremor → Asterixis

Ⓒ Coarse tremor that increases in amplitude → Consider Wilson's disease

PARKINSON'S DISEASE

Erwin B. Montgomery, Jr., M.D.

Parkinson's disease is a common disorder of the elderly, affecting nearly 2% of the population >65 years of age. As the baby boom generation enters the age of greatest risk, there may be a marked increase in Parkinson's disease. In the past, treatment provided only symptomatic relief; if symptoms did not cause disability or embarrassment, there was little reason for medical treatment. A new medication, selegiline (Eldepryl), has been introduced that may slow progression of the disease. This emphasizes the need for early diagnosis.

A. The diagnosis of Parkinson's disease requires the presence of at least three of the major symptoms: resting tremor, lead pipe or cogwheel rigidity, bradykinesia/akinesia, or abnormal posture. However, any of these symptoms may be variable between and within individuals, which may cause diagnostic confusion. As many as 30% of parkinsonian patients may not have tremor. Although parkinsonism has its greatest onset in the sixth and seventh decades of life, it may occur in the young. In about 7% of patients onset is at <40 years of age.

B. This decision requires adequate trial of levodopa. Levodopa/carbidopa compounds should be titrated until a satisfactory response or limiting side effect is encountered.

C. The use of selegiline as protective therapy is aimed at slowing the progression of the disease. Two placebo-controlled studies have shown that selegiline delays worsening of symptoms to the point where symptomatic therapy is necessary. These studies have been complicated because selegiline may have a symptomatic benefit. As such, this agent may have delayed reaching an end point independent of any effect on the natural history of the disease. However, both studies include wash-in and wash-out periods that either showed no symptomatic benefit or delayed progression in those who did have symptomatic benefit.

D. The division between young or mildly affected and older or more severely affected patients is based on two issues. First is the relative risk of significant side effects. Older patients generally, do not tolerate anticholinergics, amantadine, or direct dopaminergic agonists (bromocriptine or pergolide) as well as levodopa/carbidopa compounds. The second issue is the long-term risks of complications such as involuntary movements (dyskinesias) or postures (dystonias) and marked fluctuations in clinical response. The controversy centers on whether these long-term complications are a consequence of the natural history of the disease or of exposure to levodopa. The controversy is further complicated by the nature of levodopa exposure. It may be that the pulsatile administration rather than a more continuous application increases the risk of long-term complications. The algorithm is based on the assumption that exposure to levodopa should be minimized and when levodopa is needed, more continuous application that is desired (as can be accomplished with Sinemet CR). However, owing to the high incidence of side effects from anticholinergics, amantadine, bromocriptine, and pergolide relative to levodopa, the latter is the first choice in the elderly.

E. Amantadine can be added, but it has significant anticholinergic properties that could be synergistic with anticholinergics already used and thus increase the risk of side effects.

F. Rarely, patients may not respond to levodopa/carbidopa compounds but may respond to direct dopaminergic agonists. In elderly patients who fail to respond to levodopa/carbidopa, direct dopaminergic agonists should be tried.

References

Montgomery EB Jr. Treatment of Parkinson's disease. In: Bressler R, ed. Geriatric pharmacology. New York: McGraw-Hill, 1992.

Tetrud JW, Langston JW. The effect of deprenyl (selegiline) on the natural history of Parkinson's disease. Science 1989; 245:519.

Parkinson Study Group. Effect of deprenyl on the progression of disability in early Parkinson's disease. N Engl J Med 1989; 321:1364.

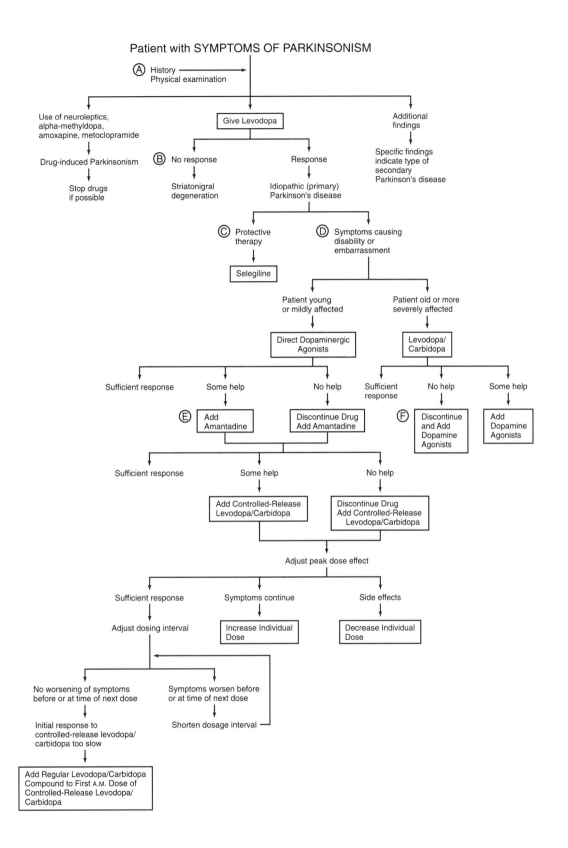

Patient with SYMPTOMS OF PARKINSONISM

Ⓐ History ——→ Physical examination

Use of neuroleptics, alpha-methyldopa, amoxapine, metoclopramide
↓
Drug-induced Parkinsonism
↓
Stop drugs if possible

Give Levodopa

Ⓑ No response
↓
Striatonigral degeneration

Response
↓
Idiopathic (primary) Parkinson's disease

Additional findings
↓
Specific findings indicate type of secondary Parkinson's disease

Ⓒ Protective therapy
↓
Selegiline

Ⓓ Symptoms causing disability or embarrassment

Patient young or mildly affected
↓
Direct Dopaminergic Agonists

Patient old or more severely affected
↓
Levodopa/ Carbidopa

Sufficient response

Some help
↓
Ⓔ Add Amantadine

No help
↓
Discontinue Drug Add Amantadine

Sufficient response

No help
↓
Ⓕ Discontinue and Add Dopamine Agonists

Some help
↓
Add Dopamine Agonists

Sufficient response

Some help
↓
Add Controlled-Release Levodopa/Carbidopa

No help
↓
Discontinue Drug Add Controlled-Release Levodopa/Carbidopa

Adjust peak dose effect

Sufficient response
↓
Adjust dosing interval

Symptoms continue
↓
Increase Individual Dose

Side effects
↓
Decrease Individual Dose

No worsening of symptoms before or at time of next dose
↓
Initial response to controlled-release levodopa/ carbidopa too slow
↓
Add Regular Levodopa/Carbidopa Compound to First A.M. Dose of Controlled-Release Levodopa/ Carbidopa

Symptoms worsen before or at time of next dose
↓
Shorten dosage interval

PERIPHERAL NEUROPATHY

Lynn M. Tolander, M.D.

A. Peripheral neuropathies (PNs) are disorders of the peripheral nerves and occasionally nerve roots or cranial nerves as well. They usually involve a mixture of motor, sensory, and autonomic dysfunction and rarely affect a single fiber type. The typical distribution of weakness and numbness is distal and symmetric, the feet being affected first in a stocking distribution followed by the hands in a glove distribution. The most distal deep tendon reflex, the Achilles, is the first to disappear. Spontaneous tingling sensations (paresthesias) or burning, unpleasant sensations (dysesthesias) may also occur distally. Atrophy may develop and is usually eventually proportional to the degree of weakness. The most common causes of PN are diabetes and alcoholism. When those risk factors are absent, obtain additional historical information, including occupation, family history, drug and toxin exposure, nutritional status, medical history, travel history, and a review of systems. The next step is classification as symmetric PN, mononeuropathy, or multifocal mononeuropathy, also termed mononeuritis multiplex. This is accomplished by examination and electrophysiologic testing with nerve conduction studies (NCS) and electromyography (EMG).

B. NCS/EMG confirms mononeuropathy and rules out a more widespread peripheral nerve disorder. Consider conditions that predispose to the development of a mononeuropathy, such as pregnancy, diabetes, collagen vascular disease, trauma, myxedema, and amyloid. Mechanisms of focal nerve damage include compression, entrapment, severance, infiltration, and ischemia. Common cranial neuropathies include idiopathic facial (Bell's) palsy and oculomotor palsy. The latter typically spares the pupil in diabetic or hypertensive patients. Common mononeuropathies of the upper extremity are radial (Saturday night) palsy, ulnar palsy, and median palsy (carpal tunnel syndrome). Nerves commonly affected in the lower extremity are the sciatic, femoral, lateral femoral cutaneous, and peroneal. Treatment depends on the nerve affected and the cause. For example, diabetic mononeuropathies and Bell's palsy tend to recover spontaneously; a short course of prednisone hastens recovery in the latter. Compression neuropathies often improve with removal of the offending behavior or underlying condition. Carpal tunnel syndrome is treated with rest and splinting. Surgery is reserved for refractory cases.

C. Multifocal mononeuropathy (MM) is suggested when two or more peripheral nerves are involved in an asymmetric manner. Confirm the pattern of involvement by NCS/EMG. Most cases are of the axonal type. Axonal damage results from various mechanisms, including ischemia, inflammation, compression, and infiltration. The two most important causes are diabetes and collagen vascular disease. Diabetes produces a painful MM that is probably ischemic in origin. Vasculitic neuropathies are seen in association with polyarteritis nodosa (PAN), rheumatoid arthritis (RA), systemic lupus erythematosus (SLE), allergic angiitis, and Wegener's granulomatosis. Leprosy is notable for its ability to cause widespread sensory loss without loss of reflexes. Sarcoid has a predilection for the facial and other cranial nerves. MM has also been reported in Lyme disease and AIDS. The multifocal variant of chronic inflammatory demyelinating polyradiculoneuropathy (CIDP) may be idiopathic or associated with myeloma, other malignancies, or dysproteinemias. Although similar in presentation to MM, multiple cranial nerve palsies and radiculopathies should alert one to the possibility of leptomeningeal metastases. The above-mentioned causes of MM have distinctive findings on nerve biopsy, making nerve biopsy extremely helpful in etiologic diagnosis. The importance of etiologic diagnosis is that treatment is available for most causes of MM. For example, both vasculitic neuropathies and CIDP may dramatically improve with steroid therapy.

(Continued on page 334)

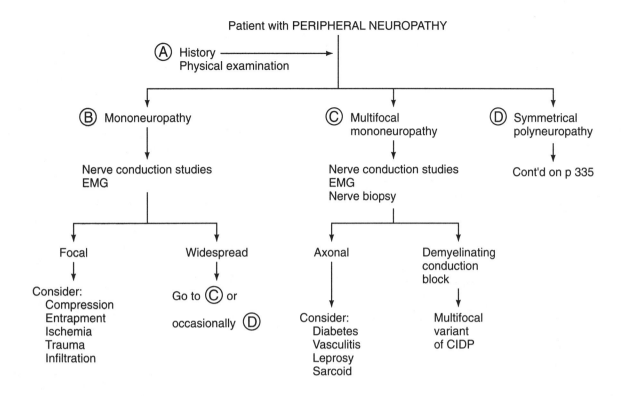

Patient with PERIPHERAL NEUROPATHY

Ⓐ History ——————→
Physical examination

Ⓑ Mononeuropathy

Nerve conduction studies
EMG

Focal

Consider:
Compression
Entrapment
Ischemia
Trauma
Infiltration

Widespread

Go to Ⓒ or

occasionally Ⓓ

Ⓒ Multifocal
mononeuropathy

Nerve conduction studies
EMG
Nerve biopsy

Axonal

Consider:
Diabetes
Vasculitis
Leprosy
Sarcoid

Demyelinating
conduction
block

Multifocal
variant
of CIDP

Ⓓ Symmetrical
polyneuropathy

Cont'd on p 335

D. Attempt to classify the type of PN, or polyneuropathy, and the cause in all cases. Electrical studies differentiate predominantly axonal from predominantly demyelinating neuropathies: The former are characterized by decreased amplitude and to a lesser extent slowing on NCS; the latter show more marked slowing of the nerve conduction velocity. The most common type of axonal PN, a distal, symmetric, and predominantly sensory type, is referred to as a "dying-back" neuropathy.

E. Causes of acute axonal neuropathies include porphyria, tick paralysis, and certain toxins. Acute intermittent porphyria is autosomal dominantly inherited with an adolescent onset. Attacks are characterized by abdominal pain, unusual behavior, seizures, sympathetic overactivity, and bibrachial weakness. They may be precipitated by drugs, particularly barbiturates, and alcohol. High urine porphobilinogen is diagnostic. Toxins causing acute axonal neuropathies include triorthocresylphosphate and thallium. There is considerable overlap between subacute and chronic axonal neuropathies. However, subacute generally refers to onset over weeks to months, while chronic neuropathies begin insidiously over years. The category of subacute axonal neuropathies is vast and is led by patients with underlying metabolic disease, including diabetes, renal failure, and hypothyroidism. Toxins known to cause axonal PN include alcohol, industrial solvents, organophosphates, and heavy metals (arsenic, thallium, mercury). Drugs known to cause PN include nitrofurantoin, isoniazid, hydralazine, vincristine, cisplatin, disulfiram, suramin, amiodarone, and dapsone. Nutritional deficiencies of thiamine and vitamins E, B_6, and B_{12} cause treatable neuropathies. (B_{12} deficiency may also cause myelopathy and dementia.) Vasculitic causes include SLE, PAN, RA, allergic angiitis, and Wegener's granulomatosis. Infectious causes include Lyme disease and AIDS. Neuropathies associated with dysproteinemias and paraproteinemias include multiple myeloma, macroglobulinemia, cryoglobulinemia, ataxia-telangiectasia, and benign monoclonal gammopathy. Amyloid may be inherited, sporadic, or associated with myeloma and has a characteristic appearance on biopsy. Carcinomas may cause PNs via paraneoplastic syndromes or in association with nutritional deficiencies or chemotherapy. It is not uncommon for the PN to appear months to years before the tumor is found. Chronic axonal PNs include those entities listed under the subacute heading plus hereditary motor and sensory neuropathy (HMSN), type II. Etiologic investigation of axonal PN includes vitamin B_{12} level, CBC, serum protein electrophoresis, ESR, ANA, rheumatoid factor, fasting glucose, BUN, thyroid stimulating hormone, urine heavy metal screen, HIV titer, Lyme titer, and a chest film. Consider nerve biopsy if the etiology is difficult to determine.

F. Demyelinating neuropathies can be classified according to the pattern of slowing on NCS and mode of onset. Those of insidious onset are generally either hereditary neuropathies or inherited metabolic disorders affecting nerves. Nerves are often enlarged, and biopsy is often helpful. HMSN, type I, also known as Charcot-Marie-Tooth disease or peroneal muscular atrophy, is characterized by autosomal dominant inheritance, pes cavus, distal atrophy, weakness and numbness, and profound slowing on NCS. HMSN type III, or Déjérine-Sottas, is characterized by autosomal recessive inheritance, palpable nerves, severe weakness, and scoliosis. HMSN, type IV, or Refsum's disease, is also inherited in an autosomal recessive pattern and causes elevated serum phytanic acid and multisystem dysfunction. Metachromatic leukodystrophy and abetalipoproteinemia are other inherited metabolic disorders affecting peripheral nerves. Acute segmental demyelinating neuropathies include the common Guillain-Barré syndrome and the now uncommon diphtheria. Guillain-Barré is preceded by a viral syndrome in 60–70% of cases. It begins with mild paresthesias followed by a rapid ascending paralysis and diffuse areflexia. Patients must be hospitalized or followed very closely, as 10–25% require artificial ventilation. Autonomic and cranial nerve involvement are common. Patients with a rapid, severe course should be considered for plasmapheresis. Chronic or relapsing segmental demyelinating neuropathies include CIDP, dysproteinemias, osteosclerotic myeloma, and lead toxicity. CIDP may begin similarly to Guillain-Barré but has a more protracted and often relapsing course. Diagnosis is made clinically and with aid of lumbar puncture, NCS/EMG, and nerve biopsy. Current treatment is with steroids, plasmapheresis, and other forms of immunosuppressive therapy. Dysproteinemias and paraproteinemias may be isolated or may occur in the context of myeloma, Waldenström's macroglobulinemia, cryoglobulinemia, POEMS syndrome, or ataxia-telangiectasia. Lead toxicity in adults is characteristically manifested by a motor neuropathy, particularly bilateral wrist drop. It is uncertain whether lead exerts its toxic effect on myelin, the anterior horn cell, or both.

References

Adams RD, Victor M. Principles of neurology. 4th ed. New York: McGraw-Hill, 1989.

Autoimmune neuropathies. Guillain-Barré syndrome. Proceedings of a Symposium. Bethesda, MD, November 1989. Ann Neurol 1990; 27 (Suppl):S1.

Dyck PJ, Thomas PK, Griffin JW, et al, eds. Peripheral neuropathy. 3rd ed. Philadelphia: WB Saunders, 1992.

Greene DA, et al. Diabetic neuropathy. Annu Rev Med 1990; 41:303.

Schaumburg HH, Spencer PS, Thomas PK. Disorders of peripheral nerves. Philadelphia: FA Davis, 1983.

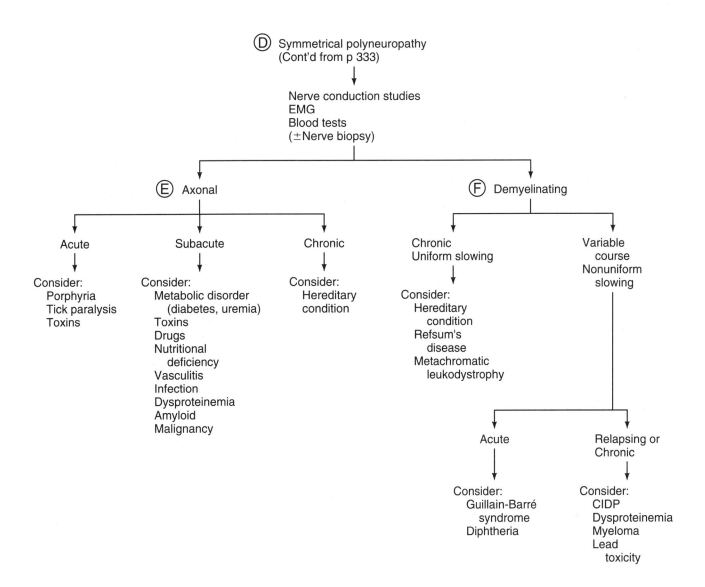

D Symmetrical polyneuropathy
(Cont'd from p 333)

Nerve conduction studies
EMG
Blood tests
(±Nerve biopsy)

E Axonal

Acute

Consider:
  Porphyria
  Tick paralysis
  Toxins

Subacute

Consider:
  Metabolic disorder
    (diabetes, uremia)
  Toxins
  Drugs
  Nutritional
    deficiency
  Vasculitis
  Infection
  Dysproteinemia
  Amyloid
  Malignancy

Chronic

Consider:
  Hereditary
  condition

F Demyelinating

Chronic
Uniform slowing

Consider:
  Hereditary
    condition
  Refsum's
    disease
  Metachromatic
    leukodystrophy

Variable
course
Nonuniform
slowing

Acute

Consider:
  Guillain-Barré
    syndrome
  Diphtheria

Relapsing or
Chronic

Consider:
  CIDP
  Dysproteinemia
  Myeloma
  Lead
    toxicity

HYPERKINESIAS

Erwin B. Montgomery, Jr., M.D.

Hyperkinesias refer to a group of involuntary movements from which rhythmic movements such as tremor are excluded. Also generally excluded are myoclonic jerks, fasciculations, asterixis, restless leg syndrome, and seizures. The different entities that make up the hyperkinetic disorders are united by the association with disorders of the basal ganglia, whether documented or presumed. Akathisia also is generally excluded, although thought to be related to abnormal dopamine function in the basal ganglia. Akathisia is the subjective complaint of feeling the need to move in order to be comfortable. The manifestations of the hyperkinetic syndromes are divided into dystonia, chorea, athetosis, choreoathetosis, ballismus, tics, and mannerisms. While the division gives the impression of discrete categories, they actually represent a continuum. The poles of the continuum are measured by coarseness versus gracefulness, proximal versus distal, and slow versus fast. There is not a one-to-one correspondence between the different hyperkinesias and disease entities. A single disease may be associated with a variety of hyperkinesias, and different types of hyperkinesias may co-exist in the same individual.

A. Ballismus tends to be a coarse, rapid, violent, and proximal involuntary movement. Treatment is directed at the underlying cause.

B. Athetosis tends to be a slow, graceful, and distal involuntary movement. Chorea is less graceful, faster, and more proximal than athetosis while more so than ballismus. Treatment of chorea, choreoathetosis, and athetosis is first directed at the underlying cause. Symptomatic benefit can be provided by use of drugs that deplete presynaptic dopamine stores (e.g., reserpine) or drugs that block postsynaptic dopamine receptors (e.g., phenothiazines, pimozide, haloperidol).

C. Levodopa in Parkinson's disease patients can produce a dose-related hyperkinesia.

D. Any drug that blocks postsynaptic dopamine receptors or depletes presynaptic stores of dopamine can produce a tardive dyskinesia or dystonia. Treatment of tardive dyskinesia and dystonia is problematic, since medications that can control the symptoms cause the disorder in the first place. While many cases of tardive dyskinesias or dystonias do not improve, some may take years to resolve. Thus, make every effort to avoid drugs associated with tardive dyskinesias or dystonias. However, the symptoms of tardive dyskinesia and dystonia sometimes may be severe enough to warrant treatment.

E. Tics and mannerisms are distinguished from the remaining groups by the patient's ability to suppress or be distracted from having them.

(Continued on page 338)

Patient with HYPERKINESIA

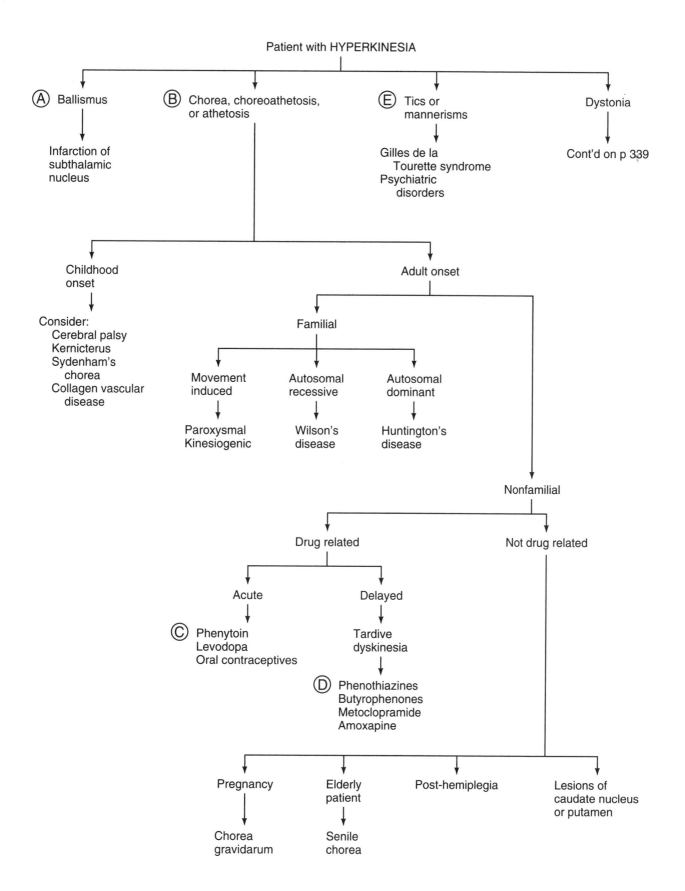

A. Ballismus → Infarction of subthalamic nucleus

B. Chorea, choreoathetosis, or athetosis

E. Tics or mannerisms → Gilles de la Tourette syndrome / Psychiatric disorders

Dystonia → Cont'd on p 339

Childhood onset → Consider: Cerebral palsy, Kernicterus, Sydenham's chorea, Collagen vascular disease

Adult onset

Familial
- Movement induced → Paroxysmal Kinesiogenic
- Autosomal recessive → Wilson's disease
- Autosomal dominant → Huntington's disease

Nonfamilial
- Drug related
  - Acute → C. Phenytoin, Levodopa, Oral contraceptives
  - Delayed → Tardive dyskinesia → D. Phenothiazines, Butyrophenones, Metoclopramide, Amoxapine
- Not drug related

Pregnancy → Chorea gravidarum

Elderly patient → Senile chorea

Post-hemiplegia

Lesions of caudate nucleus or putamen

F. Dystonia tends to be the slowest of these types of involuntary movements, giving the appearance of an abnormal posture rather than an involuntary movement.

G. Treatment of dystonias is difficult. Many varied medications have been tried with varying sucess. High-dose anticholinergics generally have been the most successful, particularly in childhood generalized dystonia. Occasionally, levodopa may produce significant benefit, especially in childhood generalized dystonias.

H. Intramuscular injections of botulinum toxin may produce dramatic benefits in focal dystonias. The benefits may last for several months and the injections may need to be repeated.

I. Surgical treatments in the past have included surgical ablations of thalamic nuclei. In torticollis, selective lesions of muscles or nerves may produce temporary benefit. However, dystonia is a dynamic process and the pattern of muscular involvement changes. It may be possible to identify the muscles involved, cut them, and produce benefit. Later, other muscles become involved and the torticollis returns. The same phenomena may occur with botulinum injections, but the pattern of injections can be adjusted.

J. Early morning foot cramping or dystonia is commonly seen in Parkinsonism.

References

Fahn S, Marsden CD. The treatment of dystonia. In: Marsden CD, Fahn S, eds. Movement disorders 2. London: Butterworths, 1987:359.

Fahn S, Marsden CD, Calne DB. Classification and investigation of dystonia. In: Marsden CD, Fahn S, eds. Movement disorders 2. London: Butterworths, 1987:332.

Jankovic J. The neurology of tics. In: Marsden CD, Fahn S, eds. Movement disorders 2. London: Butterworths, 1987:359.

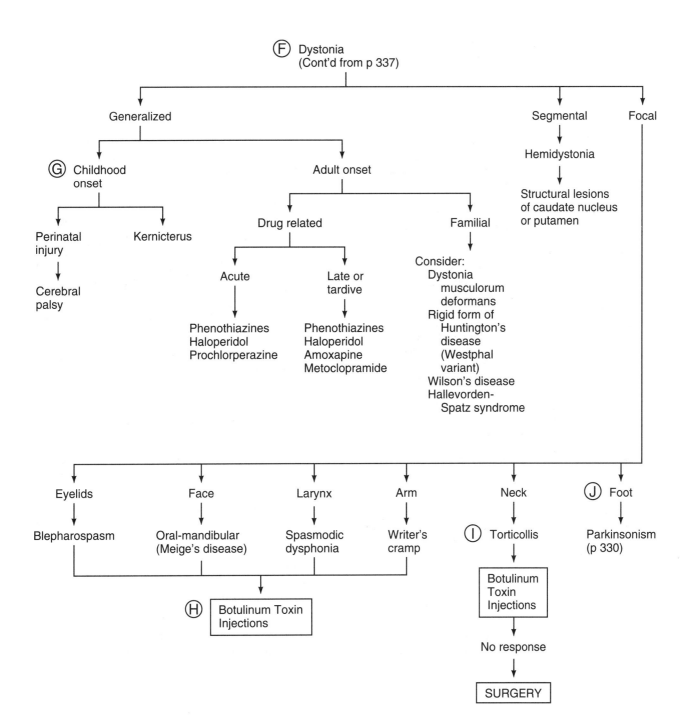

F Dystonia
(Cont'd from p 337)

Generalized

Segmental

Focal

G Childhood onset

Adult onset

Hemidystonia

Structural lesions of caudate nucleus or putamen

Perinatal injury

Kernicterus

Cerebral palsy

Drug related

Familial

Acute

Late or tardive

Consider:
  Dystonia
    musculorum
    deformans
  Rigid form of
    Huntington's
    disease
    (Westphal
    variant)
  Wilson's disease
  Hallevorden-
    Spatz syndrome

Phenothiazines
Haloperidol
Prochlorperazine

Phenothiazines
Haloperidol
Amoxapine
Metoclopramide

Eyelids

Face

Larynx

Arm

Neck

J Foot

Blepharospasm

Oral-mandibular (Meige's disease)

Spasmodic dysphonia

Writer's cramp

I Torticollis

Parkinsonism (p 330)

H Botulinum Toxin Injections

Botulinum Toxin Injections

No response

SURGERY

339

MUSCLE CRAMPS AND ACHES

Lawrence Z. Stern, M.D.

Cramps are sudden, episodic, involuntary, painful contractions of a muscle or part of a muscle that last from seconds to several minutes. Ordinary cramps may occur spontaneously at rest, but more often they are precipitated by a brief muscle contraction. They are caused by a hyperexcitability of the motor neurons supplying the muscle. Such cramps are distinguished from those more correctly termed contractures, seen in certain metabolic myopathies such as phosphorylase deficiency (McArdle disease). Contractures are usually associated with intense or ischemic exercise and are due to depletion of muscle energy stores. They are often associated with myoglobinuria. In many cases the reason for recurrent cramps remains unclear even after a complete diagnostic evaluation. Treatment with quinine sulfate is often helpful in controlling nocturnal cramps. Frequent daytime cramps may respond to carbamazepine or phenytoin. The initial history should elicit whether the cramps occur with exercise or at rest.

A. In children and pregnant women, leg cramps tend to occur at rest, often at night, after unusual daytime activity, and especially when the feet are cold. The neurologic examination and serum enzyme levels (creatine kinase and aldolase) are normal. These usually require no treatment.

B. Cramps occurring at rest or precipitated by minor exercise increase in frequency under certain conditions and in certain diseases. These should be excluded by appropriate inquiries and laboratory examinations. The cramps usually respond well to correction of the underlying problem.

C. Frequent cramps occurring during or after exercise require detailed investigation, including a complete history, neurologic examination, and serum enzyme level tests. Muscle biopsy should include histochemistry, electron microscopy, and appropriate biochem-

ical studies. It should be preceded by electromyography and a forearm ischemic exercise test, including determinations of serum lactate, pyruvate, and ammonia.

D. Exercise intolerance, along with cramps or myalgia, characterizes this group of hereditary disorders. All but the last two listed involve abnormalities of glycogen or glucose metabolism. Carnitine palmityl transferase deficiency results in a disorder of lipid metabolism more frequently associated with muscle soreness or aching than with cramps. With the exception of myoadenylate deaminase deficiency, all these disorders commonly result in myoglobinuria after especially strenuous exercise.

E. Cramps, and other entities that may be confused with cramps, occur in a variety of neurologic and neuromuscular disorders. Because investigations required to evaluate the diagnostic possibilities vary from patient to patient, such cases are usually best handled by a neurologist. Many of the conditions are treatable.

F. Leg pain and cramps in adults that are precipitated by exercise and promptly relieved by rest are often due to peripheral vascular disease. When surgical treatment is feasible, results are usually excellent.

References

Joekes AM. Cramp: a review. J R Soc Med 1982; 75:546.
Layzer RB. Motor unit hyperactivity states. In: Vinken PJ, Bruyn GW, eds. Handbook of clinical neurology. Amsterdam: North Holland, 1979; 41:295.
Layzer RB, Rowland LP. Cramps. N Engl J Med 1971; 285:31.
Sumi SM, Ruff RL, Swanson PD. Motor disturbances. In: Swanson PD, ed. Signs and symptoms in neurology. Philadelphia: JB Lippincott, 1984:168.

Patient with MUSCLE CRAMPS AND ACHES

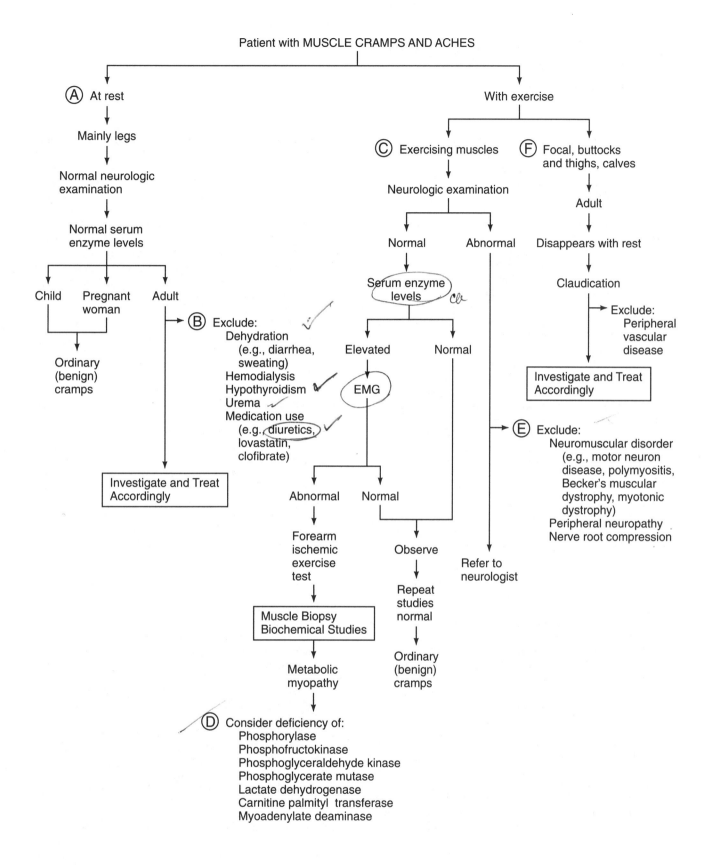

(A) At rest

Mainly legs

Normal neurologic examination

Normal serum enzyme levels

Child   Pregnant woman   Adult

Ordinary (benign) cramps

(B) Exclude:
Dehydration (e.g., diarrhea, sweating)
Hemodialysis
Hypothyroidism
Urema
Medication use (e.g., diuretics, lovastatin, clofibrate)

Investigate and Treat Accordingly

(C) Exercising muscles

Neurologic examination

Normal   Abnormal

Serum enzyme levels

Elevated   Normal

EMG

Abnormal   Normal

Forearm ischemic exercise test

Muscle Biopsy Biochemical Studies

Metabolic myopathy

(D) Consider deficiency of:
Phosphorylase
Phosphofructokinase
Phosphoglyceraldehyde kinase
Phosphoglycerate mutase
Lactate dehydrogenase
Carnitine palmityl transferase
Myoadenylate deaminase

Observe

Repeat studies normal

Ordinary (benign) cramps

Refer to neurologist

(E) Exclude:
Neuromuscular disorder (e.g., motor neuron disease, polymyositis, Becker's muscular dystrophy, myotonic dystrophy)
Peripheral neuropathy
Nerve root compression

(F) Focal, buttocks and thighs, calves

Adult

Disappears with rest

Claudication

Exclude:
Peripheral vascular disease

Investigate and Treat Accordingly

ACUTE BEHAVIOR CHANGE

Geoffrey L. Ahern, M.D., Ph.D.

Acute behavior change is often considered synonymous with the term acute confusional state. Other labels encountered include delirium, toxic-metabolic encephalopathy, and organic brain syndrome. The dominant feature of these states is a combination of confusion and inattention. Other higher-cortical functions can also be impaired. The most common causes of acute confusional states lie outside the CNS, such as metabolic derangements, toxins, drugs and medications. Pathologic processes in the CNS can also produce the syndrome, as may primary psychiatric illnesses that impair higher-order attention and concentration.

The approach to patients with acute behavioral change should begin with a careful history, although many patients are so confused that little or no useful information can be obtained. In this circumstance, one must depend on clinical examination and laboratory testing and history obtained from family or other observers. The mental status examination should focus on the attentional matrix (e.g., digit span, reciting days of the week or months of the year forward and backward, word list generation). Particularly pertinent aspects of the neurologic examination include looking for evidence of metabolic derangement, such as asterixis, myoclonus, or exaggerated postural tremor. Pay attention also to findings such as hemiparesis, visual field defects, asymmetric reflexes, upgoing toes, or hemineglect, indicative of focal CNS lesions that may produce confusional states. When the history is virtually unobtainable and the clinical examination does not point to a clear precipitant, one may have to resort to laboratory tests to find the cause(s) of the presenting condition.

A. Vascular disease may cause acute changes in mental status. Focal lesions in higher-order association cortex may result in confusion and agitation; specific sites of pathology include right frontal and parietal lobes, as well as mesial temporal-occipital lesions in either hemisphere. Mass lesions of different types (e.g., tumors, subdural hematomas, abscesses) may produce a picture similar to that of a cerebrovascular event. Also keep in mind the possibility of transient global amnesia (p 312). In young patients, migraine may present with confusion, with or without headache or other focal neurologic findings.

B. Patients with mild traumatic brain injury may present with transient loss of consciousness (concussion) with or without residual problems with higher-order attention, concentration, and memory (postconcussion syndrome). When brain tissue has been damaged (e.g., by contusion), more permanent deficits may obtain; the profile of cognitive deficits will depend on which areas are involved. More severe cases may result in coma; in these, early intervention should center on intensive care issues. Especially in the elderly, even trivial injuries may result in subdural hematoma.

C. Exogenous substances may cause a toxic confusional state. Medications (particularly those with prominent anticholinergic effects) may adversely affect cognitive function. Street drugs should be considered in appropriate populations or circumstances. Alcohol's effects on mentation may result from chronic intoxication, alcoholic dementia, alcohol withdrawal, Wernicke's encephalopathy, and/or Korsakoff's psychosis. Elimination of alcoholic intake is important, but do not forget to administer thiamine and benzodiazepines in the acute period to prevent the emergence of Wernicke-Korsakoff syndrome and alcoholic withdrawal symptoms, respectively. Toxic agents include organic chemical substances (e.g., insecticides), heavy metals, and carbon monoxide. Reduction of further environmental exposure and of the body's burden of toxic agent should be the therapeutic goal.

D. Confusional states may be secondary to metabolic derangements resulting from systemic illness. The potential causes are legion and include thyroid, hepatic, renal, and endocrine dysfunction. Any condition leading to hypoxia or ischemia may also lead to a confusional state. A chronic confusional state may result if the underlying illness cannot be brought under control. A related concept is that of beclouded dementia, in which a patient with a known dementing illness becomes acutely worse during periods of intercurrent systemic illness. In both cases, make a vigorous attempt to find the underlying cause and treat it.

E. Signs and symptoms compatible with systemic or CNS infection should prompt a search for the cause(s). Bacterial and viral agents are more likely to cause acute behavioral changes than fungal agents. CNS abscesses and infected subdurals should also be considered in certain instances. Perform lumbar puncture when indicated.

F. When a patient with a known seizure disorder presents with confusion, consider the possibility of a postictal state. Medication effects may also be responsible for confusion. Alterations in consciousness may result from absence or complex partial seizures. In the extreme case (e.g., nonconvulsive status epilepticus), full consciousness may not be regained and a state resembling a fugue may result. If there is doubt about the diagnosis, obtain an EEG.

G. Patients with known psychiatric conditions may present with confusion or inattention as the main feature. Diagnoses such as anxiety, depression, and psychotic disorders, especially acute mania, may produce inattention. Appropriate consultation and treatment is indicated.

Patient with ACUTE BEHAVIOR CHANGE

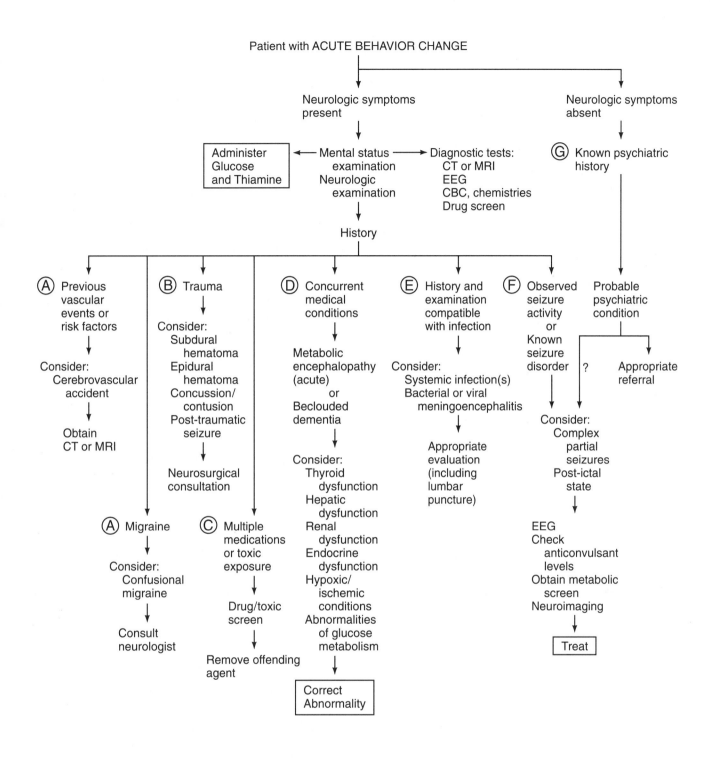

References

Cummings JL. Dissociative states, depersonalization, multiple personality, and episodic memory lapses. In: Cummings JL, ed. Clinical neuropsychiatry. Orlando: Grune & Stratton, 1985:117.

Lipowski ZJ. Delirium: acute confusional states. New York: Oxford University Press, 1990.

Mesulam MM. Attention, confusional states, and neglect. In: Mesulam MM, ed. Principles of behavioral neurology. Philadelphia: FA Davis, 1985:125.

CHRONIC BEHAVIOR CHANGE

Geoffrey L. Ahern, M.D., Ph.D.

Chronic behavior change may in many instances be considered synonymous with dementia. Dementia itself may be defined as a progressive deterioration in mental function that interferes with activities of daily living appropriate for one's age and background. Any or all areas of mental function may be affected (e.g., language, memory, visuospatial skills, calculation, praxis, gnosis, judgment, behavioral comportment). The persistence of the deficits differentiates dementia from acute confusional state or delirium (see p 342). While many of the dementias are progressive, some are not (e.g., post-traumatic and other static lesion etiologies, psychiatric causes). The list of potential causes of chronic behavior change is lengthy, but it is important to arrive at a correct diagnosis, as some dementing illnesses are treatable. Intelligent use of the mental status and neurologic examinations, in conjunction with a good history and judicious use of laboratory tests, should allow the clinician to reach a reasonably firm diagnosis in many cases.

A. Laboratory evaluation of patients with chronic behavior change goes hand in hand with the history and neurologic examination. Avoid a "shotgun" approach; rather, select tests based on the most likely causes, given the history and examination. Nevertheless, the elements of what might constitute a dementia screening battery are presented for the sake of completeness. Abnormalities in some of these tests may point to a potentially reversible cause of dementia.

B. If mental status testing reveals deficits in specific higher-cortical functions, one may be dealing with senile dementia of the Alzheimer type (SDAT). This is the most commonly diagnosed form (approximately 50%) of dementia. It usually presents in the sixth to eighth decades with an insidious and steady progression, usually starting with problems in memory (especially short-term), language (especially anomia), and orientation/judgment (e.g., getting lost, behaving inappropriately). It then progresses over 6–10 years to ultimately involve all areas of mental function. The elemental neurologic examination is relatively preserved until late in the illness. The far less common Pick's disease may present with inappropriate and bizarre behavior or apathy in the absence of amnesia, aphasia, or agnosia. This may lead to erroneous primary psychiatric diagnoses. The neuropathologic process in SDAT preferentially affects the parietotemporal regions (and the frontal lobes to a lesser extent), while in Pick's disease the frontal and temporal lobes bear the brunt of the damage. These changes may be reflected in atrophy seen in these regions in either CT or MRI scans. There is no cure for either of these entities, but low-dose neuroleptics, benzodiazepines, or other psychopharmacologic agents may help achieve behavioral control.

C. When the clinical presentation is characterized by slowed mental processes, forgetfulness (rather than true amnesia), dilapidated cognition, hypophonic or dysarthric speech, and apathetic or depressed appearance, the two principal diagnostic entities to consider are depression or the dementia that may be associated with one of the extrapyramidal syndromes such as Parkinson's disease (PD), Huntington's disease (HD), or progressive supranuclear palsy (PSP). Some useful points in differentiating the two groups are a compatible history and clinical signs (e.g., vegetative signs) and a relatively nonfocal neurologic examination in depression, contrasted with the characteristic motor system findings in the extrapyramidal syndromes (e.g., bradykinesia, rigidity, and tremor in PD; choreoathetosis in HD; and eye movement abnormalities in PSP). In certain instances, however, the differentiation may be difficult, and one may have to resort to a trial of empiric therapy with antidepressants or agents that affect the extrapyramidal system (e.g., amantadine, levodopa, bromocriptine, and selegiline in PD; neuroleptics in HD).

D. When elements of both B and C are present, the differential diagnosis includes a number of possible entities. In younger patients, consider demyelinating diseases (e.g., multiple sclerosis), degenerative diseases (usually genetic), and vasculitic syndromes (e.g., systemic lupus erythematosus). Appropriate laboratory studies, in conjunction with the clinical history and presentation, should lead to a diagnosis. In older patients the neurologic examination may lead to the correct diagnosis. Multi-infarct dementia may show elements characteristic of SDAT, the extrapyramidal dementias, or both, depending on the areas involved. Stepwise progression, a pseudobulbar syndrome, and focal neurologic deficits are sometimes found. Mass lesions may produce focal neurologic deficits as well as signs of increased intracranial pressure (ICP). Myoclonus may suggest Jakob-Creutzfeldt disease, a slow viral infection; the EEG, which may demonstrate periodic discharges, may be useful in these cases. The triad of dementia, incontinence, and ataxic gait should raise the question of normal-pressure hydrocephalus. Neuroimaging may demonstrate enlarged ventricles; cisternography may show ventricular reflux and retarded clearance of the radioisotope. Removal of CSF by spinal tap may result in transient improvement in the symptoms. Obtain neurosurgical consultation to see whether a shunt procedure is indicated.

(Continued on page 346)

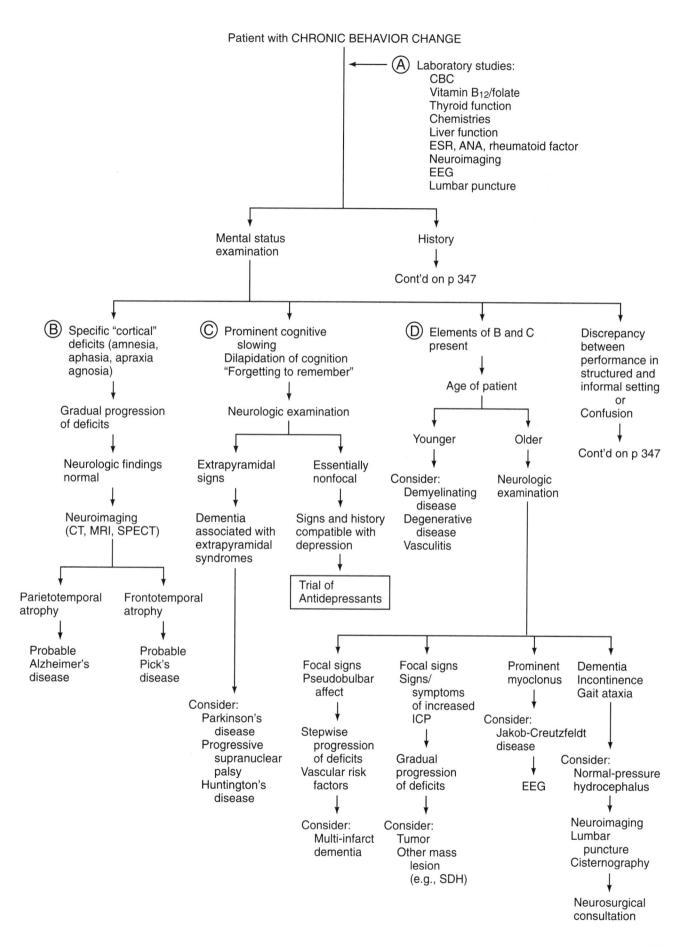

Patient with CHRONIC BEHAVIOR CHANGE

A Laboratory studies:
　　CBC
　　Vitamin B$_{12}$/folate
　　Thyroid function
　　Chemistries
　　Liver function
　　ESR, ANA, rheumatoid factor
　　Neuroimaging
　　EEG
　　Lumbar puncture

Mental status examination

History

Cont'd on p 347

B Specific "cortical" deficits (amnesia, aphasia, apraxia agnosia)

Gradual progression of deficits

Neurologic findings normal

Neuroimaging (CT, MRI, SPECT)

Parietotemporal atrophy

Probable Alzheimer's disease

Frontotemporal atrophy

Probable Pick's disease

C Prominent cognitive slowing
Dilapidation of cognition
"Forgetting to remember"

Neurologic examination

Extrapyramidal signs

Dementia associated with extrapyramidal syndromes

Consider:
　Parkinson's disease
　Progressive supranuclear palsy
　Huntington's disease

Essentially nonfocal

Signs and history compatible with depression

Trial of Antidepressants

D Elements of B and C present

Age of patient

Younger

Consider:
　Demyelinating disease
　Degenerative disease
　Vasculitis

Older

Neurologic examination

Focal signs
Pseudobulbar affect

Stepwise progression of deficits
Vascular risk factors

Consider:
　Multi-infarct dementia

Focal signs
Signs/symptoms of increased ICP

Gradual progression of deficits

Consider:
　Tumor
　Other mass lesion (e.g., SDH)

Prominent myoclonus

Consider:
　Jakob-Creutzfeldt disease

EEG

Dementia
Incontinence
Gait ataxia

Consider:
　Normal-pressure hydrocephalus

Neuroimaging
Lumbar puncture
Cisternography

Neurosurgical consultation

Discrepancy between performance in structured and informal setting
or
Confusion

Cont'd on p 347

E. In hysterical dementia, the examiner may observe a marked discrepancy between the patient's relatively normal performance in informal settings and poor performance in structured testing situations. Ganser's syndrome is a related variant in which patients may respond to questions with ridiculous or approximate answers. Make appropriate referral to a behavioral neurologist or neuropsychiatrist.

F. When the dominant clinical picture is one of confusion, look for signs of systemic illness or the ingestion of toxic substances. Confusional states may be secondary to systemic illness leading to metabolic derangements. The potential causes are legion (see p 342). A chronic confusional state may result if the underlying illness is not, or cannot be, brought under control. A related concept is that of beclouded dementia, in which a patient with a known dementing illness becomes acutely worse during periods of intercurrent systemic illness. In both cases a vigorous attempt should be made to find the underlying cause and treat it. Exogenous substances may also result in a toxic confusional state. Medications and drugs (prescription or otherwise) may frequently cause cognitive difficulties; agents known to do this should be eliminated from the patient's regimen, if at all possible. Alcohol's effects on mentation may result from chronic intoxication, alcoholic dementia, alcohol withdrawal, Wernicke's encephalopathy, or Korsakoff's psychosis. Elimination of alcoholic intake is important, but do not forget to administer thiamine and benzodiazepines in the acute period to prevent the emergence of the Wernicke-Korsakoff syndrome and alcoholic withdrawal symptoms, respectively. Also, do not overlook the effects of trauma (e.g., subdural hematoma (SDH), contusion, post-traumatic epilepsy) in this population. Other classes of agents capable of inducing cognitive changes include heavy metals (e.g., arsenic, lead, thallium, manganese, mercury), organic agents (e.g., solvents and organophosphate insecticides), and carbon monoxide. Reduction of further environmental exposure and the body's burden of toxic agent should be the therapeutic goal.

G. Elements of the history may be particularly useful in arriving at a diagnosis. If trauma has occurred, consider the possibility of SDH. Contusions of the brain substance may occur as a result of trauma; the frontal and temporal regions of the brain are the most likely to be affected. Dementia pugilistica is a form of post-traumatic dementia that may be seen in boxers. If a history and examination compatible with CNS infection is obtained, consider meningoencephalitis. Nonbacterial forms (e.g., cryptococcal, tuberculous, neurosyphilis) may present with a relatively indolent course. Also, consider the AIDS dementia complex, if appropriate risk factors are present. Do not forget that HIV infection in the CNS may be accompanied by a number of "fellow travelers," including progressive multifocal leukoencephalopathy (PML), toxoplasmosis, and *Cryptococcus*.

References

Cummings JL, ed. Subcortical dementia. New York: Oxford, 1990.

Cummings JL, Benson DF. Dementia: a clinical approach. 2nd ed. Boston: Butterworth-Heinemann, 1992.

Joynt RJ, Shoulson I. Dementia. In: Heilman KM, Valenstein E, eds. Clinical neuropsychology. 2nd ed. New York: Oxford, 1985:453.

Signoret JL. Memory and amnesias. In: Mesulam MM, ed. Principles of behavioral neurology. Philadelphia: FA Davis, 1985:169.

Strub RL, Black FW. The mental status examination in neurology. 2nd ed. Philadelphia: FA Davis, 1985.

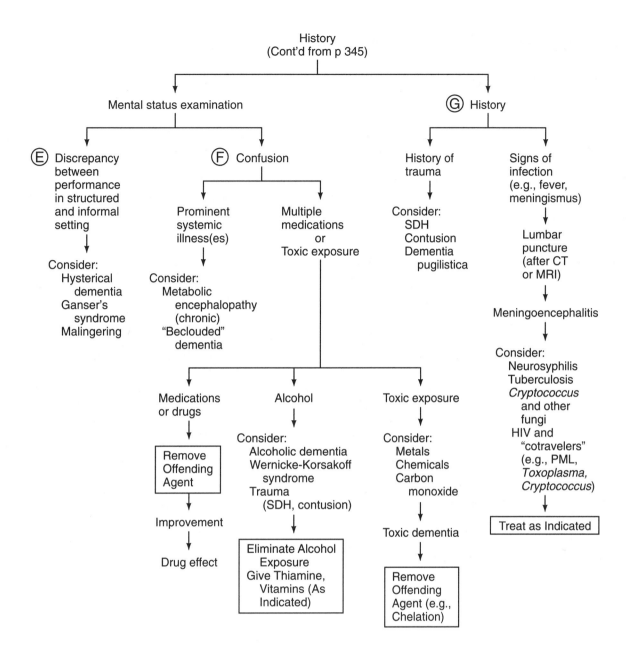

History
(Cont'd from p 345)

Mental status examination

Ⓔ Discrepancy between performance in structured and informal setting

Consider:
Hysterical dementia
Ganser's syndrome
Malingering

Ⓕ Confusion

Prominent systemic illness(es)

Consider:
Metabolic encephalopathy (chronic)
"Beclouded" dementia

Multiple medications or Toxic exposure

Medications or drugs

Remove Offending Agent

Improvement

Drug effect

Alcohol

Consider:
Alcoholic dementia
Wernicke-Korsakoff syndrome
Trauma (SDH, contusion)

Eliminate Alcohol Exposure
Give Thiamine, Vitamins (As Indicated)

Toxic exposure

Consider:
Metals
Chemicals
Carbon monoxide

Toxic dementia

Remove Offending Agent (e.g., Chelation)

Ⓖ History

History of trauma

Consider:
SDH
Contusion
Dementia pugilistica

Signs of infection (e.g., fever, meningismus)

Lumbar puncture (after CT or MRI)

Meningoencephalitis

Consider:
Neurosyphilis
Tuberculosis
Cryptococcus and other fungi
HIV and "cotravelers" (e.g., PML, *Toxoplasma*, *Cryptococcus*)

Treat as Indicated

DISTURBANCES OF SMELL AND TASTE

Eugenie A.M.T. Obbens, M.D.

Dysfunction of smell or taste usually is not a disease entity in itself, but part of a disease process. Both are somewhat obscure symptoms; loss of taste often is not noticed by the patient, especially when the onset is gradual. Loss of smell, on the other hand, may be attributed to changes in taste. Anosmia is the absence of smell sensation; dysosmia or parosmia is a distorted smell perception, either with or without an odorant stimulus present. Abnormalities in taste sensation are classified into ageusia (absence of taste perception) and dysgeusia (distortion of taste resulting in a persistent metallic, bitter, sour, sweet, or salty taste).

A. Congenital anosmia appears to be due to absence of olfactory epithelium. The most common congenital disorder is Kallmann's syndrome, in which there is agenesis of the olfactory bulbs in combination with hypogonadism and other developmental abnormalities.

B. Tumors implicated as a cause of anosmia are olfactory groove meningiomas, frontal lobe gliomas, and pituitary adenomas with suprasellar extension. Another cause is an aneurysm of the anterior cerebral or anterior communicating artery. Cigarette smoking has been demonstrated to cause progressive loss of smell in a dose-related manner, with a gradual restoration of smell perception once patients have stopped smoking. Medications affecting the sense of smell include opiate analgesics, beta blockers, and some antithyroid medications. Diseases such as chronic rhinitis and sinusitis, or conditions leading to nasal obstruction, are a common cause of decreased smell. Anosmia caused by these conditions is most amenable to treatment; if untreated, it may steadily worsen.

C. Anosmia may occur after even mild head trauma, especially after a blow to the occiput. It is thought to be caused by shearing of the olfactory filaments as they course through the cribriform plate. Although there is no treatment for post-traumatic loss of smell, gradual recovery of smell function occurs in about one third of patients. The olfactory bulbs and its nerves can be damaged during subfrontal craniotomy, or as the result of a subarachnoid hemorrhage, meningitis at the base of the skull, or a frontal lobe abscess. Sudden loss of smell, and sometimes also of taste, may occur after an upper respiratory infection. This is more common in older patients and is thought to be due to viral damage of the olfactory mucosa. Recovery, if it occurs at all, may take years.

D. Uncinate fits, a form of temporal lobe seizures, consist of brief periods of unpleasant or foul odor perception, together with an alteration of consciousness. The diagnosis can be confirmed with EEG, and the seizures treated with anticonvulsant medication. Olfactory hallucinations have also been described with psychiatric illness such as endogenous depression, schizophrenia, Alzheimer's dementia, and alcohol withdrawal.

E. A unilateral loss of taste on the anterior two thirds of the tongue can be found in Bell's palsy and is due to involvement of the chorda tympani. Loss of taste due to head injury is less common than loss of smell. It may be unilateral or bilateral, presumably caused by damage to the chorda tympani. Patients with diabetes mellitus frequently have a decreased sensation of sweet, bitter, and sour flavors. This is more common in patients with long-standing diabetes and in those with associated diabetic neuropathy.

F. Oral disorders causing taste disturbances include oral candidiasis, lichen planus, leukoplakia, carcinoma of the tongue, and other tongue afflictions; xerostomia and sialoadenitis; and palatal clefts and facial hypoplasia. Periodontal disease and other infectious processes may produce abnormal oral secretions, resulting in taste changes. Dental restorations or prostheses can give a metallic taste, while dentures may block taste reception. Medications responsible for taste changes are numerous: antibiotics, antifungal agents, anti-inflammatory drugs, cytotoxic agents, and many cardiovascular drugs. Gustatory hallucinations may be part of a temporal lobe seizure, as well as manifestations of other temporoparietal dysfunctions.

References

Barwick MC. Neurological evaluation of taste and smell disorders. Ear Nose Throat J 1989; 68:354.

Frye RE, Schwartz BS, Doty RL. Dose-related effects of cigarette smoking on olfactory function. JAMA 1990; 263:1233.

Jafek BW, Gordon ASD, Moran DT, Eller PM. Congenital anosmia. Ear Nose Throat J 1990; 69:331.

Kadi J, Greer RO, Jafek BW. Oral evaluation of patients with chemosensory disorders. Ear Nose Throat J 1989; 68:373.

Le Floch J-P, Le Lievre G, Sadoun J, et al. Taste impairment and related factors in type I diabetes mellitus. Diabetes Care 1989; 12:173.

Scott AE. Clinical characteristics of taste and smell disorders. Ear Nose Throat J 1989; 68:297.

Scott AE. Medical management of taste and smell disorders. Ear Nose Throat J 1989; 68:386.

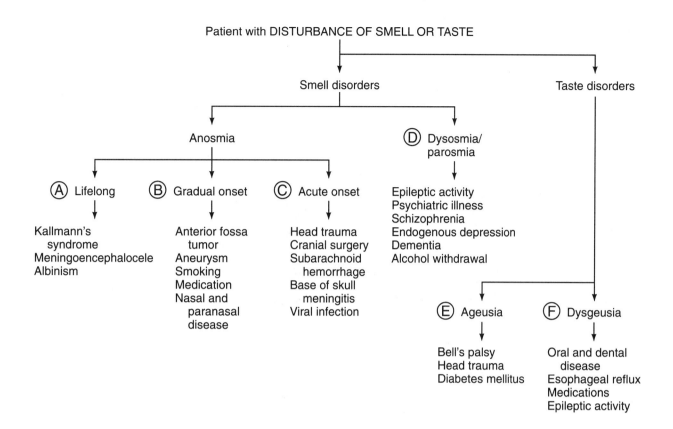

Patient with DISTURBANCE OF SMELL OR TASTE

Smell disorders

Taste disorders

Anosmia

Ⓓ Dysosmia/
parosmia

Epileptic activity
Psychiatric illness
Schizophrenia
Endogenous depression
Dementia
Alcohol withdrawal

Ⓐ Lifelong

Ⓑ Gradual onset

Ⓒ Acute onset

Kallmann's
    syndrome
Meningoencephalocele
Albinism

Anterior fossa
    tumor
Aneurysm
Smoking
Medication
Nasal and
    paranasal
    disease

Head trauma
Cranial surgery
Subarachnoid
    hemorrhage
Base of skull
    meningitis
Viral infection

Ⓔ Ageusia

Ⓕ Dysgeusia

Bell's palsy
Head trauma
Diabetes mellitus

Oral and dental
    disease
Esophageal reflux
Medications
Epileptic activity

SLEEP DISTURBANCE

Colin R. Bamford, M.D.

Sleep disorders can be conveniently divided into those that alter the quantity of sleep during the 24-hour day and those that alter the characteristics of sleep without affecting its quantity.

The decision trees provided are not intended to be all-inclusive. Further details about diagnostic possibilities can be obtained by referring to the ASDC's Diagnostic Classification of Sleep and Arousal Disorders.

A. Although not carried out in this order, the most to the least productive components of the sleep evaluation are history taking, polysomnography (PSG), multiple sleep latency tests (MSLTs), the sleep diary, a formal psychological evaluation, and finally the physical examination. History taking, aside from eliciting details of the presenting complaint, should include a description of a typical night of sleep, daytime performance, intercurrent illnesses, and the ingestion of psychoactive drugs.

B. The complaint of getting too little sleep is called insomnia and the respective diagnosis should generally be listed under the category "Disorders of initiation and maintenance of sleep." Appropriate questions to ask are: "Does your sleep disturbance decrease the number of hours you sleep?" and "Does your sleep disturbance disrupt the quality of your sleep?"

(Continued on page 352)

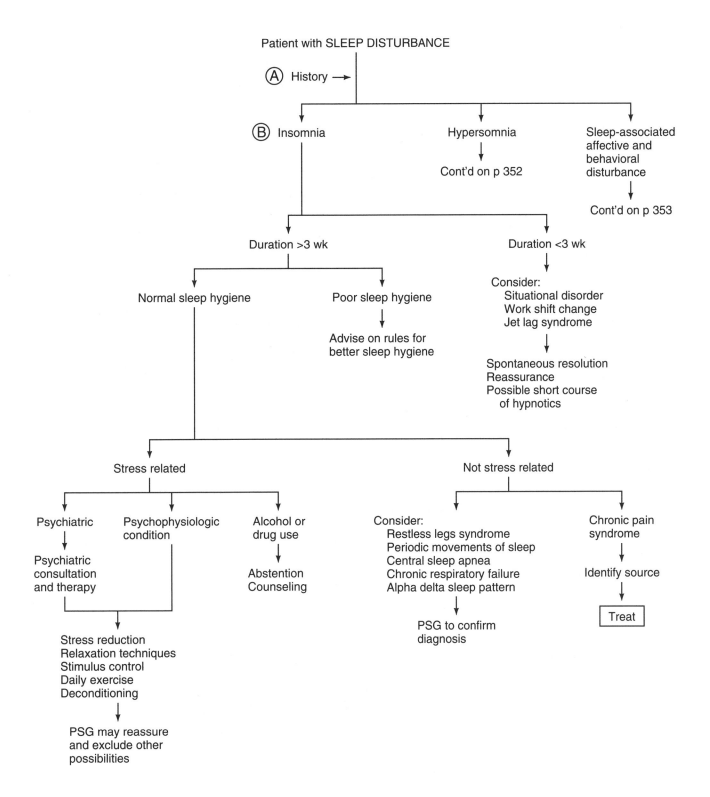

Patient with SLEEP DISTURBANCE

(A) History →

(B) Insomnia

Hypersomnia

Cont'd on p 352

Sleep-associated
affective and
behavioral
disturbance

Cont'd on p 353

Duration >3 wk

Duration <3 wk

Normal sleep hygiene

Poor sleep hygiene

Advise on rules for
better sleep hygiene

Consider:
   Situational disorder
   Work shift change
   Jet lag syndrome

Spontaneous resolution
Reassurance
Possible short course
   of hypnotics

Stress related

Not stress related

Psychiatric

Psychophysiologic
condition

Alcohol or
drug use

Psychiatric
consultation
and therapy

Abstention
Counseling

Stress reduction
Relaxation techniques
Stimulus control
Daily exercise
Deconditioning

PSG may reassure
and exclude other
possibilities

Consider:
   Restless legs syndrome
   Periodic movements of sleep
   Central sleep apnea
   Chronic respiratory failure
   Alpha delta sleep pattern

PSG to confirm
diagnosis

Chronic pain
syndrome

Identify source

Treat

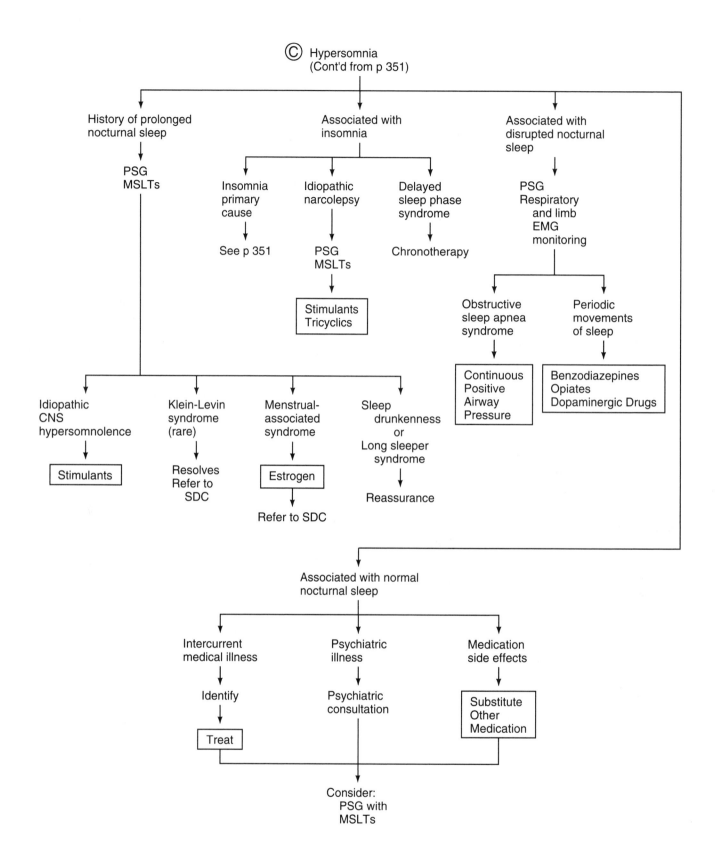

C. The complaint of excessive daytime sleepiness is called hypersomnia and the appropriate diagnosis should be listed under the category "Disorders of excessive sleepiness." Ask patients whether the sleepiness impairs their daytime performance, safety, or emotional state. Although insomnia is the most common sleep disorder in the general population, hypersomnia is the predominant problem seen in a sleep disorders clinic (SDC).

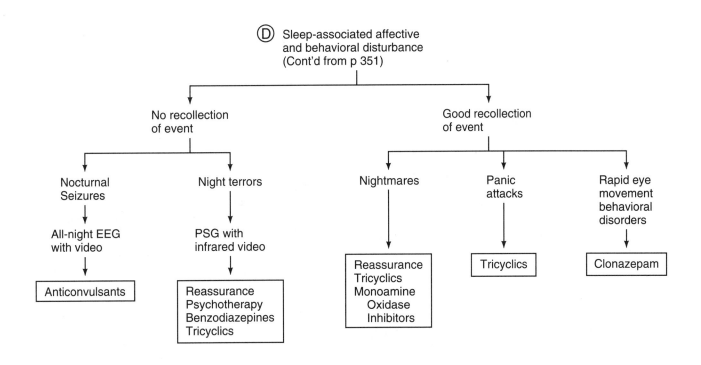

D. Conditions that do not affect the quantity of sleep include those that affect the timing of sleep (disorders of the sleep-wake schedule) and those that alter sleep behavior (dysfunctions that are associated with sleep, sleep stages, or partial arousals—parasomnias).

References

Association of Sleep Disorders Centers. Diagnostic classification of sleep and arousal disorders. 1st ed. Sleep Disorders Classification Committee, HP Roffwarg, chairman. Sleep 1979; 2:1.

Bixler EO, Kales A, Soldatos CR. Sleep disorders encountered in medical practice: a national survey of physicians. Behav Med 1979; 6:1.

Kales A, Soldatos CR, Kales JD. Sleep disorders: evaluation and management in the office setting. In: Arieti S, ed. American handbook of psychiatry. 2nd ed. Vol 7. New York: Basic Books 1981:423.

COMA

Geoffrey L. Ahern, M.D., Ph.D.

The causes of coma may be broadly categorized into four main groups: (1) supratentorial lesions (including subarachnoid hemorrhage and meningitis) that produce increased intracranial pressure and thereby cause dysfunction of the reticular activating system, (2) infratentorial lesions that affect the reticular activating system directly, (3) toxic-metabolic encephalopathies that affect the neuraxis diffusely, and (4) status epilepticus. The roles of the primary care physician include stabilizing patient's vital functions, initiating evaluation with the aim of being able to characterize the coma into one of the four groups, and instituting appropriate treatment.

A. The primary goal is to stabilize the patient. This involves the ABCs (airway, breathing, circulation) of basic life support. Place IV, nasogastric, and urinary catheters. Endotracheal intubation may be necessary. Glucose (with thiamine) and naloxone should be administered after blood is drawn for CBC, chemistries, toxic screen, and blood gases.

B. Next, assess the depth of coma, using the Glasgow Coma Scale (Table 1).

C. A history or signs of trauma can provide useful information. Palpate the skull for fractures/hematomas and look for Battle's sign (ecchymosis over the mastoid), raccoon eyes (ecchymosis around the eyes), hemotympanum, and CSF leaks from the nose or ears. From the very beginning, neck trauma *must* be considered and evaluated. This pertains not only to the performance of the examination, but to such manipulations as moving the patient and endotracheal intubation. If trauma is present, obtain neuroimaging. CT may be preferable to MRI for its ability to detect acute blood and bone abnormalities. Obtain neurosurgical consultation. The presence of trauma does not preclude the possibility of other concurrent processes (vide infra).

D. A nonfocal examination should raise suspicion of a toxic or metabolic etiology. Dysfunction in virtually any bodily system may lead to acute and chronic confusional states or even coma. Also, consider drug ingestion and toxic exposure. In most cases, metabolic dysfunction does not result in nonreactive pupils or focal signs. However, atropine-like substances and gluthethimide abolish pupillary reactivity; in opiate overdose, the pupils may be so constricted that a very bright light and a magnifying glass may be needed to observe any reactivity. Toxic-metabolic insults may also result in seizures and lateralizing neurologic signs that wax and wane or even shift from side to side. Extensor plantar responses may also be seen. On the other hand, metabolic causes of coma (especially intoxication) may obscure signs of an underlying focal

lesion. In practice, therefore, neuroimaging is performed in most patients presenting with coma.

E. When a focal lesion is responsible for coma, it may be useful to try to localize the lesion to a supratentorial or infratentorial location. The examination should emphasize appendicular movement (e.g., symmetric versus asymmetric responses, decorticate/decerebrate posturing), stretch reflexes, pupillary response (size, asymmetry, reactivity), eye movement abnormalities (including doll's eyes), brain-stem reflexes (e.g., corneal reflex), and respiratory pattern (e.g., Cheyne-Strokes, central neurogenic hyperventilation, ataxic and apneustic breathing, "fish mouthing"). Rostro-caudal deterioration of CNS function is reflected in a characteristic set of responses in each of these areas. A complete exposition of the abnormalities observed with lesions in different areas is beyond the scope of this chapter (any of the texts listed below provide the information necessary to interpret these findings). The key is to have the examination information available for consultations with neurologists and/or neurosurgeons.

F. Signs of meningism include nuchal rigidity and Kernig's and Brudzinski's signs. Such findings may accompany either a nonfocal or focal examination. In the former, they may reflect subarachnoid hemorrhage or meningitis. In the latter, mass lesions may lead to meningismus either because of meningeal irritation per se (e.g., parenchymal hemorrhage with rupture into the subarachnoid space) or because they produce increased intracranial pressure, which in turn may lead to herniation of the cerebellar tonsils (e.g., cerebellar hemorrhage). Perform lumbar puncture (probably after a CT scan), looking for evidence of blood, xanthochromia, or infection. Note that up to 15% of subarachnoid hemorrhages are missed by CT. Further, signs of meningismus may be absent in deep coma, so consider lumbar puncture if the history suggests an infectious etiology.

G. Prolonged or sustained seizure activity (i.e., status epilepticus) may lead to impaired consciousness. Seizures may also reflect an underlying process that itself leads to coma. Observe patients carefully for evidence of seizure activity. Focal seizures suggest a focal source. Generalized seizures or myoclonus may be caused by toxic-metabolic abnormalities. These rules are not absolute. Laboratory investigation should consider anticonvulsant levels as well as metabolic parameters. EEG may be useful not only to assess seizure activity, but to look for abnormalities compatible with metabolic abnormalities or focal lesions. Neuroimaging is useful to look for underlying focal lesions. For treatment of status epilepticus, see page 320.

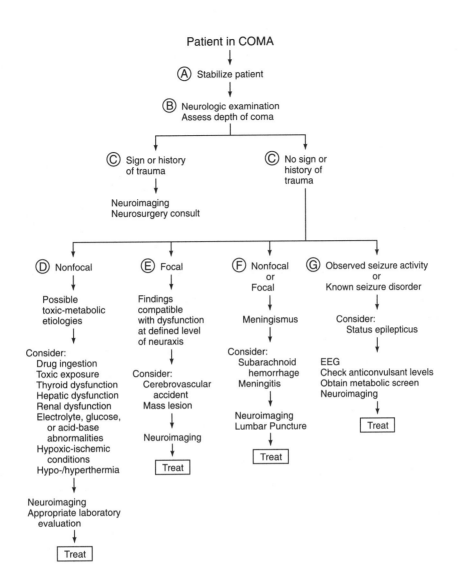

Patient in COMA

(A) Stabilize patient

(B) Neurologic examination
Assess depth of coma

(C) Sign or history
of trauma

Neuroimaging
Neurosurgery consult

(C) No sign or
history of
trauma

(D) Nonfocal

Possible
toxic-metabolic
etiologies

Consider:
Drug ingestion
Toxic exposure
Thyroid dysfunction
Hepatic dysfunction
Renal dysfunction
Electrolyte, glucose,
or acid-base
abnormalities
Hypoxic-ischemic
conditions
Hypo-/hyperthermia

Neuroimaging
Appropriate laboratory
evaluation

Treat

(E) Focal

Findings
compatible
with dysfunction
at defined level
of neuraxis

Consider:
Cerebrovascular
accident
Mass lesion

Neuroimaging

Treat

(F) Nonfocal
or
Focal

Meningismus

Consider:
Subarachnoid
hemorrhage
Meningitis

Neuroimaging
Lumbar Puncture

Treat

(G) Observed seizure activity
or
Known seizure disorder

Consider:
Status epilepticus

EEG
Check anticonvulsant levels
Obtain metabolic screen
Neuroimaging

Treat

TABLE 1   Glasgow Coma Scale

Function	Score*
Motor response	
Obeys	6
Localizes	5
Withdraws	4
Abnormal flexion	3
Extensor response	2
No response	1
Verbal response	
Oriented	5
Confused conversation	4
Inappropriate words	3
Incomprehensible sounds	2
No response	1
Eye opening	
Spontaneous	4
To command	3
To pain	2
No response	1

*The best score from each of the three areas is summed. Scores can range from 15 (essentially a normal examination) to 3 (no response in any area).

References

Adams RD, Victor M. Coma and related disorders of consciousness. In: Adams RD, Victor M, eds. Principles of Neurology. 4th ed. New York: McGraw-Hill, 1989:273.

Aquino TM, Samuels MA. Coma and other alterations in consciousness. In: Samuels MA, ed. Manual of neurology: diagnosis and therapy. 4th ed. Boston: Little, Brown, 1991:3.

Brust JCM. Coma. In: Rowland LP, ed. Merritt's textbook of neurology. 8th ed. Philadelphia: Lea & Febiger, 1989:21.

Gilroy J. Coma. In: Gilroy J, ed. Basic neurology. 2nd ed. New York: Pergamon, 1990:48.

Plum F, Posner J. The diagnosis of stupor and coma. 3rd ed. Philadelphia: FA Davis, 1980.

Teasdale G, Jennett B. Assessment of coma and impaired consciousness. A practical scale. Lancet 1974; 2:81.

BRAIN DEATH

William M. Feinberg, M.D.

Over the last 20 years the concept of brain death has become accepted by both medical and legal professions. In 1981 the President's Commission for the Study of Ethical Problems in Medicine and Biomedical and Behavioral Research issued a report on "Guidelines for the Determination of Death." This included a model statute called the "Uniform Determination of Death Act." This states: "An individual who has sustained either (1) irreversible cessation of circulatory and respiratory functions, or (2) irreversible cessation of all functions of the entire brain, including the brain stem, is dead. A determination of death must be made in determination with accepted medical standards." Most states now have statutes or judicial decisions recognizing this concept. Criteria given in the decision tree are valid for adults and children over 5 years of age.

A. Rule out reversible causes of cerebral depression. Body temperature must be >90° F (32.2° C). Profound metabolic or electrolyte disturbance cannot be present. Depressant drugs should not be present. Toxicology screens or measurement of serum drug levels may be required.

B. There should be no spontaneous respiration despite arterial P_{CO_2} >60 mm Hg. A suggested protocol for establishment of apnea follows: (1) There should be a stable hemodynamic and ventilatory status. The patient should be preoxygenated using an inspired oxygen tension of 100% for 15 minutes. Arterial P_{CO_2} should be adjusted to 40–45 mm Hg. (2) After an initial blood gas determination, place the patient on a T-piece with 6 L O_2/min via an endotracheal cannula. Monitor pulse oximetry. (3) After 2, 4, and 6 minutes, obtain an arterial blood gas. After 6 minutes return the patient to mechanical ventilation. The test should be terminated if spontaneous ventilation returns, if there is a fall in systolic blood pressure of >20 mm Hg, if heart rate increases by >20 bpm, or if arterial saturation falls below 80%. (4) An apnea test is positive if the patient achieves spontaneous ventilation. It is negative if the patient is apneic for the entire time and an arterial P_{CO_2} >60 mm Hg is achieved. The test is indeterminate if it is terminated early without achieving a P_{CO_2} of 60 mm Hg.

C. Ancillary studies such as EEG or cerebral radionuclide angiography may be confirmatory but are not required for the diagnosis of brain death.

References

Belsh JM, Blatt R, Schiffman PL. Apnea testing in brain death. Arch Intern Med 1986; 146:2385.

Benzel EC, Gross CD, Hadden TA, et al. The apnea test for the determination of brain death. J Neurosurg 1989; 71:191.

Guidelines for the determination of death: report of the medical consultants on the diagnosis of death to the President's Commission for the Study of Ethical Problems in Medicine and Biomedical and Behavioral Research. JAMA 1981; 246:2184.

Joynt RJ. A new look at death. JAMA 1984; 252:680.

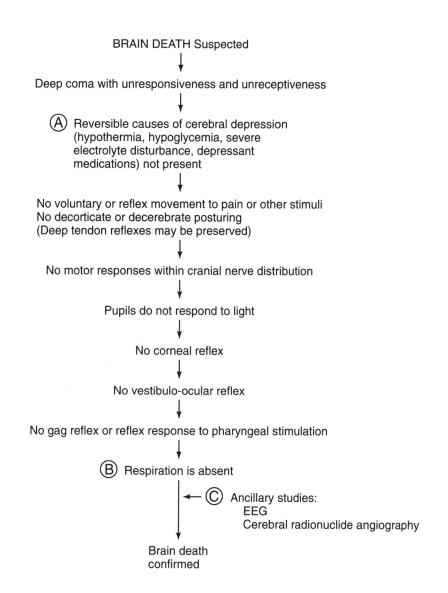

BRAIN DEATH Suspected

↓

Deep coma with unresponsiveness and unreceptiveness

↓

(A) Reversible causes of cerebral depression
(hypothermia, hypoglycemia, severe
electrolyte disturbance, depressant
medications) not present

↓

No voluntary or reflex movement to pain or other stimuli
No decorticate or decerebrate posturing
(Deep tendon reflexes may be preserved)

↓

No motor responses within cranial nerve distribution

↓

Pupils do not respond to light

↓

No corneal reflex

↓

No vestibulo-ocular reflex

↓

No gag reflex or reflex response to pharyngeal stimulation

↓

(B) Respiration is absent

← (C) Ancillary studies:
EEG
Cerebral radionuclide angiography

↓

Brain death
confirmed

PULMONARY DISEASE
HEMOPTYSIS

Anthony Camilli, M.D.

Hemoptysis is the expectoration of blood from the tracheobronchial tree. It ranges from trivial to life threatening in severity and has numerous causes. Disease processes that may result in hemoptysis include those of the pulmonary parenchyma and the airways, and infectious, inflammatory, and malignant disorders.

A. The history may suggest likely causes of hemoptysis. Patients with known bronchiectasis may have a history of a recent infective exacerbation. A history of valvular heart disease may indicate elevated pulmonary capillary pressure as a likely cause. Hemoptysis in an older smoker suggests the likelihood of a malignant lesion.

B. The chest film provides two important pieces of information in this setting. First, it may strongly suggest the bleeding source by showing a lesion with bleeding potential, such as a cavitary mass in the lower left lobe. It may also show the amount of associated hemorrhage into the lung via associated infiltrate.

C. The basic approach to hemoptysis depends on prompt assessment of its severity; this can range from a medical emergency to a problem that can be handled on an outpatient basis. Mild intermittent hemoptysis such as blood-streaked sputum can be evaluated by bronchoscopy, which should include the entire respiratory tract. Patients presenting with active bleeding but without impaired respiratory function can be treated for infection during quantitation of hemoptysis, reversal of coagulopathy, and optimizing the timing of bronchoscopy. Massive hemoptysis, usually defined as >600 ml in 24 hours, requires an emergent diagnostic/therapeutic approach. This may involve rigid bronchoscopy and protection of the nonhemorrhaging lung with a Fogarty catheter or endotracheal tube.

D. If hemoptysis is persistent despite treatment of presumed infection and supportive care, perform bronchial arteriography with embolization or resection of the involved segment or lobe if the source can be clearly identified. Bronchial artery embolization carries the risk of spinal cord infarction and the risk: benefit ratio must be carefully weighed.

References

Garzon AA, Gourin A. Surgical management of massive hemoptysis: a ten year experience. Ann Surg 1978; 187:267.

Poe RH, Isreal RH, Mari MG, et al. Utility of fiberoptic bronchoscopy in patient with hemoptysis and a nonlocalizing chest roentgenogram. Chest 1988; 93:70.

Wolfe JD, Simmons DH. Hemoptysis: diagnosis and management. West J Med 1977; 127:383.

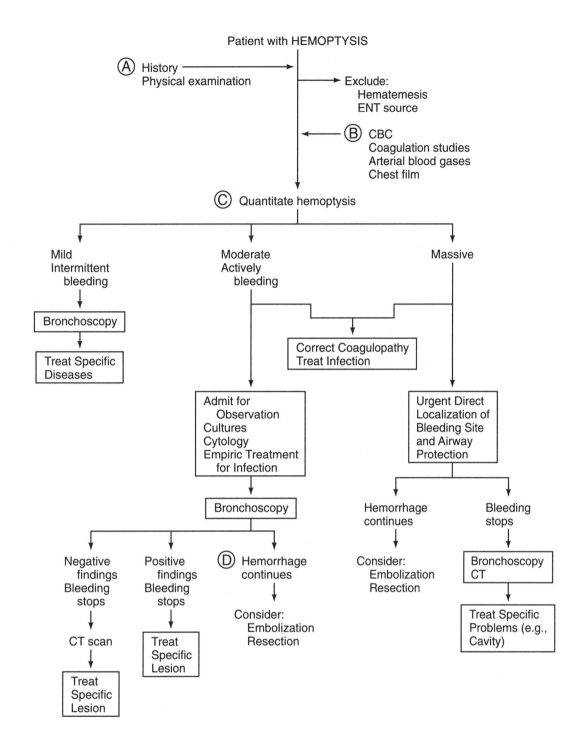

Patient with HEMOPTYSIS

Ⓐ History
Physical examination

Exclude:
Hematemesis
ENT source

Ⓑ CBC
Coagulation studies
Arterial blood gases
Chest film

Ⓒ Quantitate hemoptysis

Mild
Intermittent
bleeding

Bronchoscopy

Treat Specific
Diseases

Moderate
Actively
bleeding

Correct Coagulopathy
Treat Infection

Admit for
Observation
Cultures
Cytology
Empiric Treatment
for Infection

Bronchoscopy

Negative
findings
Bleeding
stops

CT scan

Treat
Specific
Lesion

Positive
findings
Bleeding
stops

Treat
Specific
Lesion

Ⓓ Hemorrhage
continues

Consider:
Embolization
Resection

Massive

Urgent Direct
Localization of
Bleeding Site
and Airway
Protection

Hemorrhage
continues

Consider:
Embolization
Resection

Bleeding
stops

Bronchoscopy
CT

Treat Specific
Problems (e.g.,
Cavity)

359

STRIDOR

Neil C. Clements, Jr., M.D.

Stridor is a continuous, monophonic upper airway sound heard predominantly during inspiration. Because it indicates upper airway obstruction, expedient management is essential.

A. Initial history should elicit the duration (minutes, hours, or days) and the severity of symptoms. Clinical evidence of impending respiratory failure (fatigue, cyanosis, poor chest wall excursion, mental status changes) mandates intubation or tracheostomy (see D below) before further diagnostic evaluation. All other patients with acute or subacute stridor also require constant observation in the intensive care unit. Provide symptomatic relief in these patients by administration of an inhaled mixture of helium and oxygen (heliox), during which specific diagnosis and treatment should be aggressively pursued.

B. Acute laryngospasm or laryngeal edema must be suspected after exposure to allergens; treat by subcutaneous injection of 0.5 ml of 0.1% epinephrine. Inhaled racemic epinephrine may also be useful and is also indicated in inhalation airway injury, along with intubation and surgical repair. Tracheal stenosis (e.g., from previous airway intubation) may respond to racemic epinephrine if there is coexistent inflammation or edema.

C. Consider foreign body aspiration in alcoholics, in those with neuromuscular or cerebral disorders that impair swallowing or airway protective reflexes, and in children. Inspection of the oropharynx may reveal obstructions that can easily be removed with forceps or by suction. When it is determined that the patient is stable, soft tissue roentgenography and CT of the chest may complement the chest roentgenographic diagnosis.

D. In severe cases, laryngoscopy and bronchoscopy in the operating room or intensive care unit may facilitate diagnosis. Intubation over the bronchoscope may be required when there is marked airway edema or when neck injury is suspected. Intubation by bronchoscopy, light wand, or laryngoscopy should always be performed by the most skilled available personnel.

E. Personnel skilled at tracheostomy should be present in case intubation cannot be successfully performed. Specific therapies include appropriate antibiotics or indicated surgery for infectious upper airway disorders. Achalasia may often be decompressed by nasogastric tube suction.

F. To localize the site of obstruction, stable patients may undergo chest and soft tissue neck radiography with continued cardiopulmonary monitoring, and a physician skilled in airway management in constant attendance.

References

Baughman RP, Loudon RG. Stridor: differentiation from asthma or upper airway noise. Am Rev Respir Dis 1989; 139:1407.

Hollingworth HM. Wheezing and stridor. Clin Chest Med 1987; 8:231.

Koster ME, Baughman RP, Loudon RG. Continuous adventitious lung sounds. J Asthma 1990; 27:237.

Miller RD, Hyatt RE. Evaluation of obstructing lesions of the trachea and larynx by flow volume loops. Am Rev Respir Dis 1973; 108:475.

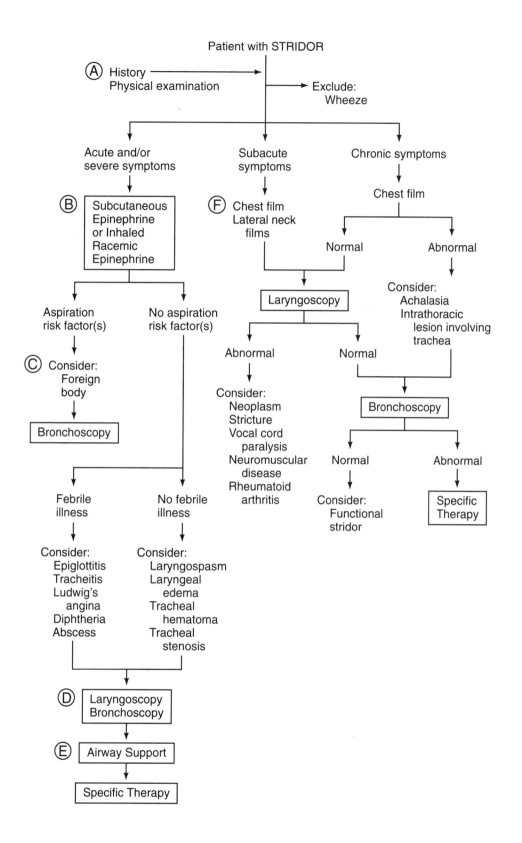

Patient with STRIDOR

Ⓐ History
Physical examination → Exclude: Wheeze

Acute and/or severe symptoms

Subacute symptoms

Chronic symptoms

Ⓑ Subcutaneous Epinephrine or Inhaled Racemic Epinephrine

Ⓕ Chest film Lateral neck films

Chest film

Aspiration risk factor(s)

No aspiration risk factor(s)

Normal

Abnormal

Ⓒ Consider: Foreign body

Bronchoscopy

Laryngoscopy

Consider: Achalasia Intrathoracic lesion involving trachea

Abnormal

Normal

Febrile illness

No febrile illness

Consider: Neoplasm Stricture Vocal cord paralysis Neuromuscular disease Rheumatoid arthritis

Bronchoscopy

Consider: Epiglottitis Tracheitis Ludwig's angina Diphtheria Abscess

Consider: Laryngospasm Laryngeal edema Tracheal hematoma Tracheal stenosis

Normal

Abnormal

Consider: Functional stridor

Specific Therapy

Ⓓ Laryngoscopy Bronchoscopy

Ⓔ Airway Support

Specific Therapy

WHEEZING

Neil C. Clements, Jr., M.D.

Wheezes are continuous, high-pitched, mono- or polyphonic sounds that occur when airway caliber narrows sufficiently to produce oscillation of airway walls. Asthma is the most common cause. Nonasthmatic causes of wheezing may also produce stridor (p 360).

A. Initial evaluation of the wheezing patient should determine the degree of respiratory impairment (see B). Important diagnostic clues include a personal or family history of asthma, cigarette use, medical ailments predisposing to aspiration (e.g., alcoholism or neuromuscular or cerebral disorders that impair swallowing or airway protective reflexes), previous intubation or tracheostomy, or recent foreign travel. Seek signs and symptoms of infection, congestive heart failure (CHF), deep venous thrombosis, pulmonary embolism, or vasculitic or granulomatous disease (e.g., erythema nodosum or multiforme).

B. Endotracheal intubation is indicated emergently if there is clinical evidence of respiratory failure (e.g., refractory cyanosis, respiratory paradox) or refractory hypoxia and/or hypercarbia with acidosis. In patients with impending respiratory failure, give empiric antiasthmatic therapy with nebulized beta-agonists. IV steroids may require several hours to have a significant effect.

C. Drug-induced asthma may be caused by systemic or ophthalmic beta blockers and nonsteroidal anti-inflammatory drugs. A trial of elimination of these should be made.

D. An obstructive spirometric pattern reversible by bronchodilators implies an asthmatic diathesis. Equivocal cases may be clarified by bronchoprovocation, exercise testing, or empiric courses of bronchodilators. Poorly reversible obstructive spirometric patterns suggest chronic obstructive pulmonary disease. Adjunctive diagnostic information may be provided by a history of excessive sputum (bronchitis, bronchiectasis), sweat chloride testing (cystic fibrosis), and CT scan (bronchiectasis, emphysema). An elevated urinary 5-hydroxyindoleacetic acid (5-HIAA) level in the presence of diarrhea, wheezing, and flushing may be found in carcinoid syndrome. Abnormally frequent and prolonged intraesophageal pH lowering is often present in reflux-associated bronchospasm. Large airway obstructions may be suggested by flattening of the inspiratory or expiratory limbs of the spirometric flow-volume loop.

E. Several atypical pneumonias, diffuse interstitial lung disease (DILD), autoimmune disorders, or vasculitis may present with wheezing. The optimal diagnostic approach depends on the clinical setting and specific x-ray findings. Rarely, pulmonary embolism presents with wheezing despite normal chest x-ray findings.

F. Previous chest radiographs are extremely useful in determining the duration and rapidity of evolution of existing abnormalities. Mass lesions and many infiltrates require invasive techniques of diagnosis (see D).

G. Invasive diagnostic techniques include bronchoscopy with bronchoalveolar lavage, Wang needle, or forceps bronchial biopsies; mediastinoscopy; transthoracic needle aspiration; and open lung biopsies. Determine the ideal approach by consultation with pulmonologists, radiologists, and surgeons. Decision making is often facilitated by CT scanning.

References

Holden DA, Mehta AC. Evaluation of wheezing in the nonasthmatic patient. Cleve Clin J Med 1990; 57:345.

Hollingsworth HM. Wheezing and stridor. Clin Chest Med 1987; 8:231.

Koster ME, Baughman RP, Loudon RG. Continuous adventitious lung sounds. J Asthma 1990; 27:237.

Miller RD, Hyatt RE. Evaluation of obstructing lesions of the trachea and larynx by flow-volume loops. Am Rev Respir Dis 1973; 108:475.

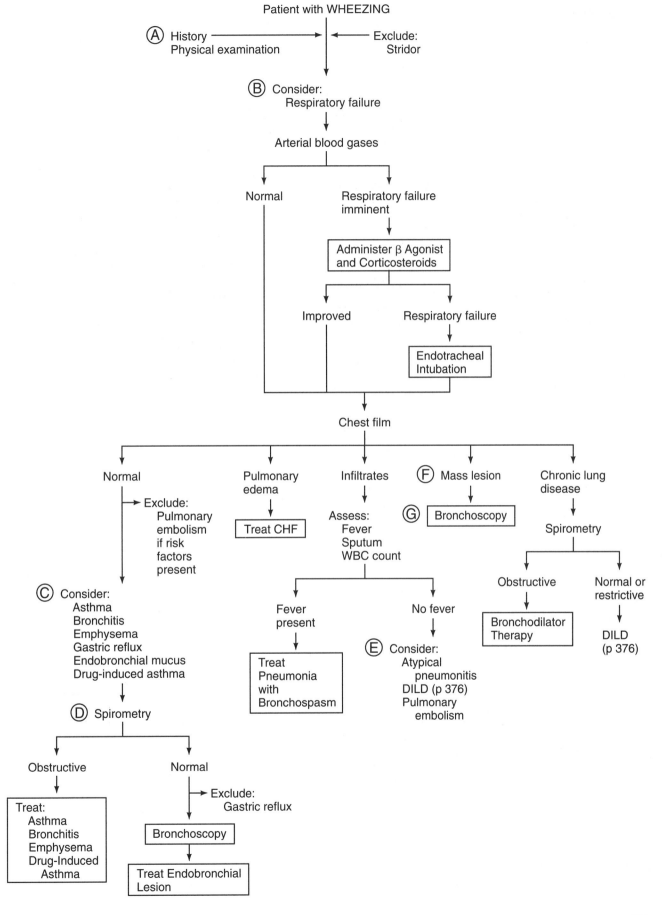

Patient with WHEEZING

A History
Physical examination → ← Exclude: Stridor

B Consider: Respiratory failure

Arterial blood gases

Normal — Respiratory failure imminent

Administer β Agonist and Corticosteroids

Improved — Respiratory failure

Endotracheal Intubation

Chest film

Normal — Pulmonary edema — Infiltrates — F Mass lesion — Chronic lung disease

Exclude: Pulmonary embolism if risk factors present

Treat CHF

Assess: Fever Sputum WBC count

G Bronchoscopy

Spirometry

C Consider:
Asthma
Bronchitis
Emphysema
Gastric reflux
Endobronchial mucus
Drug-induced asthma

Fever present — No fever

Obstructive — Normal or restrictive

Treat Pneumonia with Bronchospasm

E Consider:
Atypical pneumonitis
DILD (p 376)
Pulmonary embolism

Bronchodilator Therapy

DILD (p 376)

D Spirometry

Obstructive — Normal

Treat:
Asthma
Bronchitis
Emphysema
Drug-Induced Asthma

Exclude: Gastric reflux

Bronchoscopy

Treat Endobronchial Lesion

363

COUGH

Steven R. Knoper, M.D.

In most instances, cough is beneficial. Generated by mechanical, thermal, or chemical stimulation of afferent receptors in the external auditory canal, paranasal sinuses, nose, pharynx, larynx, tracheobronchial tree, pleura, diaphragm, and stomach: Cough acts as one of the main pulmonary defense mechanisms. Its importance increases when other defense mechanisms are impaired, such as in the absence of a gag reflex or the abnormal mucociliary clearance seen in chronic bronchitis. Nevertheless, in many patients it either is pathologic by itself or is the manifestation of underlying disease that requires attention.

A. The history and physical examination assume overwhelming importance. Inquire about chronicity, frequency, whether it is productive and if so the quality and amount of phlegm, the existence or absence of sinusitis or rhinitis with attendant postnasal drip, heartburn, and smoking history. Factors that ameliorate or precipitate cough (e.g., positional or temporal) are important. Concomitant signs such as hemoptysis should be elicited (p 358). Chronic cough generally requires radiography; consider neoplastic, inflammatory, and immunologic etiologies. Acute cough is usually secondary to an infectious process, and if the history and physical are in concordance with this, radiography is not warranted unless symptoms persist or hemoptysis is present. Thick, discolored, purulent, and abundant phlegm is consistent with bronchiectasis, pulmonary abscess, acute bronchitis and pneumonia, or occasionally chronic bronchitis. The last-named frequently has a mucoid but noninfectious-appearing phlegm. The definition of chronic bronchitis is cough, with or without phlegm, for 3 months in two consecutive years. Positional change in cough occurs in pulmonary abscess, chronic bronchitis, bronchiectasis, postnasal drip, reflux esophagitis, and endobronchial tumor. If there is nocturnal cough, consider asthma, postnasal drip, or reflux esophagitis. Lastly, a medication history is important, especially in regard to angiotensin converting enzyme inhibitors, which carry a high incidence of cough-related side effects.

B. Occasional patients with a presumed upper respiratory infection do not improve over time or after what is deemed appropriate therapy. This may be because there was no infection per se but rather an allergic or immunologic cause. Against the background of a now chronic process, new information may become available with a repeated history and physical examination. Chest radiography or a nasal smear for eosinophils may be helpful. Spirometry, with and without bronchodilators, may reveal occult asthma, or (rarely) bronchoprovocation with methacholine is necessary to yield the diagnosis. In the latter case, consider repeating the study in 2 to 3 months, as postviral patients frequently have increased reaction to bronchoprovocation. Postviral cough may require both oral and inhaled steroids for prolonged periods.

C. Chest radiography is necessary in all patients in whom there is no clear etiology or who have a chronic cough, hemoptysis, or a new cough without an upper airway abnormality. Abnormalities may include pneumonia, pleural effusion, parenchymal mass such as neoplasm, bronchiectasis, interstitial lung disease, congestive heart failure (CHF), and signs of emphysema. The chest radiograph may be normal in the presence of a foreign body, endobronchial neoplasia, airway hyperresponsiveness, pulmonary hypertension, pulmonary embolic disease, and sinus problems.

D. If there are otolaryngologic symptoms such as hoarseness, referral is appropriate. The chest radiograph may have revealed hilar or aortopulmonary window fullness, suggesting recurrent laryngeal nerve paralysis. Chronic rhinitis or sinusitis, nasal or laryngeal polyposis, thyroiditis, laryngeal paralysis, cricoarytenoid arthritis, external auditory canal foreign bodies, or primary tumor may be discovered.

E. In patients with a normal chest radiograph, chronic cough, and a normal otolaryngologic examination, explore the possibility of occult asthma with pulmonary function testing. Usually this means spirometry, with and without bronchodilators, but in occasional patients bronchoprovocation, testing with methacholine or postexercise spirometry is necessary to confirm a diagnosis of airway hyperresponsiveness that is responsible for the cough. Examination of the inspiratory and expiratory flow loops may point to intra- or extrathoracic obstruction.

F. Patients in whom there is still no diagnosis after the above work-up may benefit from bronchoscopy. Endobronchial tumor, broncholith, tracheal web, or foreign body may be seen. In addition, if the preceding examination has suggested interstitial disease, transbronchial biopsies may be warranted. A negative work-up at this point should lead to patient reassurance, reanalysis over time, and symptomatic therapy.

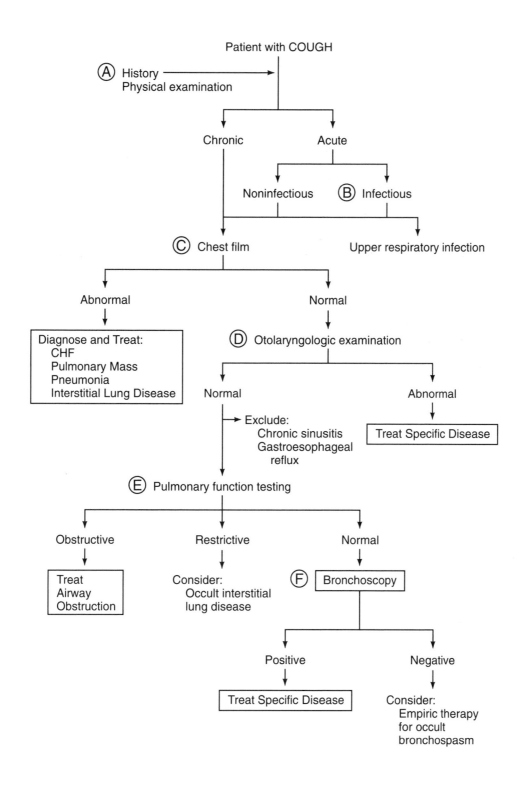

Patient with COUGH

(A) History
Physical examination

Chronic · Acute

Noninfectious · (B) Infectious

(C) Chest film · Upper respiratory infection

Abnormal · Normal

Diagnose and Treat:
CHF
Pulmonary Mass
Pneumonia
Interstitial Lung Disease

(D) Otolaryngologic examination

Normal · Abnormal

Exclude:
Chronic sinusitis
Gastroesophageal
reflux

Treat Specific Disease

(E) Pulmonary function testing

Obstructive · Restrictive · Normal

Treat
Airway
Obstruction

Consider:
Occult interstitial
lung disease

(F) Bronchoscopy

Positive · Negative

Treat Specific Disease

Consider:
Empiric therapy
for occult
bronchospasm

References

Fuller RW, Jackson DM. Physiology and treatment of cough. Thorax 1990; 45(6):425.

Irwin RS, Carley FJ. The treatment of cough: a comprehensive review. Chest 1991; 99(6);1477.

Parks DP, Ahrens RC, Humphries T, Weinberger MM. Chronic cough in childhood: approach to diagnosis and treatment. J Pediatr 1989; 115 (5, Pt 2):856.

Poe RH, Israel RH, Utell MJ, Hall WJ. Chronic cough: bronchoscopy or pulmonary function testing. Am Rev Respir Dis 1982; 126(1):160.

PULMONARY DYSPNEA

Anthony Camilli, M.D.

Chronic dyspnea usually has a cardiac or pulmonary cause. Information elicited during the history and physical examination may strongly suggest a particular etiology, but laboratory studies are often required.

A. The chest film suggests an etiology not suspected by physical examination in some patients and will direct a specific work-up. Obvious congestive heart failure (CHF) can be treated while the etiology is clarified. A chest film showing chronic interstitial lung disease requires a specific diagnosis from sputum, bronchoscopy, or biopsy. A pleural effusion necessitates thoracentesis as the initial diagnostic test. Mass lesions of the mediastinum, pleura, and lung often require biopsy after further imaging.

B. Dyspnea in the context of a normal chest film suggests many pulmonary and cardiac etiologies. Airway obstructive disease may be easily detected with spirometry. Arterial blood gases may suggest neuromuscular problems or occult pulmonary interstitial disease by high P_{CO_2} or increased arterial-alveolar gradient.

C. Dyspnea in the context of a normal chest film, normal arterial blood gases, and normal spirometry can be approached with exercise testing and echocardiography. Occult interstitial disease can be detected by arterial desaturation; an ischemic response would explain dyspnea on a cardiac basis.

References

Mahler DA. Dyspnea: diagnosis and management. Clin Chest Med 1987; 8:215.

Seaton A, Seaton D, Leitch AG, Blackwell. The clinical manifestations of respiratory disease. In: Seaton A, et al, eds. Douglas respiratory diseases. 4th ed. St Louis: Mosby–Year Book, 1989.

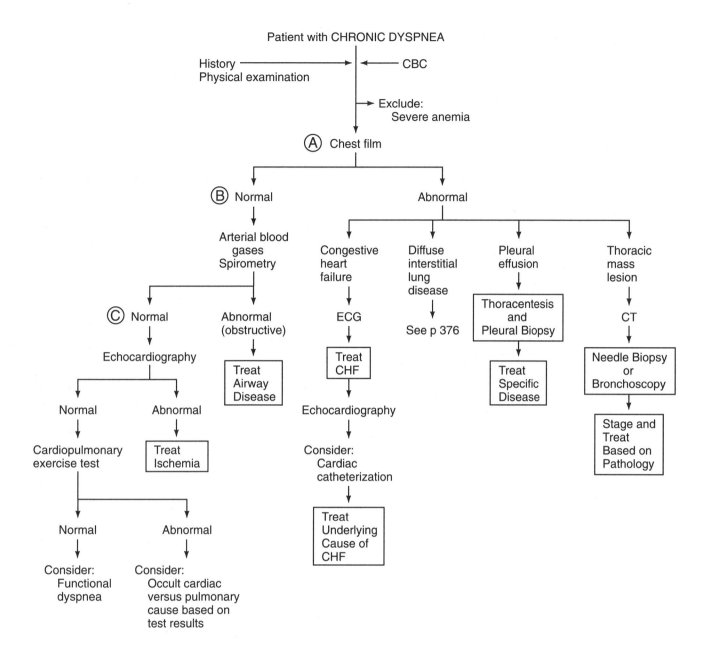

Patient with CHRONIC DYSPNEA

History ——————————→ ←—————— CBC
Physical examination

→ Exclude:
Severe anemia

Ⓐ Chest film

Ⓑ Normal   Abnormal

Arterial blood   Congestive   Diffuse   Pleural   Thoracic
gases   heart   interstitial   effusion   mass
Spirometry   failure   lung   lesion
                                      disease

Ⓒ Normal   Abnormal   ECG   See p 376   Thoracentesis   CT
            (obstructive)   and
                                                   Pleural Biopsy

Echocardiography Treat   Treat   Needle Biopsy
                  Airway   CHF   Treat   or
                  Disease   Specific   Bronchoscopy
                                                    Disease
Normal   Abnormal   Echocardiography   Stage and
                                                                      Treat
                  Treat   Based on
Cardiopulmonary   Ischemia   Consider: Pathology
exercise test   Cardiac
                              catheterization

Normal   Abnormal   Treat
                              Underlying
Consider: Consider: Cause of
Functional Occult cardiac   CHF
dyspnea   versus pulmonary
          cause based on
          test results

PLEURAL EFFUSION

Steven R. Knoper, M.D.

An estimated 1 million patients per year in the United States develop a pleural effusion. Symptoms include dyspnea, cough, and or pain. Many patients have no symptoms. In any one individual the symptoms usually reflect the causative disease. Radiographically, pleural effusions usually collect in dependent spaces, occasionally hide subpulmonically, and if loculated may appear as pseudotumors in the major fissure or as unusual pleural-based masses.

A. Examination of the thorax may reveal hemithoracic asymmetry, intercostal bulging or indentation, and occasionally subcutaneous edema as evidenced by pressure indentations. However, in many patients it is normal. Tactile fremitus over the effusion is reduced, percussion is dull, egophony at the superior margin is frequently elicited, and occasionally a pleural rub is heard on auscultation. Depending on the cause of the effusion, other organ systems may be abnormal; look for signs of pulmonary parenchymal disease, congestive heart failure (CHF), adenopathy, abdominal disease, arthritis, and other abnormalities.

B. The need for thoracentesis must be assessed individually and is guided by one's medical judgment. For instance, if the effusion occurs in the setting of a pneumonia, thoracentesis is not necessary if the height of freely flowing fluid on a lateral decubitus film is <1 cm, as these rarely become complicated. Before attempting the procedure, one should ascertain the free-flowing nature with decubitus views. If the amount of fluid is small or loculated, aspiration with ultrasound guidance can be helpful.

C. The appearance is important. Most effusions are straw colored, but only 1 ml of blood per 0.5L of effusion (assuming a normal hematocrit [Hct]) gives the fluid a bloody appearance. A pleural to blood Hct ratio <50% but a RBC count >100,000/mm^3 usually indicates pulmonary embolism, trauma, or malignancy—but not exclusively. If the fluid is purulent, an empyema is present and tube thoracostomy is indicated, although a chylous effusion can mimic a purulent appearance for those who have not seen one before. These can be differentiated by centrifugation or a fluid triglyceride level.

D. The effusion is considered an exudate if one of the following three conditions is met: (1) pleural to serum lactate dehydrogenase (LDH) ratio >0.6, (2) pleural LDH value more than two thirds the upper normal value for the serum, and (3) the pleural to serum total protein ratio >0.5. Transudative effusions require no further work-up; treat the underlying condition. Some diseases may appear in some patients as transudates and others as exudates; this is true of myxedema, and pulmonary embolism-effusion from the latter diagnosis occurs as a transudate 25% of the time.

E. The sensitivity of cytologic examination is 40–87%. Usually, if three samples are submitted from three different thoracenteses separated by a day or more, the sensitivity is about 80%. Add heparin to the collection container before obtaining the sample to prevent clotting. Occasionally, the pathologist can examine cell blocks cut from a centrifuged "button" specimen to increase the yield. Pleural biopsy usually only adds 10% additional sensitivity to that of cytology alone when the underlying cause is malignancy.

F. Most physicians do not proceed through the decision process outlined in this decision tree to decide that a parapneumonic effusion is present, but instead decide on the basis of the history and physical examination that a pneumonia is present. Following Occam's razor, the effusion usually is a result of the pneumonia. The major decision in managing a parapneumonic effusion is whether to place a thoracostomy tube, and if so when. Gram's stain, fluid pH (as measured from an iced, heparinized sample collected in the same fashion as that for an arterial blood gas analysis), fluid glucose, and fluid LDH are the criteria by which the need for a thoracostomy tube is judged. In borderline pH values, for example, a low glucose or high LDH level indicate that the effusion is likely to become complicated over time and that earlier thoracostomy tube placement is appropriate.

G. Not all laboratories differentiate small lymphocytes from mononuclear cells, which consist of mesothelial cells, macrophages, plasma cells, malignant cells, and lymphocytes. Their presence in transudates has no significance. When seen in exudates, malignancy or tuberculosis was the diagnosis 94% of the time (90/96) when two series were added (present in 96/211 exudates). Since the ability to diagnose these two diseases is increased with pleural biopsy, consider this procedure when small lymphocytes are seen.

References

Light RW. Pleural diseases. Philadelphia: Lea & Febiger, 1983.
Light RW. Clin Chest Med 1985; 1:1.

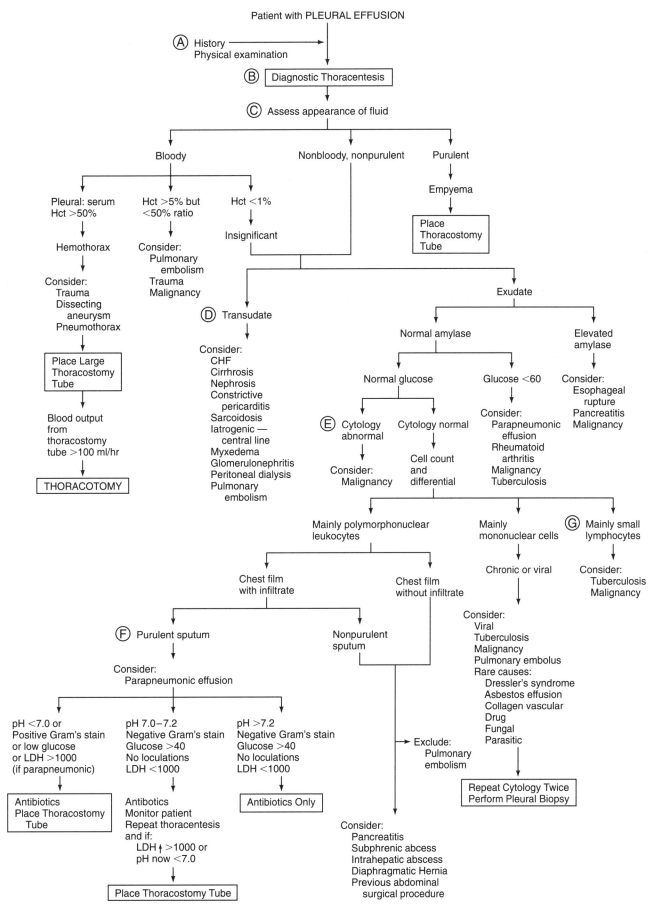

Patient with PLEURAL EFFUSION

Ⓐ History
Physical examination

Ⓑ Diagnostic Thoracentesis

Ⓒ Assess appearance of fluid

Bloody · Nonbloody, nonpurulent · Purulent

Bloody

Pleural: serum
Hct >50%

Hct >5% but
<50% ratio

Hct <1%

Hemothorax

Consider:
Pulmonary
embolism
Trauma
Malignancy

Insignificant

Consider:
Trauma
Dissecting
aneurysm
Pneumothorax

Place Large
Thoracostomy
Tube

Blood output
from
thoracostomy
tube >100 ml/hr

THORACOTOMY

Purulent

Empyema

Place
Thoracostomy
Tube

Ⓓ Transudate

Consider:
CHF
Cirrhosis
Nephrosis
Constrictive
pericarditis
Sarcoidosis
Iatrogenic —
central line
Myxedema
Glomerulonephritis
Peritoneal dialysis
Pulmonary
embolism

Exudate

Normal amylase

Elevated
amylase

Consider:
Esophageal
rupture
Pancreatitis
Malignancy

Normal glucose

Glucose <60

Consider:
Parapneumonic
effusion
Rheumatoid
arthritis
Malignancy
Tuberculosis

Ⓔ Cytology
abnormal

Cytology normal

Consider:
Malignancy

Cell count
and
differential

Mainly polymorphonuclear
leukocytes

Mainly
mononuclear cells

Ⓖ Mainly small
lymphocytes

Chronic or viral

Consider:
Tuberculosis
Malignancy

Consider:
Viral
Tuberculosis
Malignancy
Pulmonary embolus
Rare causes:
Dressler's syndrome
Asbestos effusion
Collagen vascular
Drug
Fungal
Parasitic

Chest film
with infiltrate

Chest film
without infiltrate

Ⓕ Purulent sputum

Nonpurulent
sputum

Consider:
Parapneumonic effusion

→ Exclude:
Pulmonary
embolism

Repeat Cytology Twice
Perform Pleural Biopsy

pH <7.0 or
Positive Gram's stain
or low glucose
or LDH >1000
(if parapneumonic)

pH 7.0–7.2
Negative Gram's stain
Glucose >40
No loculations
LDH <1000

pH >7.2
Negative Gram's stain
Glucose >40
No loculations
LDH <1000

Antibiotics
Place Thoracostomy
Tube

Antibiotics
Monitor patient
Repeat thoracentesis
and if:
LDH ↑ >1000 or
pH now <7.0

Antibiotics Only

Place Thoracostomy Tube

Consider:
Pancreatitis
Subphrenic abcess
Intrahepatic abscess
Diaphragmatic Hernia
Previous abdominal
surgical procedure

369

MEDIASTINAL ADENOPATHY

Anthony Camilli, M.D.

The differential diagnosis of lesions causing mediastinal adenopathy includes malignancies (primary and secondary), and granulomatous disease.

A. Detection of peripheral adenopathy in a patient with suspected mediastinal adenopathy may provide a diagnosis by biopsy of the superficial lesion. Risk factors such as age, smoking history, or area of incidence may suggest malignant versus benign disease. A history of risk factors for HIV infection may suggest AIDS-related adenopathy.

B. The chest CT scan allows one to distinguish between masses, nodes, and vascular structures in the hilum and mediastinum. The diagnosis of vascular lesions such as thoracic aneurysms and enlarged pulmonary arteries can be easily confirmed by CT. CT more precisely defines the anatomic location and size of masses, or the distribution and size of nodes, and often shows more extensive adenopathy than revealed by chest radiography.

C. After exclusion of thromboembolism and other vascular lesions of the hilum, the principal differential diagnosis of unilateral hilar adenopathy is between fungal infection and carcinoma or lymphoma. Skin tests and fungal serologic studies may suggest a diagnosis of coccidioidomycosis or histoplasmosis. Bronchoscopy often leads to a diagnosis with biopsy of an endobronchial lesion. If bronchoscopy is negative, attempt needle biopsy of the hilum with CT guidance. Thoracotomy is rarely required for diagnosis.

D. In patients with bilateral hilar adenopathy, the chest film or chest CT (particularly with thin-section technique) may confirm or demonstrate pulmonary parenchymal disease. Sarcoidosis frequently presents with bilateral hilar adenopathy and may include involvement of the lung parenchyma or airways. Bronchoscopy with transbronchial biopsy may confirm the diagnosis, particularly if there is evidence of parenchymal involvement.

References

Lillington GA. Bilateral hilar enlargement. In: Lillington GA, ed. A diagnostic approach to chest dieseases. 3rd ed. Baltimore: Williams & Wilkins, 1987:283.

Lillington GA. Unilateral hilar enlargement. In: Lillington GA, ed. A diagnostic approach to chest diseases. 3rd ed. Baltimore: Williams & Wilkins, 1987:274.

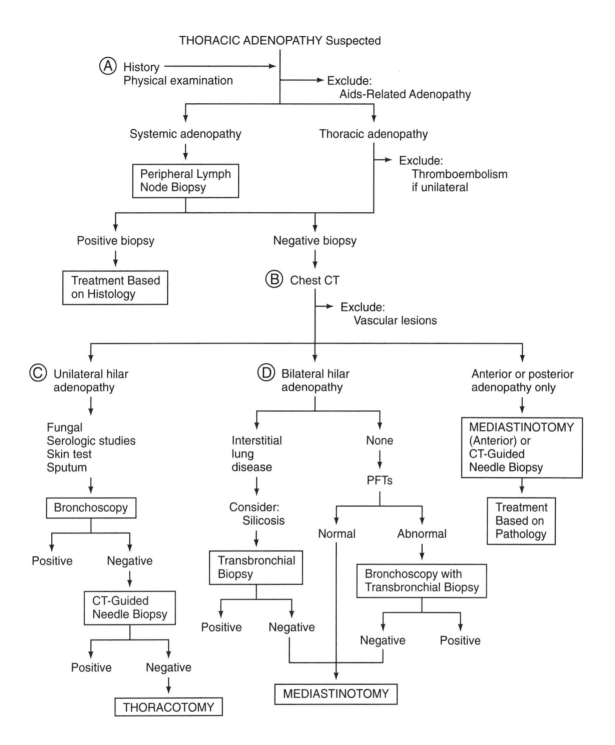

THORACIC ADENOPATHY Suspected

(A) History
Physical examination → Exclude:
Aids-Related Adenopathy

Systemic adenopathy ———— Thoracic adenopathy

Exclude:
Thromboembolism
if unilateral

Peripheral Lymph
Node Biopsy

Positive biopsy ———— Negative biopsy

Treatment Based
on Histology

(B) Chest CT

Exclude:
Vascular lesions

(C) Unilateral hilar
adenopathy

(D) Bilateral hilar
adenopathy

Anterior or posterior
adenopathy only

Fungal
Serologic studies
Skin test
Sputum

Interstitial
lung
disease

None

MEDIASTINOTOMY
(Anterior) or
CT-Guided
Needle Biopsy

PFTs

Bronchoscopy

Consider:
Silicosis

Normal

Abnormal

Treatment
Based on
Pathology

Positive   Negative

Transbronchial
Biopsy

Bronchoscopy with
Transbronchial Biopsy

CT-Guided
Needle Biopsy

Positive   Negative

Negative   Positive

Positive   Negative

MEDIASTINOTOMY

THORACOTOMY

371

SOLITARY PULMONARY NODULE

John Lace, M.D.

A. A solitary pulmonary nodule is a common abnormality seen on radiography. It is defined as a pulmonary opacity surrounded completely by lung, <4 cm in diameter, and without associated atelectasis or adenopathy. Malignant causes include primary lung neoplasms and metastases from distant primary tumors. Benign causes include infectious and noninfectious inflammatory lesions, as well as benign tumors such as hamartomas. Perform physical examination with careful attention to the skin, lymphatic system, and upper respiratory tract in addition to the chest.

B. Exclude pseudonodules due to intralobar fluid collections, nipple shadows, or other extrathoracic opacities.

C. Radiographic characteristics of solitary pulmonary nodules may suggest an underlying etiology. The presence of certain patterns of calcification is the most reliable radiographic criterion of benignity. A diligent search for old chest radiographs is warranted.

D. Pulmonary nodules usually show a constant growth rate throughout their clinical course unless altered by therapeutic intervention. The growth rate is expressed as a doubling time (the time it takes for the nodule to double in volume), which is determined on radiography to be an increase in diameter by a factor of 1.27. Malignant nodules usually show doubling times of 20–400 days. Nodules that show stability for >2 years do not require further follow-up.

E. Further imaging studies may include standard tomography or CT. These techniques are more sensitive in detection of calcification or multiple nodules. CT is preferred to assess for mediastinal enlargement. The type of calcification observed when present is useful in further risk stratification of patients.

F. The yield of fiberoptic bronchoscopy in the diagnosis of solitary pulmonary nodules is modest, and it is less effective in confirmatory diagnosis of benign lesions, which is the main goal of the procedure in avoiding unnecessary thoracotomy. Larger, more central lesions are more amenable to bronchoscopic diagnosis, which also allows inspection of the central airways and detection of endobronchial lesions as well as extrinsic compression due to nodal enlargement. Risks of the procedure include pneumothorax and pulmonary hemorrhage. Always take into account the preference and clinical status of the patient.

G. Transthoracic needle aspiration is simple to perform and has a low complication rate in experienced hands. Positive and negative predictive values >90% are achievable. Risks include pneumothorax and pulmonary hemorrhage. Chest tubes are required in 5–10% of patients. Again, always consider the preference and clinical status of the patient.

H. Mediastinoscopy is useful in the staging of malignancy once the diagnosis is established and there is radiographic evidence of hilar or mediastinal involvement.

I. Thoracotomy was often the first diagnostic procedure in the past, before the advent of less invasive means of obtaining tissue for examination. Immediate thoracotomy may yet be an appropriate choice in a male smoker >45 years of age with a large nodule, all of which factors indicate a high probability of neoplasm. The pulmonary reserve of the patient is an important consideration when planning a pulmonary resection.

References

Goodwin JD. The solitary pulmonary nodule. In: Sperber M, ed. Radiologic diagnosis of chest disease. New York: Springer-Verlag, 1990.

Lillington GA. The solitary circumscribed pulmonary nodule. In: Lillington GA, ed. A diagnostic approach to chest diseases. 3rd ed. Baltimore: Williams & Wilkins, 1987.

Lillington GA. Systematic diagnostic approach to pulmonary nodules. In: Fishman AP, ed. Pulmonary diseases and disorders. 2nd ed. San Francisco: McGraw-Hill, 1988.

Swensen SJ, et al. An integrated approach to evaluation of the solitary pulmonary nodule. Mayo Clin Proc 1990; 65:173.

Patient with SOLITARY PULMONARY NODULE ON CHEST FILM

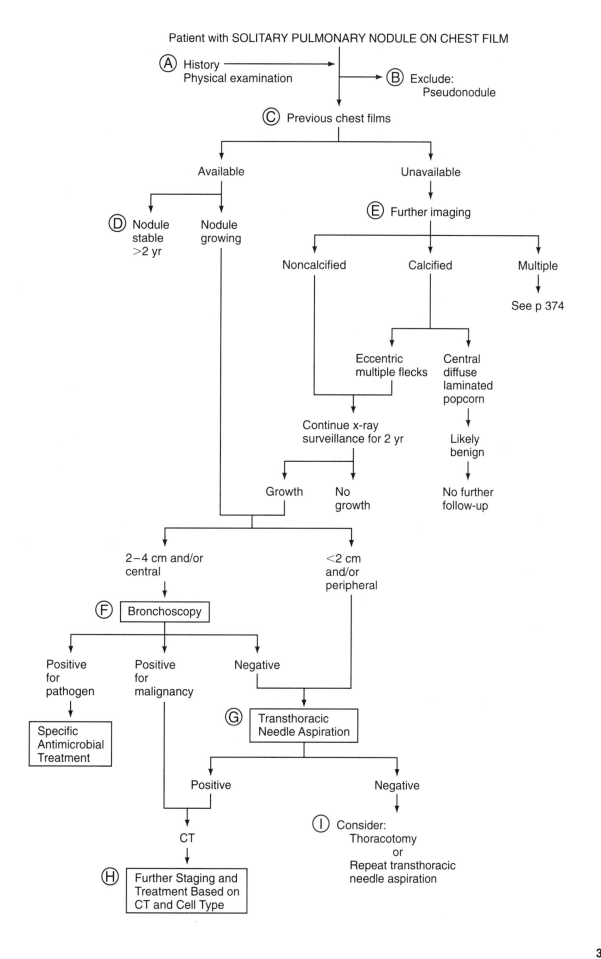

MULTIPLE PULMONARY NODULES

John Lace, M.D.

A. Multiple pulmonary nodules are usually defined as multiple discrete lesions discovered on chest roentgenography, at least two being >8 mm in diameter. Metastatic carcinoma to the lungs is a common cause of multiple pulmonary nodules. Others to consider include alveolar cell carcinoma; pulmonary lymphoma; multiple primary lung neoplasms; benign neoplasms; other benign conditions, including granulomas, both infectious and noninfectious; and arteriovenous malformations (AVMs). Combinations of lesions may occur and serial radiography may show that these lesions have appeared at different times. The presence of combinations is particularly important in the case of a potentially resectable lung carcinoma together with other benign nodular lesions. The history may reveal a geographic predisposition to histoplasmosis, coccidioidomycosis, or parasitic infestations. Physical examination should include careful examination of the upper respiratory tract, eyes, skin, lymphatics and (in young males) testicles. The radiographic appearance of the lesions on chest roentgenography, standard tomography, or CT scans can narrow the differential diagnosis. Additional imaging studies such as CT may demonstrate additional nodules more accessible by a particular diagnostic technique.

B. Patients are best classified into three groups: those with known extrapulmonary malignancy, those with extrapulmonary malignancy suggested by history, and those with no evidence of extrapulmonary malignancy. In the first group, the nodules are highly likely to be metastases. Obtaining a tissue diagnosis by invasive studies is warranted if the therapy would be changed or if there is doubt as to the diagnosis.

C. When an extrapulmonary malignancy is suspected but not confirmed, make a vigorous search for the primary lesion. Transthoracic needle aspiration may assist in the search for the primary lesion and establish the pulmonary lesions as metastases.

D. Infections may at times be diagnosed by cultures of appropriate samples or by serologic studies. If septic emboli are suspected, start appropriate empiric antimicrobial therapy after cultures are taken. AVMs may be suggested by radiographic criteria and diagnosed by angiography.

E. Transthoracic needle aspiration is simple to perform and has a low complication rate in experienced hands. High positive predictive values are achievable. Risks include pneumothorax and pulmonary hemorrhage. Chest tubes are required in 5–10% of patients. Always consider the patient's clinical status.

F. The yield of fiberoptic bronchoscopy in the diagnosis of multiple pulmonary nodules is modest, and it is less effective in confirmatory diagnosis of benign lesions. Larger, more central lesions are more amenable to bronchoscopic diagnosis, which also allows inspection of the central airways. Risks of the procedure include pneumothorax and pulmonary hemorrhage. Always consider the patient's clinical status.

G. If only two nodules are present and there is evidence that one of these is old and stable, the second nodule may be a bronchogenic carcinoma that is potentially resectable for cure. The patient's pulmonary reserve is an important consideration when planning a pulmonary resection. Thoracotomy may also be indicated for localized hydatid cysts, for symptomatic multiple AVMs, and for diagnosis of opportunistic infections in immunocompromised hosts. Mediastinoscopy may be indicated before thoracotomy if there is evidence of mediastinal enlargement on imaging studies.

H. Miliary tuberculosis produces smaller nodules than the classic form. It usually presents as a diffuse pattern of 1- to 2-mm nodules throughout the lung fields. Diagnosis is made by examination of transbronchial, liver, or bone marrow biopsies.

References

Lillington GA. Multiple nodular lesions. In: Lillington GA, ed. A diagnostic approach to chest diseases. 3rd ed. Baltimore: Williams & Wilkins, 1987.

Lillington GA. Systematic diagnostic approach to pulmonary nodules. In: Fishman AP, ed. Pulmonary diseases and disorders. 2nd ed. San Francisco: McGraw-Hill, 1988.

Patient with MULTIPLE PULMONARY NODULES ON CHEST FILM

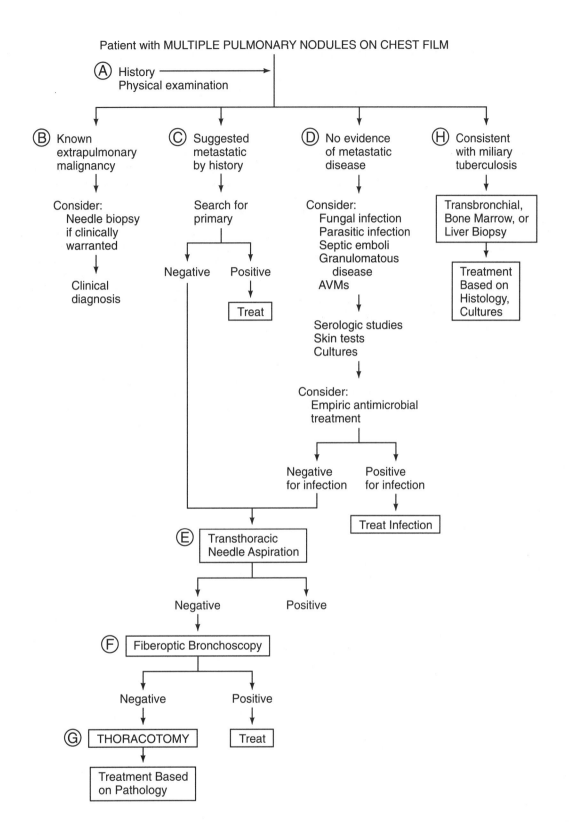

Ⓐ History
Physical examination

Ⓑ Known
extrapulmonary
malignancy

Consider:
Needle biopsy
if clinically
warranted

Clinical
diagnosis

Ⓒ Suggested
metastatic
by history

Search for
primary

Negative   Positive

Treat

Ⓓ No evidence
of metastatic
disease

Consider:
Fungal infection
Parasitic infection
Septic emboli
Granulomatous
disease
AVMs

Serologic studies
Skin tests
Cultures

Consider:
Empiric antimicrobial
treatment

Negative   Positive
for infection   for infection

Treat Infection

Ⓗ Consistent
with miliary
tuberculosis

Transbronchial,
Bone Marrow, or
Liver Biopsy

Treatment
Based on
Histology,
Cultures

Ⓔ Transthoracic
Needle Aspiration

Negative   Positive

Ⓕ Fiberoptic Bronchoscopy

Negative   Positive

Ⓖ THORACOTOMY   Treat

Treatment Based
on Pathology

DIFFUSE INTERSTITIAL LUNG DISEASE

Anthony Camilli, M.D.

A. The clinical history (with attention to exposures), together with the chest film and other clinical findings, suggest a clinical diagnosis of diffuse interstitial lung disease in many cases. Such working diagnosis includes the pneumoconioses, congestive heart failure (CHF), post-adult respiratory distress syndrome, viral infections, and collagen vascular disease and may require further confirmation. Atypical findings or other considerations may require further tests, including biopsy.

B. Perform skin tests, sputum cultures, and, where the diagnosis is not strongly suggested, serologic studies to establish diagnoses of mycobacterial and fungal disease. If these tests are negative, pulmonary function tests (PFTs) to assess obstructive versus restrictive physiology are helpful.

C. Many obstructive diseases (e.g., bronchitis, asthma, bronchiectasis) show changes on chest films representing fibrosis associated with the underlying disease.

These diagnoses often can be made clinically. Biopsy confirmation in typical presentations of interstitial disease with airway obstruction may be necessary to diagnose conditions such as bronchiolitis obliterans or lymphangiomyomatosis.

D. Some patients with restrictive physiology may be diagnosed by bronchoscopy with bronchoalveolar lavage and transbronchial biopsy. Some of these require a more extensive tissue diagnosis with open lung biopsy. Careful consideration of clinical history, chest films, and bronchoscopic findings should determine the need for thoracotomy.

Reference

Lillington GA. Diffuse interstitial patterns. In: Lillington GA, ed. A diagnostic approach to chest diseases. 3rd ed. Baltimore: Williams & Wilkins, 1987.

DIFFUSE INTERSTITIAL LUNG DISEASE
(Nonimmunosuppressed) Suspected

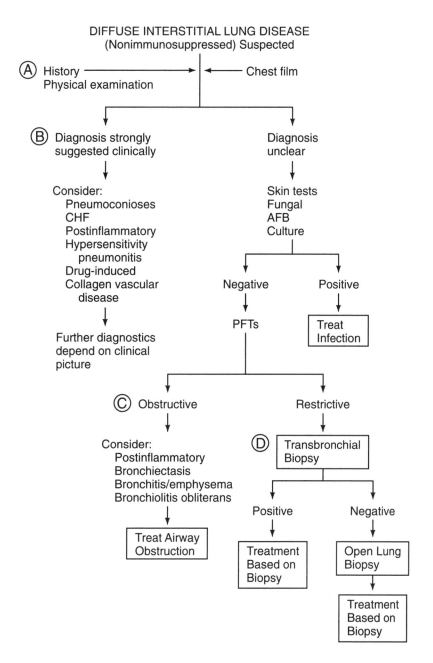

Ⓐ History ——————→ ←—— Chest film
Physical examination

Ⓑ Diagnosis strongly
suggested clinically

Diagnosis
unclear

Consider:
  Pneumoconioses
  CHF
  Postinflammatory
  Hypersensitivity
    pneumonitis
  Drug-induced
  Collagen vascular
    disease

Skin tests
Fungal
AFB
Culture

Negative

Positive

PFTs

Treat
Infection

Further diagnostics
depend on clinical
picture

Ⓒ Obstructive

Restrictive

Consider:
  Postinflammatory
  Bronchiectasis
  Bronchitis/emphysema
  Bronchiolitis obliterans

Ⓓ Transbronchial
Biopsy

Positive

Negative

Treat Airway
Obstruction

Treatment
Based on
Biopsy

Open Lung
Biopsy

Treatment
Based on
Biopsy

PULMONARY INFILTRATES IN PATIENTS WITH AIDS

John W. Bloom, M.D.

The approach to patients with pulmonary symptoms who have or are at risk for AIDS is directed by our knowledge of pulmonary involvement in AIDS patients. Opportunistic infections are common in these patients, and *Pneumocystis carinii* pneumonia (PCP) is by far the predominant pulmonary complication. In addition to opportunistic infections, pyogenic bacteria such as *Streptococcus pneumoniae* and *Haemophilus influenzae* cause pneumonia in AIDS patients. There also appears to be a recent increase in the incidence of pulmonary and extrapulmonary infection with *Mycobacterium tuberculosis*. Noninfectious pulmonary complications of AIDS include Kaposi's sarcoma, lymphoid interstitial pneumonitis, and non-Hodgkin's lymphoma. Empiric therapy for patients with HIV-related pulmonary disease is probably not appropriate except when awaiting the results of diagnostic procedures. This is especially important in patients who are at risk for, but are not diagnosed with, AIDS.

A. Patients with PCP usually present with dyspnea, which may be accompanied by cough and fever. Cough productive of purulent sputum suggests bacterial pneumonia. There are no specific pulmonary physical findings. Evidence of cutaneous Kaposi's sarcoma raises the possibility of pulmonary involvement with Kaposi's sarcoma.

B. If chest radiography shows a typical lobar pneumonia in a patient with a consistent clinical picture of cough, fever, and purulent sputum, a reasonable approach is to obtain a sputum Gram's stain and culture. If a diagnosis of pyogenic bacterial pneumonia can be made, fiberoptic bronchoscopy is not necessary.

C. The typical radiographic picture of PCP is a bilateral diffuse interstitial pattern, often more prominent in the lower lung fields. Later in the course of the illness, the radiographic picture may progress to diffuse air-space consolidation.

D. When the radiographic picture is consistent with PCP, examination of induced sputum is a reasonable initial step. Proper technique is essential; possible variations include sputum induction technique, sputum processing, and staining techniques.

E. When the clinical and radiographic picture is consistent with PCP, fiberoptic bronchoscopy with broncho-alveolar lavage (BAL) is a reasonable approach. If the clinical picture is less clear or if the patient has been receiving prophylaxis for *P. carinii* infection, perform transbronchial biopsy in addition to BAL unless there is a contraindication to transbronchial biopsy (e.g., uncorrectable coagulopathy, respiratory failure).

F. If bronchoscopy is nondiagnostic, the options are observation, repeat bronchoscopy, and open lung biopsy. Patients with normal chest radiography may be observed, but if symptoms are progressive, repeat bronchoscopy is necessary. If chest radiography is abnormal, carry out repeat bronchoscopy. If the patient's clinical condition is deteriorating, open lung biopsy is an option, but these usually do not reveal treatable causes undetected by bronchoscopy.

G. In patients at risk for AIDS with respiratory symptoms and normal chest radiography, a noninvasive evaluation with one of several "indirect" tests is a reasonable initial approach. These tests include rest and exercise arterial blood gas analysis with calculation of the alveolar-arterial P_{O_2} gradient, diffusing capacity, and gallium scanning. If no abnormalities are detected, observation is appropriate unless symptoms progress.

References

Fitzgerald W, Bevelaqua FA, Garay SM, Aranda CP. The role of open lung biopsy in patients with the acquired immunodeficiency syndrome. Chest 1987; 91:659.

Golden JA, Hollander H, Stulbarg MS, Gamsu G. Bronchoalveolar lavage as the exclusive diagnostic modality for *Pneumocystis carinii* pneumonia. Chest 1986; 90:18.

Hopewell PC, Luce JM. Pulmonary involvement in the acquired immunodeficiency syndrome. Chest 1985; 87:104.

Luce JM. Sputum induction in the acquired immunodeficiency syndrome. Am Rev Respir Dis 1986; 133:513.

Murray JF, Garay SM, Hopewell PC, et al. Pulmonary complications of the acquired immunodeficiency syndrome: an update. Am Rev Respir Dis 1987; 135:504.

Zaman MK, Wooten OJ, Suprahmanya B, et al. Rapid noninvasive diagnosis of *Pneumocystis carinii* from induced liquefied sputum. Ann Intern Med 1988; 7.

Patient with AIDS,
Patient with positive HIV,
or
Patient at risk for AIDS
with RESPIRATORY SYMPTOMS

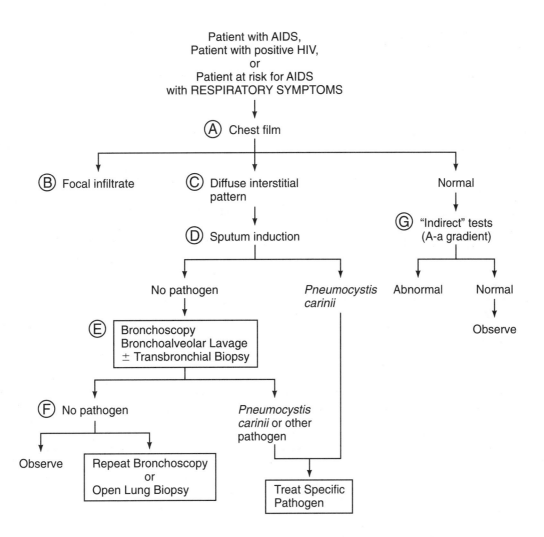

Ⓐ Chest film

Ⓑ Focal infiltrate

Ⓒ Diffuse interstitial
pattern

Ⓓ Sputum induction

No pathogen

*Pneumocystis
carinii*

Ⓔ Bronchoscopy
Bronchoalveolar Lavage
± Transbronchial Biopsy

Ⓕ No pathogen

*Pneumocystis
carinii* or other
pathogen

Observe

Repeat Bronchoscopy
or
Open Lung Biopsy

Treat Specific
Pathogen

Normal

Ⓖ "Indirect" tests
(A-a gradient)

Abnormal   Normal

Observe

POSITIVE TUBERCULIN SKIN TEST

Anthony Camilli, M.D.

The tuberculin skin test is particularly useful to identify persons with infection due to *Mycobacterium tuberculosis* who do not have clinical disease. The intradermal test (Mantoux) must be properly administered using 5 tuberculin units and properly interpreted at 48–72 hours to achieve best results. The American Thoracic Society and Centers for Disease Control recommend that the criteria for positivity of the Mantoux test be based on risk group to improve sensitivity: 5-mm induration for those with HIV infection, close contact with an active case of tuberculosis (TB), and chest films showing healed TB; 10-mm induration for those from countries with a high prevalence of TB, IV drug abusers, medically underserved populations, residents of long-term care facilities, and those with co-morbid medical conditions; and 15-mm induration for all others.

A. Chest films help determine whether the evidence of tuberculous infection is associated with active clinical disease, healed TB, or a normal chest film. Obtain multiple sputum smears and cultures if there are any x-ray abnormalities. Treat patients with active disease with at least two antituberculous drugs, and consider the possibility of isoniazid (INH) resistance when appropriate.

B. Prevention of tuberculous disease in those with tuberculous infection can be achieved by treatment with INH for 6–12 months. Patients with positive tuberculin tests and the highest risk of tuberculous disease include those (1) with close contact with infectious cases, (2) with a recent skin test conversion, (3) with previous tuberculosis who never received chemotherapy, (4) with stable radiographic changes of "healed" tuberculosis and negative sputum, (5) with silicosis, diabetes mellitus, hematologic or reticuloendothelial malignancy, HIV positivity, end-stage renal disease, or chronic undernutrition, and (6) who have received steroids, immunosuppressives, or gastrectomy.

C. The benefits of INH preventive therapy must be weighed against the risk of INH toxicity in the form of hepatitis. Studies show a clear relationship between age and INH hepatotoxicity and recommend that, in patients with no special risks, preventive therapy be limited to those <35 years of age.

D. In young people with no risk factors and those without comorbid conditions or other risks, those with adverse reactions to INH or active liver disease are excluded from preventive therapy.

E. Clinical monitoring at monthly intervals for liver damage or other adverse effects is essential. Those >35 years of age or with other risks of INH toxicity (possible drug interactions, continual alcohol use) should receive initial and subsequent monitoring of transaminase or other relevant clinical measures during preventive therapy. For those in whom resistant organisms are suspected (such as an INH resistant source case) several alternatives have been proposed. Options include a different or additional drug, INH alone, or observation. Consider the risks of INH resistance, tuberculosis disease, and potential drug toxicity when deciding on alternatives.

References

American Thoracic Society. Treatment of tuberculosis and tuberculosis infection in adults and children. Am Rev Respir Dis 1986; 1134:325.

American Thoracic Society. Diagnostic standards and classification of tuberculosis. Am Rev Respir Dis 1990; 142:725.

Patient with POSITIVE TUBERCULIN SKIN TEST

History
Physical examination

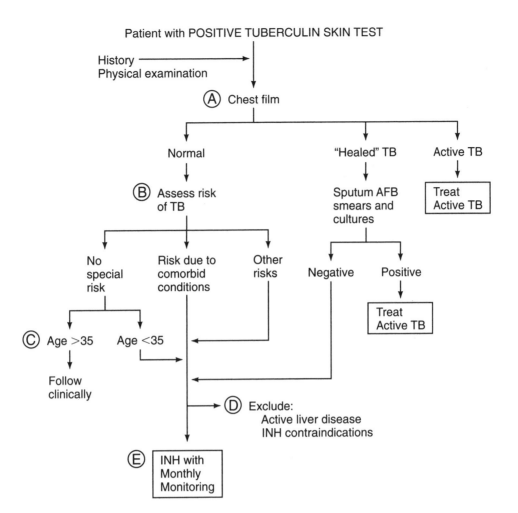

Ⓐ Chest film

Normal

Ⓑ Assess risk of TB

No special risk

Risk due to comorbid conditions

Other risks

Ⓒ Age >35   Age <35

Follow clinically

Ⓓ Exclude:
Active liver disease
INH contraindications

Ⓔ INH with Monthly Monitoring

"Healed" TB

Sputum AFB smears and cultures

Negative   Positive

Treat Active TB

Active TB

Treat Active TB

RESPIRATORY SYMPTOMS AND OCCUPATIONAL EXPOSURE TO ASBESTOS

Anthony Camilli, M.D.

Asbestos-related disease of the thorax includes both benign and malignant disorders of the lung parenchyma and the pleura.

A. An occupational history of asbestos exposure may be described by the patient or may be suggested by specific work situations, including use of insulating materials, automotive brake repair, or shipyard employment.

B. A lung mass in an older asbestos-exposed smoker is likely to be malignant. The size and location of the lesion suggest needle biopsy or bronchoscopy as the initial diagnostic test. Staging for possible resection follows consideration of cell type, resectability, and operability.

C. Interstitial lung disease due to asbestos is a diffuse process radiographically characterized by small, irregular opacities primarily in the bases. If exposure history, latency, physical and chest x-ray findings, and pulmonary function test changes are consistent, a clinical diagnosis of asbestosis can be made. Atypical presentations may require a tissue diagnosis.

D. Pleural lesions may show the characteristic shape, location, and calcification of plaques or may be otherwise. CT scanning may help identify noncalcified plaques from masses. Pleural mass lesions due to mesothelioma are difficult to diagnose by needle biopsy and may require thoracotomy.

E. Pleural plaques are characteristically seen on the diaphragm and chest wall. The raised lesions of the parietal pleura are more easily identified when viewed tangentially. Oblique films or chest CT improve sensitivity.

F. Diffuse pleural thickening occurs as a sequence of asbestos exposure and may restrict lung function due to a "trapped lung." Lung volume tests help identify this restriction.

G. A pleural effusion in an asbestos-exposed person may be due to occult malignancy (lung cancer or mesothelioma), a non–asbestos-related condition, or a benign asbestos effusion (a diagnosis of exclusion). Repeat radiography after thoracentesis; CT scans can help identify an associated mass.

Reference

Becklake MR. Asbestos-related diseases of the lung and other organs: their epidemiology and implications for clinical practice. Am Rev Respir Dis 1976; 114:187.

Patient with RESPIRATORY SYMPTOMS AND OCCUPATIONAL EXPOSURE TO ASBESTOS

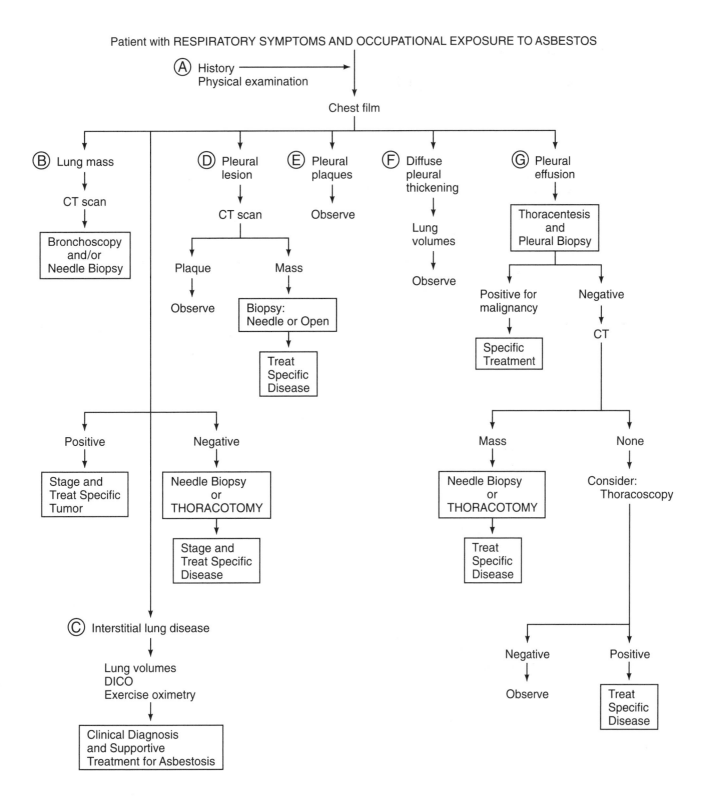

RHEUMATOLOGY

MONOARTICULAR ARTHRITIS

Deborah Doud, M.D.

A. A complete history is vital. Monarthritis of acute onset usually indicates trauma, infection, or crystal-induced arthropathies. Monarthritis persisting >4–6 weeks suggests chronic conditions such as tuberculosis, fungal infection, osteoarthritis, or tumor. A complete physical examination is necessary to determine whether an articular or a periarticular disorder is present and whether a systemic process is involved.

B. Aspiration of the affected joint with subsequent synovial fluid analysis is always indicated in the evaluation of monarticular arthritis. The synovial fluid WBC is the single most important quantitative measurement of synovial inflammation. If >5000, an inflammatory process is present; if <2000, the effusion is noninflammatory. Clinical correlation, however, is mandatory.

C. If analysis of fluid, including Gram's stain, culture, sensitivity, and examination for crystals, does not reveal a diagnosis, perform radiography and a repeat synovial fluid analysis, including cultures and smears for acid-fast bacteria and fungus.

D. When chronic monarthritis persists for >4–6 weeks without a definite diagnosis, a synovial biopsy is indicated. This can reliably diagnose tuberculosis or fungal synovitis, amyloid (prevalent in dialysis patients), pigmented villonodular synovitis, and other tumors. If no diagnosis is obtained from synovial biopsy, follow the patient closely for development of new symptoms.

E. If analysis of fluid reveals monosodium urate crystals intracellularly, the diagnosis of gouty arthritis is established (p 386). Rhomboid-shaped, positively birefringent calcium pyrophosphate crystals indicate calcium pyrophosphate deposition disease (CPPD) or pseudogout. Consider disorders associated with CPPD, such as hyperparathyroidism, hemochromatosis, ochronosis, and Wilson's disease in a patient <60 years of age with pseudogout. Calcium hydroxyapatite crystals can be identified only by electron microscopy or alizarin red stain. Identification of crystals in joint fluid does not negate the possibility of coexistent infection, although this would be rare.

F. Acute bacterial arthritis is a true medical emergency. The most common cause of septic arthritis is disseminated gonococcal infection (DGI). Synovial fluid cultures from patients with DGI are positive <50% of the time. If DGI is suspected, other sites (blood, genitourinary, pharyngeal, rectal, and skin lesions) should be cultured. The most common nongonococcal infectious arthritis is due to *Staphylococcus aureus*. Two thirds of persons with nongonococcal infectious arthritis show evidence of a primary focus of infection elsewhere. Thus patients with an unexplained arthritis associated with pneumonia, genitourinary infection, etc., should be presumed to have an infectious arthritis.

G. Hemarthrosis may result from trauma, excessive anticoagulant, inherited coagulopathies, or a neuropathic joint. It must be distinguished from a traumatic tap. The effusion of hemarthrosis is uniformly bloody throughout the aspiration, and the fluid will not spontaneously clot.

H. Persistent bloody effusions in the absence of trauma, anticoagulation, or a coagulopathy should lead to consideration of a tumor, particularly pigmented villonodular synovitis. In such cases, a synovial biopsy is indicated for accurate diagnosis.

I. Osteoarthritis may be present when there is little synovial inflammation in proportion to the degree of destruction of bone and cartilage, and the synovial fluid count is <2000. In neuropathic arthropathy the loss of pain and proprioceptive responses allows joints to exceed normal ranges of motion and develop significant joint instability. Ultimately, dislocation and deformity occur. Diabetes mellitus is the most commonly associated disease, but neuropathic arthropathy may occur in a variety of neurologic diseases. Avascular necrosis is a common cause of monarthritis of the hip, shoulders, and knees in young people with systemic disease requiring corticosteroid therapy. It occurs in a variety of other conditions such as alcoholism, barotrauma, hemoglobinopathies, diabetes, hyperlipidemia, hyperuricemia, and systemic lupus erythematosus.

References

McCarty DJ. Differential diagnosis of arthritis: analysis of signs and symptoms. In: McCarty DJ, ed. Arthritis and allied conditions. Philadelphia: Lea & Febiger, 1989.

Schmid FR. Approach to monoarticular arthritis. In: Kelley WN, Harris ED, Ruddy S, Sledge CB, eds. Textbook of rheumatology. Philadelphia: WB Saunders, 1989.

Patient with MONOARTICULAR ARTHRITIS

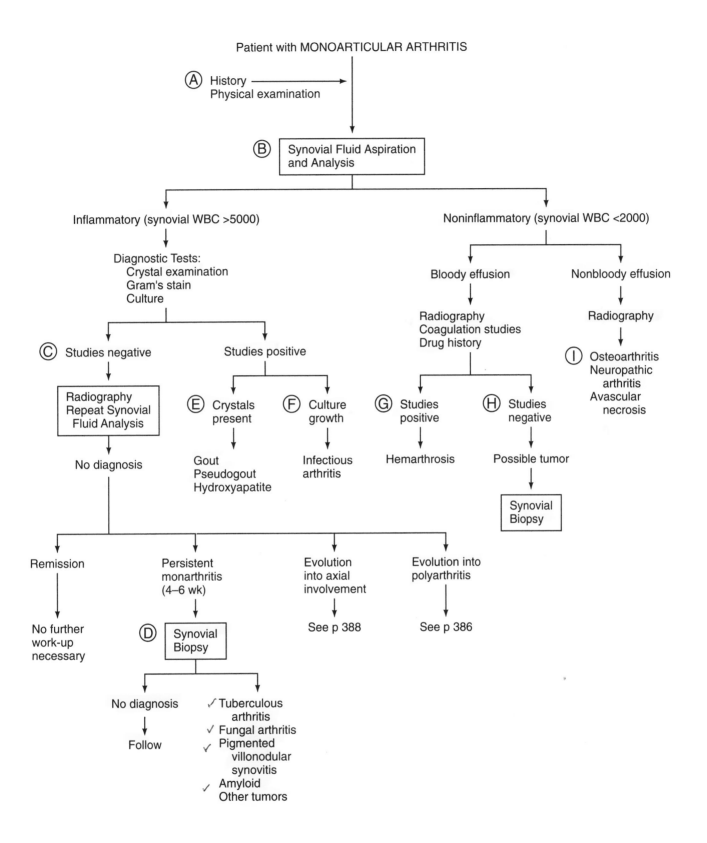

Ⓐ History ——————→
Physical examination

Ⓑ Synovial Fluid Aspiration
and Analysis

Inflammatory (synovial WBC >5000)

Noninflammatory (synovial WBC <2000)

Diagnostic Tests:
    Crystal examination
    Gram's stain
    Culture

Bloody effusion

Nonbloody effusion

Radiography
Coagulation studies
Drug history

Radiography

Ⓒ Studies negative

Studies positive

Ⓘ Osteoarthritis
    Neuropathic
        arthritis
    Avascular
        necrosis

Radiography
Repeat Synovial
Fluid Analysis

Ⓔ Crystals
    present

Ⓕ Culture
    growth

Ⓖ Studies
    positive

Ⓗ Studies
    negative

No diagnosis

Gout
Pseudogout
Hydroxyapatite

Infectious
arthritis

Hemarthrosis

Possible tumor

Synovial
Biopsy

Remission

Persistent
monarthritis
(4–6 wk)

Evolution
into axial
involvement

Evolution into
polyarthritis

No further
work-up
necessary

Ⓓ Synovial
    Biopsy

See p 388

See p 386

No diagnosis

✓ Tuberculous
    arthritis
✓ Fungal arthritis
✓ Pigmented
    villonodular
    synovitis
✓ Amyloid
    Other tumors

Follow

POLYARTICULAR ARTHRITIS

Deborah Doud, M.D.

A. The history in polyarticular arthritis is crucial. Joint distribution, axial involvement, symmetry, and morning stiffness must be delineated. Because many systemic diseases present with polyarthritis, a complete physical examination is necessary.

B. Historical features supporting inflammation include prolonged morning stiffness, fever, weight loss, and spontaneous joint swelling. Physical examination may reveal local warmth, erythema, or effusions. Laboratory findings supporting inflammation include anemia and elevated ESR. Radiographs of affected joints may show uniform cartilage loss, periarticular osteopenia, or erosions of subchondral bone. If synovial fluid is present, evaluation may be helpful; reduced viscosity and an elevated WBC count (>2000) exist in most inflammatory conditions. Crystal examination should also be made to determine if a crystal-induced arthritis is present.

C. Inflammatory polyarthritis with axial involvement includes the seronegative spondyloarthropathies: ankylosing spondylitis, Reiter's syndrome, psoriatic arthritis, and enteropathic arthritis (p 388). Radiographs of the sacroiliac joints may detect the presence of early axial involvement.

D. Inflammatory polyarthritis without axial involvement includes polyarthritis limited to peripheral joints. One must then determine if the polyarthritis is symmetric or asymmetric.

E. Rheumatoid arthritis (RA) typically begins in multiple small joints in a symmetric pattern. The earliest involved joints are the small joints of the hands and feet, sparing the distal interphalangeal (DIP) joints. The arthritis of RA is typically additive and destructive. Systemic lupus erythematosus (SLE) often presents as a chronic polyarthritis and may be misdiagnosed as RA. This arthritis typically is mildly inflammatory and nondestructive. Subacute bacterial endocarditis (SBE) may cause a chronic polyarthritis resembling RA; positive rheumatoid factor is often found in SBE and can cause serious diagnostic errors. Psoriatic arthritis, typically pauciarticular and asymmetric, can present in a polyarticular fashion, resembling RA. Scleroderma often presents with painful swollen hands with early contractures.

F. Psoriatic arthritis may precede skin disease. There is a good correlation between nail involvement and psoriatic arthritis, but overall correlation with skin disease is not as strong. This condition usually begins as an asymmetric pauciarticular arthritis including the DIP joints, or it may include all the joints of a digit, producing a "sausage" digit. Reiter's syndrome may entirely spare the axial skeleton and present with an arthritis similar to psoriatic arthritis, but with greater predilection for lower extremity joints. Enteropathic arthritis may present with only peripheral pauciarticular arthritis. The arthritis usually involves the lower extremity joints and generally parallels the activity of the bowel disease. Ankylosing spondylitis may present initially without axial involvement, especially in juveniles. The most common peripheral joints involved are the knees and hips. Adult rheumatic fever is rare; it causes very painful pauciarticular disease, most prominent in the larger joints of the lower extremities. Carditis, chorea, rash and subcutaneous nodules are rarely found. Gout may be misdiagnosed in its early stages and may progress to its polyarticular form, which can resemble RA (p 384). Polyarticular gout is common in the elderly. Calcium pyrophosphate deposition (CPPD, pseudogout) may present as polyarticular arthritis, mainly affecting the knees, wrists, and metacarpophalangeal (MCP) joints. Other rare causes of pauciarticular arthritis that may need to be considered include amyloidosis, sarcoidosis, Lyme disease, AIDS, relapsing polychondritis, polymyositis, and Behçet's disease.

G. If there is no clinical evidence of inflammation, and radiographs show changes such as bony hypertrophy and asymmetric cartilage loss, the patient may be presumed to have osteoarthritis (OA).

H. Secondary OA includes several polyarticular syndromes. Obesity causes a number of joint problems, the most characterisitic being bilateral OA of the knees, especially in women. Chondromalacia of the patella has multiple causes but is usually seen in physically active young and middle-aged women. Hemophilia causes a severe destructive arthritis following repeated episodes of intra-articular hemorrhage.

I. Particular patterns of OA have been described in association with several metabolic disorders, including hemochromatosis, ochronosis, acromegaly, hypothyroidism, and hyperparathyroidism.

J. OA of the hands, a hereditary disease much more prevalent in women, typically develops within a few years of the menopause and is often associated with mild inflammation for the first year or two. The disease is symmetric and involves the proximal interphalangeal and DIP joints, with development of the typical osteophytes of Heberden's and Bouchard's nodes. This disease spares the MCP joints and the wrists except the first carpometacarpal joint. Primary generalized OA is a rare hereditary disease with a high frequency of OA of multiple joints. It usually begins in middle age and involves typical joints (hips, knees, hands) early; eventually it may involve other joints such as the shoulders and ankles.

Patient with POLYARTICULAR ARTHRITIS

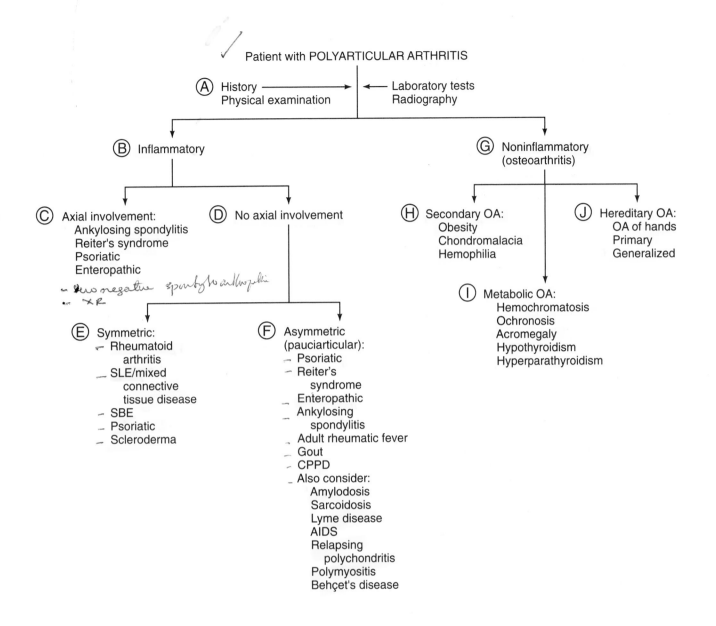

(A) History ———→ ←— Laboratory tests
Physical examination   Radiography

(B) Inflammatory

(G) Noninflammatory
(osteoarthritis)

(C) Axial involvement:
Ankylosing spondylitis
Reiter's syndrome
Psoriatic
Enteropathic

- sero negative spondyloarthropathic
- XR

(D) No axial involvement

(H) Secondary OA:
Obesity
Chondromalacia
Hemophilia

(J) Hereditary OA:
OA of hands
Primary
Generalized

(I) Metabolic OA:
Hemochromatosis
Ochronosis
Acromegaly
Hypothyroidism
Hyperparathyroidism

(E) Symmetric:
- Rheumatoid
arthritis
- SLE/mixed
connective
tissue disease
- SBE
- Psoriatic
- Scleroderma

(F) Asymmetric
(pauciarticular):
- Psoriatic
- Reiter's
syndrome
- Enteropathic
- Ankylosing
spondylitis
- Adult rheumatic fever
- Gout
- CPPD
- Also consider:
Amylodosis
Sarcoidosis
Lyme disease
AIDS
Relapsing
polychondritis
Polymyositis
Behçet's disease

References

Anderson RJ. Polyarticular arthritis. In: Kelley WN, Harris ED, Ruddy S, Sledge CB. Textbook of rheumatology. Philadelphia: WB Saunders, 1989.

McCarty DJ. Differential diagnosis of arthritis: analysis of signs and symptoms. In: McCarty DJ, ed. Arthritis and allied conditions. Philadelphia: Lea & Febiger, 1989.

SERONEGATIVE ARTHRITIS

Michael J. Maricic, M.D.

A. The seronegative arthritides (ankylosing spondylitis, Reiter's disease, psoriatic arthritis, and arthritis associated with inflammatory bowel disease) may or may not involve the spine. When they do, they are commonly referred to as the seronegative spondyloarthropathies.

B. Laboratory tests are usually not helpful. HLA-B$_{27}$ is positive in over 95% of cases of ankylosing spondylitis but is usually unnecessary. This test is neither specific nor sensitive enough to be useful for the other diseases. Consider AIDS in a patient with risk factors for HIV: in some patients, severe Reiter's disease has been reported as the initial manifestation.

C. Spinal involvement is usually categorized by inflammatory low back pain with morning stiffness and pain, improving with exercise. Physical examination should include Schober's test to examine lumbosacral mobility. This involves making two marks on the patient (one at the dimple of Venus and one 10 cm above the first) and asking the patient to flex at the waist. Normally, the marks should stretch 10–15 cm. Thoracic expansion at the nipple line (normal = >3 cm) and occiput to wall distance (normal = 0) should also be measured.

D. Radiographic examination should begin with plain radiographs of the sacroiliac (SI) joints and lumbosacral spine. Technetium bone scans, CT, or MRI may be helpful in more subtle cases, depending on the need to establish a firm diagnosis. Ankylosing spondylitis usually involves both SI joints and ascends continuously up the spine, whereas the other diseases frequently involve only one SI joint and may skip areas of the spine.

E. Look for peripheral arthritis and determine the joint distribution. Common to all the seronegative arthritides is asymmetric involvement of the joints of the lower extremities. Involvement of two or more joints of the same digit (sausaging) may be found, especially in Reiter's disease or psoriatic arthritis.

F. Search meticulously for skin changes throughout the body and for clues to the type of arthritis. Nail changes such as pitting or onycholysis may be a clue to psoriatic arthritis or Reiter's disease. Psoriatic plaques may be subtle but may be the only clue to psoriatic arthritis. Keratoderma blennorrhagica, found in Reiter's disease, may be clinically and histologically indistinguishable from psoriasis, but it tends to occur more often on the palms and soles. Balanitis circumscripta, a circular, plaque-like lesion on the head of the penis, may be found in Reiter's disease. Pyoderma gangrenosum may be seen with either ulcerative colitis or Crohn's disease.

G. Other organ systems may be involved. Iritis or conjunctivitis, urethritis, prostatitis, and aortic or mitral regurgitation may be seen with any of the seronegative arthritides. Apical pulmonary fibrosis may be seen with ankylosing spondylitis.

References

Arnett FC. Seronegative spondylarthropathies. Bull Rheum Dis 1987; 37:1.
Keat A. Reiter's syndrome and reactive arthritis in perspective. N Engl J Med 1983; 309:1606.

Patient with SERONEGATIVE ARTHRITIS

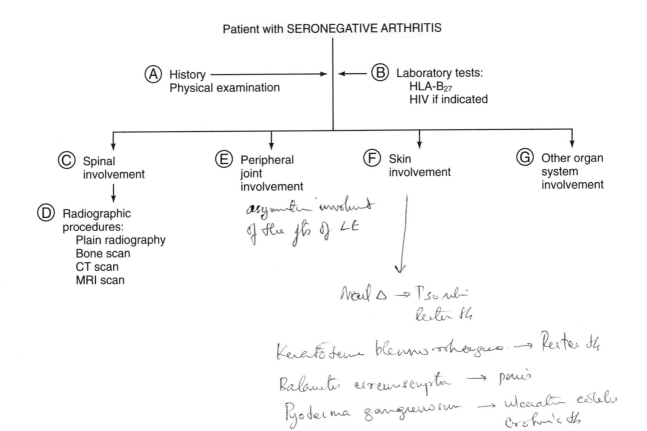

(A) History —— Physical examination

(B) Laboratory tests:
HLA-B$_{27}$
HIV if indicated

(C) Spinal involvement

(D) Radiographic procedures:
Plain radiography
Bone scan
CT scan
MRI scan

(E) Peripheral joint involvement

(F) Skin involvement

(G) Other organ system involvement

asymmetr involvemt
of the jts of LE

Nail Δ → Psorbi
Reiter th

Keratoderm blennorrhagco → Reiter th

Balanitis circumscripta → penis

Pyoderma gangrenosum → ulcerative colitis
Crohn's dh

SOFT TISSUE PAIN

Michael J. Maricic, M.D.

A. Soft tissue pain (nonarticular rheumatism) is a common problem in patients presenting with musculoskeletal symptoms. The history and physical examinations are vital in differentiating soft tissue pain from true arthritis. Although the suffix *-itis*, implying inflammation, is used with terms such as tendinitis, bursitis, and fibrositis, pain and tenderness are usually not accompanied by redness, heat, and swelling.

B. The first step is to determine whether the pain is intra- or extra-articular. This may be done by testing active and passive motion of the joint nearest the pain. Extra-articular problems cause pain on active but not passive movement of the joint. Intra-articular pain (true arthritis) is present on both active and passive motion.

C. If the pain is extra-articular, determine whether it is generalized or localized. If localized, it may be due to inflammation of a number of different tendons, bursae, or soft tissue structures. Bicipital tendinitis (in the long head of the biceps within the bicipital groove of the humerus), subdeltoid bursitis (in the lateral aspect of the shoulder), lateral epicondylitis (at the proximal attachment of the brachioradialis muscle on the lateral epicondyle of the humerus), trochanteric bursitis (superior to the greater trochanter), and anserine bursitis (over the medial aspect of the knee) are some of the more common causes of localized soft tissue pain.

D. If pain is generalized, consider systemic disorders such as early rheumatoid arthritis, systemic lupus erythematosus, polymyalgia rheumatica, and hyper-

or hypothyroidism. History and physical examination should exclude these. If they are suspected, confirmatory testing may be done with antinuclear antibody, rheumatoid factor, ESR, and thyroid function tests. In general, these tests should not be conducted if the history and physical examination are otherwise normal. Also, question the patient about symptoms of depression, which may present as generalized pain.

E. If there is no evidence of another systemic disorder in patients with generalized soft tissue pain, consider fibrositis or fibromyalgia. Generalized aches and pains, stiffness, fatigue, and difficulty in staying asleep in a patient who is usually a young to middle-aged female suggest this diagnosis. The physical examination is usually remarkable only for multiple, symmetric "trigger" points over the occiput, neck, trapezium, paraspinous muscles, elbows, shoulder, trochanters, and knees. Laboratory tests and radiographs are normal.

References

Boyer JT. Nonarticular rheumatism. In: Riggs GK, Gall EP, eds. Rheumatic disease: rehabilitation and management. Boston: Butterworth, 1984.

Campbell SM, Clark S, Tindall EA, et al. Clinical characteristics of fibrositis. Arthritis Rheum 1983; 26:817.

Smythe H. "Fibrositis" and other diffuse musculoskeletal syndromes. In: Kelley WN, Harris ED, Ruddy S, Sledge CB, eds. Textbook of rheumatology. Philadelphia: WB Saunders, 1989.

Patient with SOFT TISSUE PAIN

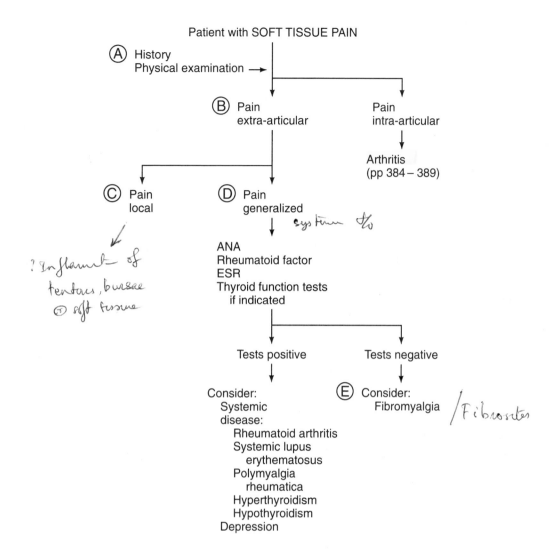

(A) History
Physical examination →

(B) Pain
extra-articular

Pain
intra-articular

Arthritis
(pp 384 – 389)

(C) Pain
local

(D) Pain
generalized

system to

? Inflamm— of
tendons, bursae
or soft tissue

ANA
Rheumatoid factor
ESR
Thyroid function tests
if indicated

Tests positive

Tests negative

Consider:
Systemic
disease:
Rheumatoid arthritis
Systemic lupus
erythematosus
Polymyalgia
rheumatica
Hyperthyroidism
Hypothyroidism
Depression

(E) Consider:
Fibromyalgia

/Fibrositis

NECK PAIN

Michael J. Maricic, M.D.

The neck as a functional unit is composed of a variety of structures that may individually or in combination give rise to both local and radicular pain. These structures include the vertebrae, intervertebral discs, uncovertebral and apophyseal joints, spinal cord and nerve roots, paracervical muscles, and anterior and posterior longitudinal ligaments.

A. In taking a history, any recent trauma is of foremost importance. Fractures of the odontoid, C1, C2, and fracture dislocations of C3-C7 may occur and demand immediate neurologic and radiographic evaluation, immobilization, and orthopedic referral. A history of inflammatory arthritis such as rheumatoid arthritis, psoriatic arthritis, Reiter's syndrome, or ankylosing spondylitis may suggest that the pain is due to synovitis (usually worse in the morning, relieved by motion). More important, a history of inflammatory arthritis should alert one to the possibility of a wide variety of axial and subaxial subluxations that may give rise to local pain, long tract symptoms, and vertebrobasilar symptoms (due to compression of the vertebral arteries). Acute onset of neck pain may suggest nerve root irritation or muscle spasm. Chronic pain is more common with discogenic disc disease. Local pain may be due to involvement of any of the structures listed above. Radicular pain is most commonly secondary to nerve root compression by foraminal encroachment or a herniated intervertebral disc. Neurologic symptoms may include paresthesias radiating to the arm and weakness of the arm, hand, or fingers secondary to nerve impingement. Paresthesias and weakness of the legs, with or without bladder or bowel symptoms, may indicate cord compression.

B. Local physical signs of spasm and tenderness may occur with involvement of any of the above structures. Weakness of the biceps and wrist extensors, decreased biceps reflex, and sensory loss in the thumb and index finger suggest C5-C6 root involvement. Weakness of the triceps muscle, wrist flexors, and finger extensors along with a decreased triceps reflex suggest a C6-C7 nerve root condition. Weakness of the intrinsic musculature of the hand and finger flexors and decreased triceps reflex suggests C7-C8 root involvement. Bilateral weakness, spasticity, and hyperreflexia in the lower extremities suggest cervical cord compression.

C. Perform radiography in the anteroposterior, lateral, and oblique views. Open-mouth views of the odontoid may give information about odontoid fractures and also allow visualization of the C1-C2 facet joints. Flexion and extension views in the lateral projection are necessary when subluxation is suspected.

D. Electromyography may help document nerve root compression in cases of chronic radicular pain. Myelography may be performed in patients suspected of having cervical spinal stenosis or in those with intractable neck pain due to nerve root compression. CT is useful for the same indications. MRI may be useful for the same indications as myelography and CT. It is also the procedure of choice in cases of suspected subluxation in inflammatory arthritis, since soft tissue (including pannus) delineation is superior with this technique. Technetium bone scans may be helpful in cases of suspected infection when the radiograph is negative. MRI is probably superior where available.

References

Jackson R. The cervical syndrome. Springfield, IL: Charles C Thomas, 1979.

Maricic MJ. The spine. In: Schumacher HR, Gall EP, eds. Rheumatoid arthritis—an illustrated guide to pathology, diagnosis and management. Philadelphia: JB Lippincott, 1988:12.1.

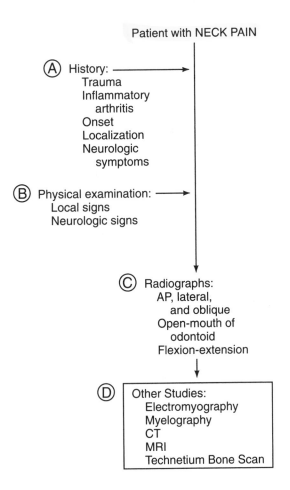

Patient with NECK PAIN

Ⓐ History:
    Trauma
    Inflammatory
      arthritis
    Onset
    Localization
    Neurologic
      symptoms

Ⓑ Physical examination:
    Local signs
    Neurologic signs

Ⓒ Radiographs:
    AP, lateral,
      and oblique
    Open-mouth of
      odontoid
    Flexion-extension

Ⓓ Other Studies:
    Electromyography
    Myelography
    CT
    MRI
    Technetium Bone Scan

SHOULDER PAIN

James B. Benjamin, M.D.

A. Standard radiographs should include an anteroposterior view of the shoulder with internal rotation and external rotation of the humerus, and an axillary view. A tangential "Y" view is often helpful in evaluating the position of the humeral head in relationship to the glenoid if an axillary view is unobtainable.

B. With a history of trauma, consider fracture of the humeral neck, distal clavicle, and scapula (decreasing incidence). Anterior dislocation of the glenohumeral joint is by far the most common (>90%) and is usually obvious on physical examination and radiography. Posterior dislocations are often missed radiographically if an axillary view is not obtained; these occur classically with seizures or electrical shocks and are the result of violent muscular contractions rather than direct trauma. The most salient physical finding with a posterior glenohumeral dislocation is the patient's inability to externally rotate the shoulder. Acromioclavicular separations usually result from a fall on the point of the shoulder with the arm adducted. Pain that is localized at the acromioclavicular joint can be severe even with minimal displacement of the clavicle. Standing views of the shoulder with the patient holding weights are of little additional value, as muscle spasm can prevent displacement of the clavicle. Falls on the point of the shoulder can also result in tears of the rotator cuff that, if large enough, can prevent active shoulder abduction. Patients can often compensate with the deltoid, and physical findings are limited to pain and weakness with abduction. Although MRI is gaining popularity in evaluation of rotator cuff tears, shoulder arthrography is a more cost-effective means of diagnosing this injury.

C. Inflammatory conditions about the shoulder are often precipitated by recreational or occupational overuse. Although often diffuse, pain can be localized to specific tendons by careful palpation. Radiographs are most often unremarkable except with calcific rotator cuff tendinitis. In this case, calcium deposition in the supraspinatus tendon at its insertion into the greater tuberosity of the humerus is pathognomonic for this condition.

D. Most inflammatory conditions about the shoulder resolve with conservative care in 6–8 weeks. If symptoms persist beyond this time, consider rotator cuff tear and undertake further evaluation as in acute traumatic tears.

E. Rule out cervical radiculopathy in any patient with radiating upper extremity pain. If physical examination demonstrates evidence of cervical spine pathology, begin work-up with radiographic evaluation and proceed as indicated.

References

Evancho AM, et al. MR imaging diagnosis of rotator cuff tears. 1988; 151:751.

Hawkins RJ. Cervical spine and the shoulder. In: Stauffer ES, ed. Instructional course lectures. Vol XXXIV. St Louis: Mosby–Year Book, 1985:191.

Norwood LA, Barrack R, Jacobson KE. Clinical presentation of complete tears of the rotator cuff. J Bone Joint Surg 1989; 21A:499.

Resnick D, Niwayama G. Diagnosis of bone and joint disorders. Vol 1. 2nd ed. Philadelphia: WB Saunders, 1988:343.

Rowe CR. Calcific tendonitis In: Stauffer ES, ed. Instructional course lectures. Vol XXXIV. St Louis: Mosby–Year Book, 1985:196.

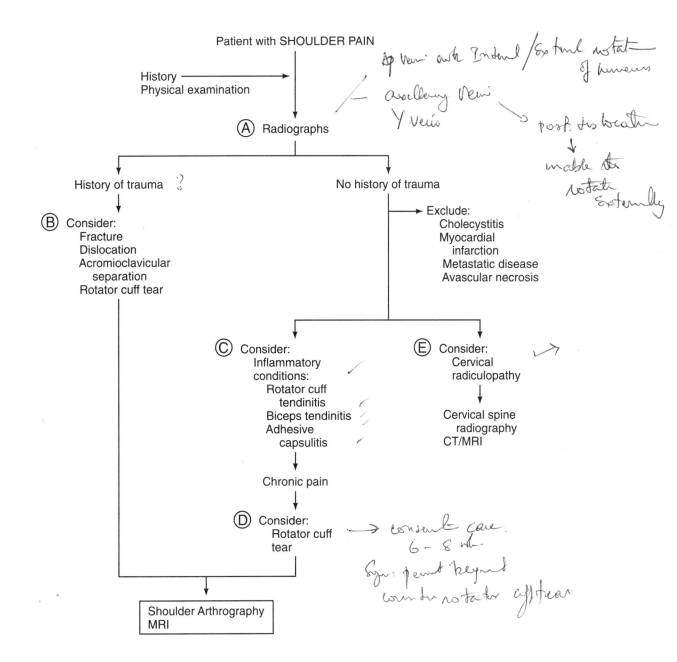

Patient with SHOULDER PAIN

History ———————→
Physical examination

Ⓐ Radiographs

History of trauma ?

Ⓑ Consider:
    Fracture
    Dislocation
    Acromioclavicular
      separation
    Rotator cuff tear

No history of trauma

→ Exclude:
    Cholecystitis
    Myocardial
      infarction
    Metastatic disease
    Avascular necrosis

Ⓒ Consider:
    Inflammatory
    conditions:
      Rotator cuff
        tendinitis
      Biceps tendinitis
      Adhesive
        capsulitis

Chronic pain

Ⓓ Consider:
    Rotator cuff
    tear

Ⓔ Consider:
    Cervical
    radiculopathy

Cervical spine
radiography
CT/MRI

Shoulder Arthrography
MRI

Handwritten annotations:
Ap view with Internal/External rotation of humerus
axillary view
Y view
→ post. dislocation ↓ unable to rotate Externally

→ conservative care
6 – 8 wk
Sym. persist beyond consider rotator cuff tear

LOW BACK PAIN

Barbara Bode, M.D.

Low back pain accounts for approximately one third of rheumatic complaints and affects 80% of adults at some time during their life. It most frequently is self-limiting; even a herniated disc rarely requires surgery. Typically, diagnoses are nonspecific; a precise pathoanatomic cause is identified in only 10–20% of patients. This positive outcome should be considered in the evaluation and treatment of all patients with low back pain.

A. A thorough history and physical examination are crucial to obtain an accurate assessment of low back pain. History taking should fully characterize the pain to differentiate local from radicular or referred pain. The relationship of pain to activity associated with postural changes is important. The pain of spinal stenosis is exacerbated by walking and relieved by rest and spinal flexion. Sitting frequently worsens symptoms of disc herniation. Determine bowel, bladder, and sexual function, as they may be involved in central midline herniations of the disc and spinal stenosis. Inspect the back for normal curvature and palpate it for local spasm, sacroiliac joint tenderness, or sciatic notch tenderness. Physical examination should also include evaluation of gait, back range of motion, leg length determination, straight leg raising, a thorough neurologic examination, chest expansion, and Schober's test.

B. Approximately 1% of patients with low back pain have sciatica, which is defined as pain in the distribution of a lumbar root, often associated with motor or sensory deficits. This frequently is the first indication of a herniated disc. Of lumbar disc herniations, 95% occur at the L4-L5 or L5-S1 levels. There is a 10% incidence of two-level herniations. Typically, L5 nerve root involvement results in extensor hallucis longus weakness with medial foot sensory loss, and there is no loss of reflex. S1 nerve root involvement causes loss of the ankle jerk, weakness of the plantar flexors of the foot, and sensory loss of the posterior calf and lateral foot. The knee reflex is lost with involvement at the L4-L5 level.

C. Multiple nerve root entrapment may result in symptoms of neurogenic claudication. Presentation typically occurs in the sixth decade. Spinal stenosis may be congenital or acquired secondary to degenerative changes, spondylolysis, or spondylolisthesis, and may be postsurgical or post-traumatic. It may involve either the lateral recesses or the central canal.

D. The inflammatory spondyloarthropathies affect 2% of the population. Patients frequently present <40 years of age with insidious onset of low back pain relieved by exercise and associated with morning stiffness. These diseases are characterized by sacroiliitis, inflammatory peripheral arthritis, and enthesopathy.

Evaluate these patients for ocular, pulmonary, and cardiovascular disease.

E. Target the early diagnostic work-up of low back pain toward identifying neurologic abnormalities, factors that may influence conservative treatment, and signs of systemic disease. Plain radiography is rarely useful in the definitive diagnosis of low back pain, although it can be important in identifying tumor, infection, fracture, spondylolisthesis, or sacroiliitis. Immediate additional imaging studies are indicated in patients with a cauda equina syndrome (bowel and bladder dysfunction with bilateral leg weakness and numbness), a progressive neurologic deficit, or evidence of tumor or infection. In patients with a suspected herniated disc, 1–2 weeks of conservative therapy before further diagnostic work-up is suggested. Disc herniation is common in asymptomatic persons, and this isolated test finding without the corresponding clinical signs may initiate unnecessary clinical interventions. In patients who have clinical signs to suggest a herniated disc and have failed conservative therapy, the diagnosis must be confirmed on CT scan, MRI, or myelography. The sensitivities and specificities of CT and myelography are similar (90–95% and 65–85% respectively). It is as yet unknown how MRI compares with these. EMG may be useful in differentiating radicular pain from peripheral neuropathy. Bone scan may help the diagnosis of tumor, infection, or early inflammatory disease. Depression, substance abuse, and excessive somatization are poor prognostic features that may warrant psychological testing.

F. If a patient presents writhing in pain, suspect an intra-abdominal or vascular process. Suspect cancer or an infectious process, such as an epidural abscess or spinal osteomyelitis, in a patient with constant pain at rest or fever. Acute pain in a patient at risk for osteoporosis should suggest a vertebral compression fracture. Paget's disease is another metabolic bone condition that may give rise to low back pain.

References

Deyo RA, Diehl AK, Rosenthal M. How many days of bed rest for acute low back pain? A randomized clinical trial. N Engl J Med 1986; 315:1064.

Deyo RA, Loeser JD, Bigos SJ. Herniated lumbar intervertebral disc. Ann Intern Med 1990; 112:598.

Fast A. Low back disorders: conservative management. Arch Phys Med Rehabil 1988; 69:880.

Frymoyer JW. Back pain and sciatica. N Engl J Med 1988; 318:291.

Lipson SJ. Low back pain. In: Kelley WN, Harris ED, Ruddy S, Sledge CB, ed. Textbook of rheumatology. 3rd ed. Philadelphia: WB Saunders, 1989.

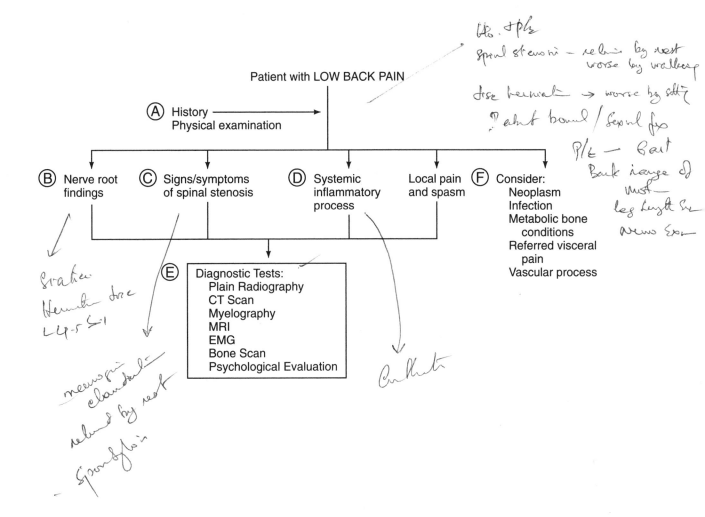

Patient with LOW BACK PAIN

(A) History
Physical examination

(B) Nerve root findings

(C) Signs/symptoms of spinal stenosis

(D) Systemic inflammatory process

Local pain and spasm

(F) Consider:
Neoplasm
Infection
Metabolic bone conditions
Referred visceral pain
Vascular process

(E) Diagnostic Tests:
Plain Radiography
CT Scan
Myelography
MRI
EMG
Bone Scan
Psychological Evaluation

Handwritten annotations:

Hx. Sx
Spinal stenosis - relived by rest worse by walking

disc herniation → worse by sitting
? abnt bowel / sexual fn

P/E — Gait
Back range of mvmt
leg length Sx
Neuro Exam

Sciatica
Hernia disc
L4-5 S-1

neurogenic claudication
relieved by rest
Spondylosis

Arthritis

HIP PAIN

James B. Benjamin, M.D.

A. For evaluation of hip pain, radiographs should include an anteroposterior (AP) view of the pelvis in addition to AP and lateral views of the hip. The pelvis view provides valuable additional information, including views of the sacroiliac joints, sacrum and opposite hip for comparison.

B. Judet or lateral oblique views of the pelvis are extremely valuable for evaluating pelvic fracture. The posterior elements of the pelvis can best be evaluated with CT.

C. Stress fractures of the proximal femur and pelvis can be difficult to diagnose on plain radiography. These injuries are commonly seen in patients who are long distance runners or who do aerobic exercise with repetitive impact loading. A bone scan often assists the diagnosis.

D. Perform a joint aspirate if the diagnosis of inflammatory arthropathy is suspected. Often this procedure is diagnostic, as in cases of infectious etiology and crystalline arthropathy. Fluid should be analyzed for cell count with differential, the presence or absence of crystals, and Gram's stain and culture if indicated. Glucose level is of benefit only if a serum glucose level is obtained at the same time for comparison.

E. Early avascular necrosis may not show any changes on plain radiography. MRI has evolved as the most sensitive tool in diagnosing this disorder.

F. Lumbar spine disorders can mimic hip pathology and should be considered if pain is localized to the buttock. Although osteoarthritic changes can be easily seen on routine radiography, nerve root compression and spinal stenosis are best evaluated with alternative imaging techniques.

G. Trochanteric bursitis is one of the most common problems in patients presenting with "hip pain". The pain is classically localized to the lateral aspect of the hip over the greater trochanter.

References

Hauzeur JP, Pasteels JL, Schoutens A, et al. The diagnostic value of magnetic resonance imaging in nontraumatic osteonecrosis of the femoral head. J Bone Joint Surg 1989; 71A:641.

Kirkaldy-Willis WH, Wedge JH, Yong-Hing K, Reily J. Pathology and pathogenesis of lumbar spondylosis and stenosis. Spine 1978; 3:319.

Pavlov H, Nelson TL, Warren RF, et al. Stress fractures of the pubic ramus. J Bone Joint Surg 1982; 65A:1020.

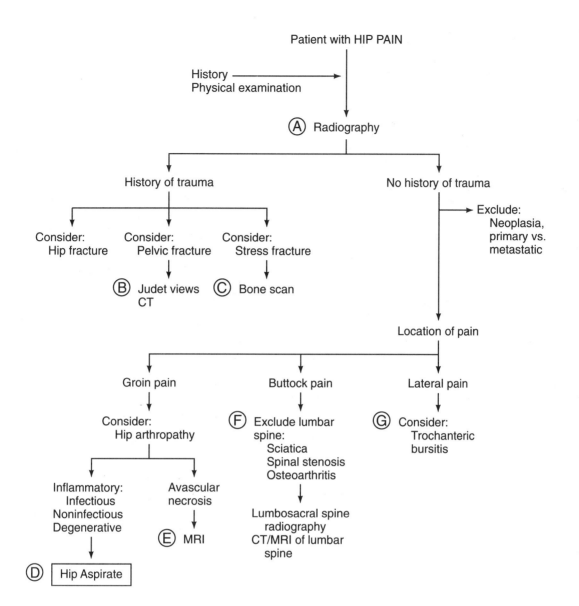

Patient with HIP PAIN

History ──────→
Physical examination

Ⓐ Radiography

History of trauma

Consider:
Hip fracture

Consider:
Pelvic fracture

Consider:
Stress fracture

Ⓑ Judet views
CT

Ⓒ Bone scan

No history of trauma

→ Exclude:
Neoplasia,
primary vs.
metastatic

Location of pain

Groin pain

Consider:
Hip arthropathy

Inflammatory:
Infectious
Noninfectious
Degenerative

Avascular
necrosis

Ⓔ MRI

Ⓓ Hip Aspirate

Buttock pain

Ⓕ Exclude lumbar
spine:
Sciatica
Spinal stenosis
Osteoarthritis

Lumbosacral spine
radiography
CT/MRI of lumbar
spine

Lateral pain

Ⓖ Consider:
Trochanteric
bursitis

HAND AND WRIST PAIN

Michael J. Maricic, M.D.

Pain in the hands or wrists may have a variety of causes. Pain may originate from the bones or joints or from extra-articular tissues such as the muscles or tendons, or may be due to vascular or neural compromise. The history and physical examination often provide the diagnosis without the need for further studies.

A. If the pain is articular (pain on active and passive motion of the joint), note symmetry and joint distribution. Degenerative joint disease (DJD) may be asymmetric, but often affects the first carpometacarpal, distal interphalangeal (DIP), and proximal interphalangeal (PIP) joints in a symmetric fashion. There is usually a lack of inflammation. Gout or pseudogout (calcium pyrophosphate deposition disease [CPPD]) may involve any of the small joints of the hands or wrist in a symmetric or asymmetric fashion. CPPD has a predilection for the wrists and index and middle metacarpophalangeal (MCP) joints. Rheumatoid arthritis (RA) is always symmetric and involves the wrists and MCP and PIP joints.

B. Extra-articular causes of pain may be acute or chronic. Acute causes of pain include tenosynovitis, tendon rupture, and infection. The pain in De Quervain's tenosynovitis is usually near the anatomic snuffbox and is due to inflammation of the abductor pollicis longus and extensor pollicis brevis. Adduction of the thumb while the wrist is held in ulnar deviation (Finkelstein's test) exacerbates the pain. Rupture of the extensor or flexor tendons may occur after trauma or in conditions such as RA. In RA, rupture of the ring and little finger extensors may result from dorsal subluxation and radial displacement of the ulnar styloid. Infections such as cellulitis, abscesses, felons (infections of the distal pulp of the fingertip), and paronychias (infections of the soft tissue around the nail) are usually obvious to the observer. Chronic soft tissue pain may be caused by ganglions (soft tissue tumors most commonly found over the dorsum of the wrist) or Dupuytren's contractures (thickening and contracture of the palmar aponeurosis). The latter is most commonly found in patients with diabetes, alcoholism, and a family history of these contractures.

C. Vascular problems in the hand are uncommon. Bilateral vascular spasm and discoloration should suggest Raynaud's syndrome (p 410). Unilateral or digital problems should suggest thoracic outlet syndrome, vasculitis, and thromboembolic disease. Doppler flow studies and angiography may be necessary in the latter disorders.

D. Neural pain may be due to dysfunction of the radial, ulnar, or median nerves. Ulnar nerve dysfunction is suggested by weakness in the intrinsic muscles of the hand and numbness of the ulnar nerve distribution. Radial nerve dysfunction results in weakness of the wrist and finger extensors and numbness of the dorsum of the hand. The median nerve supplies innervation to the thenar muscles (except the adductor) and the lumbricales of the index and long fingers. It provides sensation to the palmar aspect of the thumb, index, and middle and radial half of the ring finger. Carpal tunnel syndrome is caused by compression of the median nerve at the wrist. It is commonly seen in diabetes, pregnancy, hypothyroidism, repetitive trauma, and any inflammatory arthropathy of the wrist (RA, gout, CPPD). Tinel's (tapping the median nerve over the wrist) and Phalen's (sustained hyperflexion of the wrists) signs may reproduce the symptoms. Nerve conduction velocities (NCVs) may document the involved nerves and sites of compression.

References

Kendall D. Aetiology, diagnosis and treatment of paraesthesiae in the hands. Br Med J 1960; 2:1663.

Phalen GS. Soft tissue affection of the hand and wrist. Hosp Med 1971; 7:47.

RA is always symmetric

De Quervain's tenosynovitis
- near anatomical snuff box
- inflam of abductor pollicis longus and extensor a pollicis brevis

Finkelstein's test → Adduction of thumb while the wrist is held in ulnar deviation exacerbate the pain

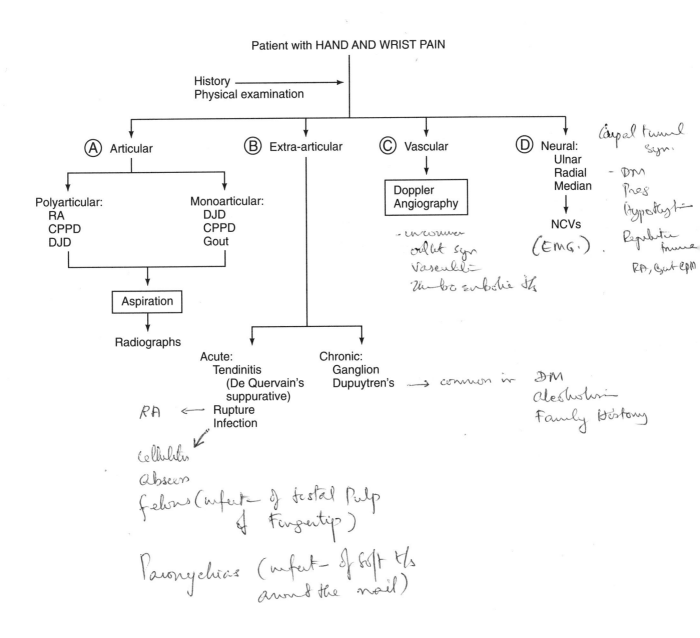

Patient with HAND AND WRIST PAIN

History ⟶
Physical examination

A Articular   **B** Extra-articular   **C** Vascular   **D** Neural:
Ulnar
Radial
Median

Polyarticular: Monoarticular:
RA   DJD
CPPD   CPPD
DJD   Gout

Aspiration

Radiographs

Doppler
Angiography

NCVs

Carpal tunnel
syn.

- DM
Pres
Hypothyroid

Replative
trauma

RA, Gout RPM

- increased
oulet syn
Vasculitis
Umbo embolie Th

(EMG.)

Acute: Chronic:
Tendinitis   Ganglion
(De Quervain's   Dupuytren's ⟶ common in   DM
suppurative)   Alcoholism
RA ⟵ Rupture   Family History
Infection

Cellulitis

Abscess

felons (infect— of distal Pulp
of Fingertip)

Paronychias (infect— of soft t/s
around the nail)

Carpal tunnel syndrome

Tinel's sign ⟶ tapping of median n/s over the wrist
Phalen's sign ⟶ sustained hyper flexion of wrist
may reproduce symptoms

KNEE PAIN

Michael J. Maricic, M.D.

A. The history and physical examination are crucial to establishing the proper diagnosis of knee pain. The first step is to determine whether the pain is intra-articular (which may involve any or all of the five joints in the knee: patellofemoral, fabellofemoral, medial tibiofemoral, lateral tibiofemoral, or tibiofibular) or extra-articular. Pain on both active and passive range of motion of the joint suggests intra-articular disease, whereas pain on active but not passive motion of the joint suggests extra-articular disease.

B. Pain worse in the morning, improved with motion, and associated with signs of inflammation (redness, heat, swelling) suggests inflammatory arthritis. Bilateral inflammation of the knees associated with inflammation of the small joints of the hands and feet is consistent with rheumatoid arthritis (most common), psoriatic arthritis, and systemic lupus erythematosus. Unilateral inflammatory arthritis of the knee could be due to crystals (gout, pseudogout), a seronegative spondyloarthropathy (Reiter's, psoriatic arthritis, ankylosing spondylitis) arthritis associated with inflammatory bowel disease, or infection (bacterial, mycobacterial, fungal). Lyme arthritis should also be considered in endemic areas. A Baker's (popliteal) cyst may be present in any type of inflammatory arthritis. These sometimes rupture and simulate an acute deep venous thrombosis. Chronic pain worse on weight bearing and with activity, and not associated with morning stiffness or signs of inflammation, suggests degenerative arthritis. Consider avascular necrosis of the knee when there is acute onset of pain in a patient with predisposing factors (glucocorticoid use, alcoholism, sickle cell disease, infiltrative marrow disorders). Consider neoplastic disorders, especially in children or adolescents. Night pain and periarticular soft tissue swelling are diagnostic clues suggesting neoplasm. Meniscal tears are often preceded by a history of a twisting injury. Mild inflammation of the knee may be present. McMurray's test (internal and external rotation of the knee with the knee brought from full flexion into extension) may produce pain or an audible click. Chondromalacia patellae is suggested by the history of anterior knee pain that is worse during climbing or descending stairs or squatting. Physical examination may reveal crepitus of the patellofemoral joint or subluxation/dislocation of the patella.

C. In the case of monoarticular joint swelling, synovial fluid examination is mandatory (p 384).

D. Arthrography may be performed to demonstrate meniscal and cruciate tears or a popliteal cyst. Ultrasonography is a less invasive method for this purpose.

E. Technetium bone scanning may be useful for demonstrating infectious arthritis of avascular necrosis. MRI is preferable when available.

F. MRI is the procedure of choice when considering the diagnosis of meniscal or ligamentous tears, tumor, infection, or avascular necrosis.

G. The prepatellar bursa (anterior) and anserine bursa (medial) may cause localized pain and swelling. The pes anserinus tendons (sartorius, gracilis, semitendinous) located medially and the quadriceps and patellar tendons located anteriorly may be the source of localized pain. Osgood-Schlatter disease refers to pain at the insertion of the patellar tendon into the tibial tubercle in adolescents; it is believed to be due to a mild avulsion. Ligamentous pain may arise from a strain of the medial collateral, lateral collateral, anterior cruciate, or posterior cruciate ligaments. Perform tests for valgus and varus stability and the anterior and posterior Drawer signs to test for laxity.

References

Helfet A. Disorders of the knee. Philadelphia: JB Lippincott, 1974.

Stoller DW, Genant HK. Magnetic resonance imaging of the knee and hip. Arthritis Rheum, 1990; 33:441.

Patient with KNEE PAIN

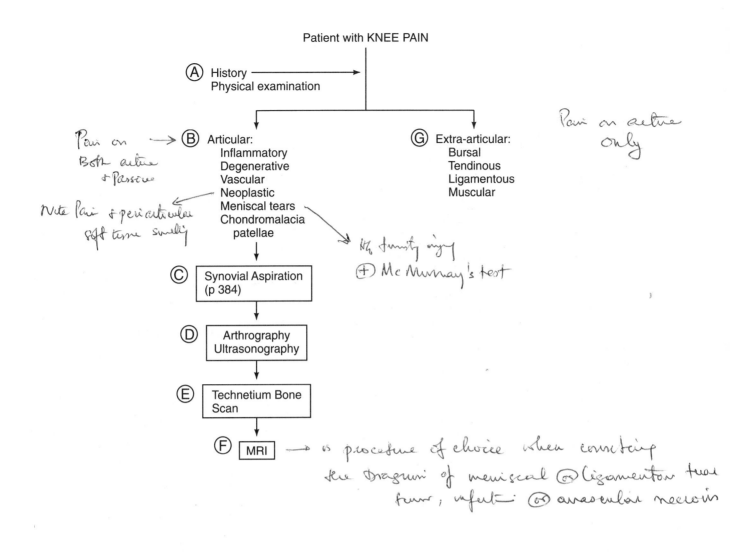

Ⓐ History ——————→
Physical examination

Pain on ——→ Ⓑ Articular:
Both active   Inflammatory
+ Passive   Degenerative
                     Vascular
Note Pain + periarticular   Neoplastic
soft tissue swelly   Meniscal tears
                     Chondromalacia
                       patellae

Ⓖ Extra-articular:
    Bursal
    Tendinous
    Ligamentous
    Muscular

Pain on active
only

Hx twisting injury
⊕ McMurray's test

Ⓒ Synovial Aspiration
   (p 384)

Ⓓ Arthrography
   Ultrasonography

Ⓔ Technetium Bone
   Scan

Ⓕ MRI —→ is procedure of choice when correcting
        the Diagnosis of meniscal or ligamentous tear
        tear, infection or avascular necrosis

avascular Necrosis of knee — steroid use
                              alcohol
                              Sickle cell Its
                              infiltrative marrow disorder

Lat   med
) ◯ (—→ pre petellar Bursa
         —→ anserine Bursa

403

FOOT PAIN

Martin Snyder, D.P.M.

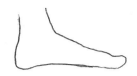

A. A careful history and thorough physical examination provide many clues to the cause of foot pain. The onset of pain, aggravating and relieving factors, and the conditions in which pain occurs are important subjective information. Objective signs are also crucial. Radiography, laboratory values, muscle testing, vascular and neurologic examinations, ranges of motion, and comparison of one side with the other help in the differential diagnosis. Also consider simple skin patterns of discoloration, edema, warmth, and texture.

B. Trauma may be the result of a simple sprain, an athletic injury, or an accidental slip or fall in walking or running. There may be microtrauma, as seen in occupational injuries when a worker uses one foot to operate a lever or press. The mechanism of the injury should explain the trauma. Radiography is essential to rule out fractures. Edema and discoloration reflect the internal trauma to the vascular system. Pressure from the injured part on nerves and blood vessels must be reduced to prevent permanent damage. Trauma to the foot or toes may also result from improperly fitted footgear. Tight shoes may cause corns or toe contractures, with resultant metatarsal depression.

C. Systemic factors are probably the most common, and most disabling, cause of foot pain. These may also become the most chronic lesions of the foot, since they encompass rheumatologic, vascular, and neurologic systems. Many systemic causes begin in areas remote from the feet. Because major systems are involved, consider such causes carefully in the differential diagnosis.

D. Rheumatologic causes are numerous. Some basic questions will help to classify the pain as one of the many arthritides that affect the feet: Is the condition inflammatory (swollen, red, and warm)? Is the condition symmetrical and bilateral? Is the pain greater at one time of day? How long does it take the patient to gain some relief from stiffness and aching? Since inflammatory arthritic changes are superimposed on a biomechanically weak structure, osseous articulations are destroyed and major digital deformities result. Even noninflammatory conditions affect weight distribution in the feet during the stance and propulsive phases of gait, and cause pain and disability.

E. Vascular pain may be acute and potentially destructive. Arterial emboli may lead to limb-threatening situations. If the lesion is spastic, as in Raynaud's disease affecting the arterial trunk, the prognosis is not as devastating as organic clot or blockage. Temperature variations have a bearing on spasticity. Firm clots or emboli are not subject to outside temperature, although cold weather causes some vasoconstriction. Arteriography may be required to distinguish spastic from fixed stenosis. In venous problems, edema ulcerations and phlebitis may be end results of venous failure or congestion. Varicose veins usually do not cause foot pain per se, but reflect the inadequate return of the vascular system and can break down over bony prominences and ulcerate.

F. Neurologic pain generally falls within two major areas. Pain in the distal part of the foot, especially around the toes and commonly in the third intermetatarsal space, is common and may be due to Morton's neuroma. Pain in the medial plantar portion of the heel is due to a compression neuropathy in the tarsal tunnel. The pain from this condition may mimic other symptoms around the heel, e.g., plantar fasciitis, neuroma of the medial calcaneal nerve, or pain secondary to the seronegative arthritides such as in Reiter's disease, ankylosing spondylitis, or even psoriasis. Diabetes mellitus and the complication of peripheral neuropathy cause a burning pain that is greater when the foot is not weight bearing.

G. Biomechanical causes are not always evident to casual observation. Be attuned to both obvious and subtle variations in gait. Whether the primary complaint is in the forefoot or rear foot, the entire axial and appendicular skeleton must be observed and measurements obtained that detail any decrease in motion, strength, or size compared with the opposite side. Paddings, strapping, special shoes, orthoses made to casts, and physical medicine may alleviate symptoms and help to re-establish normal foot function.

H. Infectious diseases that cause foot pain are usually related to trauma that permits the introduction of organisms into broken skin. A common infection is that of an ingrowing toenail that produces exudate and proud flesh and causes sharp, lancinating pain. The resultant paronychia, abscess, or even cellulitis may necessitate surgery. Other infections need not penetrate the skin but may lodge in the superficial cells and create the common verruca plantaris. Mycotic toenails with heavy deposits of subungual debris are uncomfortable with simple shoe pressure. Eventually, onychogryphotic nails develop from fungal infestation and neglect, and their very thickness may cause pain. While tinea pedis in itself may not be especially painful, the use of very aggressive medications and delay in proper treatment may result in overlay infections secondary to loss of skin protection.

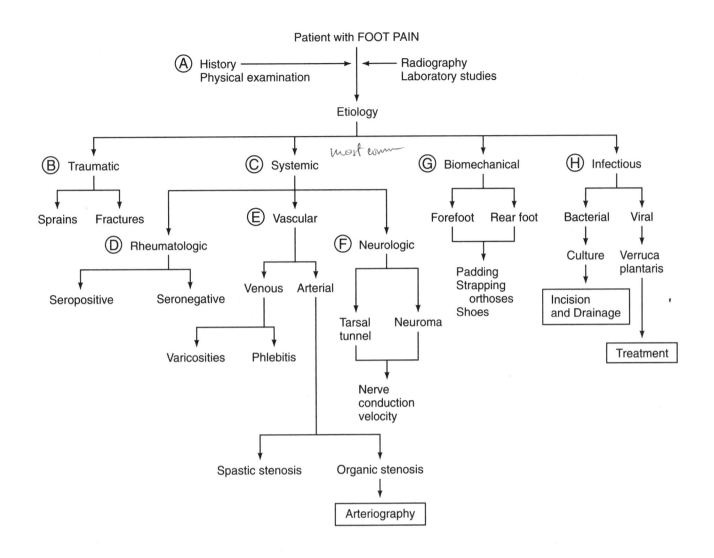

Patient with FOOT PAIN

Ⓐ History
Physical examination → ← Radiography
Laboratory studies

Etiology

most comm

Ⓑ Traumatic   Ⓒ Systemic   Ⓖ Biomechanical   Ⓗ Infectious

Sprains Fractures

Ⓓ Rheumatologic

Ⓔ Vascular

Ⓕ Neurologic

Seropositive Seronegative

Venous Arterial

Tarsal tunnel Neuroma

Varicosities Phlebitis

Nerve conduction velocity

Spastic stenosis Organic stenosis

Arteriography

Forefoot Rear foot

Padding
Strapping
orthoses
Shoes

Bacterial Viral

Culture Verruca plantaris

Incision and Drainage

Treatment

Tarsal tunnel → Pain in medial plantar portion of heel
d/t compression neuropathy

Pain in distal Part of Foot & 3°/2° intra metatarsal space
d/t Morton's Neuroma

References

Hoppenfeld S. Physical examination of the foot by complaint. In: Jahss MH; ed. Disorders of the foot. Philadelphia: WB Saunders, 1982.

Cailliet R. Foot and ankle pain. 2nd ed. Philadelphia: 1983.

Snyder, M. Disorders of the foot. In: Riggs, Gall. Rheumatic diseases Rehabilitation and Management. Butterworth, 1984.

Root M, Orien W, Weed J. Normal and abnormal function of the foot. Los Angeles: Clinical Biomechanics Corporation, 1977.

SCLERODERMA

Barbara Bode, M.D.

Scleroderma is a variable disease with several clinical presentations, each having differing prognoses. Progressive systemic sclerosis is considered the most severe and is characterized by diffuse inflammatory and proliferative vascular lesions with atrophy and fibrosis of skin, muscle, and involved organs (primarily GI tract, lung, and kidneys). The cause and pathogenesis are unknown. Disease onset is usually 30–50 years of age, with an increased incidence in women.

The sclerodermatous disorders frequently present with skin thickening. This usually involves the fingers and hands and may begin as painless swelling with pitting edema. The skin appears shiny and erythematous and eventually becomes indurated and "bound-down."

A. Patients with limited scleroderma typically have CREST syndrome (calcinosis, *R*aynaud's phenomenon, *e*sophageal dysfunction, *s*clerodactyly, and *t*elangiectasia). Calcinosis is most frequently found over the hands and fingers or over the olecranon bursa. Sclerodactyly is defined as skin involvement distal to the metacarpophalangeal joints; telangiectasia is seen on the palms of the hands or over the face and lips. Patients with limited scleroderma and CREST syndrome may also have internal organ involvement, but this is usually delayed in comparison to diffuse scleroderma.

B. After the skin thickening of hands and fingers, the face and neck usually become involved next. The patient may develop pinched facies and pursed lips. The skin changes progress at variable rates to involve the arms, legs, and trunk. Hyper- and hypopigmentation frequently develop.

C. Patients with extensive skin involvement may develop digital skin ulcerations and joint contractures with inability to fully extend the fingers or form a fist. Skin tightening about the mouth may limit the oral aperture. In approximately 70% of patients, Raynaud's phenomenon is part of the initial presentation. GI complaints are the third most common symptom. Dysmotility of the lower two thirds of the esophagus may cause dysphagia and odynophagia as well as symptoms of reflux. Constipation and malabsorption may signify colonic dysmotility or small bowel involvement, respectively. Generalized arthralgias and morning stiffness frequently occur, although clinical synovitis is rare. Symptoms related to pulmonary involvement, such as progressive dyspnea on exertion, are usually insidious.

D. Antinuclear antibodies are present in >90% of patients with systemic sclerosis, usually with a nucleolar pattern. Anticentromere antibodies are present in most patients with CREST syndrome and in <10% of patients with systemic sclerosis. Chest radiographs may reveal increased bi-basilar interstitial markings but are relatively insensitive as a screening test. Pulmonary function testing reveals restriction with decreased vital capacity and compliance. The most frequent abnormality, however, is diminished diffusing capacity. Gallium lung scanning has proved relatively insensitive. Bronchoalveolar lavage has been used recently with increased frequency and reveals increased neutrophils and lymphocytes. Holter monitoring may detect atrial and ventricular tachyarrhythmias, which occur in 50% of patients. Skin biopsy may be helpful, but obviously the differentiation between the limited and diffuse forms of scleroderma is made clinically.

E. Eosinophilic fasciitis is a scleroderma-like disease characterized by inflammation and thickening of the deep fascia. The skin may have an "orange-peel" appearance. Raynaud's and internal organ involvement are usually absent. Eosinophilic myalgia syndrome is a recently described disease characterized by eosinophilia and myalgias. It has been associated with ingestion of the amino acid health food supplement tryptophan. In overlap syndromes, patients may present with features of both scleroderma and SLE, inflammatory arthritis, or rheumatoid arthritis. Chronic graft-versus-host disease, a common complication of the allogeneic bone marrow transplant, may clinically appear very similar to scleroderma, skin induration being the most frequent manifestation. Drugs that may induce skin thickening are bleomycin and pentazocine.

F. Localized scleroderma differs from systemic scleroderma in that there is no involvement of internal organs. Localized scleroderma may occur in at least two different clinical variants: morphea and linear scleroderma.

G. Morphea is characterized initially by well-circumscribed superficial plaques with subsequent development of ivory-colored centers and violaceous borders. Plaques may range in size from 1–30 cm; they may be few in number or multiple. Typically, they are asymmetric, although patients can present with extensive involvement referred to as "generalized morphea." The disease course is variable, but not infrequently there is spontaneous improvement or resolution over several months to years.

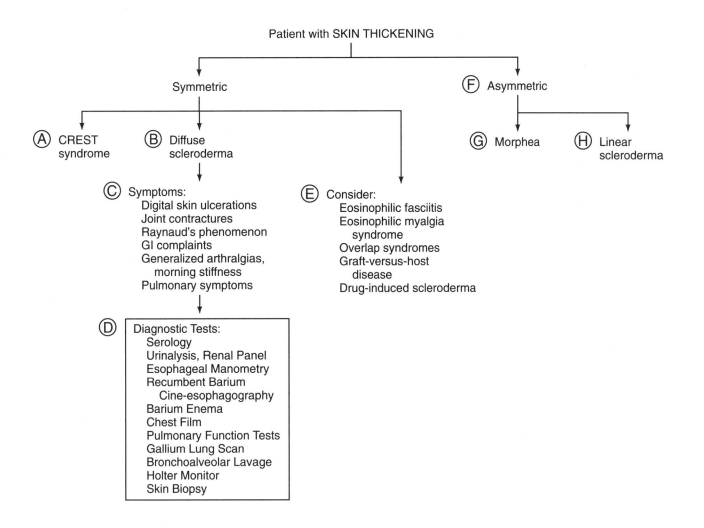

Patient with SKIN THICKENING

Ⓐ CREST syndrome

Ⓑ Diffuse scleroderma

Ⓒ Symptoms:
Digital skin ulcerations
Joint contractures
Raynaud's phenomenon
GI complaints
Generalized arthralgias, morning stiffness
Pulmonary symptoms

Ⓓ Diagnostic Tests:
Serology
Urinalysis, Renal Panel
Esophageal Manometry
Recumbent Barium
Cine-esophagography
Barium Enema
Chest Film
Pulmonary Function Tests
Gallium Lung Scan
Bronchoalveolar Lavage
Holter Monitor
Skin Biopsy

Ⓔ Consider:
Eosinophilic fasciitis
Eosinophilic myalgia syndrome
Overlap syndromes
Graft-versus-host disease
Drug-induced scleroderma

Ⓕ Asymmetric

Ⓖ Morphea

Ⓗ Linear scleroderma

H. Linear scleroderma, unlike morphea, tends to involve deeper layers of the skin, frequently with fixation to underlying muscle and bone and occasionally causing fibrous contractures. It commonly occurs in a linear, bandlike distribution on the head, trunk, or extremities. When linear scleroderma involves the face and scalp, it may develop a depressed appearance and is referred to as "en coup de sabre."

References

Falanga V. Localized scleroderma. Med Clin North Am 1989; 73:1143.

Lally EV, Jimenez SA, Kaplan SR. Progressive systemic sclerosis: mode of presentation, rapidly progressive disease course, and mortality based on an analysis of 91 patients. Semin Arthritis Rheum 1988; 18:1.

Masi AT, Rodnan GP, Medsger TA, et al. Preliminary criteria for the classification of systemic sclerosis (scleroderma). Arthritis Rheum 1980; 23:581.

Seibold JR. Scleroderma. In: Kelley WN, Harris ED, Ruddy S, Sledge CB, eds. Textbook of rheumatology. 3rd ed. Philadelphia: WB Saunders, 1989: 1215.

KERATOCONJUNCTIVITIS SICCA (SJÖGREN'S SYNDROME)

Marcia Ko, M.D.

A. Symptoms of keratoconjunctivitis sicca (KCS) result from decreased tear formation. Patients most often complain of gradual onset of "dry eyes" characterized as a foreign body sensation, grittiness, or sandy sensation, with or without visual changes or photophobia. Xerostomia or dry mouth secondary to salivary gland atrophy is often described as difficulty chewing or swallowing dry foods such as crackers or bread, or difficulty talking secondary to dryness. There may also be a complaint of fissures or ulcers on mucosal surfaces or lips and the need to drink liquids to enable speech and eating. "Dryness" related to other exocrine gland dysfunction occurs (nose, tracheobronchial tree, skin).

B. Examination to confirm KCS may include a Schirmer test as a measure of tear formation. In this test, Schirmer filter paper is placed in the conjunctival sac. After 5 minutes the strips are removed to determine the extent of wetness (<15 mm of wetness is abnormal). A 1% rose bengal solution application and slit-lamp examination may demonstrate areas of corneal or conjunctival epithelial damage secondary to dryness. Another cause of diminished tear secretion is senile atrophy of the lacrimal glands.

C. Confirmation of dry mouth secondary to labial gland atrophy is difficult. Mild dryness may be normal or secondary to drugs such as anticholinergic medications. Salivary flow (volume) may be measured. Biopsy of minor salivary glands in the lip has also been used to support a clinical diagnosis, since there is a characteristic histopathologic picture associated with Sjögren's syndrome characterized by a lymphocytic infiltration of the glands. Lack of salivary pooling in the floor of the mouth may be a sign of xerostomia.

D. Primary Sjögren's syndrome is diagnosed when other connective tissue disease is not present.

E. Other rheumatic diseases associated with Sjögren's syndrome ("secondary" Sjögren's) include rheumatoid arthritis, systemic lupus erythematosus, scleroderma, polyarteritis nodosa, and polymyositis.

F. Other clinical findings are related to exocrine gland dysfunction (mucous membrane dryness of the nose and upper airway, skin dryness, genital dryness). Pancreatic disease may also be seen. Atrophic gastritis has been described, but pernicious anemia is rare. Nonexocrine organs may also be involved, including peripheral nerves, joints, skin, and blood. Vasculitis and Raynaud's phenomenon may be found. Renal involvement is manifested most often as interstitial nephritis and type II renal tubular acidosis.

G. There are no specific laboratory tests for the diagnosis of Sjögren's syndrome. Rheumatoid factor is present in approximately 75–95% of patients; antinuclear antibodies may be found in 50–80%. Anti-La (SS-B) and anti-Ro (SS-A) may be found. Other nonspecific laboratory tests include a normochromic, normocytic anemia; leukopenia, and elevated ESR. Serum protein electrophoresis may demonstrate diffuse elevation in all immunoglobulin classes. A fall in the rheumatoid factor may signify a malignant transformation to lymphoma, which has a 44-fold increased incidence in patients with primary Sjögren's syndrome.

References

Talal N. Sjögren's syndrome. In: Schumacher HR, ed. Primer on rheumatic diseases. 9th ed. Atlanta: Arthritis Foundation, 1988: 136.

Whaley K, Alspaugh MA, Kelley WN, et al. Sjögren's syndrome. In: Kelley WN, Harris ED Jr, Ruddy S, Sledge CB, eds. Textbook of rheumatology. 3rd ed. Philadelphia: WB Saunders, 1989.

Youinov P, Mousopoulos HM, Pennec YL. Clinical features of Sjögren's syndrome. Curr Opinion Rheumatol 1990; 2:687.

KERATOCONJUNCTIVITIS SICCA Suspected

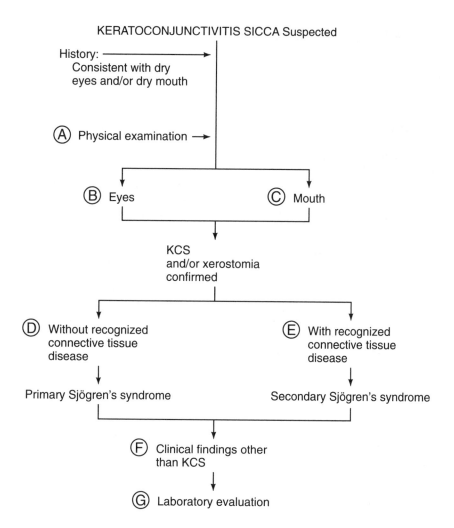

History: ──────────────→
Consistent with dry
eyes and/or dry mouth

Ⓐ Physical examination ──→

Ⓑ Eyes   Ⓒ Mouth

KCS
and/or xerostomia
confirmed

Ⓓ Without recognized   Ⓔ With recognized
connective tissue   connective tissue
disease   disease

Primary Sjögren's syndrome   Secondary Sjögren's syndrome

Ⓕ Clinical findings other
than KCS

Ⓖ Laboratory evaluation

RAYNAUD'S PHENOMENON

Patricia Mayer, M.D.

Raynaud's phenomenon is characterized by intermittent vasoconstriction of the digits, usually triggered by cold or stress. Three classic stages are recognized: blanching, cyanotic, and ruborous. Raynaud's phenomenon may be mild and only minimally uncomfortable or may be severe, involving digital ulceration and/or gangrene. The phenomenon may be idiopathic (primary) or related to underlying abnormality (secondary).

A. A thorough history and a meticulous physical examination are essential to the evaluation and reveal most secondary causes.

B. Raynaud's phenomenon is almost always bilateral. Unilateral complaints should prompt an evaluation for neurogenic (thoracic outlet syndrome, carpal tunnel syndrome, reflex sympathetic dystrophy) or vascular (arteriosclerosis, embolic phenomenon, thromboangiitis obliterans) disease.

C. Raynaud's phenomenon may be seen in pneumatic hammer operators, in patients with repetitive wrist and finger motion (pianists, computer operators, typists), and after injury from trauma or cold. Environmental agents such as heavy metals and polyvinyl chloride have also been implicated.

D. Multiple drugs and medications are associated with Raynaud's phenomenon. These include beta-blocking agents, ergotamine preparations, various chemotherapeutic agents, oral contraceptives, nicotine, caffeine, and various antihistamines and decongestants.

E. Multiple underlying abnormalities may be associated with Raynaud's phenomenon, including most commonly any of the connective tissue disorders (e.g., systemic lupus erythematosus, Sjögren's syndrome, rheumatoid arthritis, dermatomyositis, scleroderma). If an underlying condition is suspected from the history and physical examination, further laboratory testing or other evaluations may be needed as the situation requires.

F. In patients in whom a thorough history and physical examination reveal no clues for further work-up or associated conditions, undertake a minimal laboratory work-up to rule out serious underlying causes, including occult malignancy, hematologic disease, and rheumatic disease. Raynaud's phenomenon may precede the development of connective tissue disease by months or years.

References

Campbell PM, LeRoy EC. Raynaud phenomenon. Semin Arthritis Rheum 1986; 19:92.

Greenberger NJ, Agee KR, King TM, Nelson M. The medical book of lists. Chicago: Year Book, 1990.

Grisanti JM. Raynaud's phenomenon. Am Fam Physician 1990; 41:134.

Langevitz P, Buskila D, Lee P, Urowitz MB. Treatment of refractory ischemic skin ulcers in patients with Raynaud's phenomenon with PGE infusions. J Rheumatol 1989; 16:1433.

Patient with RAYNAUD'S PHENOMENON

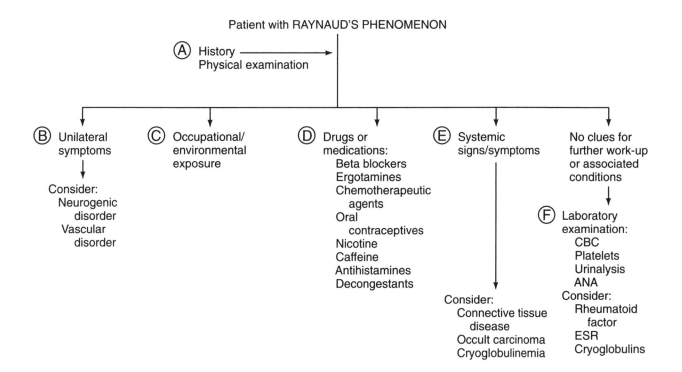

(A) History ——————→ Physical examination

(B) Unilateral symptoms

Consider:
Neurogenic
disorder
Vascular
disorder

(C) Occupational/
environmental
exposure

(D) Drugs or
medications:
Beta blockers
Ergotamines
Chemotherapeutic
agents
Oral
contraceptives
Nicotine
Caffeine
Antihistamines
Decongestants

(E) Systemic
signs/symptoms

Consider:
Connective tissue
disease
Occult carcinoma
Cryoglobulinemia

No clues for
further work-up
or associated
conditions

(F) Laboratory
examination:
CBC
Platelets
Urinalysis
ANA
Consider:
Rheumatoid
factor
ESR
Cryoglobulins

OSTEOPENIA

Michael J. Maricic, M.D.

A. The initial evaluation of patients suspected of being osteopenic begins with historical evaluation of their risk factors. These include estrogen deficiency, family history, small body frame, calcium deficiency, inactivity, tobacco or alcohol abuse, or use of medications such as corticosteroids. A history of vitamin D deficiency, malabsorption, gastrectomy, anticonvulsant use, or renal disorders such as renal tubular acidosis may alert one to the possibility of osteomalacia. If these are all negative and there is no history of fractures or loss of height, further work-up is probably not necessary.

B. Osteopenia, meaning "poverty of bone," is the radiographic appearance of diminished bone density. It is not possible to distinguish osteoporosis (decreased bone mass) from osteomalacia (decreased mineralization of bone) or osteitis fibrosa cystica (the bone lesion that occurs in hyperparathyroidism characterized by increased osteoclastic resorption and fibrosis) radiographically. Early radiographic signs of osteopenia may include preferential loss of horizontal striations in vertebral bodies or Schmorl's nodules (herniation of the nucleus pulposus into softened vertebral bodies). Often, 30–40% of bone density must be lost before osteopenia may be apparent on radiographs. Bone density scanning (such as dual energy x-ray absorptiometry) gives much more exact estimations of bone density and should be considered in high-risk patients.

C. If osteopenia is present, perform screening laboratory tests for calcium, phosphorus, and alkaline phosphatase. A low phosphorus and high alkaline phosphatase level should alert one to the possibility of osteomalacia. Normal values do not exclude osteomalacia, however, and the vigor with which this is pursued depends on the presence of risk factors for osteomalacia mentioned above. A dual-labeled tetracycline bone biopsy is necessary for the definitive diagnosis of osteomalacia. High calcium with low phosphorus and elevated alkaline phosphatase levels should alert one to hyperparathyroidism.

D. If osteomalacia is excluded, the patient may have type I (postmenopausal), type II (senile), or secondary osteoporosis. Type I osteoporosis is characterized by estrogen deficiency and early vertebral (trabecular) bone loss. Type II occurs at a later age, presumably as a result of the combination of estrogen deficiency and decreased 1,25-dihydroxy vitamin D production by the aging kidney. Both cortical and trabecular bone loss are present. Secondary causes of osteoporosis include neoplasia (multiple myeloma, lymphoma), drugs (corticosteroids), and endocrine disorders (hyperthyroidism, hyperparathyroidism, and primary or secondary gonadal failure such as in prolactin-secreting tumors). Besides a detailed history and physical examination to seek these disorders, consider laboratory screening with serum calcium, phosphate, alkaline phosphatase, complete blood count, thyroid function tests, ESR, and urinanalysis.

References

Frame B, Parfitt AM. Osteomalacia: current concepts. Ann Intern Med 1978; 89:966.

Mundy GR. Differential diagnosis of osteopenia. Hosp Pract 1978; 65–72.

Riggs BL, Melton LJ. Involutional osteoporosis. N Engl J Med 1986; 314:1676.

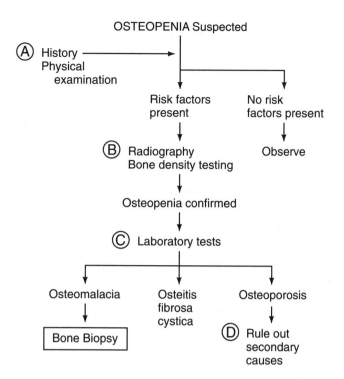

OSTEOPENIA Suspected

(A) History
Physical
examination

Risk factors
present

No risk
factors present

(B) Radiography
Bone density testing

Observe

Osteopenia confirmed

(C) Laboratory tests

Osteomalacia

Osteitis
fibrosa
cystica

Osteoporosis

Bone Biopsy

(D) Rule out
secondary
causes

HYPERURICEMIA AND GOUT

Eric P. Gall, M.D.

A. Hyperuricemia may be caused by many mechanisms, including overproduction of uric acid (20–25% of patients) and inability of the kidneys to excrete uric acid (75–80%). Overproduction may be caused by a congenital enzyme defect, but other clinical problems, including hemolytic anemia, myeloproliferative disease, and psoriasis, should be excluded. Underexcretion of uric acid may be due to renal failure, drug action on the kidney, or idiopathic mechanisms. Hyperuricemia is generally defined as a serum uric acid level >8 mg/dl.

B. The decision whether to treat asymptomatic hyperuricemia is controversial. Most physicians treat uric acid levels >10 mg/dl if the patient has only one kidney; hyperuricosuria (>1000 mg/day), placing the kidney at risk for stones; or extreme serum levels (>12–13 mg/dl). If these criteria are satisfied, treatment with allopurinol may be begun. If these conditions are not present, observation of the patient will suffice.

C. The acute attack of gout can occur in any joint. Commonly, it occurs nocturnally in the first metatarsophalangeal (MTP) joint, but any joint may be involved. The definitive diagnosis of gout is made by demonstration of sodium urate crystals under polarized light microscopy. The crystals are negatively birefringent and needle shaped. A polarizing microscope with a first-order red compensator is necessary. The definitive diagnosis is made when six or more of the following criteria are present: (1) more than one attack of arthritis, (2) development of maximum inflammation within 1 day, (3) oligoarthritis attack, (4) redness over the joint, (5) painful or swollen first MTP, (6) unilateral attack in the first MTP, (7) unilateral attack in the tarsal joint, (8) tophus, (9) hyperuricemia, (10) asymmetric swelling within a joint, and (11) termination of the attack with colchicine therapy.

D. The acute attack is treated before the underlying hyperuricemia. If there is no peptic ulcer disease or other contraindication to nonsteroidal anti-inflammatory drugs (NSAIDs), these are the treatment of choice. One usually uses a short-acting NSAID such as ibuprofen, but long-acting agents will work. The drugs should be started in relatively high dose. Continue NSAID treatment until the acute arthritis is resolved. If peptic ulcer disease or other disease contraindicates the use of NSAIDs, alternative therapy is required.

E. The use of alternative therapy depends on whether there is renal failure, hepatic insufficiency, or bone marrow depression. If none of these conditions are present, IV colchicine can be used in an initial dose of 2 mg in 50–100 ml of saline or glucose, infused by IV catheter over 15–30 min. It should not be pushed because it can cause cardiovascular collapse. Extravasation of colchicine can cause tissue necrosis. Doses of 1 mg may be repeated, if necessary, every 6 hrs until a total daily dose of 4 mg is given. Higher doses may cause GI toxicity and marrow aplasia, and therefore are contraindicated.

F. If there is significant impairment of kidney, liver, or bone marrow function, give corticosteroids orally or parenterally in a dose of 40–60 mg prednisone equivalent per day until the acute attack is resolved.

G. Before initiating chronic treatment for gout, measure serum and urine uric acid and creatinine. This should be done after the acute attack resolves. Patients are divided into overproducers of uric acid (24-hr uric acid >800 mg or a spot urinary uric acid/creatinine ratio >0.7) and underexcretors (24-hr urine uric acid <600 mg or a urinary uric acid/creatinine ratio <0.7).

H. In patients who are overproducers of uric acid, give allopurinol along with colchicine. Begin with a single daily dose of 200–300 mg along with 0.5 mg colchicine twice a day. If the patient has significant renal disease, use allopurinol as the drug of choice, since uricosuric drugs will not be effective.

I. In patients who are underexcretors of uric acid and have no renal disease, uricosuric agents are the treatment of choice. The reason for using these drugs in this situation is because of allopurinol's significant toxicity, including skin rash and systemic vasculitis. Start probenecid 500 mg twice a day orally and adjust according to the serum uric acid. Adequate urinary volume with good fluid intake should be assured. Patients who have had renal calculi should not take uricosuric agents. Those on probenecid should be given colchicine in a low dose initially.

J. With either allopurinol or probenecid, adjust the serum uric acid level to <6 mg/dl. This is done by instituting therapy and ensuring compliance. Gradual adjustments are made until the serum uric acid level drops to <6 mg/dl. Colchicine in a low dose is maintained until 6 weeks after the required serum level is reached, or until all recurrent acute attacks have resolved, or, if the patient has tophaceous gout, until the tophi disappear. If acute attacks recur, treatment is similar to that earlier, without a change in uric acid–lowering drugs during the initial acute treatment.

References

Liang MH, Fries JF. Asymptomatic hyperuricemia: the case for conservative management. Ann Intern Med 1978; 88: 666.

Simkin PA. Management of gout. Ann Intern Med 1979; 90:812.

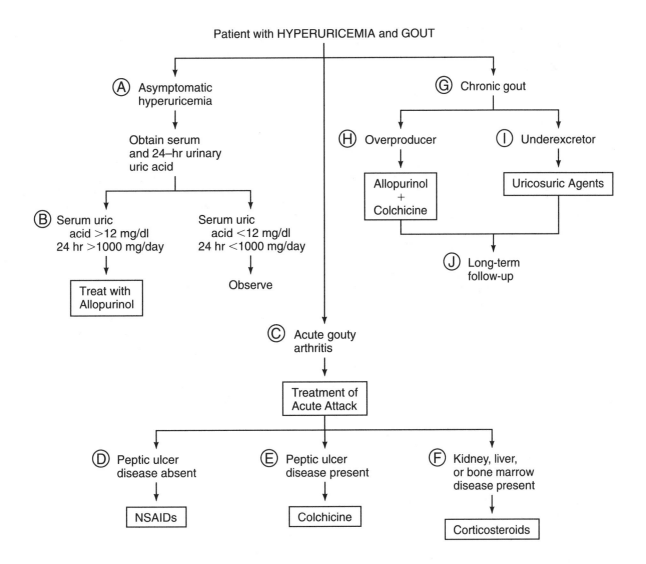

Patient with HYPERURICEMIA and GOUT

(A) Asymptomatic hyperuricemia

Obtain serum and 24–hr urinary uric acid

(B) Serum uric acid >12 mg/dl 24 hr >1000 mg/day

Serum uric acid <12 mg/dl 24 hr <1000 mg/day

Treat with Allopurinol

Observe

(C) Acute gouty arthritis

Treatment of Acute Attack

(D) Peptic ulcer disease absent

NSAIDs

(E) Peptic ulcer disease present

Colchicine

(F) Kidney, liver, or bone marrow disease present

Corticosteroids

(G) Chronic gout

(H) Overproducer

Allopurinol + Colchicine

(I) Underexcretor

Uricosuric Agents

(J) Long-term follow-up

DIFFUSE MUSCLE PAIN AND STIFFNESS: POLYMYALGIA RHEUMATICA AND GIANT CELL ARTERITIS

Michael J. Maricic, M.D.

A. Diffuse muscle pain and stiffness are usually manifestations of systemic disease and therefore necessitate a complete history and physical examination. It is important initially to determine if weakness is present or absent, and whether the patient complaints suggest a neuropathy (distal weakness, dropping things, tripping, such as over curbs) or a myopathy (proximal weakness, such as inability to get out of a chair or to comb one's hair). Early in the disease, there may be mild overlap between the disorders that cause true weakness and those that do not.

B. If myopathic weakness is present, consider endocrine (hyperthyroid, hypothyroid, hyperparathyroid, acromegaly, diabetes mellitus), electrolyte (hypophosphatemia, hypokalemia), neoplastic (Eaton-Lambert), drug-induced (alcohol, corticosteroids), inflammatory (poly- or dermatomyositis) disorders, and muscular dystrophy. Appropriate laboratory testing for the endocrine and electrolyte disorders, electromyographic (EMG) studies showing incremental response to repetitive muscle stimulation in the Eaton-Lambert syndrome and characteristic rash, and EMG and biopsy findings in polydermatomyositis help lead to the appropriate diagnosis. A family history is usually present in the various types of muscular dystrophy.

C. If true muscle weakness is absent, yet the patient complains of severe pain and stiffness, consider polymyalgia rheumatica (PMR) (in patients >50 years old), viral syndromes, fibromyalgia, depression, and hypothyroidism as potential causes. Appropriate laboratory testing in such patients having chronic symptoms includes ESR and thyroid function tests.

D. PMR is most commonly seen in patients >60 years old with occasional onset in those >50. The onset is usually abrupt, with severe morning stiffness relieved by activity. True weakness of the muscles is absent, although patients may develop some disuse atrophy and flexion contractures of the shoulders over time owing to severe pain. The ESR is usually greatly elevated, although a normal ESR does not rule out the diagnosis. Once the diagnosis of PMR is entertained, and since 20% of patients with PMR have or will develop giant cell arteritis (GCA), question and examine them extensively for symptoms and signs of GCA. These include headache, visual changes, jaw claudication, scalp numbness, tender temporal arteries, and signs of ischemic retinopathy on funduscopic examination. Nonspecific systemic symptoms such as fever, night sweats and weight loss should also alert one to the possibility of a systemic vasculitis.

E. If there is any suspicion of GCA, begin therapy with high-dose prednisone immediately and schedule the patient for temporal artery biopsy. If there are no signs or symptoms of GCA, low-dose prednisone may be begun.

References

Bohan A, Peter JB, Bowman RL, et al. A computer assisted analysis of 153 patients with polymyositis and dermatomyositis. Medicine (Baltimore) 1977; 56:255.

Hall S, Persellin S, Lie JT, et al. The therapeutic impact of temporal artery biopsy. Lancet 1983; 2:1217.

Huston KA, Hunder GG, Lie JT, et al. Temporal arteritis. A 25-year epidemiologic, clinical, and pathologic study. Ann Intern Med 1978; 88:162.

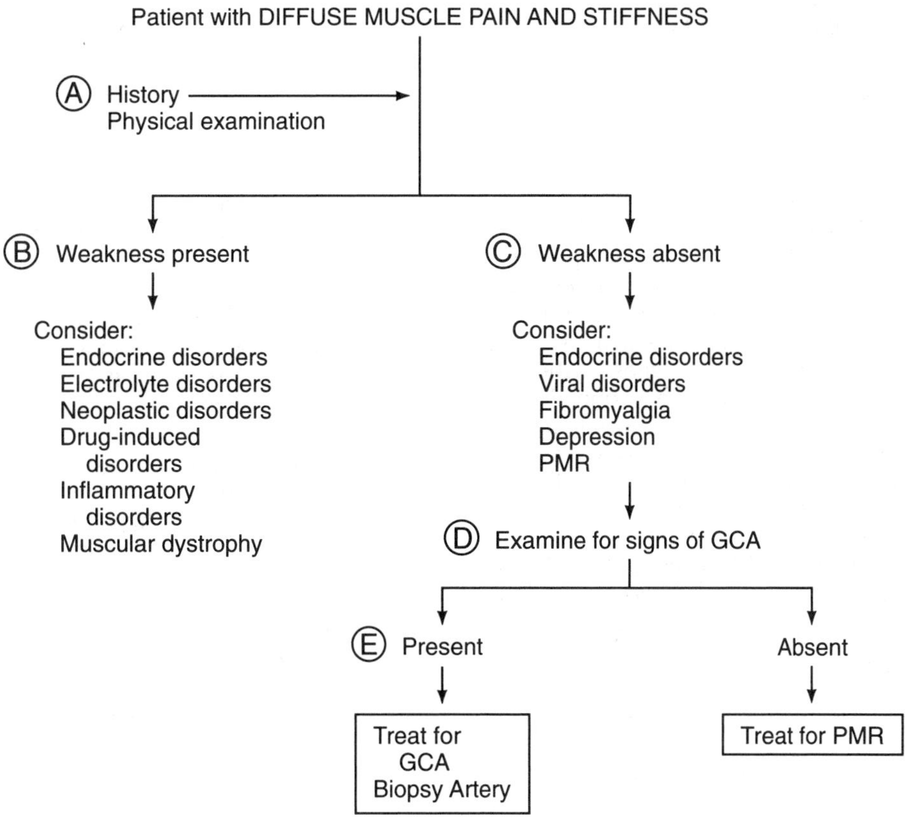

Patient with DIFFUSE MUSCLE PAIN AND STIFFNESS

(A) History ———————→
    Physical examination

(B) Weakness present

Consider:
    Endocrine disorders
    Electrolyte disorders
    Neoplastic disorders
    Drug-induced
        disorders
    Inflammatory
        disorders
    Muscular dystrophy

(C) Weakness absent

Consider:
    Endocrine disorders
    Viral disorders
    Fibromyalgia
    Depression
    PMR

(D) Examine for signs of GCA

(E) Present

Absent

┌──────────────┐
│ Treat for   │
│   GCA   │
│ Biopsy Artery│
└──────────────┘

┌──────────────┐
│ Treat for PMR│
└──────────────┘

JOINT HYPERMOBILITY

Patricia Mayer, M.D.

A. The congenital disorders causing joint hypermobility can usually be diagnosed with a careful history and physical examination. Family history may provide a diagnosis, but spontaneous mutations do occur and are responsible for many cases. Since family history may be unhelpful or unavailable, the algorithm relies on clinical characteristics for diagnosis whenever possible. Patients with true joint hypermobility are able to perform at least four of the following maneuvers: hyperextend the elbow 10 degrees or more past neutral; extend the metacarpophalangeal (MCP) joints to 90 degrees or more; flex the thumb to touch the wrist, digits (hyperextension of the proximal interphalangeal with flexion of the distal interphalangeals); flex the trunk forward so that the palms rest on the floor.

B. Evaluate the patient for evidence of Marfan's syndrome. A patient with all the cardinal manifestations (ocular, skeletal, and cardiac) or two of the major manifestations in the presence of a positive family history can be considered to meet the criteria. The most common ocular manifestation is ectopia lentis with upward displacement of the lens. Cardiovascular involvement includes dilation of the ascending aorta, aortic dissection, aortic regurgitation, and mitral valve prolapse. Skeletal features include abnormally tall stature, dolichostenomelia, arachnodactyly, high arched palate, and anterior chest deformities.

C. If criteria are met, consider the differential diagnosis of Marfan's syndrome. It is especially important to consider the possibility of homocystinuria, a recessively inherited inborn error of metabolism that is treatable. Erdheim's disease (annuloaortic ectasia) and Stickler's syndrome (hereditary arthro-ophthalmopathy) may also mimic Marfan's syndrome.

D. An evaluation of skin texture allows categorization of most disorders into one of three groups: normal skin, hyperextensible skin with dystrophic scarring, or lax or wrinkled skin. A few disorders do not fit this classification (see R).

E. If the skin is normal, evaluate stature. Most patients with short stature have frank characteristics of dwarfism and are less than the 5th percentile in height for their age and sex.

F. Abnormally short patients with joint hypermobility generally suffer from one of the skeletal dysplasias associated with joint hypermobility. Prominent spinal involvement with malalignment and dislocation is a hallmark of spondyloepimetaphyseal dysplasia with joint laxity (SEMDJL). Larsen's syndrome (flattened nasal bridge and broad terminal phalanges) and Desbuquois' syndrome (prominent eyes, broad terminal phalanges, and supernumerary phalanges) generally lack features of spinal malalignment or dislocation.

G. Recurrent dislocations are the cardinal feature of familial joint hypermobility of the so-called "dislocating" type. Dislocations are most prominent at the knees, hips, and elbows. Larsen's syndrome is also characterized by recurrent dislocations, and may be associated with normal, as well as short, stature.

H. Ehlers-Danlos syndrome (EDS) type X may show striae distensae or prominent bruising or petechiae on skin with otherwise normal texture and extensibility. Patients with joint hypermobility unrelated to skin or stature abnormalities, and without recurrent dislocations, may have either familial hypermobility, so-called "uncomplicated" type, or EDS III. Although EDS III usually has some skin hyperextensibility, it may be so mild that it is overlooked.

(Continued on page 420)

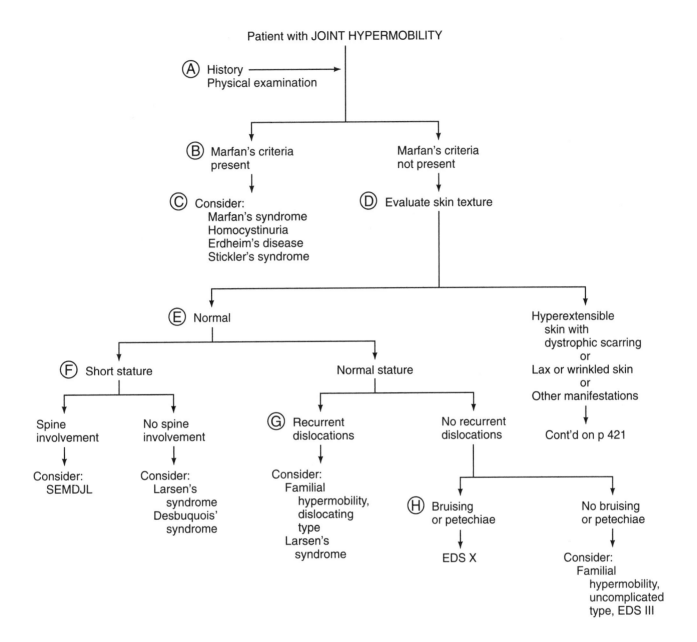

Patient with JOINT HYPERMOBILITY

(A) History
Physical examination

(B) Marfan's criteria present

Marfan's criteria not present

(C) Consider:
Marfan's syndrome
Homocystinuria
Erdheim's disease
Stickler's syndrome

(D) Evaluate skin texture

(E) Normal

Hyperextensible skin with dystrophic scarring
or
Lax or wrinkled skin
or
Other manifestations

Cont'd on p 421

(F) Short stature

Normal stature

Spine involvement

No spine involvement

(G) Recurrent dislocations

No recurrent dislocations

Consider:
SEMDJL

Consider:
Larsen's syndrome
Desbuquois' syndrome

Consider:
Familial hypermobility, dislocating type
Larsen's syndrome

(H) Bruising or petechiae

No bruising or petechiae

EDS X

Consider:
Familial hypermobility, uncomplicated type, EDS III

I. Hyperextensible skin is usually associated with dystrophic scarring, as evidenced by the so-called cigarette paper scars, and may also be associated with tissue fragility and easy bruising. Such "loose skin" is a cardinal manifestation of several types of EDS.

J. Some of the Ehlers-Danlos syndromes are distinguished primarily by their dramatic extradermal/extra-articular involvement. EDS VIII is characterized by the early onset of severe periodontitis associated with gingival recession and early tooth loss. Short stature and micrognathia accompany severe skin and joint involvement in EDS VII. Ocular involvement and scoliosis are seen in EDS VI. Stickler's syndrome can mimic both EDS VI and Marfan's syndrome.

K. The severity of joint involvement in the EDS syndromes associated with characteristic hyperextensible skin with dystrophic scarring can be gauged as either severe to moderate or moderate to mild.

L. Severely affected skin and severely affected joints are seen in the X-linked EDS V as well as the autosomal dominant EDS I, or "gravis" type.

M. EDS III, also referred to as benign hypermobility, may have mild or even undetectable (see H) skin changes associated with severe joint hypermobility.

N. Both EDS II and EDS V may have moderate or mild joint involvement and are then distinguished by their inheritance. EDS II or "mitis" type is autosomal dominant; EDS V is X-linked.

O. The lax and wrinkled skin syndromes are generally not associated with hyperextensibility, scarring, or the fragility described above.

P. Menkes' syndrome, formerly called Menkes' kinky hair syndrome, is characterized by abnormal hair as well as vascular rupture and brain dysfunction. It is caused by an X-linked disorder of copper transport and can be seen in both classic (severe) and mild forms.

Q. Wrinkled skin over the hands and feet associated with low birth weight characterizes wrinkly skin syndrome. Diffuse wrinkly or lax skin is seen in both occipital horn syndrome and the variant of cutis laxa referred to as cutis laxa with joint hypermobility and developmental delay. The classic form of cutis laxa is not associated with joint hypermobility.

R. Disorders with characteristic skin manifestations not described in other groups include the yellow infiltrated flexural lesions of pseudoxanthoma elasticum (PXE) and the striae distensae of EDS X.

References

Beighton P, dePaepe A, Danks D, et al. International nosology of heritable disorders of connective tissue, Berlin, 1986. Am J Med Genet 1988; 00:581.

Beighton P, McKusick VA, eds. McKusick's heritable disorders of connective tissue. 5th ed. St. Louis: Mosby-Year Book, 1992.

Finsterbush A, Pogrund H. The hypermobility syndrome. Clin Orthop 1982; 168: 124.

Pyeritz RE. The Marfan syndrome. Am Fam Physician 1986; 34:83.

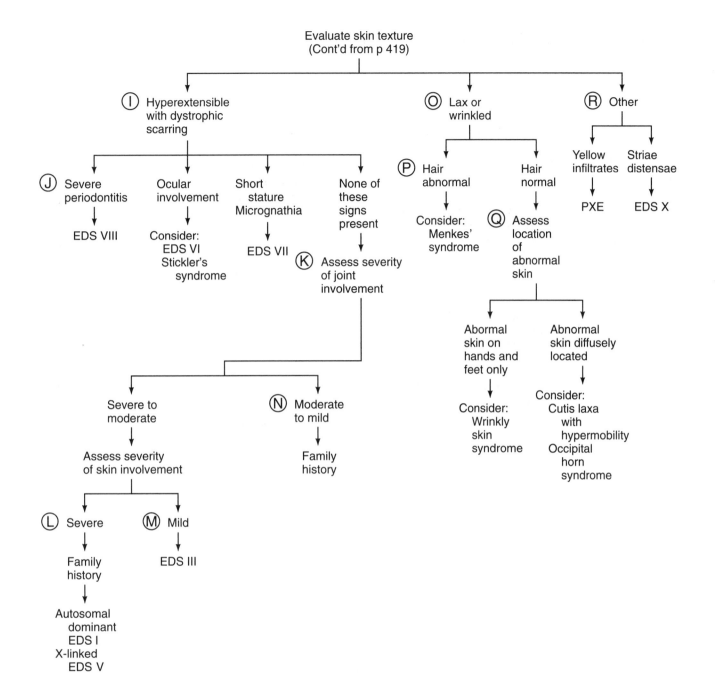

Evaluate skin texture
(Cont'd from p 419)

Ⓘ Hyperextensible with dystrophic scarring

Ⓙ Severe periodontitis → EDS VIII

Ocular involvement → Consider: EDS VI Stickler's syndrome

Short stature Micrognathia → EDS VII

None of these signs present → Ⓚ Assess severity of joint involvement

Severe to moderate → Assess severity of skin involvement

Ⓛ Severe → Family history → Autosomal dominant EDS I X-linked EDS V

Ⓜ Mild → EDS III

Ⓝ Moderate to mild → Family history

Ⓞ Lax or wrinkled

Ⓟ Hair abnormal → Consider: Menkes' syndrome

Hair normal → Ⓠ Assess location of abnormal skin

Abormal skin on hands and feet only → Consider: Wrinkly skin syndrome

Abnormal skin diffusely located → Consider: Cutis laxa with hypermobility Occipital horn syndrome

Ⓡ Other

Yellow infiltrates → PXE

Striae distensae → EDS X

TEMPOROMANDIBULAR PAIN

Michael J. Maricic, M.D.

A. A thorough history and physical examination are required to exclude pain not originating in the temporomandibular joint (TMJ).

B. Plain radiographs should be taken in the panoramic and transcranial views in both open and closed positions. Tomography may also be helpful. Radiography may reveal roughened and irregular bony cortices and flattening and anterior lipping of the condyle in degenerative joint disease. Radiographs may be normal in internal derangement, and in this case arthrography and/or MRI may be necessary to establish a definitive diagnosis.

C. Nonarticular causes of pain in the TMJ region include otitis, pain of dental origin, sinusitis, neuralgia, and temporal arteritis. Myofascial pain and dysfunction of the muscles of mastication may be present. Pain present on palpation of the muscle, no pain on palpation of the TMJ, and normal radiographs may be clues to this latter diagnosis.

D. Internal derangement of the TMJ occurs because of an abnormal relationship of the fibrous connective tissue disc with the condyle when the teeth are in maximal occlusion. Pain on palpation of the condyle and popping and clicking in the TMJ are common signs.

E. Degenerative joint disease generally has an insidious onset. Pain is usually continuous and increases with activity. Coarse crepitus may be present.

F. Other systemic arthritides such as rheumatoid arthritis, systemic lupus, and gout, as well as developmental deformities and neoplasia, may also affect the TMJ joint, necessitating a complete history and physical examination.

References

Dolwick MF, Katzberg RW, Helms CA, Bales DJ. Arthrotomographic evaluation of the temporomandibular joint. J Oral Surg. 1979; 37:793.

Ryan DE. Painful temporomandibular joint. In: McCarthy DJ, ed. Arthritis and allied conditions. Philadelphia: Lea & Febiger, 1989.

Patient with TEMPOROMANDIBULAR PAIN

(A) History ──────────→ ←────── (B) Radiographic studies:
    Physical examination   Plain films
                                            Arthrography
                                            MRI

(C) Nonarticular: (D) Pain on palpation of   (E) Continuous   (F) Other
    Otitis   condyle   pain, increasing   systemic
    Dental   Popping and clicking   with activity   arthritides
    Sinusitis   in TMJ   Coarse crepitus   Developmental
    Neuralgia   Radiographic findings: deformities
    Temporal arteritis   Roughened,   Neoplasia
                                                           irregular
                            Internal derangement   bony
                                                            cortices
                                                         Flattening
                                                           and anterior
                                                           lipping of
                                                           condyle

                                                         Degenerative
                                                         joint disease

POSITIVE ANTINUCLEAR ANTIBODY TEST

Marcia Ko, M.D.

A. Order the antinuclear antibody (ANA) test only if there is a strong clinical suspicion of rheumatic disease based on history and physical examination. The ARA criteria may be helpful in focusing in an organized manner, specifically on clinical symptoms and signs suggesting systemic lupus erythematosus (SLE).

B. The titer of ANA may be helpful. Low titers of 1:40 may be seen in up to 5% of normal individuals and increase with age.

C. The pattern of antinuclear antibodies may help direct further laboratory evaluation of ANA-related diseases. The four recognized patterns of ANA immunofluorescence are (1) homogeneous (suggests antibodies to nuclear proteins); (2) speckled (antibodies to nonhistone nuclear antigens, such as Smith [SM] and ribonucleoprotein [RNP]), (3) rim (antibodies to DNA) and (4) nuclear (antibodies to nuclear RNA). For example, the rim patterns may be seen in SLE and may suggest follow-up testing for antibody to double-stranded DNA. A speckled ANA immunofluorescence pattern may warrant further evaluation with testing for extractable nuclear antigens such as SM or RNP.

D. Antibodies to double-stranded DNA are measured via the Farr assay (radioimmunoassay) or using *Crithidia luciliae* as a substrate for indirect immunofluorescence. These antibodies are thought to be fairly specific for SLE and the titer may be used to follow disease activity.

E. Many extractable nuclear antigens are recognized. In clinical practice, the most commonly measured include anti-SM, anti-RNP, anti-RO (SSA), and anti-LA (SSB).

F. The SM antigen is saline extractable and although not very sensitive (20–35% of patients with SLE) is considered very specific for SLE.

G. Antibody to RNP is nonspecific and found in many connective tissue diseases, including SLE, rheumatoid arthritis, Sjögren's syndrome, scleroderma, and polymyositis. The presence of high-titer anti-RNP in the absence of other ANA and typical clinical picture may suggest mixed connective tissue disease (MCTD).

H. Anti-RO and anti-LA are antibodies to the extractable nuclear antigens SS-A and SS-B. These antibodies may be detected in several rheumatic diseases, including Sjögren's syndrome (approximately 60–70%), SLE, and subacute cutaneous lupus. The neonatal lupus syndrome has been associated with the presence of RO or anti-SS-A in the mothers of affected infants.

I. The anticentromere antibody, directed against the centromere of chromosomes, appears as a speckled ANA and may be helpful if other clinical features of the CREST syndrome are not fully apparent. The test is reported to be 57–96% positive in patients with this diagnosis.

J. Antihistone antibodies have been reported to be a helpful adjunct in the diagnosis of drug-induced lupus syndromes. Multiple drugs have been incriminated, including sulfonamides, penicillin, procainamide, alpha-methyldopa, anticonvulsants, isoniazid, antithyroid agents, and quinidine.

K. A negative ANA does not completely exclude the diagnosis of SLE: 10–15% of SLE patients may have a negative ANA, depending on the methods used. A negative ANA may also be interpreted as unsupportive of a diagnosis of SLE if other criteria are absent.

References

Fritzler MJ. Antinuclear antibodies in the investigation of rheumatic diseases. Bull Rheum Dis 1985: 35:00.

Robin R. Drug-induced lupus. Clin Asp Autoimmun 1988; 2:16.

Schumacher HR, ed. Primer on rheumatic disease. 9th ed. Atlanta, Arthritis Foundation, 1988.

Tan EM. Antinuclear antibodies: diagnostic markers for autoimmune disease and probes for cell immunology. Adv Immunol 1989; 44:93.

Tan EM, Cohen AS, Fries JF, et al. The 1982 revised criteria for the classification of systemic lupus erythematosus. Arthritis Rheum 1982; 25:1271.

Watson RM, et al. Neonatal lupus erythematosus. Medicine 1984; 63:362.

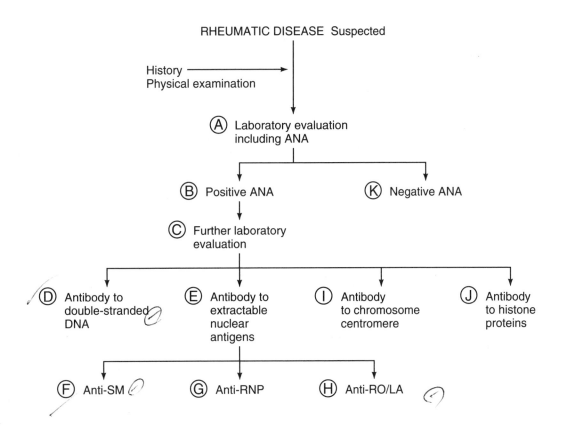

RHEUMATIC DISEASE Suspected

History ⟶
Physical examination

Ⓐ Laboratory evaluation
including ANA

Ⓑ Positive ANA   Ⓚ Negative ANA

Ⓒ Further laboratory
evaluation

Ⓓ Antibody to   Ⓔ Antibody to   Ⓘ Antibody   Ⓙ Antibody
double-stranded   extractable   to chromosome   to histone
DNA   nuclear   centromere   proteins
                       antigens

Ⓕ Anti-SM   Ⓖ Anti-RNP   Ⓗ Anti-RO/LA

ELEVATED ALKALINE PHOSPHATASE LEVEL

Michael J. Maricic, M.D.

A. An isolated elevated alkaline phosphatase level is a common finding with the widespread use of chemistry screening. A complete history and physical examination may point toward the cause of the elevation and preclude the need for further extensive evaluation. Although alkaline phosphatase may be derived from any organ, an elevation is most commonly seen in biliary tract and bone disease.

B. The first step in the laboratory work-up should be to obtain a serum GGPT and other liver function tests (LFTs) to determine whether there is biliary tract or liver disease. The alkaline phosphatase may also be fractionated, the heat-stable portion being derived from liver and the heat-labile portion from bone.

C. If these tests are abnormal, a work-up of liver and biliary tract disease is indicated, including ultrasonography.

D. If these tests point toward bone as the source of the elevation, check serum calcium and phosphorus to screen for metabolic bone disease.

E. An elevated calium and low phosphorus may suggest osteomalacia.

F. If the calcium and phosphorus are normal in an asymptomatic patient, Paget's disease of bone is the most common cause in this subset. Metastatic disease to bone, healing fractures, and inflammatory arthritis may also cause an elevated alkaline phosphatase level but these should be apparent clinically.

G. Direct plain radiographic evaluation toward areas of pain or deformity when present. When these are not evident, obtain radiographs of the skull and pelvis, which are areas of frequent involvement in Paget's disease. If these are negative, obtain a technetium bone scan, always correlating areas of increased uptake with plain radiographs.

References

Resnick D. Paget disease of bone: current status and a look back to 1943 and earlier. AJR 1988; 150:249.

Siris ES, Canfield RE. Paget's disease of bone: current concepts as to its nature and management. Orthop Rev 1982; 11:43.

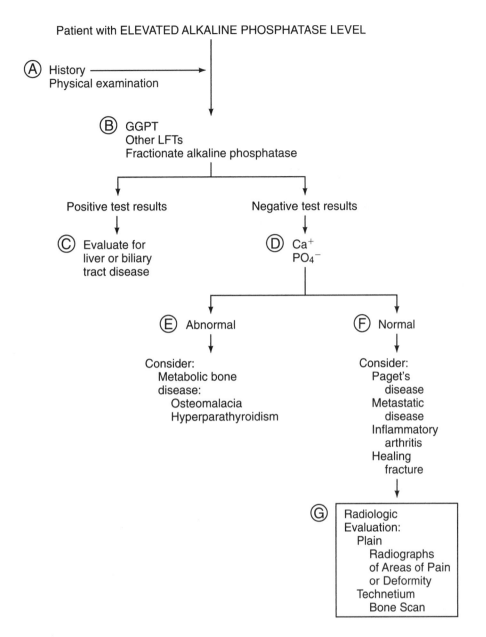

Patient with ELEVATED ALKALINE PHOSPHATASE LEVEL

(A) History
Physical examination

(B) GGPT
Other LFTs
Fractionate alkaline phosphatase

Positive test results

Negative test results

(C) Evaluate for
liver or biliary
tract disease

(D) Ca$^+$
PO$_4^-$

(E) Abnormal

(F) Normal

Consider:
Metabolic bone
disease:
Osteomalacia
Hyperparathyroidism

Consider:
Paget's
disease
Metastatic
disease
Inflammatory
arthritis
Healing
fracture

(G) Radiologic
Evaluation:
Plain
Radiographs
of Areas of Pain
or Deformity
Technetium
Bone Scan

ELEVATED CREATINE KINASE LEVEL

Patricia Mayer, M.D.

A. An elevated creatine kinase (CK) level may be detected on routine panel testing or may be ordered in a variety of clinical settings, most commonly in the work-up of musculoskeletal or cardiac complaints. This chapter focuses on the elevated CK seen incidentally and in the work-up of musculoskeletal complaints. Several causes of elevated CK are obvious on presentation (malignant hyperthermia, severe hypo- or hyperthermia, acute crushing trauma causing rhabdomyolysis) and are not discussed here.

B. When assessing an elevated CK, it is essential to first determine the origin of the enzyme: cardiac (represented by the MB isoenzyme fraction), brain (BB), or muscle (MM). This may be clinically apparent, as in a patient with acute chest pain and ECG changes, or with severe proximal muscle weakness. However, if the origin of the enzyme is in question, particularly if there is any suspicion of cardiac injury, perform isoenzyme tests on at least one occasion.

C. If the CK elevation is of cardiac origin, appropriate cardiac evaluation and therapy should be immediately undertaken (see p 80).

D. Infrequently, cerebral disease causes elevated CK, with a significant percentage of the BB isoenzyme. This situation is virtually always clinically apparent (acute cerebral trauma).

E. Most noncardiac elevations of CK are due to enzyme release from muscle. The remainder of the algorithm is designed for use in distinguishing the various causes of muscle-related CK elevations.

F. A thorough history and detailed physical examination are essential and reveal the cause of the CK elevation in many cases. The history should specifically cover family history (positive in the inherited myopathies), trauma history (including vigorous exercise, contusions, intramuscular injections, surgery, eletromyography [EMG] studies, and ischemia), and drug/medication history (IV drugs, amphetamines, alcohol, corticosteroids, cholesterol-lowering drugs, excessive licorice ingestion). Explore all musculoskeletal complaints, especially muscle weakness or tenderness, in detail. The physical examination must include a complete neurologic evaluation and musculoskeletal examination that includes muscle strength testing.

G. If there are musculoskeletal symptoms or findings, perform CBC, electrolyte, and thyroid function studies before proceeding further. Again, underlying conditions should be treated.

H. If the preliminary examinations are unrevealing, perform specific muscle testing via EMG. This should distinguish normal muscle from muscle that exhibits either myopathic or neuropathic changes. Since most muscle diseases are bilateral and symmetric, a unilateral EMG is recommended.

I. If the EMG is completely normal when done on symptomatic muscle, the patient should be followed. If symptoms resolve, no further work-up is needed. If symptoms worsen or persist, consider a muscle biopsy.

J. If the EMG reveals myopathic changes, a muscle biopsy is performed to determine the underlying pathology.

K. A muscle biopsy should be done on clinically involved muscle on the side opposite the EMG site to avoid possible artifact in the biopsy from the EMG needle. In addition to routine histology, histochemical staining, ultrastructural studies, or other special tests may be required for a pathologic diagnosis.

L. If the muscle biopsy is normal, the patient may be followed. However, many muscle diseases are patchy and a single biopsy may miss the involved site. Therefore, if symptoms persist, consider repeat biopsy.

M. Treat inflammatory myopathies such as polymyositis primarily with corticosteroids.

N. The inherited and congenital myopathies are most often treated symptomatically. The muscular dystrophies in particular require appropriate neurologic follow-up.

O. A variety of other conditions may be revealed on biopsy, including other collagen vascular disorders, vasculitis, and steroid myopathy. Direct treatment specifically toward these entities.

P. If the EMG reveals neuropathic changes, consider motor neuron disease, peripheral neuropathies, or other neurologic disease. Further work-up of these conditions may be required (p 332).

Q. If the history and physical examination are completely normal, consider a minimal laboratory study, including a CBC (to evaluate possible occult infection), electrolytes (with special attention to potassium), and thyroid tests. If any of the tests are positive, the underlying abnormality should be corrected. If negative, no further work-up is recommended and the patient can be followed.

References

Bradley WG, Fries TJ. Neuromuscular testing. In: Kelley WN, Harris ED, Ruddy S, Sledge CG, eds. Textbook of rheumatology. 3rd ed. Philadelphia: WB Saunders, 1989.

Patient with ELEVATED CREATINE KINASE LEVEL

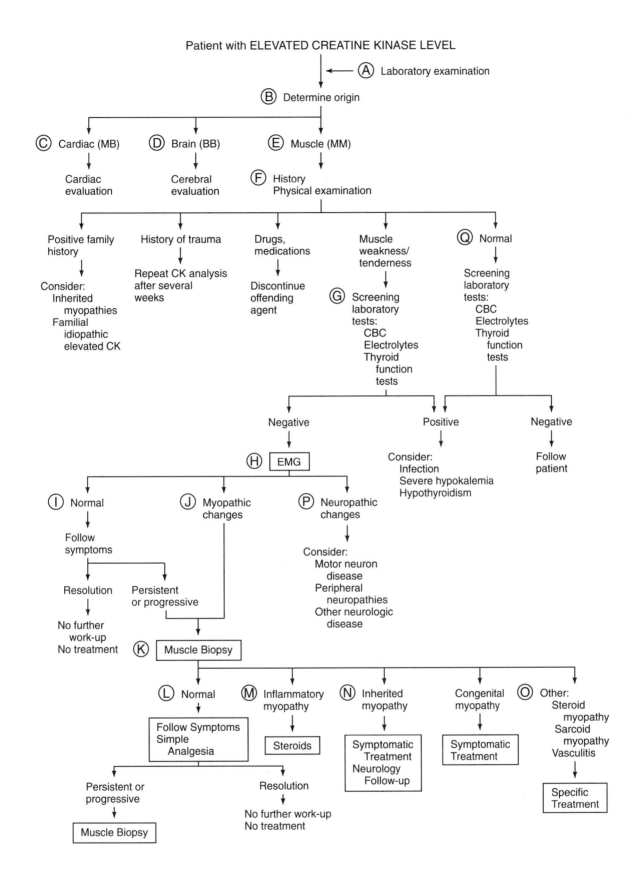

Chutkow JG. Diagnosis: muscular dystrophy. Hosp Med 1989;
     138.
Dubowitz V. Muscle biopsy: a practical approach. 2nd ed.
     Philadelphia: Bailliere Tindall, 1985.

Kagen LJ. Approach to the patient with myopathy. Bull Rheum
     Dis 1983; 33:8–10.
Nanji AA. Serum creatine kinase isoenzymes: a review.
     Muscle Nerve 1983; 6:83.

EMERGENCY MEDICINE, GYNECOLOGY, UROLOGY, BEHAVIORAL MEDICINE, AND PHARMACOLOGY

EMERGENCY MEDICINE
ACUTE PULSELESS EXTREMITY

Kenneth E. McIntyre, Jr., M.D.

A. The history and physical examination are of paramount importance. The onset is usually abrupt and may strike any time. Acute lower extremity ischemia may occur in patients with myocardial infarction, ventricular aneurysm, valvular heart disease, arrhythmia or arterial occlusive disease. One must inquire about the cardiac history. It is also important to establish whether previous vascular occlusive disease has been diagnosed or vascular reconstructive operations have been performed in the past.

B. Abrupt onset of severe unremitting pain is the classic symptom of acute ischemia. In patients with a known history of vascular occlusive disease of the lower extremities, pain may be less severe if there are abundant collaterals still open. Ischemic pain is generally not relieved by narcotics. There are no pulses below the level of obstruction and the foot is generally white or pallorous.

C. The acute pulseless extremity may result from trauma that has injured an artery, thrombosis, or embolism. In patients who have previously undergone a vascular bypass operation, thrombosis of the bypass conduit may cause acute ischemia.

D. It may be difficult to differentiate thrombosis from embolism as the cause of an acute pulseless extremity. Thrombosis tends to occur in younger patients than those with embolism and in patients with a known history of vascular occlusive disease or previous vascular surgery. Embolism usually occurs in patients with known heart disease (mitral stenosis or regurgitation, atrial fibrillation, acute myocardial infarction). Patients with embolism may have had an earlier embolic event but usually have no history of chronic circulatory impairment. Physical examination of the uninvolved extremity usually demonstrates normal pulses in patients with embolism.

E. Early heparinization helps to preserve the patency of needed collateral blood vessels. Time is of the essence for salvage of the acutely ischemic extremity. Except in trauma, heparin is always indicated as soon as the diagnosis of acute circulatory impairment is made. Give heparin as an IV bolus of 10,000 U followed by a minimum dose of 1000 U/hr to prolong the activated partial thromboplastin time to more than 2½ times control.

F. Arteriography is a luxury that may aid the vascular surgeon but should not be performed in any patient who has already developed paresthesia or paralysis. Monitor the patient during arteriography; if signs and symptoms of nerve ischemia develop, terminate the procedure and pursue operative intervention. Arteriography is especially helpful in patients with blunt injury who present with an acute pulseless extremity, because an injury requiring repair can be differentiated from the arterial vasospasm often associated with fractures. Moreover, arteriography may help distinguish thrombosis from embolism. Patients who have sustained an embolism from a cardiac source often have normal peripheral vessels. Emboli tend to lodge where vessels taper or branch and are most commonly seen in the external iliac, superficial femoral, and popliteal arteries. With acute thrombosis, there is usually evidence of significant disease in other lower extremity arteries. During the angiographic contrast injection, late films are needed to demonstrate the patency of the distal circulation below the level of obstruction.

G. If the leg is viable, one has time to pursue intra-arterial thrombolysis using urokinase. The catheter is placed directly in the clot by the radiologist, and a bolus infusion of 500,000–1,000,000 U of urokinase is given directly into the clot. After this initial bolus, urokinase is continued at 80,000–250,000 U/hr through the catheter. During thrombolytic therapy, the patient is monitored in the ICU and serum fibrinogen levels are drawn every 6 hours to monitor the systemic effect of the infusion. As long as the serum fibrinogen is >100 mg/dl and there are no signs of bleeding, the infusion may continue at the stated dose. Also, monitor the perfusion of the foot and the status of pulses during the intra-arterial urokinase infusion. After several hours, perform repeat arteriography through the catheter to measure the amount of lysis. If thrombolysis is complete, continue the patient on IV heparin until a definitive cause for the acute ischemia has been determined. If the cause is definitely cardiac embolism, institute warfarin. If the cause is thrombosis, the patient may be observed or considered for elective surgical revascularization. Intra-arterial urokinase is usually continued for a maximum of 2 days. If no or minimal thrombolysis has occurred and the foot remains viable, elective vascular surgery may be undertaken. If the leg deteriorates and becomes nonviable, an urgent operation must be performed for limb salvage.

H. If paresthesia or paralysis is present, the limb soon becomes unsalvageable without operative intervention. It is important to distinguish sensitivity to light touch from that of pressure, pain, and temperature. Pressure, pain, and temperature sensations are carried by larger nerves that are more resistant to ischemia and therefore may remain intact when sensation

Patient with ACUTE PULSELESS EXTREMITY

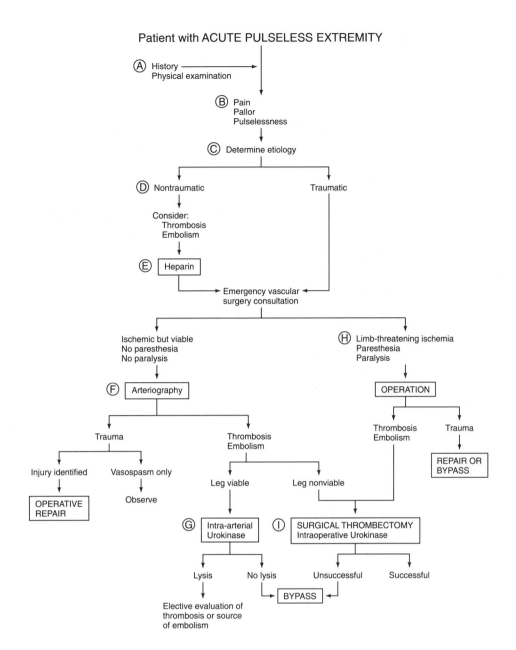

tolight touch has diminished. If there are no sensory or motor deficits, a more elective work-up may proceed. After the abrupt onset of perfusion impairment, the clock begins ticking. If the collateral circulation is not well developed, one usually has <4–6 hr to restore the circulation. Attempts to provide revascularization after 8–12 hr are seldom successful.

I. When the leg is nonviable, as evidenced by paresthesia and/or paralysis, undertake an emergent operation to facilitate limb salvage. Surgical thrombectomy is usually performed through a groin incision overlying the common femoral artery. This enables the surgeon to pass balloon thrombectomy catheters proximally and distally to extract thrombus. Although the surgeon passes the balloon thrombectomy catheter until no clot is returned, distal clot remains in as many as 30% of patients. In addition, the balloon catheter may cause intimal injury to the arteries. For these reasons, intraoperative intra-arterial urokinase is used as an

adjunct to facilitate the opening of arteries occluded by thrombus.

References

Abbott WM, Maloney RD, McCabe CC, et al. Arterial embolism: a 44 year perspective. Am J Surg 1982; 143:460.

Brewster DC, Chin AK, Fogarty TJ. Arterial thromboembolism. In: Rutherford RB, ed. Vascular surgery. 3rd ed. Philadelphia: WB Saunders, 1989.

Meier GH, Brewster DC. Acute arterial thrombosis. In: Bergan JJ, Yao JST, eds. Vascular surgical emergencies Orlando: Grune & Stratton, 1987.

Perry MO. Acute limb ischemia. In: Rutherford RB, ed. Vascular surgery. 3rd ed. Philadelphia: WB Saunders, 1989.

Quinones-Baldrich WJ, Zierler RE, Hiatt JC. Intraoperative fibrinolytic therapy: an adjunct to catheter thromboembolectomy. J Vasc Surg 1985; 2:319.

FOREIGN BODY INGESTION

Riemke Brakema, M.D.

A. The type of foreign body ingested and the site of obstruction determine the treatment approach. Try to determine what type of foreign body was ingested. This should be obtained from the patient, family members, or bystanders. A patient unable to talk likely has an airway problem that should be addressed immediately.

The most common ingested foreign bodies in children are coins, chicken or fish bones, buttons, tacks, screws, marbles, beads, button batteries, and pins. In adults, one might expect a food bolus (meat especially), bones, fruit pits, pins, dentures, or toothpicks.

All foreign bodies lodged in the airway must be removed. Complications may be related to perforation with pneumothorax or hemorrhage, pneumonia, or lung abscess. On the other hand, a missed foreign body ingestion in a bronchus may present as an atypical or recurrent pneumonia. In general, 80–85% of all foreign bodies in the GI tract pass spontaneously. Complications are usually related to perforations or obstruction and include mediastinitis, esophagogastric fistula, aortic perforation, cardiac tamponade, and peritonitis.

Certain foreign bodies deserve specific mention. Button or disc batteries may contain the alkaline potassium hydroxide, as well as a number of heavy metals such as lithium, nickel, zinc, cadmium, or mercury. Most batteries are not biologically sealed. Disc batteries lodged in the esophagus should be removed because the alkaline solution may cause liquefaction necrosis and subsequent perforation of the esophageal wall. If they are passed into the stomach, spontaneous passage from the body is likely to follow and may be documented by radiologic studies every 24 hrs. If x-ray films show that the battery has come apart, obtain heavy metal levels and follow up for consideration of chelation.

Sharp objects such as fish or chicken bones, pins, and needles deserve special mention. If lodged in the esophagus and causing symptoms, remove these expediently. If lodgment is determined by diagnostic studies but the patient is asymptomatic, exercise expectant observation for 24 hrs. Many such foreign bodies pass spontaneously. After either removal or spontaneous passage, perform esophagography to look for perforation.

Physical examination is generally brief. The ABC approach determines the general status of the patient, and interventions should be made as indicated by evaluation. This should be followed by a detailed examination of the oral and nasal pharynx for erythema, abrasions, or cuts. Evaluate the neck and soft tissues for subcutaneous emphysema. Auscultate and percuss the chest for breath sounds, wheezing, hyperresonance, or dullness to percussion.

B. Use topical anesthesia for the mucosa to facilitate examination of the pharynx and hypopharynx with the indirect laryngoscope. If the foreign body cannot be visualized in this manner, use direct laryngoscopy. If the foreign body is visualized and no sharp or jagged edges are known to be present, it may be removed with forceps.

(Continued on page 436)

Patient with INGESTED FOREIGN BODY

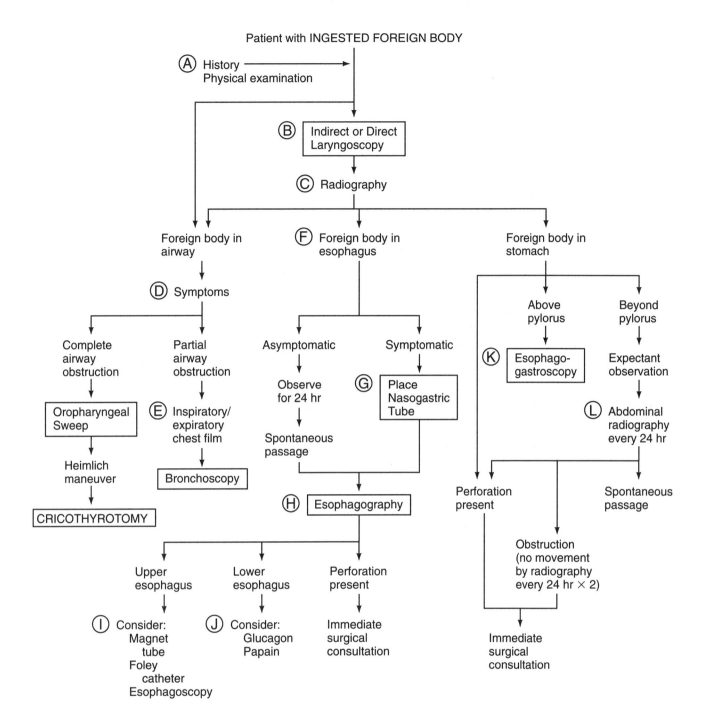

Ⓐ History
Physical examination

Ⓑ Indirect or Direct Laryngoscopy

Ⓒ Radiography

Foreign body in airway

Foreign body in esophagus

Foreign body in stomach

Ⓓ Symptoms

Complete airway obstruction

Partial airway obstruction

Asymptomatic

Symptomatic

Above pylorus

Beyond pylorus

Oropharyngeal Sweep

Ⓔ Inspiratory/expiratory chest film

Observe for 24 hr

Ⓖ Place Nasogastric Tube

Ⓚ Esophago-gastroscopy

Expectant observation

Heimlich maneuver

Bronchoscopy

Spontaneous passage

Ⓛ Abdominal radiography every 24 hr

CRICOTHYROTOMY

Ⓗ Esophagography

Perforation present

Spontaneous passage

Upper esophagus

Lower esophagus

Perforation present

Obstruction (no movement by radiography every 24 hr × 2)

Ⓘ Consider:
Magnet tube
Foley catheter
Esophagoscopy

Ⓙ Consider:
Glucagon
Papain

Immediate surgical consultation

Immediate surgical consultation

C. Use radiologic studies to determine radiolucency and the lodgment site of the foreign body. Soft tissue neck films may reveal air in the subcutaneous tissues indicating perforation. Also look to see whether the foreign body is in the tracheal air or esophageal column. Coins lodged in the trachea tend to align in the sagittal plane; those in the esophagus usually appear in coronal alignment. An anteroposterior view of the chest may reveal a pneumothorax, the foreign body, a lung abscess, or lobar atelectasis. Finally, if indicated by lack of findings on the first two radiographs, obtain a flat and upright plate of the abdomen to determine if the foreign body is indeed radiolucent and has already passed beyond the pylorus. If the patient complains of abdominal pain, look for signs of obstruction or perforation, such as free air under the diaphragm.

D. If the foreign body was aspirated, symptoms may range from throat pain and persistent cough to episodes of cyanosis or apnea and acute respiratory distress. Interventions should be directed by examination of the patient before further evaluation. Wheezes may be present in partial obstruction of a bronchus, and the absence of breath sounds may be noted on the side of a completely obstructed lung.

E. If a foreign body acts as a one-way valve in a main stem bronchus, air can get in but not out. Expiratory wheezes would be present on physical examination while the involved partially obstructed lung might appear overexpanded and hyperlucent on an expiratory chest radiograph. The diaphragm may appear fixed and flat and the heart and mediastinum may be shifted to the opposite, uninvolved side. When the obstruction becomes complete, air cannot get in or out and the involved lung may appear atelectatic on radiography, with the heart and mediastinum shifted to the involved side.

F. Inability to swallow, trouble with secretions, and refusal to eat are common symptoms of a foreign body in the esophagus. Patients may also be vomiting and gagging and may complain of neck, throat, or chest pain. They are often able to point exactly to the site of obstruction. The most common such sites are those where physiologic narrowing occurs at the cricopharyngeus muscle, the cardioesophageal junction, and Schatzki's ring in the lower esophagus.

G. A nasogastric tube may be gently placed just above the site of obstruction to manage and control secretions.

H. If esophageal perforation is suspected, use a water-soluble contrast medium to perform esophagography, as this is less irritative to surrounding tissues. In other cases barium sulfate may be used, especially if aspiration is a concern, since barium has minimal reactivity on the lung tissue. To determine the exact site of obstruction, a barium-soaked cotton ball may be swallowed. The radiolucent cotton ball will show up on the radiograph at the site of obstruction.

I. The magnet tube may be employed for removal of pins, rings, and disc batteries in the upper esophagus, although very few physicians still resort to this method of removal. Patient cooperation, especially with children, is difficult to obtain and makes this method prone to complications. Anticipate aspiration of vomit or the foreign body once it is dislodged, be prepared to deal with subsequent complications. A Foley catheter for removal of a foreign body in the esophagus is also considered controversial by many physicians, although few complications have been reported with those versed in this skill. Advantages include avoidance of general anesthesia and the complications of endoscopy. Significant disadvantages include complete or incomplete airway obstruction if the foreign body is dislodged into the oro- or nasopharynx. Missed esophageal damage or perforation and distress and pain to the patient are also a detriment to this procedure. A Foley catheter is passed orally past the foreign body with the patient in the upright position. Place the patient in the Trendelenburg position and inflate the balloon with contrast media. The catheter is then, under fluoroscopic guidance, gently and steadily withdrawn. Grasp the foreign body with forceps in the hypopharynx. Physicians performing this method of removal should be well versed in resuscitation and airway management.

J. Glucagon may be used to try to advance a food bolus lodged in the upper esophagus. Glucagon relaxes esophageal smooth muscles and the lower esophageal sphincter without inhibiting peristalsis. After a test dose to exclude hypersensitivity to this drug, give a 1-mg dose of IV glucagon with the patient in the upright position. Give it slowly, as rapid IV administration of glucagon may cause nausea and vomiting. Give a second dose of 2 mg if the patient experiences no relief 20 minutes after the first injection. Each dose should be followed by swallowing of water. If the obstruction is relieved, repeat esophagography to confirm passage. Papain is a digestive enzyme used in meat tenderizer. Its use to dissolve a meat bolus lodged in the esophagus has fallen into disfavor after a number of case reports described esophageal perforation after its use. Although normal, healthy esophageal tissue is not affected by papain, it is thought that perforation may occur secondary to impaired circulation of the esophageal wall from compression of the food bolus.

K. Most foreign bodies that find their way into the stomach pass through the remainder of the GI system spontaneously, but there are several instances in which esophagogastroscopic removal may be considered (e.g., for batteries, open pins, needles, or objects with sharp jagged edges).

L. Most foreign bodies that pass the pylorus are excreted per rectum without complication within 24–72 hr. Expectant observation may or may not include daily radiography to document advancement of the foreign body. In case abdominal pain develops, obtain radiologic studies to determine the presence of obstruction or perforation. Drug-filled condoms are generally observed to pass spontaneously without complications unless the condom perforates, in which case immediate intervention is necessary because of toxic drug exposure.

References

Krome R. Swallowed foreign bodies. In: Tintanalli JE, et al, eds. Emergency medicine: a comprehensive study guide. 2nd ed. New York: McGraw-Hill, 1988:304.

Kuhns D, Dire D. Button battery ingestions. Ann Emerg Med 1989; 18:293.

Pons PT. Foreign bodies. In: Rosen P, Barkin R, eds. Emergency medicine: concepts and clinical practice. 3rd ed. St. Louis: Mosby-Year Book, 1992:319.

Suita S, et al. Management of pediatric patients who have swallowed foreign objects. Am Surg 1989; 55:585.

Taylor R. Esophageal foreign bodies. Emerg Med Clin North Am 1987; 5:301.

CAUSTIC INGESTION AND EXPOSURE

Cynthia Madden, M.D.
Richard C. Dart, M.D., Ph.D.

Caustic exposure refers to all forms of chemical injury, alkali being more common than acid. Most exposures are in children (1–4 years old) and are accidental. Adult ingestions are usually due to a suicide attempt.

A. Determine the patient's age, the time of ingestion in relation to the last meal, and the type, physical form, and concentration of material ingested. Alkaline chemicals are in lye, drain cleaners, oven cleaners, Clinitest tablets, and button batteries; acids are found in swimming pool cleaners, rust removers, and battery acid. Examine the oropharynx for ulcerations or eschar; however, up to 20% of patients without oropharyngeal burns show endoscopic esophageal wall damage. Be alert for signs of respiratory compromise: stridor, hoarseness, aphonia. Check for Hamman's sign (a crunchy sound synchronous with the heart beat) on the chest examination and for subcutaneous emphysema when examining the neck. The pH of the patient's saliva can help determine whether an acid or alkali has been ingested.

B. Alkali burns cause liquefaction necrosis in the esophagus, involving the mucosa, submucosa, and longitudinal muscle. The stomach is affected in 20% of cases.

C. Alkali burns to the cornea are an ophthalmologic emergency and require continuous irrigation for at least 3 hours.

D. Symptoms of battery ingestion include vomiting, refusal to eat, increased salivation, and pain on swallowing. Emetics are contraindicated. Leave the patient NPO until radiographs of the entire GI tract have been obtained.

E. Cathartics may be administered to facilitate evacuation; emesis should not be attempted. Endoscopic removal is indicated if the battery does not pass in 36–48 hr or if the patient develops symptoms.

F. Acids cause coagulation necrosis with eschar formation and mainly affect the stomach, leading to pylorospasm and eventual full-thickness necrosis and perforation.

G. Patients without a reliable history and with no symptoms (e.g., oral burns, dysphagia, vomiting) can be monitored in the emergency room and discharged after 3–4 hr. Acid ingestion poses a higher risk of perforation and all such patients should be admitted.

H. First-degree burns cause hyperemia with superficial mucosal desquamation; second-degree burns cause blistering and shallow ulcers; third-degree burns suggest total loss of esophageal epithelium.

I. It is generally accepted that patients with first-degree burns rarely develop strictures; third-degree burns develop strictures regardless of steroid treatment. Steroids may delay stricture development in second-degree burns and should be used with an antibiotic to offset the increase in infection rate caused by steroid use. The dose of methylprednisone is 2 mg/kg daily; 1 g of ampicillin every 6 hr or 100 mg/kg every 24 hr in children may be used.

J. Hydrofluoric acid (HF) is a common agent in the home and industry and is capable of producing life-threatening toxicity with minimal exposure. HF dissociates in tissue and affects metabolism in three ways: liquefaction necrosis, bone destruction, and production of insoluble salts. Inhalation exposures to concentrated HF for 5 min are usually fatal.

K. Initial management for HF burns includes deactivating the fluoride ion. For severe burns, inject intradermally 10% calcium gluconate into, and for a distance of 0.5 cm around, the burn. For mild to moderate burns, apply calcium gluconate gel locally.

L. For unknown amounts of HF ingestion, administer 300 ml magnesium citrate. If the concentration of HF is known, administer oral magnesium on a milliequivalent-for-milliequivalent basis.

M. Monitor the QT interval for signs of hypocalcemia, and make frequent evaluations of acid-base status, electrolytes, and calcium. Burn care includes cleansing and parenteral analgesics.

References

Crain EF, Gershel JC, Mezey AP. Caustic ingestions: symptoms as predictors of esophageal injury. Am J Dis Child 1984; 138:863.

Hoffman RS, Goldfrank LR, Howland MA. Caustics and batteries. In: Goldfrank LR, Flomenbaum NE, Lewin NA, et al., eds, Goldfrank's toxicologic emergencies. 4th ed. E Norwalk, CT: Appleton & Lange, 1990.

Karkal SS, ed, Wason S, consulting ed. Coping swiftly and effectively with caustic ingestions. Emerg Med Rep 1989; 10:25.

CAUSTIC INGESTION AND EXPOSURE Suspected

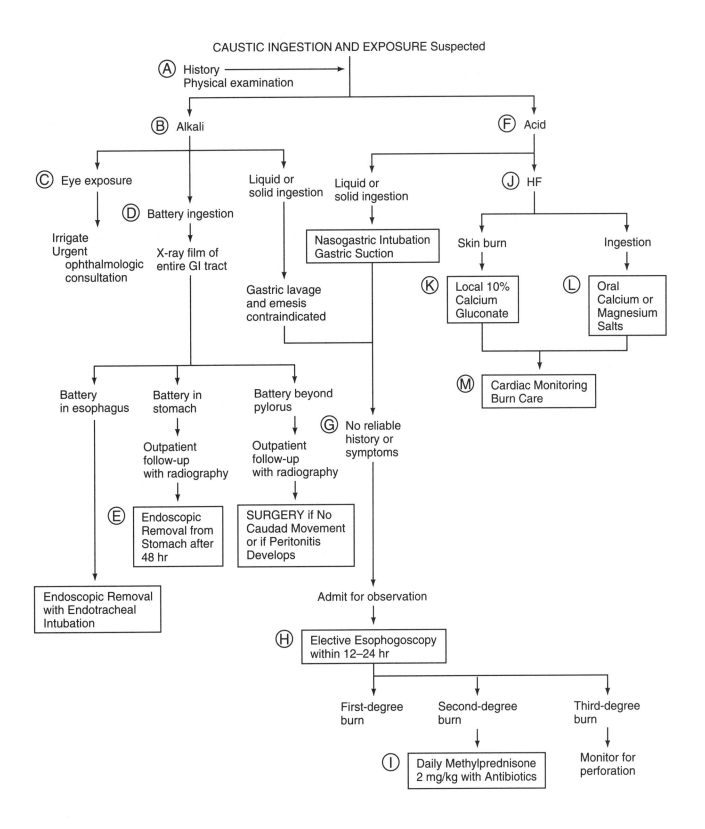

HUMAN AND ANIMAL BITES

Douglas Lindsey, M.D., Dr. P.H.

Humans make up a subset of animals. Specificity of speciation notwithstanding, the boundary between humans and other animals is flexible when defined by value judgments of behavior. The only clinical distinction is in differences of dentition and musculature of mastication. The author is not aware of any valid data to support the common premise that anatomically comparable wounds require different management depending on species.

A. Every break of the skin demands attention to the prevention of tetanus. There is no such thing as a "clean minor wound": all wounds are tetanus prone.

B. With very rare exceptions, rabies is transmitted by the saliva of mammalian species. Humans are not excluded, but in many parts of the U.S. rodents, squirrels, and rabbits are not a threat. Report all animal exposures to the local animal control authorities, follow their advice, and administer rabies prophylaxis exactly by CDC guidelines and those in the package insert.

C. Many patients present with wounds that are already infected. Make a Gram's stain, obtain a culture, and prescribe 4 days of an oral antimicrobial with the narrowest reasonable spectrum, most often a first-generation cephalosporin. Any cat bite, cat scratch, or dog bite that shows a sign of inflammation within 24 hours of the wounding is infected with *Pasteurella multocida* until proved otherwise, and the preferable agent is penicillin. Four days suffice for most simple wound infections and will allow time for culture results to suggest a better choice if the patient is not improving.

D. If a patient steps on a nail or a similar object, any attempt to debride or irrigate the simple wound is unnecessary. The surface of the wound can be gently cleaned for aesthetic purposes.

E. Some puncture wounds require opening for visual inspection. The "knuckle sandwich" or "clenched fist injury" (CFI) is a prime example. Since the pre-antimicrobial days of Kanavel the CFI has been recognized as a special problem, but it is one of human anatomy, not human oral flora. Tissue planes punctured in CFI do not permit drainage when the hand returns to its normal position of function. Return the hand to the clenched fist position, open the wound (with a transverse, not longitudinal, incision over the joint), and take a good look. If penetration of the joint capsule cannot be excluded, refer the patient to a specialist.

F. The canine tooth of canines is made for tearing meat, not for punching holes. Some canine tooth punctures are deeply undermined. The author has seen such punctures on the scalp of a child where the puncture into the cranium was 3 cm distant from the entrance wound. Probe punctures of bites by animals (nonhuman) larger than house cats. If the wound is undermined, irrigate and place a drain. A sterile rubber band is advisable. Remove the drain at 48 hours.

G. Repair bite wounds that are lacerations or avulsions in the same manner as comparable wounds from noninanimate instruments.

H. Although the profession of surgery has a sound database to support codified recommendations for perioperative prophylaxis, there is no such support for the use of systemic antimicrobial prophylaxis in accidental wounds. On the other hand, there is sound evidence to support the use of topical antimicrobials. For an undermined bite wound, flush the wound with a 10% solution of benzyl penicillin. A vial of 1 million units contains 0.6 g. Dilute with 6 ml of water, not saline. Even if the wound edges are infiltrated with anesthetic, the instillation causes significant, but transient, aching pain. A reasonable alternative is 1 g of a first-generation cephalosporin in 10 ml of water.

References

Lindsey D. Tetanus prophylaxis—do our guidelines assure protection? J Trauma 1984; 24: 1063.

Lindsey D, Christopher M, Hollenbach J, et al. Natural course of the human bite wound: incidence of infection and complications in 434 bites and 803 lacerations in the same group of patients. J Trauma 1987; 27:45.

Lindsey D, Nava C, Marti M. Effectiveness of penicillin irrigation in control of infection in sutured lacerations. J Trauma 1982: 22:186.

Lindsey D, Nava C, Silva F. Intra-incisional penicillin versus cephaloridine. J Antimicrob Chemother 1984; 14:196.

Mann JM. Systematic decision-making in rabies prophylaxis. Pediatr Infect Dis J 1983; 2:162.

Sacks T. Prophylactic antibiotics in traumatic wounds. J Hosp Infect 1988; 11 (Suppl A):251.

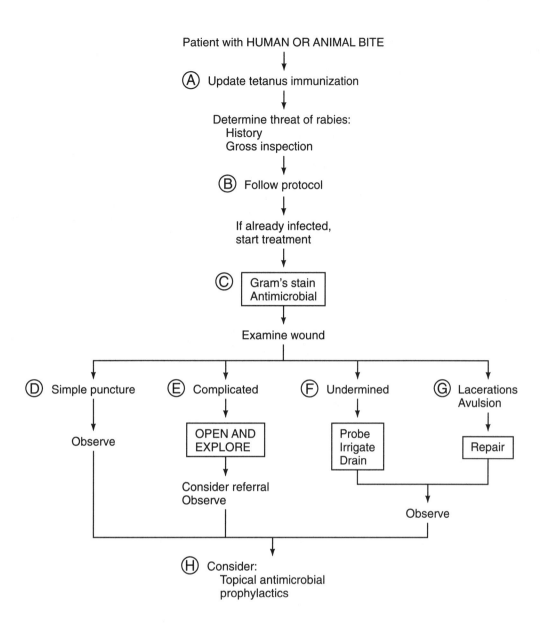

Patient with HUMAN OR ANIMAL BITE

Ⓐ Update tetanus immunization

Determine threat of rabies:
  History
  Gross inspection

Ⓑ Follow protocol

If already infected,
start treatment

Ⓒ | Gram's stain
Antimicrobial |

Examine wound

Ⓓ Simple puncture   Ⓔ Complicated   Ⓕ Undermined   Ⓖ Lacerations
                                                          Avulsion

Observe | OPEN AND
EXPLORE | | Probe
Irrigate
Drain | | Repair |

Consider referral
Observe   Observe

Ⓗ Consider:
  Topical antimicrobial
  prophylactics

SNAKE VENOM POISONING

Richard C. Dart, M.D., Ph.D.

Poisonous snakebites are caused by pit vipers (copperhead, cottonmouth, and rattlesnakes) and by coral snakes. Pit viper bites are potentially lethal and require careful medical management. Rattlesnake bites are the most dangerous, but all can cause life- or limb-threatening disease. The following management focuses on rattlesnake bites, but the algorithm can be used for all pit vipers. Coral snakebites are much rarer but can also cause life-threatening disease; their bites cause paralysis, which can be treated with antivenin and supportive care. Consult a regional poison control center for all envenomations.

A. In the United States the diagnosis of rattlesnake bite is primarily determined by a history of a bite followed by the development of symptoms. In pediatric patients an extensive history and observation of the wound must be used to differentiate snakebite wounds from puncture wounds made by insects, other animals, or inanimate objects. A snakebite may appear as one, two, or multiple puncture wounds or small lacerations. Pain, swelling, and ecchymosis usually become apparent during the first few hours.

B. The grade of envenomation is established by evaluating local wound findings, the presence of a coagulopathy, and the severity of systemic symptoms. *Minimal* envenomation consists of local pain, edema and ecchymosis with normal blood coagulation tests, and normal mental status and vital signs. *Moderate* envenomation consists of spreading pain, edema, or ecchymosis; mild to moderately abnormal coagulation studies; mild to moderate thrombocytopenia; or hemolysis. The patient may appear sleepy or lethargic but can become alert and oriented on command. *Severe* envenomation is defined as the rapid development of edema and ecchymosis, markedly abnormal coagulation studies, defibrination, disseminated intravascular coagulation—like syndromes, hemolysis, or depressed mentation. The worst findings are used to grade the envenomation. Thus, mild swelling with markedly abnormal coagulation studies or depressed mentation is classified as severe envenomation.

C. Several cases of delayed worsening of the envenomation have been reported. Observe patients for 6–8 hr with the bitten part elevated above heart level. The grade of envenomation should be changed if local or systemic symptoms signs appear or worsen.

D. Use skin test only when the decision to administer antivenin has been made. Administer antivenin (Crotalidae) polyvalent to patients with moderate or severe envenomations who demonstrate worsening of local or systemic findings. The skin test consists of 0.02 ml of the skin test material provided with the antivenin. A positive skin test consists of a wheal and flare 10 mm at the site of injection. Strong reactions to the skin test indicate a high probability of a severe reaction to antivenin infusion.

E. Most deaths caused by snakebite are caused by the patient's failure to seek medical attention or the physician's failure to recognize the severity of the envenomation. Hemodynamically unstable patients require immediate and aggressive therapy. Institute airway, breathing, and circulation (ABC) measures. Simultaneously, skin test the patient for horse serum hypersensitivity, and prepare 10–20 vials of antivenin (Crotalidae) polyvalent. After rapid evaluation of the patient, treat with antivenin. If antivenin is not immediately available, give a rapid crystalloid infusion to maintain blood pressure and reduce heart rate. If bleeding is apparent, replacement of platelets or coagulation factors should be accomplished by infusion of platelets or fresh frozen plasma until antivenin can be infused.

F. Antivenin administration consists of infusion of 5–10 vials in 250–500 ml of dextrose and water over 1–2 hr except as noted in E. The initial infusion should be slow in case an allergic reaction develops. If no reaction develops, the infusion rate can be increased to complete the infusion in 1–2 hr.

G. Up to 25% of patients develop some degree of reaction to antivenin infusion. If a reaction develops, stop the antivenin infusion immediately. Reactions take many forms, ranging from local erythema and itching to anaphylaxis. Give epinephrine, as well as H_1 and H_2 receptor blockers, to control the acute reaction. The benefits of continued antivenin infusion must be compared with the risks of restarting the infusion. In general, the antivenin can be restarted after diluting the antivenin and infusing it more slowly.

References

Burgess JL, Dart RC. Snake venom coagulopathy: use and abuse of blood products in the treatment of pit viper envenomation. Ann Emerg Med 1991; 20:795.

Hardy DL. Fatal rattlesnake envenomation in Arizona: 1969–1984. Clin Toxicol 1986; 24:1.

Kunkel DB. Treating snakebites sensibly. Emerg Med 1988; 30 June:51.

Russell FE. Snake venom poisoning. Great Neck, NY: Scholium International, 1983:235.

Wingert WA, Chan L. Rattlesnake bites in southern California and rationale for recommended treatment. West J Med 1988; 148:37.

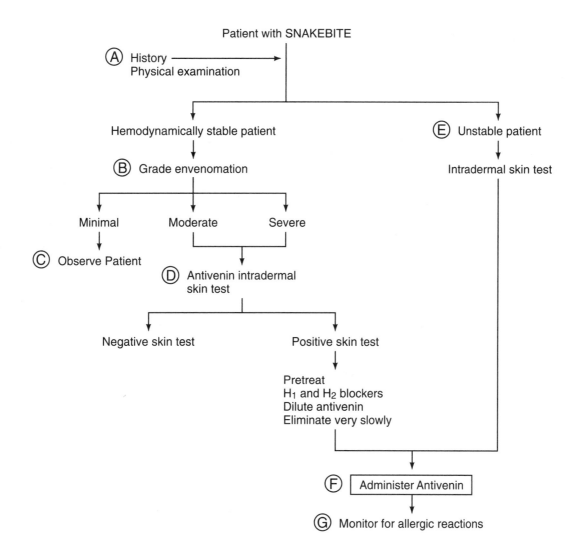

Patient with SNAKEBITE

(A) History ——————→
Physical examination

Hemodynamically stable patient

(B) Grade envenomation

Minimal   Moderate   Severe

(C) Observe Patient

(D) Antivenin intradermal
skin test

Negative skin test   Positive skin test

Pretreat
H₁ and H₂ blockers
Dilute antivenin
Eliminate very slowly

(E) Unstable patient

Intradermal skin test

(F) Administer Antivenin

(G) Monitor for allergic reactions

HYPOTHERMIA

Cynthia Madden, M.D.
John B. Sullivan, M.D.

A. Establish an airway adequate to ensure proper ventilation. Administer warm, humidified 100% O_2. Gentle intubation after preoxygenation is safe in hypothermic patients.

B. Obtain blood specimens, including CBC, blood cultures, electrolytes, BUN, creatinine, and arterial blood gases (ABGs). Temperature correction of pH and pCO_2 is not necessary when interpreting ABGs. Establish IV access with warmed normal saline.

C. Patients with stable cardiac rhythm (including sinus bradycardia) and stable vital signs may undergo passive rewarming with blankets to prevent further heat loss. Noninvasive internal modalities may be used (warmed, humidified oxygen and warmed IV fluids).

D. Patients with cardiovascular instability need to be rapidly rewarmed using a combination of methods. Core warming (warming the heart before the extremities) must be employed. Gastric/bladder/colon lavage or peritoneal lavage with warmed dialysate should be employed. Continue warmed O_2, IV fluids, and blankets. For ventricular fibrillation or asystole, defibrillate once or twice, institute CPR, and rewarm rapidly. The hypothermic myocardium is refractory to atropine, pacing, and defibrillation. Prolonged resuscitation efforts are indicated.

E. Administer 50 ml $D_{50}W$, 2 mg naloxone (Narcan), and 100 mg thiamine IV. This is therapy for drug overdose or alcohol causes of hypothermia. Obtain an ECG, which may reveal J-wave abnormalities. Continue to monitor cardiac rhythm.

F. Assess environmental exposures, spinal cord or central neurologic injuries, shock (signs of trauma, hemorrhage, or sepsis), hepatic failure, sepsis, and burns. Consider exposure to drugs and toxins (organophosphates, ethanol, opioids, beta blockers).

G. For frostbite, rapid rewarming by extremity immersion in 42° C water for 20 min is the most effective means of preserving tissue. Early surgical intervention is not indicated.

References

Danzl D, Pozos R. Multicenter hypothermia survey. Ann Emerg Med 1987; 16:1042.

Delaney K, Howland MA, Vassallo S, Goldfrank LR. Assessment of acid-base disturbances in hypothermia and their physiologic consequences. Ann Emerg Med 1989; 18:72.

Delaney K, Vassallo S, Goldfrank LR. Thermoregulatory principles. In Goldfrank LR, Flomenbaum NE, Lewin NA, et al., eds. Goldfrank's toxicologic emergencies. 4th ed. Norwalk, CT: Appleton & Lange, 1990.

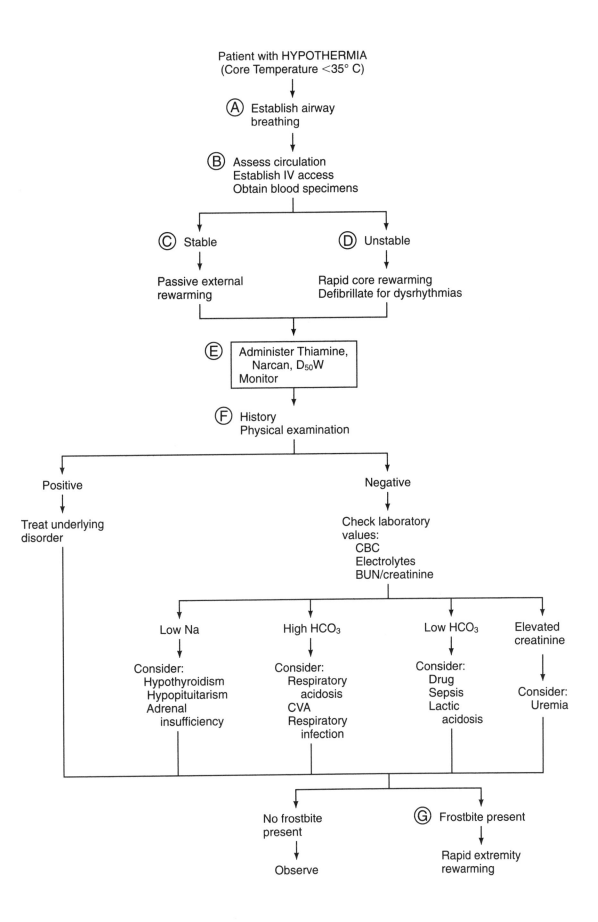

Patient with HYPOTHERMIA
(Core Temperature <35° C)

(A) Establish airway
breathing

(B) Assess circulation
Establish IV access
Obtain blood specimens

(C) Stable

Passive external
rewarming

(D) Unstable

Rapid core rewarming
Defibrillate for dysrhythmias

(E) Administer Thiamine,
Narcan, $D_{50}W$
Monitor

(F) History
Physical examination

Positive

Treat underlying
disorder

Negative

Check laboratory
values:
CBC
Electrolytes
BUN/creatinine

Low Na

Consider:
Hypothyroidism
Hypopituitarism
Adrenal
insufficiency

High HCO_3

Consider:
Respiratory
acidosis
CVA
Respiratory
infection

Low HCO_3

Consider:
Drug
Sepsis
Lactic
acidosis

Elevated
creatinine

Consider:
Uremia

No frostbite
present

Observe

(G) Frostbite present

Rapid extremity
rewarming

DROWNING AND NEAR-DROWNING

Samuel M. Keim, M.D.

Drowning is defined as death from suffocation due to submersion in a fluid. Near-drowning implies survival, at least temporarily, after such suffocation. About 10% of victims succumb to asphyxia while submerged, probably because of laryngospasm or breath holding. The other victims aspirate fluid: fresh water, salt water, contaminated water, or other liquids. The pathophysiology of drowning depends on the amount and type of fluid aspirated. Hypothermia decreases oxygen consumption and can thereby delay reversible cerebral damage. Unfortunately, hypothermia can produce lethal dysrhythmias such as ventricular fibrillation. Neurologic injury and recovery depend on the duration and degree of hypoxia, the water temperature, and the patient's underlying physical condition.

A. Some victims of near-drowning do not aspirate water, have limited laryngospasm or breath-holding, and regain effective ventilation before permanent damage occurs. These patients may appear sleepy or groggy, or completely alert. The first responder should not be lulled into a false sense of security by this presentation. Despite appearing stable, these patients may be severely hypoxic or become so quickly. Cervical spine (C-spine) precautions should be continued if neck injury is possible, and these patients should be transported with supplemental O_2 to the nearest Emergency Department (ED) or Pediatric Critical Care Center if under the age of 18 and presenting with altered mental status or shock.

B. The fundamental goal for initial resuscitation of the apneic near-drowning victim is to restore PaO_2 to normal as rapidly as possible. The victim should be extricated from the water as quickly as possible. If the victim is apneic and mouth-to-mouth ventilation in the water is possible, this should be initiated as soon as the rescuer reaches the victim. As chest compressions are not typically feasible in the water, they should be initiated as soon as the victim can be removed. C-spine precaution should be followed during extrication if a fall or diving injury is suspected. The single most important factor related to a normal recovery is the prevention of irreversible hypoxia. This usually means that the first responder must know CPR and be able to use it when necessary.

C. If the initially apneic patient has a palpable pulse, the rescuer should continue providing assisted ventilation and activate the emergency medical system by asking another person to call 911. The rescuer should continue assessing the victim's airway to ensure its patency. If necessary, the rescuer may use a Heimlich maneuver to clear the airway (with the awareness that gastric contents may be aspirated during this maneuver). The Heimlich maneuver should not be used in an attempt to empty the stomach. The apneic patient should be intubated by paramedic personnel as soon as possible and transported to the nearest ED or Pediatric Critical Care Center.

D. The apneic, pulseless patient should receive CPR (one- or two-rescuer) while C-spine precautions are maintained. The rescuer should have a bystander call 911. The patient should be intubated by paramedic personnel as soon as possible and transported with CPR and Advanced Cardiac Life Support (ACLS) in progress to the nearest ED or Pediatric Critical Care Center.

(Continued on page 448)

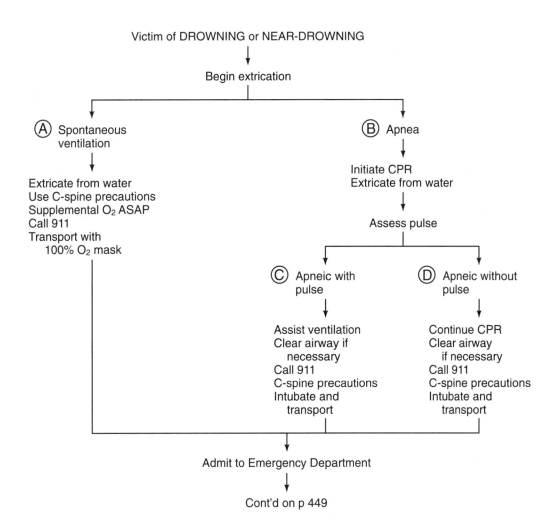

Victim of DROWNING or NEAR-DROWNING

Begin extrication

Ⓐ Spontaneous
   ventilation

Extricate from water
Use C-spine precautions
Supplemental O₂ ASAP
Call 911
Transport with
   100% O₂ mask

Ⓑ Apnea

Initiate CPR
Extricate from water

Assess pulse

Ⓒ Apneic with
   pulse

Assist ventilation
Clear airway if
   necessary
Call 911
C-spine precautions
Intubate and
   transport

Ⓓ Apneic without
   pulse

Continue CPR
Clear airway
   if necessary
Call 911
C-spine precautions
Intubate and
   transport

Admit to Emergency Department

Cont'd on p 449

E. In the ED the alert, yet hypoxic patient should be treated aggressively. If the patient is alert or easily arousable, the physician may try mask continuous positive alveolar pressure (CPAP) first. If CPAP is not readily available or cannot be implemented because of altered consciousness, the patient should be intubated via nasal or oral routes. The patient's oxygenation may then be augmented with positive end-expiratory pressure (PEEP). A nasogastric (NG) tube should be placed to aspirate stomach contents. If present, treat hypothermia, bronchospasm, and acidosis. These patients should be admitted to the ICU.

F. The spontaneously breathing patient who is extremely fortunate will present with a normal PaO_2, $PaCO_2$, and pH. Check the C-spine for injuries. If the patient is normothermic and exhibits no other abnormalities, including bronchospasm or altered consciousness, he or she may be released to a strong social support system with strict precautionary advice. The nonhypoxic hypothermic patient should be treated for hypothermia (see I). Patients exhibiting bronchospasm or acidosis should be admitted for observation.

G. The initially apneic patient with an intact circulation will likely be hypoxic on arrival at the ED. If not yet intubated by pre-hospital personnel, the patient should be intubated on arrival. Occasionally, patients begin breathing spontaneously during the initial pre-hospital resuscitation, and present without hypoxia. In this situation, they should be treated as in F. Intubated hypoxic patients benefit from PEEP. This can dramatically improve the ventilation-perfusion mismatch. An NG tube should be placed to aspirate gastric contents. If present, treat bronchospasm and acidosis (inhaled β_2-adrenergic agonists and sodium bicarbonate). Examine the patient for C-spine injuries, and obtain chest film. Treat hypothermia (see I). These patients should be admitted to the ICU.

H. The apneic and pulseless patient who arrives without previous intubation should be intubated on arrival. CPR and ACLS should be continued. Arterial blood gases (ABGs) should be drawn immediately, and acidosis treated. The evaluation of ABGs in hypothermia is controversial. In general, as temperature decreases, the oxygen-hemoglobin dissociation curve is shifted to the left, thereby decreasing the release of bound O_2. The acidosis (which shifts the curve to the right) may only partially compensate for this. Take care not to administer excessive sodium bicarbonate during resuscitation (alkalosis will shift the curve further to the left).

I. In the hypothermic patient, CPR should be continued until the core temperature is $>32°$ C. In the severely hypothermic patient (core temperature $<32°$ C), Active Core Rewarming should be implemented to prevent the phenomena of "afterdrop," which can occur when active external rewarming (e.g., warm immersion) used alone leads to reperfusion of cold peripheral tissues and subsequent cooling of the previously sequestered warm-core blood. Active Core Rewarming can include heated humidified O_2, heated peritoneal lavage, and cardiopulmonary bypass. Other methods include gastric and colonic irrigation, thoracostomy with pleural and mediastinal irrigation, and hemodialysis. Each of these techniques carries inherent risks and complications. Truncal active external rewarming may be added to augment core rewarming. For the patient with mild to moderate hypothermia (core temperature $32-37°$ C), passive external rewarming is appropriate. This includes the removal of wet clothing and prevention of further heat loss by applying blankets. The efficacy of ACLS medications is controversial in hypothermia. Bretylium has been reported to be effective in ventricular fibrillation. The efficacy of atropine in hypothermia-induced bradycardia is doubtful. The combination of hypoxia and hypothermia can lead to a marked decrease in tissue O_2 delivery. Although hypothermia may be protective via diminished metabolic rate, it is more frequently lethal. Nonetheless, the dictum "No one is dead until warm and dead" should be followed.

J. In the ICU, ventilatory management should be aggressive, including PEEP, frequent suctioning, and frequent monitoring of the ventilation-perfusion shunt. Acidosis and cardiac dysrhythmias should also be treated aggressively. Although controversial, consider intracranial pressure monitoring, pulmonary artery pressure monitoring, and barbiturate coma. These treatments contain risks and have questionable benefit. Ensure that no C-spine injury exists (if this is not already done). Treat hypothermia (see I). Treat bronchospasm and acidosis if present. Monitor electrolytes and fluid status closely. Steroids, barbiturates, and induced hypothermia have not been shown to improve survival. Psychosocial issues with the family should be addressed.

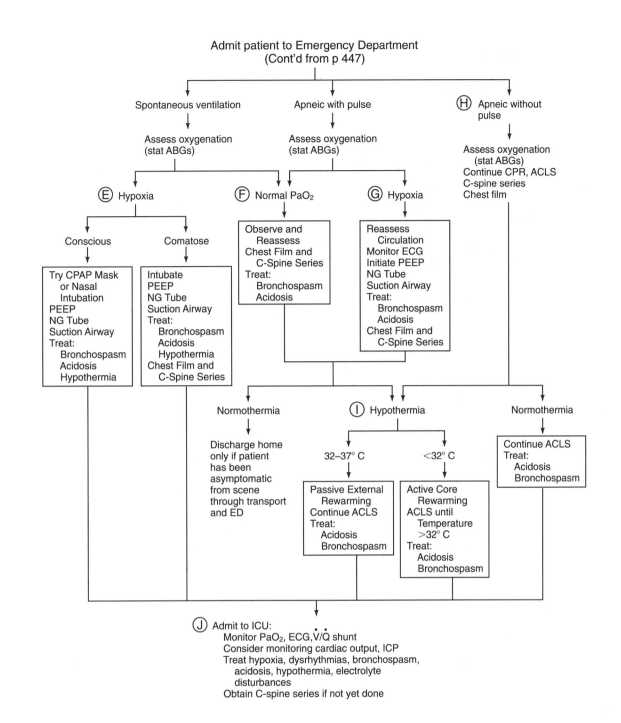

Admit patient to Emergency Department
(Cont'd from p 447)

Spontaneous ventilation | Apneic with pulse | Ⓗ Apneic without pulse

Assess oxygenation (stat ABGs) | Assess oxygenation (stat ABGs) | Assess oxygenation (stat ABGs) Continue CPR, ACLS C-spine series Chest film

Ⓔ Hypoxia | Ⓕ Normal PaO₂ | Ⓖ Hypoxia

Conscious | Comatose

Try CPAP Mask or Nasal Intubation
PEEP
NG Tube
Suction Airway
Treat:
  Bronchospasm
  Acidosis
  Hypothermia

Intubate
PEEP
NG Tube
Suction Airway
Treat:
  Bronchospasm
  Acidosis
  Hypothermia
Chest Film and C-Spine Series

Observe and Reassess
Chest Film and C-Spine Series
Treat:
  Bronchospasm
  Acidosis

Reassess Circulation
Monitor ECG
Initiate PEEP
NG Tube
Suction Airway
Treat:
  Bronchospasm
  Acidosis
Chest Film and C-Spine Series

Normothermia | Ⓘ Hypothermia | Normothermia

Discharge home only if patient has been asymptomatic from scene through transport and ED

32–37° C | <32° C

Passive External Rewarming
Continue ACLS
Treat:
  Acidosis
  Bronchospasm

Active Core Rewarming
ACLS until Temperature >32° C
Treat:
  Acidosis
  Bronchospasm

Continue ACLS
Treat:
  Acidosis
  Bronchospasm

Ⓙ Admit to ICU:
  Monitor PaO₂, ECG, V̇/Q̇ shunt
  Consider monitoring cardiac output, ICP
  Treat hypoxia, dysrhythmias, bronchospasm, acidosis, hypothermia, electrolyte disturbances
  Obtain C-spine series if not yet done

References

Bohn DJ, Biggar WD, Smith CR, et al. Influence of hypothermia, barbiturate therapy, and intracranial pressure monitoring on morbidity and mortality after near-drowning. Crit Care Med 1986; 14:529.

Boysen PG. Dispelling the myths and controversies of near-drowning. Emerg Med Rep 1984; 5:23.

Danzl DF, Sowers MB, Vicaria SJ, et al. Chemical ventricular defibrillation in severe accidental hypothermia. Ann Emerg Med 1982; 11:698.

Marin TG. Near-drowning and cold-water immersion. Ann Emerg Med 1984; 13:263.

Modell JH. Drowning vs. near-drowning: a discussion of definition. Crit Care Med 1981; 9:301.

Modell JH, Boysen PG. Drowning and near-drowning. In: Shoemaker, ed. Textbook of critical care. 2nd ed. Philadelphia: WB Saunders, 1989.

Rueler JB. Hypothermia. Ann Intern Med 1978; 89:519.

GYNECOLOGY
VAGINAL DISCHARGE

Robert N. Samuelson, M.D.

A. Vulvovaginitis is the most common complaint necessitating a gynecologic examination. It is commonly defined as inflammation of the vulva and vagina. Upon initial evaluation, obtain a thorough history of previous episodes, possible sexual exposure, and color and consistency of the discharge. Pay particular attention to factors that can change vaginal flora, thus leading to vaginitis (recent antibiotic use, oral contraceptives, spermicides, douching). Also consider systemic conditions (poorly controlled diabetes, menopause, AIDS).

B. The cause of the vaginitis can frequently be determined at the time of speculum examination. Prepare two wet mounts using 10% KOH and normal saline, and view them under low and high power. Appearance of the discharge can often be helpful in diagnosis: bacterial vaginosis gives a gray-white appearance; *Trichomonas vaginalis* a profuse, watery, white green or yellow appearance; and *Candida* a white cheesy discharge. Determining the pH of the vaginal discharge using pH indicator paper can be most useful. Normal physiologic discharge and yeast are usually <4.5; >5.0 may indicate *Trichomonas* or bacterial vaginosis.

C. In the event of a nondiagnostic wet mount, consider allergic reaction to chemical or physical irritants. These possibilities are numerous and include tight clothing, deodorants, laundry detergent, soaps, tampons, and spermicides. Obtain culture for *Neisseria gonorrhoeae* and *Chlamydia trachomatis* in sexually active patients, and base treatment on subsequent results. Viral causes of vulvovaginitis include human papillomavirus (HPV) and herpes simplex virus (HSV). These are often diagnosed by appearance but can be confirmed by biopsy and culture. Aphthous ulcers can also occur on the vulva with an appearance similar to HSV.

D. The appearance of the unicellular protozoan *Trichomonas vaginalis* is diagnostic. Culture is not necessary for confirmation. The appearance under high power is of mobile flagellated organisms slightly larger than a WBC. The smear may also have many inflammatory cells and vaginal epithelial cells. To decrease the risk of reinfection, treat both patient and partner with metronidazole, 1 g twice daily for 7 days or 2 g PO (a 2-g dose is contraindicated in the first trimester of pregnancy).

E. A thin gray-white discharge with an unpleasant odor ("musty" or "fishy") is frequently caused by *Gardnerella vaginalis*, a gram-variable coccobacillus. The normal saline wet mount often shows "clue cells": stippled epithelial cells (*Gardnerella* organisms adhered to the epithelial cells). Treat the patient with metronidazole, 500 mg twice daily for 7 days. Treatment of the partner is controversial.

F. Significant vulvar pruritus is the usual presenting symptom of vaginal yeast infections. The appearance of filamentous forms (pseudohyphae) and blastospores on KOH wet mount can confirm clinical suspicion. Many equally effective topical treatment regimens are available, including clotrimazole 1% cream, one applicatorfull (5 g) per vagina QHS for 7 nights or miconazole, 200-mg suppositories QHS for 3 nights. The cream should also be applied to the vulva for pruritus.

G. Recurrent yeast infection can be a frustrating problem for both practitioner and patient. Obtain culture of the discharge on Sabouraud's or Nickerson's medium to confirm the etiology as yeast. Evaluate for other complicating factors, including evidence of diabetes, immunodeficiency (AIDS), or reinfection from partner (10–15% of male sexual partners of women with yeast infections have had positive oral, rectal, and seminal cultures). Treatment options are varied and include topical therapy for 30 days, and ketoconazole, 200 mg PO twice daily for 14 days. *Candida albicans* is the cause of monilial vulvovaginitis in >90% of cases, but occasionally *Torulopsis glabrata* can be a cause of resistant yeast. A 3- to 7-day course of terconazole frequently eliminates the organism.

References

ACOG Technical Bulletin. Vulvovaginitis. No. 135, November 1989.

Herbst AL, Mishell DR Jr., Stenchever MA, eds. Droegemueller W, Comprehensive gynecology. 2nd ed. St. Louis: Mosby–Year Book, 1992.

Ledger W. Infection in the female. Philadelphia: Lea & Febiger, 1986.

Quilligan E, Zuspan F. Current therapy in obstetrics and gynecology. Philadelphia: WB Saunders, 1990.

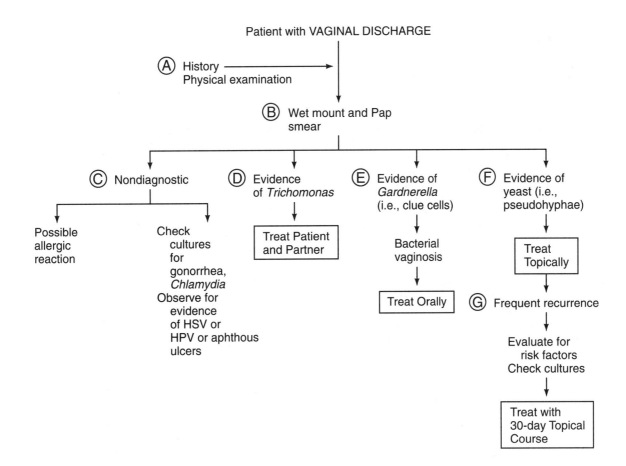

Patient with VAGINAL DISCHARGE

(A) History ———→ Physical examination

(B) Wet mount and Pap smear

(C) Nondiagnostic

Possible allergic reaction

Check cultures for gonorrhea, *Chlamydia* Observe for evidence of HSV or HPV or aphthous ulcers

(D) Evidence of *Trichomonas*

Treat Patient and Partner

(E) Evidence of *Gardnerella* (i.e., clue cells)

Bacterial vaginosis

Treat Orally

(F) Evidence of yeast (i.e., pseudohyphae)

Treat Topically

(G) Frequent recurrence

Evaluate for risk factors Check cultures

Treat with 30-day Topical Course

CERVICITIS

Hugh S. Miller, M.D.

A. Although acute cervicitis can result from trauma, malignancy, or systemic collagen vascular conditions, it is most commonly caused by infectious agents, notably *Neisseria gonorrhoeae*, *Chlamydia trachomatis*, and (to a lesser extent) herpes simplex virus (HSV). The epidemiology of these pathogens is similar, and 25–45% of patients have concomitant infections. Assessing a patient's risk for cervical infection involves taking a careful history, including age of first sexual contact, number of sexual partners, and history of previous sexually transmitted diseases (STDs) or pelvic inflammatory disease (PID). To differentiate infections of the lower genital tract (cervicitis) from those of the upper tract (PID), note signs or symptoms of systemic disease, including fever or lower abdominal pain or pressure associated with a vaginal discharge. In evaluating vaginal discharge, perform appropriate tests to exclude infections confined to the vagina.

B. Too often, complaints of lower abdominal pain in sexually active females immediately provoke the diagnosis of PID without application of criteria to substantiate the diagnosis. Hager's criteria for diagnosing acute salpingitis include a history of lower abdominal pain or tenderness, cervical motion tenderness, and adnexal tenderness. The patient must also have one of the following objective findings: (1) fever >38° C, (2) leukocytosis >10,500 WBC/mm^3, (3) culdocentesis fluid containing WBCs or bacteria, (4) inflammatory mass on pelvic examination or sonography, (5) ESR >20, and (6) evidence of gonococcus or *Chlamydia* on cervical Gram's stain. The severity of the illness determines whether outpatient care or hospitalization is appropriate. In both cases the antibiotic regimen involves a broad-spectrum cephalosporin with tetracycline.

C. Cervical ulcerations are often accompanied by inguinal or vulvar adenopathy. Pain distinguishes HSV from syphilitic lesions in primary outbreaks. Primary genital HSV often involves the vulva, urethra, and cervix, progressing from multiple painful vesicles to ulcers in the presence of a systemic viremia. First-episode nonprimary genital herpes, like recurrent HSV, occurs in the presence of circulating antibodies and is associated with an infection of muted duration and intensity. Acyclovir, the mainstay of treatment, is particularly effective in primary infections in which early intervention significantly reduces viral shedding, accelerates healing, and hastens recovery. Syphilis, by contrast, usually manifests on the cervix in a primary infection; however, since it is usually asymptomatic, it is rarely diagnosed at this stage. Identification of the stage of infection plays a major role in determining the duration of treatment. Penicillin is the drug of choice, with almost no reported resistant strains.

D. When a growth is noted on the cervix in association with cervicitis and discharge, obtain a cervical biopsy specimen from the leading edge of the tumor to exclude endophytic cervical neoplasia. More commonly a whitish exophytic lesion is associated with genital warts or human papillomavirus (HPV). These lesions by themselves usually represent an infectious process involving HPV serotypes 6 and 11. Types 16, 18, 31, 33, 35, and 56 are associated with neoplasia. Application of 3% acetic acid to the cervix, along with colposcopically directed biopsies, makes it possible to distinguish between infectious and neoplastic lesions. This difference may have an important influence on the choice of treatment. In rare instances, tuberculous cervicitis manifests as a mucopurulent discharge or fungating mass. Diagnosis is made by cervical biopsy demonstrating caseating granulomas and/or AFB stain or culture.

E. Gonoccoccal endocervicitis manifests symptoms, including mucopurulent vaginal discharge, uterine bleeding, and dysuria, in 40–60% of infections. The diagnosis is traditionally made by an endocervical culture plated on modified Thayer-Martin medium. Of more practical consideration are newer rapid-assay techniques such as the Gonozyme. Although procaine penicillin G, ampicillin, and amoxicillin continue to be effective, ceftriaxone, 250 mg IM, is the drug of choice. As a single treatment it ensures compliance while simultaneously covering penicillinase-producing and chromosomally mediated resistant *N. gonorrhoeae*. The increasing prevalence of chlamydial endocervicitis is associated with its relative "silence" compared with *N. gonorrhoeae*. Two immunoassays have emerged as rapid and accurate methods for diagnosing *Chlamydia*. Doxycycline (100 mg twice daily for 7 days) is preferred to tetracycline, which causes more side effects and is given four times a day. Since both *N. gonorrhoeae* and *Chlamydia* are reportable STDs, direct the patient to ask all of her sexual contacts to seek evaluation and treatment. In addition, it is vital to obtain a test of cure, to ensure compliance and confirm the absence of antimicrobial resistance.

References

ACOG Technical Bulletin. Gonorrhea and chlamydial infections. No. 89, November 1985.

Sweet RL, Gibbs RS. Infectious diseases of the female genital tract. 2nd ed. Baltimore: Williams & Wilkins, 1990.

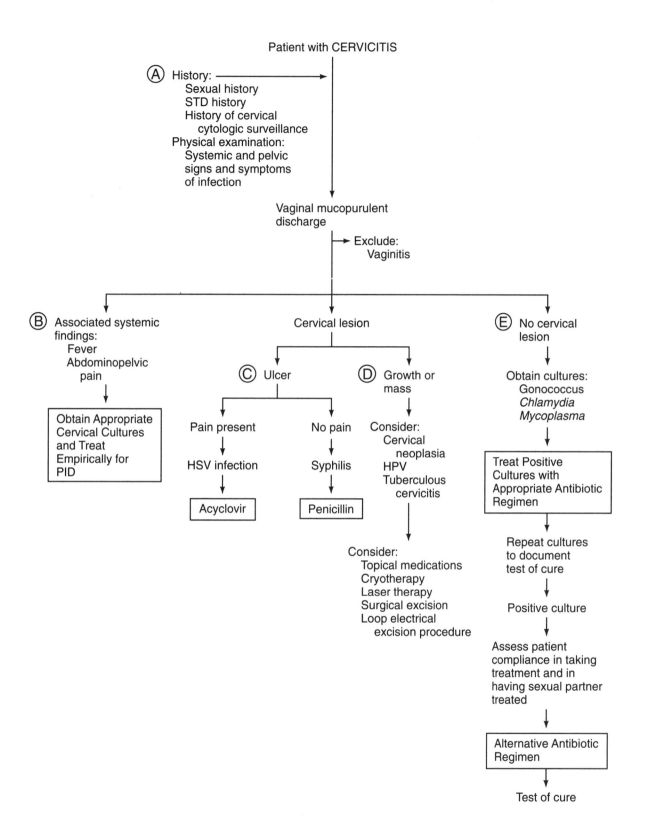

Patient with CERVICITIS

(A) History:
    Sexual history
    STD history
    History of cervical
      cytologic surveillance
    Physical examination:
    Systemic and pelvic
    signs and symptoms
    of infection

Vaginal mucopurulent
discharge

Exclude:
Vaginitis

(B) Associated systemic
findings:
    Fever
    Abdominopelvic
    pain

Obtain Appropriate
Cervical Cultures
and Treat
Empirically for
PID

Cervical lesion

(C) Ulcer

Pain present

HSV infection

Acyclovir

No pain

Syphilis

Penicillin

(D) Growth or
mass

Consider:
    Cervical
    neoplasia
    HPV
    Tuberculous
    cervicitis

Consider:
    Topical medications
    Cryotherapy
    Laser therapy
    Surgical excision
    Loop electrical
      excision procedure

(E) No cervical
lesion

Obtain cultures:
    Gonococcus
    Chlamydia
    Mycoplasma

Treat Positive
Cultures with
Appropriate Antibiotic
Regimen

Repeat cultures
to document
test of cure

Positive culture

Assess patient
compliance in taking
treatment and in
having sexual partner
treated

Alternative Antibiotic
Regimen

Test of cure

ABNORMAL VAGINAL BLEEDING

Hugh S. Miller, M.D.

Abnormal vaginal bleeding unassociated with uterine bleeding is uncommon and can often be discerned from a careful history and physical exam. When genitourinary and GI pathologies have been ruled out, concentrate on the genital etiologies, which are most often uterine. Abnormal perimenarchal and early perimenopausal bleeding is usually hormonally mediated, although the bleeding characteristics may vary widely. Conversely, late perimenopausal and postmenopausal bleeding is more likely to be related to a neoplastic process that is not necessarily malignant.

A. A detailed obstetric, gynecologic, and medical history, including menstrual pattern, contraceptive choice, exposure to sexually transmitted diseases (STDs), and blood dyscrasias will serve to distinguish between benign and malignant processes. Of paramount importance is the need to identify women at high risk for genital tract cancer, specifically those with premalignant conditions of the cervix or uterus, human papilloma virus (HPV) infection, obesity, and pre-existing malignancy.

B. The complete physical examination enables one to exclude extragenital tract etiologies while lending further support to a potential endocrinologic or hematologic cause in the presence of thyromegaly or diffuse petechiae. The pelvic examination is essential, as important as the history at localizing the source of bleeding through the identification of lesions or other significant pathology such as polyps, uterine fibroids, and pelvic masses. The Pap smear obtained before the bimanual examination is essential in screening for cervical cancer and is occasionally helpful at suggesting the presence of cervicitis or higher genital tract neoplasias. In patients at risk for STDs, take the appropriate cultures. All women of reproductive age should be evaluated for pregnancy regardless of menstrual history. Accuracy of urine human chorionic gonadotropin (hCG) testing has largely eliminated the need for qualitative serum β-hCG testing. When bleeding is significant or persistent, it is helpful to obtain a complete blood count to determine the extent of anemia and rule out occult hematologic malignancies. Other diagnostic testing should be dictated by the history and physical examination, including various endocrinologic, coagulation, and imaging studies.

C. Focus first on the source of the bleeding. The availability of the necessary equipment (including specula of various sizes and shapes), flexible lighting, and adequate assistance is important. If a lesion is identified in the genital tract, obtain a biopsy regardless of the patient's age.

D. Since various contraceptive options may lead to abnormal bleeding in premenopausal women, it is essential that the clinician addresses the contraceptive choice first. The newest contributor to this spectrum is Norplant, which has been found to cause abnormal bleeding in most patients in the first 6–9 months. In the absence of an obvious cause, the etiology is most likely to be "dysfunctional uterine bleeding," a diagnosis made by exclusion, and usually the result of anovulation. Depending on the patient's wishes, the options may include either no therapy or some hormonal manipulation. In women with no absolute contraindications who desire contraception, oral contraceptives serve as a mainstay of therapy. Persistent abnormal bleeding, refractory to hormonal manipulation, should prompt further evaluation of the uterine cavity. In patients at risk for hyperplasia, endometrial sampling may be sufficient, although more and more physicians are moving to direct visualization in the form of hysteroscopy.

E. The incidence of adenocarcinoma of the uterus in women <40 years of age is approximately 5%. As a consequence, abnormal bleeding must be evaluated by endometrial biopsy (EMB) in women 40 years or older. With the ever-increasing use of hormonal replacement therapy among women in the postmenopausal years, reports of abnormal bleeding have likewise increased and require equally diligent evaluation to rule out occult carcinomas. When histopathologic examination reveals hyperplasia with cellular atypia, medical or surgical treatment is appropriate. Treatment of endometrial carcinoma should involve consultation with a gynecologist to determine the best course of therapy.

References

ACOG Technical Bulletin. Dysfunctional uterine bleeding. No. 134, October 1989.

Carlson JM. Menorrhagia and metrorrhagia. In: Friedman EA, Borten M, Chapin DS, eds. Gynecologic decision making. 2nd ed. Toronto: BC Decker, 1988.

Herbst AL, Mishell DR Jr, Stenchever MA, Droegemueller W, eds. Comprehensive gynecology. 2nd ed. St Louis: Mosby–Year Book, 1992.

Patient with ABNORMAL VAGINAL BLEEDING

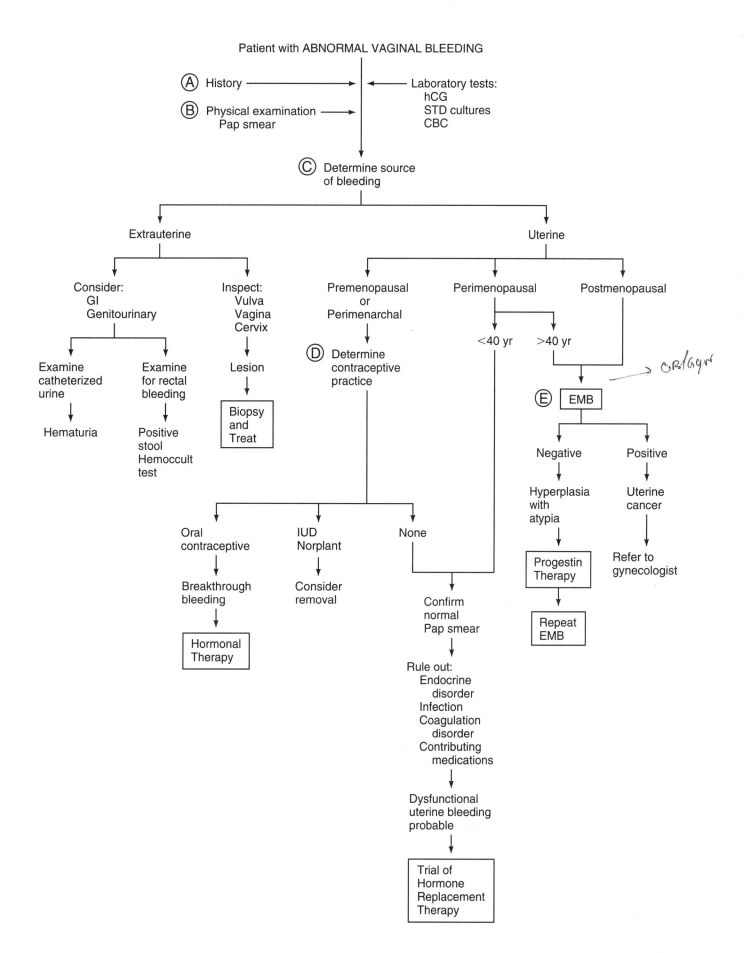

(A) History ⟶ ← Laboratory tests:
hCG
(B) Physical examination ⟶ STD cultures
Pap smear CBC

(C) Determine source
of bleeding

Extrauterine

Consider:
GI
Genitourinary

Examine
catheterized
urine

Hematuria

Inspect:
Vulva
Vagina
Cervix

Lesion

Examine
for rectal
bleeding

Positive
stool
Hemoccult
test

Biopsy
and
Treat

Uterine

Premenopausal
or
Perimenarchal

(D) Determine
contraceptive
practice

Oral
contraceptive

Breakthrough
bleeding

Hormonal
Therapy

IUD
Norplant

Consider
removal

None

Confirm
normal
Pap smear

Rule out:
Endocrine
disorder
Infection
Coagulation
disorder
Contributing
medications

Dysfunctional
uterine bleeding
probable

Trial of
Hormone
Replacement
Therapy

Perimenopausal

<40 yr   >40 yr

→ OB/Gyn

(E) EMB

Negative

Hyperplasia
with
atypia

Progestin
Therapy

Repeat
EMB

Positive

Uterine
cancer

Refer to
gynecologist

Postmenopausal

455

VAGINAL BLEEDING IN PREGNANCY

Allan R. Hartsough, M.D.

The causes of vaginal bleeding during pregnancy are protean and include obstetric, gynecologic and non–obstetric-gynecologic etiologies.

A. Urgent history and physical examination may provide clear direction in defining the cause of vaginal bleeding; moreover, some obstetric causes carry a potentially great risk to both maternal and fetal well being with advancing gestational age. An abdominal examination, quickly defining a relative gestational age, may prove valuable.

B. Evaluation by speculum may quickly define the cause of the vaginal bleeding, particularly if there is heavy bleeding. Not infrequently, products of conception may be found in the cervix. Alternatively, vulvovaginitis may be diagnosed.

C. Although sonography can clearly define the status of pregnancy and potentially the cause, determination of Doptone fetal heart tones (which may be heard by 10–12 weeks) can quickly determine fetal viability and help establish the gestational age. This may allow more circumspect evaluation for other etiologies, including gynecologic disorders (e.g., cervicitis, vaginitis) or nonobstetric gynecologic disorders (e.g., urinary tract infection, GI bleeding, trauma).

D. If the cervix appears closed on speculum examination, particularly when inflammation or discharge is present, consider culturing the cervix for gonorrhea and *Chlamydia*. Occasionally, cervical cancer presents during pregnancy with gross vaginal bleeding. Vaginitis may also be present, particularly as a serosanguineous discharge, and often associated with trichomonal infection. Sometimes, rupture of membranes, with or without contractions, causes a bloody vaginal discharge.

E. Sonography has become a very powerful tool in evaluating the gestational age of the developing embryo or fetus and in defining many gynecologic disorders.

F. If sonography reveals a viable pregnancy, loss of a second twin, a partial molar pregnancy, or more likely a threatened abortion may be the diagnosis if gynecologic and other causes have been ruled out.

G. Alternatively, if sonography shows a nonviable pregnancy, consider immaturity of the developing embryo (<5 weeks' gestation) or a condition such as a blighted ovum or molar pregnancy. Consider also a condition of potentially greatest significance to maternal well-being, an ectopic pregnancy.

H. If on speculum examination the cervix appears open, consider the diagnosis of an incompetent cervix or incomplete abortion.

I. A pregnancy of ≥20 weeks' gestation no longer falls into the category of an abortion if cervical bleeding is present. Moreover, with advancing gestational age beyond 20 weeks, fetal viability is rapidly approaching. Therefore, rapid sonographic definition of fetal age, viability, health, and particularly placental abnormalities is of paramount importance. The chief diagnosis to rule out before a vaginal digital or speculum examination is a placenta previa.

J. If no placental abnormality is defined and fetal viability is not present, an intrauterine fetal demise, or molar pregnancy is a likely diagnosis. With an intrauterine fetal demise, consider a coagulopathy; with prolonged retention of a dead fetus, this is a recognized complication.

K. With sonographic evidence of viability and no placental abnormality, perform a speculum examination.

L. If the cervix appears closed, ruptured membrane, cervicitis, vaginitis, cervical cancer, and nongynecologic disease are all possibilities.

M. If on speculum examination the cervix appears open and there are no contractions, incompetent cervix is the diagnosis.

N. Alternatively, if there are contractions and the cervix is open, consider early labor, abruption, or vasa praevia.

References

Benedetti T. Hemorrage in obstetrics. Normal and problem pregnancy. New York: Churchill Livingstone, 1990.

Disaia P, Beinau M. Cancer in pregnancy. In: Creasy RK, Resnik R, eds. Maternal-fetal medicine. Philadelphia: WB Saunders, 1984.

Green JR. Placenta abnormalities. In: Creasy RK, Resnik R, eds. Maternal-fetal medicine. Philadelphia: WB Saunders, 1984.

Wenk AC, Cartwright P. Recurrent and spontaneous abortion. In: Jones HW III, Wentz AG, Burnett LS, eds. Novak's textbook of Gynecology. 11th ed. Baltimore: Williams & Wilkins, 1988.

Pregnant Patient with VAGINAL BLEEDING

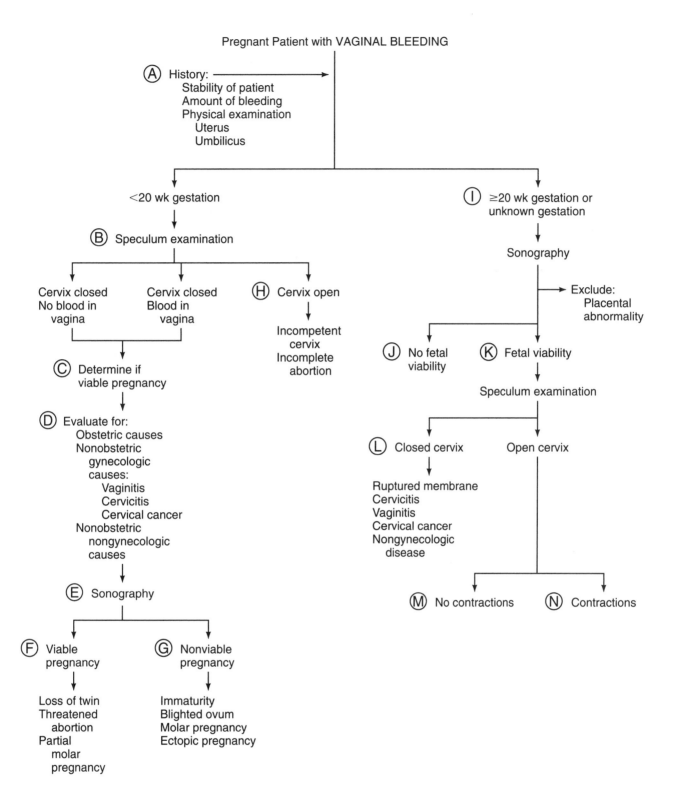

ACUTE ABDOMINAL PAIN IN WOMEN

Robert N. Samuelson, M.D.

A. The acute abdomen refers to any condition requiring an "acute" medical decision. The potential causes of acute abdominal pain in female patients are multiple. A thorough history can quickly eliminate a number of these. Information regarding menstrual cycles, previous episodes of similar pain, sexual activity, contraception, vaginal discharge, and changes in bowel, bladder, or appetite can quickly narrow the differential diagnosis. Findings in the acute abdomen frequently include severe pain, which may be caused by infection, bleeding, infarction of tissue, or obstruction of a hollow viscus (bowel, fallopian tube, ureter). Any of these conditions can irritate and inflame the peritoneum, making it very sensitive to movement. Loss of appetite, nausea, and vomiting frequently accompany the pain and tenderness. Laboratory studies necessary for adequately evaluating an acute abdomen include a CBC with differential, ESR, pregnancy test (urine or serum), urinalysis, and occasionally an amylase or lipase. Obtain cervical cultures for *Neisseria gonorrhoeae* and *Chlamydia trachomatis* at initial evaluation if the history warrants.

B. If the pregnancy test is positive, the differential diagnosis can be narrowed considerably. It is important to recognize that conditions other than pregnancy can be the source of the pain. If gestational age is <10–12 weeks, consider ectopic pregnancy, rupture or torsion of ovarian cyst, or septic or threatened abortion. If gestational age is >12–14 weeks, ectopic becomes less likely; consider other entities such as ruptured or torsed adnexa, appendicitis, septic abortion, ureteral colic, and pyelonephritis.

C. Ultrasonography continues to expand its role in the evaluation of obstetric and gynecologic patients with abdominal pain. Its use in conjunction with quantitative beta-human chorionic gonadotropin (β-hCG) can be very important. With normal pregnancy, a gestational sac is often seen at 5–6 weeks gestational age. When the β-hCG level reaches 6500 MIU/ml, an abdominal scan will be able to visualize a gestational sac; at 1500 MIU/ml a transvaginal probe will frequently visualize the pregnancy. If, on the basis of sonographic findings and quantitative β-hCG values, the possibility of an ectopic pregnancy still exists, the patient needs referral for possible surgical management (laparoscopy/laparotomy) or medical management (e.g., methotrexate) for an ectopic pregnancy. If an early intrauterine pregnancy is confirmed by sonography, other sources for the pain must be determined. Ruptured or torsed ovarian cysts, appendicitis, or an infected abortion can also present with abdominal pain.

D. If the pregnancy test is negative, history again plays an important role. Patients with a history of recurrent cyclic pain related to menses and who now have an acute exacerbation may have a ruptured endometrium. Patients with a history of fever, chills, and vaginal discharge with a recent change in sexual partners are at risk for pelvic inflammatory disease (PID). (Patients on oral contraceptives are at decreased risk for ovarian cyst formation.) If an infectious etiology is determined, admit her for IV antibiotics; if there is no improvement in 24–48 hr, consider exploration. The determination of PID versus appendicitis is frequently not resolved until laparoscopy or laparotomy is performed. Other entities that must always be considered are adnexal torsion, ovarian cyst rupture, exacerbation of endometriosis, degenerating fibroid, renal calculi, and mesenteric lymphadenitis.

E. Although many imaging modalities are available to the practitioner, the choice may need to be made in concert with the radiologist. A thin pregnant patient can be evaluated well with ultrasound; in obese postmenopausal patients more information may be obtained by CT. The need for surgical exploration often takes precedence over imaging studies. Many of the disorders in premenopausal patients apply also to postmenopausal patients. Cyst formation occurs infrequently in elderly patients, but its appearance must be evaluated carefully for the possibility of malignancy. Other processes that can cause acute pain include colonic diverticulitis (75% of these resolve with proper attention), bowel obstruction (most of these need exploration), and vascular lesions (mesenteric thrombosis), dissecting or leaking aneurysm, and acute cholecystitis or pancreatitis.

References

Harberg F. The acute abdomen in childhood. Pediatr Ann 1989; 18:117.

Jeffrey RB. CT and sonography of the acute abdomen. New York: Raven Press, 1989.

Kiernan GV, Cales RH. Acute abdominal disorders. Emerg Med Clin North Am 1989; 7:30.

Merrell RC. Gastroenterological emergencies. Gastroenterol Clin North Am 1988; 17:75.

Female Patient with ACUTE ABDOMINAL PAIN

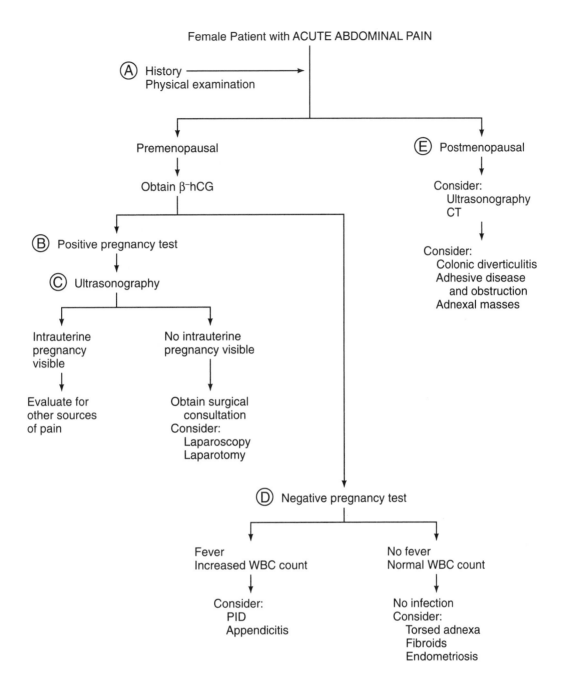

(A) History ⟶
   Physical examination

Premenopausal

Obtain β‾hCG

(E) Postmenopausal

Consider:
   Ultrasonography
   CT

Consider:
   Colonic diverticulitis
   Adhesive disease
      and obstruction
   Adnexal masses

(B) Positive pregnancy test

(C) Ultrasonography

Intrauterine
pregnancy
visible

No intrauterine
pregnancy visible

Evaluate for
other sources
of pain

Obtain surgical
consultation
Consider:
   Laparoscopy
   Laparotomy

(D) Negative pregnancy test

Fever
Increased WBC count

No fever
Normal WBC count

Consider:
   PID
   Appendicitis

No infection
Consider:
   Torsed adnexa
   Fibroids
   Endometriosis

URINARY TRACT INFECTION IN WOMEN

Michael D. Katz, Pharm.D.

A. Patients with lower urinary tract infection or cystitis complain primarily of dysuria. Frequency, nocturia, urgency, and suprapubic tenderness also may be present. Approximately one third of patients with only lower tract symptoms have an occult renal infection. Patients with overt upper tract infection or acute pyelonephritis usually present with flank, low back, or abdominal pain; fevers; chills; malaise; and nausea and vomiting. Concomitant lower tract symptoms may also be present.

B. Individuals with pyelonephritis (PN) can often be successfully treated as outpatients. However, patients with nausea and vomiting who are unable to take oral fluids and medications should be hospitalized. Enterobacteriaceae are the most common pathogens associated with acute pyelonephritis. A wide variety of antimicrobial regimens are available. Initial outpatient therapy may include ampicillin, trimethoprim/sulfamethoxazole, a cephalosporin, or a fluoroquinolone. The conventional IV regimen of ampicillin and gentamicin is effective, although trimethoprim/sulfamethoxazole and cephalosporins also may be considered. The initial choice of therapy must be based on the most likely organisms present and local susceptibility patterns. Definitive therapy must be guided by results of culture and sensitivity tests.

C. In patients with acute cystitis, certain risk factors increase the chance of an occult renal or complicated urinary tract infection (UTI). Such risk factors include nosocomial infection, pregnancy, known urinary tract abnormality or stone, indwelling catheter or recent instrumentation, previous relapse after therapy for UTI, previous UTI before age 12, acute pyelonephritis or more than three UTIs in the past year, symptoms for >7 days before therapy, recent antibiotic use, diabetes, and other immunosuppressing conditions. Treat patients with one or more of these risk factors as having an upper tract infection.

D. In acute, uncomplicated cystitis, single-dose or 3-day antibiotic therapy can be given without obtaining a pretreatment urine culture. A variety of regimens have been evaluated. Single-dose therapy is associated with a higher rate of treatment failure and relapse than 3-day therapy if an occult upper tract infection is present. Also, single-dose therapy with beta-lactam agents is less effective than 3-day therapy or single-dose therapy with other agents. Recommended short-term regimens include single dose: trimethoprim/sulfamethoxazole, 320 mg/1600 mg, trimethoprim 400 mg, ciprofloxacin 250 mg, norfloxacin 400 mg; 3 day: trimethoprim/sulfamethoxazole 160 mg/800 mg twice daily, trimethoprim 100 mg twice daily, amoxicillin/clavulanate 500 mg every 8 hr, ciprofloxacin

250 mg every 12 hr norfloxacin 400 mg every 12 hr. Many other regimens have been studied; the specific antibiotic choice must be guided by local susceptibility patterns. Post-therapy urine cultures are necessary only in patients with persisting symptoms, complicating factors, or pregnancy.

E. Sexual intercourse and use of diaphragms have been associated with an increased risk of UTI. Urination after intercourse may reduce the frequency of relapse. Postcoital antibiotic therapy is also effective. Discontinuance of a diaphragm for contraception may also reduce the frequency of relapse.

F. In patients with dysuria, a positive urine culture is considered to be $>10^2$ CFU/ml growth. Treat patients with a positive culture for 7–14 days. In acute cystitis, over 90% of cases are caused by *Escherichia coli* and other Enterobacteriaceae, *Staphylococcus saprophyticus*, and *Enterococcus*. Unless a highly resistant pathogen is present, an inexpensive agent such as trimethoprim/sulfamethoxazole should be adequate. Reserve more expensive agents such as the fluoroquinolones, cephalosporins, and amoxicillin/clavulanate for resistant infections.

G. In patients with frequent recurrences, chronic suppression can reduce this frequency by 95%. Many regimens have been evaluated. If possible, choose the least toxic, least expensive agent. Effective daily regimens include nitrofurantoin 50–100 mg, trimethoprim/sulfamethoxazole 40–80 mg/200–400 mg, and trimethoprim 100 mg. Thrice weekly administration of trimethoprim/sulfamethoxazole 40 mg/200 mg has also proved effective.

References

Hooton TM, Stamm WE. Management of acute uncomplicated urinary tract infection in adults. Med Clin North Am 1991; 75:339.

Johnson JR, Stamm WE. Urinary tract infection in women: diagnosis and treatment. Ann Intern Med 1989; 111:906.

Norrby SR. Short-term treatment of uncomplicated lower urinary tract infection in women. Rev Infect Dis 1990; 12:458.

Thomas S, Bhatia NN. New approaches in the treatment of urinary tract infection. Obstet Gynecol Clin North Am 1989; 16:897.

Tolkoff-Rubin NE, Rubin RH. Urinary tract infection: significance and management Bull NY Acad Med 1986; 62:131.

Zhanel GG, Harding GKM, Guay DRP. Asymptomatic bacteriuria, which patients should be treated? Arch Intern Med 1990; 150:1389.

Woman with DYSURIA AND FREQUENT URINATION

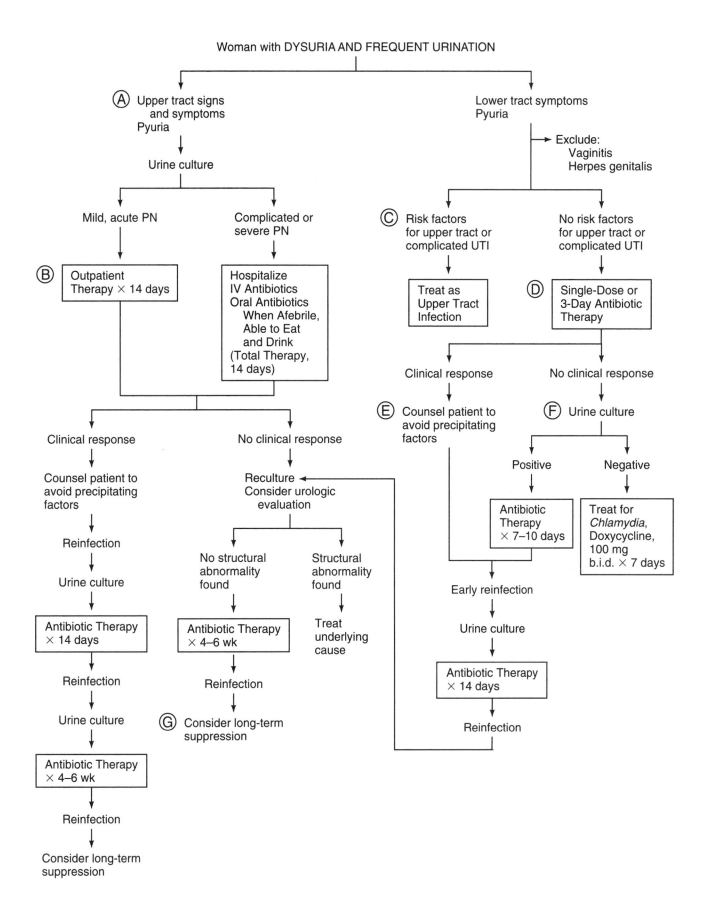

NIPPLE DISCHARGE

Allan R. Hartsough, M.D.

A. A breast discharge is a condition with potentially life-threatening consequences, but fortunately most are benign. As an initial step a careful medical history is of paramount importance, both in determining the medical significance and in directing evaluation. A medically significant breast discharge may be characterized as a spontaneous, persistent discharge in a nonpregnant and nonlactating female. Question the patient for evidence of nipple stimulation (e.g., sexual foreplay or clothing that chronically rubs the nipple). Pharmaceuticals such as estrogens, phenothiazines, reserpine, opiates, diazepam, or tricyclic antidepressants can cause galactorrhea through inhibition of PIF (dopamine). Other associated factors that can cause elevated prolactin and hence galactorrhea include chronic stress, thoracotomy scars, cervical spinal lesions, and herpes zoster.

B. It is important to differentiate between galactorrheal and nongalactorrheal discharge. Galactorrhea implies that underlying breast disease is not present. Microscopic evaluation of the nipple discharge with oil red O stain or other commercially available fat stains can identify the presence or absence of fat droplets. When there are fat droplets, a diagnosis of galactorrhea can be made. Importantly, neither the physical characteristics of the discharge nor bilaterality can be used to exclude serious causes of breast discharge.

C. In patients who present with galactorrhea, obtain prolactin and thyroid stimulating hormone (TSH) levels. If the prolactin and TSH are normal, follow the patient yearly or as dictated clinically. If the prolactin level is normal or increased with an elevated TSH, evaluate the patient further for hypothyroidism. If the prolactin level is elevated with normal TSH, continued evaluation of hyperprolactinemia is indicated.

D. An elevation of prolactin requires further evaluation to rule out a pituitary micro- or macroadenoma. However, the physician must be cognizant of diurnal variation in prolactin levels, a history of breast stimulation (such as an office breast examination) and review the medical history for pharmaceutical use when considering small elevations in prolactin levels. Prolactin levels of <100 should be repeated in the fasting state. If the repeat prolactin level is normal, observe the patient clinically with follow-up and repeat examination in 3–6 months. An elevation of the prolactin to ≥100 is highly suggestive of a pituitary adenoma; perform a CT scan to exclude this or define the nature of the tumor. If an adenoma is found, tailor treatment to the patient's needs on the basis of size, symptoms, and reproductive goals.

E. In patients who present with nongalactorrheal discharge, first perform a careful and thorough breast examination. Palpation of a mass requires immediate and complete evaluation to rule out a malignant process. If no mass is palpable, consider cytologic evaluation of the nipple discharge. While a positive cytologic evaluation may allow more rapid determination of a malignancy, its usefulness is limited and *cannot* be used to exclude a malignancy.

F. If the examination is normal, a mammogram should be obtained. Again, an abnormal mammogram requires an immediate and complete evaluation to rule out malignancy. With a normal mammographic examination and no abnormal physical findings, a repeat evaluation in 6–12 months or as clinically dictated if nipple discharge persists is recommended.

References

Borten M. Nipple discharge. In: Friedman EA, Borten M, Chapin DS, eds. Gynecological decision making. 2nd ed. Toronto: BC Decker, 1988:680.

Dickey RP, Stone SC. Drugs that affect the breast and lactation. Clin Obstet Gynecol 1975; 18:95.

Droegemueller W. Breast discharge. In: Herbst AL, Mishell DR, Stenchever MA, Droegemueller W, eds. Comprehensive gynecology. 2nd ed. St. Louis: Mosby-Year Book, 1992.

Dubuk ED, et al. Prolactin secreting pituitary adenoma. Endocr Rev 1980; 1:295.

Teitirick JE. Nipple discharge. Fam Physician 1980; 22:101.

Patient with NIPPLE DISCHARGE

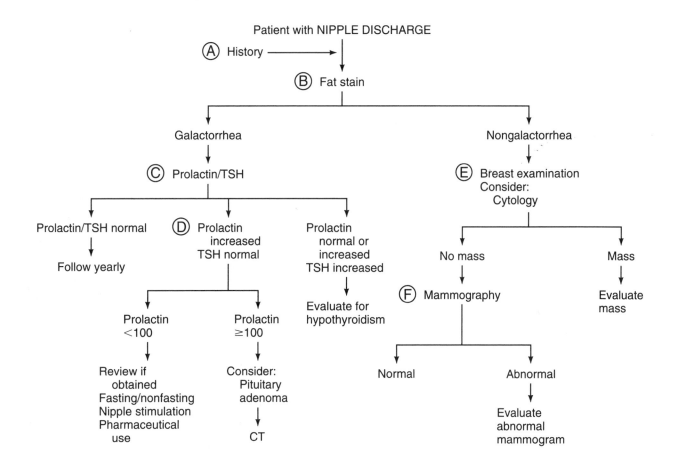

(A) History ⟶

(B) Fat stain

Galactorrhea

Nongalactorrhea

(C) Prolactin/TSH

(E) Breast examination
Consider:
Cytology

Prolactin/TSH normal

(D) Prolactin
increased
TSH normal

Prolactin
normal or
increased
TSH increased

No mass

Mass

Follow yearly

Evaluate for
hypothyroidism

(F) Mammography

Evaluate
mass

Prolactin
<100

Prolactin
≥100

Review if
obtained
Fasting/nonfasting
Nipple stimulation
Pharmaceutical
use

Consider:
Pituitary
adenoma

Normal

Abnormal

CT

Evaluate
abnormal
mammogram

ABNORMAL PAP SMEAR

Hugh S. Miller, M.D.

A. Cervical cytopathology is strongly associated with sexual activity and increasingly with human papillomavirus (HPV) as a sexually transmitted disease (STD). To identify patients' risk factors, obtain a complete gynecologic history, including a full sexual/STD history. A history of previous abnormal cervical cytopathology and associated diagnostic procedures and treatment are also of utmost importance. The Pap smear as a screening test is both sensitive and specific for pathology of the genital tract, limited neither to the cervix nor to detection of neoplasia. With the wide acceptance and use of Pap smears, the mortality rate associated with cervical cancer has steadily decreased. However, recent criticism of cervical/vaginal cytology has arisen in the wake of a poorly regulated industry that has failed to establish adequate quality assurance. The Bethesda classification system was written and adopted in 1988 in an attempt to establish national standards, recognizing that the cytopathologic report is a medical consultation and that the former Papanicolaou classification is no longer adequate. With the new system, cytopathologists are first called on to determine the adequacy of the sample, and then asked to distinguish among inflammatory, infectious and neoplastic processes. The Bethesda system adopted two new terms, low- and high-grade squamous intraepithelial lesion (SIL), to replace the spectrum of current terminology, exclusive of invasive carcinoma. Some cytopathologists may continue to use the former classifications of dysplasia, cervical intraepithelial neoplasia (CIN) 1–3. The new descriptive nomenclature also makes it possible to acknowledge the presence of the cytopathologic features of HPV with or without concurrent neoplastic changes.

B. To evaluate the female genital tract thoroughly, employ the best illumination and the proper size and shape of speculum to optimize visualization. Initially, examine the unprepared vulvar, vaginal, and cervical surfaces for whitish patches, growths, or ulcerations. Keep in mind that the use of any bactericidal/static lubricants will compromise the culture/cytopathologic results. Cervical friability, with or without an associated lesion, can represent an infectious condition as easily as a neoplastic one. In cases in which the Pap smear is judged unsatisfactory, it is usually due to the absence of endocervical cells or drying artifact. A properly obtained Pap smear seeks to obtain an extro- and endocervical scraping to maximize the probability of sampling the transformation zone. A moistened cotton-tipped applicator and a spatula generally suffice. The endocervical brush, a recent development, allows for better endocervical sampling at an increased cost with greater discomfort, and a higher risk of provoking bleeding that can obscure the cervical field.

C. Consider the "satisfactory" Pap smear that returns showing squamous atypia in the context of each patient's specific risk factors. Before the Bethesda system, many of these smears were reported as class II. One of the goals of the new system is to eliminate this wastebasket category. For patients at risk or those with straightforward SIL, proceed with colposcopy and colposcopically directed biopsies. With the recent addition of LEEF, some experienced colposcopists are collecting a surgical specimen for diagnosis while simultaneously giving treatment. For patients shown to have cellular changes associated with HPV, it remains unclear whether they derive any benefit from treatment or, for that matter, which method is best. From the standpoint of infectious disease, patients with identifiable lesions probably benefit from treatment, as do those with any degree of dysplasia. Here again, many patients with low SIL have been followed, and most regress if given sufficient time and follow-up. Regardless of the interval (every 4–6 months in the first 2 years), these patients require a thorough understanding of the nature of their condition so that they fully appreciate the need for follow-up.

D. HPV is often found in the presence of other STDs. Therefore, in evaluating an abnormal Pap smear that appears to be due to a cervicitis (p 452), remember that more than one process may be at work. In order to proceed, the necessary confirmatory cultures should be obtained, followed by appropriate antibiotic therapy.

E. Since the cervix rests in the posterior vaginal fornix, it is not uncommon to find cellular debris arising from the upper genital tract. In general, when normal endometrial or glandular cells are reported on a routine Pap smear, no further evaluation is needed. However, within the Bethesda classification, if such cells are reported as atypical or frankly cancerous, regardless of known origin, appropriate evaluation and therapy should be offered.

References

Burke L. Cervical dysplasia. In: Friedman EA, Borten M, Chapin DS, eds. Gynecological decision making. 2nd ed. Toronto: BC Decker, 1988:162.

Jones HW. Cervical cancer. Clin Obstet Gynecol 1990; 33:815.

Lundberg GD. The 1988 Bethesda System for reporting cervical/vaginal cytological diagnoses. JAMA 1989; 262:931.

Singer A. Premalignant lesions of the lower genital tract. Clin Pract Gynecol 1990; 2:2.

Patient with ABNORMAL PAP SMEAR

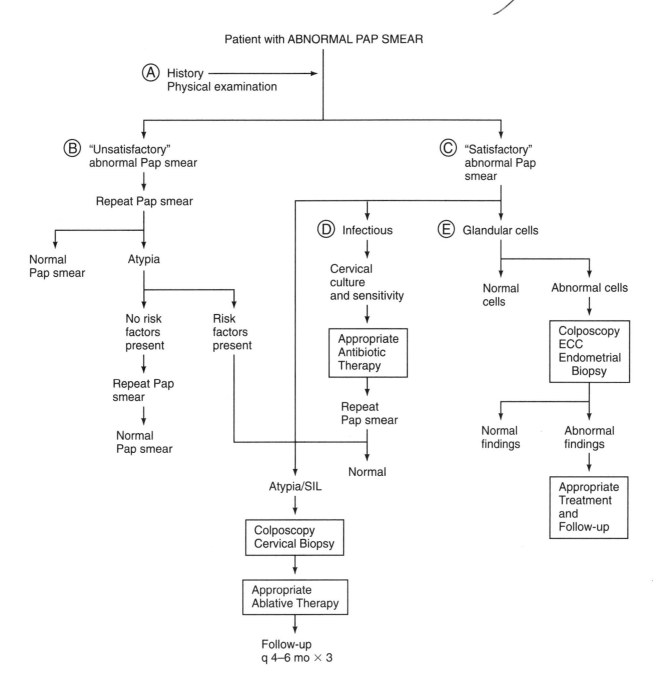

PREMENSTRUAL SYNDROME

Jessica Byron, M.D.

A. Over 50% of women experiencing cyclic menstruation report premenstrual symptoms. Manifestations may range from negligible in many women to disabling in up to 15%. Many symptoms and signs have been described as part of the syndrome and none are pathognomonic. It is the cyclic occurrence of symptoms beginning near or after ovulation, and resolving soon after the onset of menses, that is of diagnostic significance. The etiology remains unclear. The role of ovarian steroids, prolactin, prostaglandins, mineralocorticoids, neurotransmitters, endogenous opiates, vitamin and mineral deficiencies, and psychological factors is unclear.

B. Diagnostic evaluation of premenstrual syndrome (PMS) includes a complete retrospective history of the type, severity, timing, and impact of symptoms. In addition, other gynecologic problems including breast disease, endometriosis, and leiomyoma should be excluded, as they may mimic symptoms of PMS. A medical history to eliminate cardiac, renal, thyroid disease, or diabetes is important. A psychological history of major depression, panic disorder, dysthymia, or personality disorder, and information about the woman's past and current personal life, is important. Perform physical examination and laboratory examination, as needed. Investigators have been unable to document specific changes in hormone levels, prolactin, aldosterone, endorphin and glucose tolerance.

C. It is essential that the diagnosis of PMS be confirmed prospectively with the use of a daily symptom diary for at least 2 months. A variety of forms are available. The patient should document the severity in the week before the onset of menses. At least five symptoms must demonstrate a marked change during each cycle for at least two cycles, and a symptom-free week is necessary for the same cycles. If these criteria are not met, the symptoms may represent another disorder.

D. Review of treatment research fails to demonstrate consistently effective therapy, and the rates of response to placebos appear to be 50%. Numerous treatments have been advocated. The initial intervention should be to provide education and support; many women are reassured by chart review and can try to plan their schedules to avoid stress-producing activities in the premenstrual week. A diet that limits salty foods and caffeinated beverages may decrease symptoms of fluid retention, irritability, and insomnia. Moderate exercise can contribute to stress reduction and enhance self-esteem. Current research has not provided a definitive medical treatment for PMS. Progesterone has received much publicity but remains unsubstantiated in terms of efficacy. Vitamin B_6 has not proved superior to placebo; high doses have been associated with peripheral neuropathy. Anovulation therapy with oral contraceptives, danazol, and gonadotropin releasing hormone (GnRH) agonists may relieve symptoms, but unpleasant side effects frequently occur and lead to discontinuance. Psychoactive drugs may be tried to treat depression or anxiety. Referral to a mental health professional may be indicated. For symptoms that are primarily physical, treatment is symptom directed. The effectiveness of diuretics has not been proved in controlled studies. Antiprostaglandins may relieve dysmenorrhea, and this may make patients feel better even though the PMS persists. Mastodynia may be relieved by vitamin E, 400 IU daily, or bromocriptine for serious complaints. Sleep hygiene, including a regular schedule, no caffeine after noon, no alcohol, and relaxation exercises 1 hr before bedtime, may ameliorate fatigue and insomnia. Treat headaches and migraines with analgesics, vasoconstrictors, and antiemetics. A diet plan may assist with food cravings.

References

Derzko CM. Role of danazol in relieving the premenstrual syndrome. J Reprod Med 1990; 35 (1 Suppl):97.

Freeman E, Rickels K, Sondheimer SJ, Polansky M. Ineffectiveness of progesterone suppository treatment for premenstrual syndrome. A placebo-controlled, randomized, double-blind, cross-over study. JAMA 1990; 264:349.

Goodale IL, Domar AD, Benson H. Alleviation of premenstrual syndrome symptoms with the relaxation response. Obstet Gynecol 1990; 75:649.

Robinson GE. Premenstrual syndrome: current knowledge and management. Can Med Assoc J 1989; 140:605.

Patient with PREMENSTRUAL SYMPTOMS

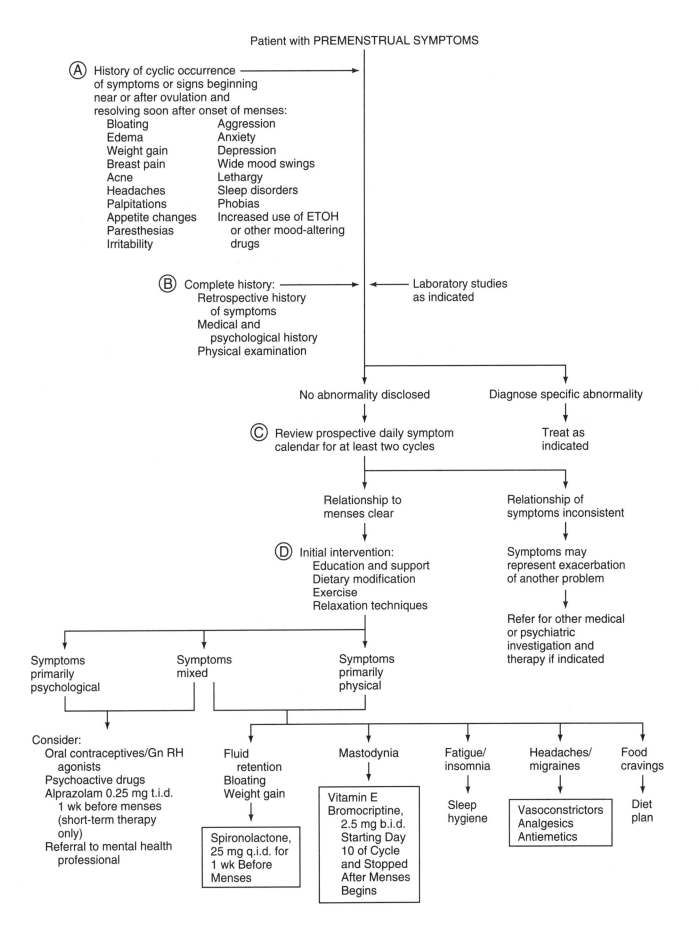

Ⓐ History of cyclic occurrence
of symptoms or signs beginning
near or after ovulation and
resolving soon after onset of menses:

Bloating	Aggression
Edema	Anxiety
Weight gain	Depression
Breast pain	Wide mood swings
Acne	Lethargy
Headaches	Sleep disorders
Palpitations	Phobias
Appetite changes	Increased use of ETOH
Paresthesias	or other mood-altering
Irritability	drugs

Ⓑ Complete history:
    Retrospective history
        of symptoms
    Medical and
        psychological history
    Physical examination

Laboratory studies
as indicated

No abnormality disclosed

Diagnose specific abnormality

Ⓒ Review prospective daily symptom
calendar for at least two cycles

Treat as
indicated

Relationship to
menses clear

Relationship of
symptoms inconsistent

Ⓓ Initial intervention:
    Education and support
    Dietary modification
    Exercise
    Relaxation techniques

Symptoms may
represent exacerbation
of another problem

Refer for other medical
or psychiatric
investigation and
therapy if indicated

Symptoms
primarily
psychological

Symptoms
mixed

Symptoms
primarily
physical

Consider:
    Oral contraceptives/Gn RH
        agonists
    Psychoactive drugs
    Alprazolam 0.25 mg t.i.d.
        1 wk before menses
        (short-term therapy
        only)
    Referral to mental health
        professional

Fluid
retention
Bloating
Weight gain

Mastodynia

Fatigue/
insomnia

Headaches/
migraines

Food
cravings

Spironolactone,
25 mg q.i.d. for
1 wk Before
Menses

Vitamin E
Bromocriptine,
2.5 mg b.i.d.
Starting Day
10 of Cycle
and Stopped
After Menses
Begins

Sleep
hygiene

Vasoconstrictors
Analgesics
Antiemetics

Diet
plan

467

CONTRACEPTIVE CHOICES

Ana María López, M.D.

The decision to conceive or not to conceive is a complicated one dependent on multiple factors. It is also one in which many patients request physician participation. To facilitate this process, the physician must be well versed in biologic factors that may influence this decision and be sensitive to patient concerns. Biologic factors that affect contraceptive choice include age, tobacco use, history of pelvic inflammatory disease (PID), and history of cardiovascular disease. Important patient issues that must be clarified include plans for future fertility, current sexual lifestyle, impact of unplanned pregnancy, history of compliance, and role of partner in birth spacing. Patients often have questions about efficacy (Table 1), safety, cost, and noncontraceptive benefits as well as the need to access the health care system to obtain or continue use of a specific birth control method (BCM). By applying active listening skills to the patient-doctor interaction, the clinician can help the patient make an informed choice.

A. Vasectomy is simple, inexpensive, and safe but does not confer immediate sterility. Sperm usually are not present after 25 ejaculations, but this can be confirmed only by microscopic examination of the semen. Although antibody formation to sperm has been noted after vasectomy, any clinically adverse implications of this are not known at this time. Bilateral tubal ligation (BLTL) is the most common BCM in the world. It is an outpatient procedure with a lower mortality rate than childbirth (3:100,000 vs. 14:100,000). If this BCM fails, the risk of ectopic pregnancy is increased. Vasectomy and BLTL may be reversed by microsurgical techniques. The success of reversals is inversely related to the amount of tissue originally damaged. Counsel patients that these are permanent methods and that their potential reversibility does not guarantee fertility.

B. Combination oral contraceptives (OCs) are second only to BLTL as the most common BCM in the world today. (They are discussed on page 472.) Long-acting progestin-only contraceptives include Depo-Provera and Norplant. The advantage of these methods is that the estrogen-associated thromboembolic complications are avoided. These methods are particularly applicable to women seeking a nonpermanent BCM who are ≥40 years old, smokers, or hypertensive. Progesterone-related side effects include increased low-density lipoprotein and decreased high-density lipoprotein with increased carbohydrate intolerance, possibly leading to diabetes. These methods act by inhibiting ovulation, maintaining thick cervical mucus

inhospitable to sperm, and producing thin atrophic endometrium subject to premature luteolysis. Depo-Provera, "the shot," consists of 150 mg of medroxyprogesterone given IM every 3 months; the most common side effect is amenorrhea. Norplant consists of six match-sized capsules surgically inserted subdermally in the woman's arm 7 days after the onset of menses. Slow hormonal release continues for the next 5 years; the failure rate is <0.57%. After 5 years the implants must be removed and a fresh set reinserted, if desired.

TABLE 1 Contraceptive Effectiveness in First Year in the United States*

	Effectiveness	
BCM	Theoretical (%)[†]	Typical (%)[‡]
Vasectomy	99.9	99.85
BLTL	99.8	99.6
Norplant	99.96	99.96
Depo-Provera	99.7	99.7
Oral contraceptives		
Combined	99.1	97
Mini-pill	99.5	80
IUD		
Cu-T 380A	99.2	97
Progestasert	98.0	93
Condom	98	88
Diaphragm	96	82
Cervical cap	94	82
Sponge		
Parous patient	91	72
Multiparous patient	94	82
Spermicides	97	80
Fertility awareness method		
Calendar	90	80
With BBT, post-ovulation coitus only	98	97
Lactation		
Breast feeding on demand with amenorrhea, 1st 6 months post partum	99	96
Chance	15	15

*Based on data in Hatcher, Trussel (1987), and Trussel (1990).
[†]Theoretical effectiveness attempts to predict the percent of contraceptive failures expected among couples using the BCM perfectly, consistently and correctly, for an entire year.
[‡]Typical effectiveness attempts to predict the percent of contraceptive failures expected among typical couples using the BCM for an entire year.

(Continued on page 470)

468

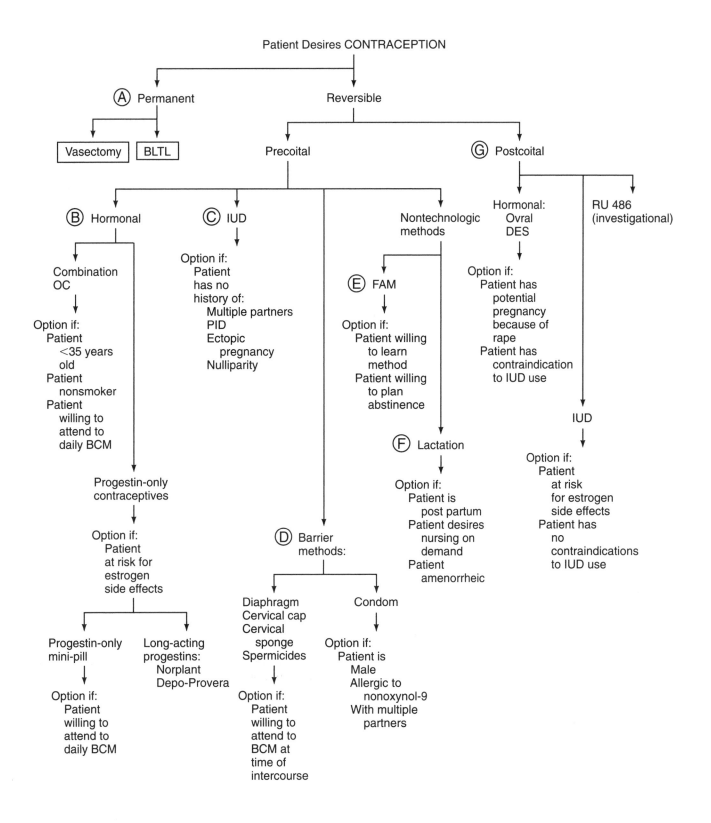

Patient Desires CONTRACEPTION

(A) Permanent

Vasectomy | BLTL

Reversible

Precoital

(B) Hormonal

Combination
OC

Option if:
Patient
<35 years
old
Patient
nonsmoker
Patient
willing to
attend to
daily BCM

Progestin-only
contraceptives

Option if:
Patient
at risk for
estrogen
side effects

Progestin-only
mini-pill

Option if:
Patient
willing to
attend to
daily BCM

Long-acting
progestins:
Norplant
Depo-Provera

(C) IUD

Option if:
Patient
has no
history of:
Multiple partners
PID
Ectopic
pregnancy
Nulliparity

(D) Barrier
methods:

Diaphragm
Cervical cap
Cervical
sponge
Spermicides

Option if:
Patient
willing to
attend to
BCM at
time of
intercourse

Condom

Option if:
Patient is
Male
Allergic to
nonoxynol-9
With multiple
partners

Nontechnologic
methods

(E) FAM

Option if:
Patient willing
to learn
method
Patient willing
to plan
abstinence

(F) Lactation

Option if:
Patient is
post partum
Patient desires
nursing on
demand
Patient
amenorrheic

(G) Postcoital

Hormonal:
Ovral
DES

Option if:
Patient has
potential
pregnancy
because of
rape
Patient has
contraindication
to IUD use

RU 486
(investigational)

IUD

Option if:
Patient
at risk
for estrogen
side effects
Patient has
no
contraindications
to IUD use

C. Intrauterine devices (IUDs) have a long history, but currently only two are available in the United States: Cu-T 380A and Progestasert, with the former being more widely used. They are thought to act by inhibiting fertilization and implantation through local foreign body inflammation and owing to the copper or progesterone effect of producing an atrophic endometrium. IUDs are contraindicated in patients with a known history of PID or ectopic pregnancy. They are inserted at the time of a woman's menses. Side effects include menorrhagia, which may result in anemia; dysmenorrhea; and uterine perforation secondary to a wandering IUD. Instruct the woman to ascertain IUD placement by checking for the IUD string.

D. Barrier methods require active patient participation. The diaphragm and cervical cap have been available for approximately 100 years and require fitting by a health care practitioner. Diaphragm use requires spermicide application before each episode of intercourse. It can be inserted up to 2 hours before intercourse and must remain in place 6–8 hours after coitus. Refitting must take place after pregnancy, pelvic surgery, or weight change of 10 pounds or more. In the U.S., the Prentif cap is the only cervical cap available. It is inserted no less than ½ hr before intercourse with a small amount of spermicide within the dome and can remain in place for 72 hr. A 24-hr limit is recommended to decrease cervical irritation and risk of toxic shock syndrome (TSS). Repeated spermicide applications are not required. The cervical cap cannot be used during menses. The cervical sponge does not require health practitioner fitting and contains 1 g of nonoxynol-9. It is available without a prescription and can be used continuously for 24 hours after moistening with tap water. All the above methods carry the risk of TSS. Spermicides can be used alone, although their efficacy is greatest when used in combination with condoms. Noncontraceptive benefits of nonoxynol 9 include prevention of sexually transmitted disease and PID. Condoms are the only male form of contraception. Problems with efficacy are associated with improper use (i.e., not leaving a ½-in. reservoir at the tip or not withdrawing carefully immediately after coitus). A female condom is under development but has not yet been approved for use.

E. Fertility awareness methods (FAMs) can be as effective as OCs in preventing pregnancy if used appropriately, with intercourse restricted to the postovulatory period. Efficacy is directly related to the employment of multiple factors to detect fertility. Owing to the complexity of these factors, formal instruction is advised before attempting use for either contraception or conception. Basal body temperature is recorded daily to detect a temperature rise of 0.4–0.8° F, indicating ovulation. Cervical mucus must also be examined daily because wet, thin mucus (as opposed to thick, dry mucus) facilitates sperm mobility. A record of the length of the patient's cycles is maintained. From this historical information and awareness that ovulation usually takes place 14 days before the onset of menses, a period of high-risk days can be defined. Some patients also note changes in cervical position and texture throughout the menstrual cycle. Finally, mittelschmerz is a sign of ovulation that some women consistently recognize.

F. World-wide, lactation has been attributed to the largest decrease in births, according to Carl Djerassi. Recent data reveal that breast feeding on demand while remaining amenorrheic in the first 6 months post partum is 98% effective as a BCM. Unfortunately, most U.S. patients are unable or do not desire to breast-feed on demand for 6 months.

G. Postcoital hormonal approaches include the use of Ovral within 72 hours of the episode of unprotected intercourse: four tablets in two doses 12 hours apart. Similarly, diethylstilbestrol (DES), 50 mg daily for 5 days, can be prescribed to prevent implantation; its most common side effect is nausea, and pregnancy termination is recommended if pregnancy does occur. Postcoital IUDs have also been used. The Cu-T may be inserted up to 5 days after intercourse; however, it is contraindicated in rape cases, in women with multiple partners, and in nulliparous patients. In prescribing postcoital OCs or IUDs, take care to screen for potential contraindications. Although these methods are part of clinical practice and are prescribed for postcoital contraception, the FDA has not approved their postcoital use. RU486, a progesterone antagonist, has been widely used in Europe to induce menses in the first 5 weeks of pregnancy and is under investigation in the U.S.

References

Affandi B, et al. Five-year experience with Norplant. Contraception 1987; 36(4):429.

Albertson BD, et al. The prediction of ovulation and monitoring of the fertile period. Adv Contracept 1987; 3(4):263.

Alderman P. The lurking sperm. JAMA 1988; 259:3142.

American College of Obstetricians and Gynecologists. Oral contraceptives. ACOG Technical Bulletin 106, July 1987.

Burnhill MS. The rise and fall and rise of the IUD. Am J Gynecol Health 1989; III(3-5):6.

Chalker R. The complete cervical cap guide. New York: Harper & Row, 1987.

Choice of contraceptives. Med Lett 1988; 30:105.

Djerassi C. The politics of contraception. Stanford, CA: Stanford Alumni Association, 1979.

Edelman DA, et al. A comparative trial of the today contraceptive sponge and diaphragm. Am J Obstet Gynecol 1984; 150:869.

Gallen ME. Men—new focus in family planning. Pop Rep 1987; Series J (33):890.

Hatcher RA, et al. Contraceptive technology 1990–1992. New York: Irvington, 1990.

Kass-Annesse B, et al. The fertility awareness notebook, Atlanta. Printed matter, 1986.

Kennedy KL, et al. Consensus statement on the use of breastfeeding as a family planning method. Contraception 1989; 39:477.

Liskin L, et al. Hormonal contraception: new long-acting methods. Popul Rep 1987; Series K (3):57.

Ory HW, et al. Making choices: evaluating the health risks and benefits of birth control methods. New York: Alan Guttmacher Institute, 1983.

Rinehart W. Post-coital contraception: an appraisal. Popul Rep 1976; Series J (9):141.

Topical spermicides. Med Lett 1980; 22:90.

Trussell J, et al. Contraceptive failure in the U.S.: an update. Stud Fam Plann 1990; 21:51.

Trussell J, et al. Contraceptive failure in the US: a critical review of the literature. Stud Fam Plann 1987; 18:237.

USE OF ORAL CONTRACEPTIVES

Terra A. Robles, Pharm.D.

Early studies found that oral contraceptives (OCs), which had a greater amount of estrogen, were associated with serious adverse outcomes. Today's low-dose formulations retain efficacy while minimizing side effects, and have an overall lower risk of cardiovascular disease. OCs contain synthetic estrogens and progestins. They differ in dosage, proportion of ingredients, and prescribed regimens. Three considerations are important in selection of OC products: effectiveness, safety, and patient acceptability. Provide a product that offers the lowest effective dose of both hormones and that minimizes side effects. Data are not available for determining which OC is "better"; cost considerations should be included in product selection.

A. Before prescribing an OC, obtain a complete history, including history of previous contraceptive use and failures or adverse effects of previously used methods; menstrual history, focusing on patterns and problems; gynecologic and obstetric history; and general medical history. Perform a complete physical examination in which risk factors are assessed and contraindications to OC use determined. Order appropriate laboratory tests as necessary.

B. Monophasic pills contain a constant estrogen and progestin dose. Biphasic products contain a constant dose of estrogen, with a lower progestin dose on days 1–10 than on days 11–21. Triphasic pills have varied amounts of hormones; Ortho-Novum 777, Tri-Levelen, and Triphasil have an increase of progestin at mid- and end-cycle; Tri-Norinyl has increased progestin only at midcycle. Ortho-Novum 777 and Tri-Norinyl have fixed amounts of estrogen; Triphasil and Tri-Levelen have increased estrogen at midcycle. These differences in triphasic pills are generally insignificant in most women who do not have specific problems or menstrual irregularities.

Ethinyl estradiol (EE) and mestranol are the two estrogen agents used in OCs. EE is pharmacologically active and mestranol is hepatically converted to EE. Progestins used in OCs include norethindrone, norethindrone acetate, ethynodiol diacetate, dl-norgestrel, norethynodrel, and levonorgestrel (norgestimate is a new progestin said to have the lowest androgenic effect). Norethindrone acetate and ethynodiol diacetate are about equal in progestational activity, endometrial support, and lipid metabolic effects. These two are metabolized to norethindrone and offer no significant advantage over norethindrone. dl-Norgestrel and levonorgestrel are isomers, levonorgestrel being the active component. Some studies suggest that dl-norgestrel has little pharmacologic activity, while others state that it prevents breakthrough bleeding (BTB) more effectively. The progestins generally considered in selection of an OC are levonorgestrel and norethindrone. Norethindrone has been shown to have the least effect on carbohydrate metabolism or on the cardiovascular system and levonorgestrel having the least effect on triglycerides.

A back-up method of birth control is recommended along with the first cycle of OCs. Compliance is important for low-dose OCs, as missed pills often lead to breakthrough ovulation.

C. Use clinical judgment in deciding whether any woman with cardiovascular disease risk factors (e.g., hypertension, diabetes mellitus, hypercholesterolemia) should use OCs. Some studies of low-dose OCs have shown no increased risk of cardiovascular complications; however, OCs are currently considered synergistic in increased risk, and each patient must be carefully evaluated for OC use. Follow and monitor patients closely and offer alternative contraceptive methods when indicated.

D. Progestin-only pills or "mini-pills" have lower effectiveness than combination OCs (COCs), as ovulation is not consistently inhibited. Progestin-only pills are taken every day of the month, without a break for withdrawal bleeding. Up to two thirds of users experience menstrual irregularities, BTB, and amenorrhea. Products with norethindrone may be safest.

E. There is some concern over infant exposure to estrogens. Some believe this exposure is not clinically significant; others advocate waiting until an infant is weaned before instituting OC use. The pill may diminish the protein content and volume of breast milk. The FDA recommends deferring the use of OCs until a baby is weaned.

F. Diabetic patients whose diabetes is controlled may take low-dose OCs. Products with norethindrone are least likely to alter glucose tolerance.

G. ACHES is a mnemonic commonly used to help remember possible adverse effects of OCs: *A*, abdominal pain (gallbladder disease, hepatic adenoma, pancreatitis, blood clot); *C*, chest pain (pulmonary embolism, myocardial infarction); *H*, headaches (stroke, migraines, hypertension); *E*, eye problems (hypertension, stroke); *S*, severe leg pain (venous thromboembolism). COCs have relative estrogen dominance, and estrogen-related side effects can be expected to predominate. Familiarization with symptoms of estrogen/progestin excess/deficiency will aid in OC adjustments. Symptoms of estrogen excess include nausea, breast tenderness, fluid retention, and cervical mucorrhea, whereas estrogen deficiency is suggested by early or midcycle BTB, increased spotting, and hypomenorrhea. Symptoms of progestin excess are increased appetite, depression, fatigue, acne, diabetogenic effects, decreased carbohydrate tolerance, increased low-density lipoprotein and decreased high-density lipoprotein; symptoms of progestin deficiency include late-cycle BTB, amenorrhea,

(Continued on page 474)

Patient Desires ORAL CONTRACEPTIVE

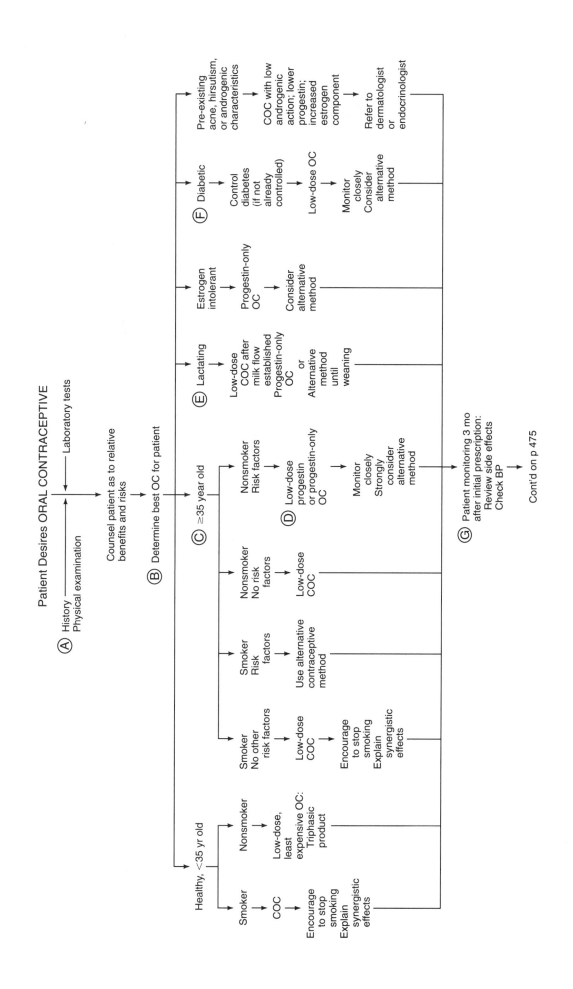

A History
Physical examination — Laboratory tests

Counsel patient as to relative benefits and risks

B Determine best OC for patient

Healthy, <35 yr old

Smoker
↓
COC
↓
Encourage to stop smoking
Explain synergistic effects

Nonsmoker
↓
Low-dose, least expensive OC: Triphasic product

≥35 year old

Smoker
No other risk factors
↓
Low-dose COC
↓
Encourage to stop smoking
Explain synergistic effects

Smoker
Risk factors
↓
Use alternative contraceptive method

Nonsmoker
No risk factors
↓
Low-dose COC

Nonsmoker
Risk factors
↓
D Low-dose progestin or progestin-only OC
↓
Monitor closely
Strongly consider alternative method

E Lactating
↓
Low-dose COC after milk flow established
Progestin-only OC
or
Alternative method until weaning

Estrogen intolerant
↓
Progestin-only OC
↓
Consider alternative method

F Diabetic
↓
Control diabetes (if not already controlled)
↓
Low-dose OC
↓
Monitor closely
Consider alternative method

Pre-existing acne, hirsutism, or androgenic characteristics
↓
COC with low androgenic action; lower progestin; increased estrogen component
↓
Refer to dermatologist or endocrinologist

G Patient monitoring 3 mo after initial prescription:
Review side effects
Check BP
↓
Cont'd on p 475

473

and hypermenorrhea. An excess of both hormones can cause headaches, weight gain, and hypertension.

H. Lowering the potency of OCs for greater safety has led to an increased incidence of BTB. BTB is common in the first few cycles of OC use.

I. Estrogens are conjugated in the liver and hydrolyzed by intestinal bacteria. Any drug that affects these two systems may lead to decreased OC efficacy.

J. The absence of withdrawal bleeding may be the result of insufficient endometrial development. Switching to an OC with greater progestin content may resolve the problem.

K. An increase in blood pressure (BP) may be seen even in normotensive patients. Increases can occur 1–36 months after initiation of the OC. The risk is lower with low-dose OCs. Patients who are started on OCs should be checked for BP changes within the first month. When hypertension is associated with an OC, it is reversible. Monitor any patient who develops hypertension while on OC closely for the development of OC-associated complications. A return to normal BP after discontinuation of OC may take 3–6 months.

L. Breast tenderness is usually due to cyclic fluid retention or growth of breast tissue. An OC with lower estrogenic activity or greater progestational activity, or an OC with less estrogen *and* less progestin, may alleviate the tenderness. If tenderness persists, a progestin-only pill may be tried.

M. Nausea may occur frequently during the first few cycles of OC use or may occur with the first few pills of each cycle. Many patients can prevent nausea by taking the pill with food or at bedtime. If nausea persists, an OC with lower estrogenic activity (as little as 20 μg in severe cases) may bring relief. Vomiting is rare. If vomiting occurs within 2 hr after taking the OC, the dose should be repeated to ensure contraception.

N. Weight loss and gain occur with equal frequency in OC users. Most weight changes are unrelated to OC use. However, estrogen can cause cyclic weight gain owing to fluid retention, and progestins can stimulate appetite and insulin release.

O. There is an increased risk of infarction in OC users with a history of migraine. Cerebrovascular accident (CVA) must be ruled out in all OC users who suffer from migraine headaches. Vascular (migraine-like) headaches generally do not improve with a change in OC; these patients need to consider alternative contraceptive methods. Headaches accompanied by fluid retention (edema, breast enlargement, cyclic weight gain) may be caused by both estrogens and progestins. Prescribe an OC with lower estrogenic and/or progestational activity and follow the patient closely to ensure resolution of symptoms after one or two cycles.

P. Depression may be caused by an excess of estrogen and/or progestin or by a deficiency of estrogen. If switching to an OC with lower estrogenic and/or progestational activity does not alleviate the depression, the pill should be discontinued for three to six cycles and re-evaluation performed at that time. Patients with severe depression unrelated to OC use should be referred to a psychiatrist.

References

Casper RF, Powell AM. Evaluation and therapy of breakthrough bleeding in women using a triphasic oral contraceptive. Fertil Steril 1991; 55:292.

Ellsworth AJ, Leversee JH. Oral contraceptives. Primary Care 1990; 17:603.

Hatcher RA, Stewart F, Trussell J, et al. Contraceptive Technology 1990–1992. 15th ed. New York: Irvington Publishers, 1990.

Orife J. Benefits and risks of oral contraceptives. Adv Contracept 1990; 6(Suppl):15.

Wall DM, Roos MP. Update on combination oral contraceptives. Am Fam Physician 1990; 42:1037.

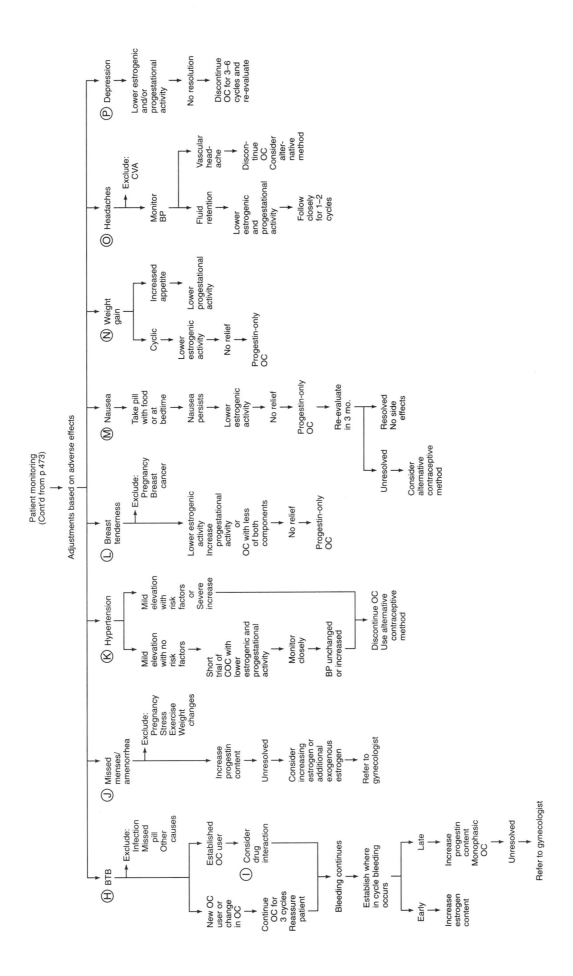

Patient monitoring
(Cont'd from p 473)

Adjustments based on adverse effects

Ⓗ BTB

Exclude:
Infection
Missed
pill
Other
causes

New OC
user or
change
in OC

Established
OC user

Continue
OC for
3 cycles
Reassure
patient

Ⓘ Consider
drug
interaction

Bleeding continues

Establish where
in cycle bleeding
occurs

Early
Increase
estrogen
content

Late
Increase
progestin
content
Monophasic
OC

Unresolved

Refer to gynecologist

Ⓙ Missed
menses/
amenorrhea

Exclude:
Pregnancy
Stress
Exercise
Weight
changes

Increase
progestin
content

Unresolved

Consider
increasing
estrogen or
additional
exogenous
estrogen

Refer to
gynecologist

Ⓚ Hypertension

Mild
elevation
with no
risk
factors

Mild
elevation
with risk
factors
or
Severe
increase

Short
trial of
COC with
lower
estrogenic and
progestational
activity

Monitor
closely

BP unchanged
or increased

Discontinue OC
Use alternative
contraceptive
method

Ⓛ Breast
tenderness

Exclude:
Pregnancy
Breast
cancer

Lower estrogenic
activity
Increase
progestational
activity
or
OC with less
of both
components

No relief

Progestin-only
OC

Ⓜ Nausea

Take pill
with food
or at
bedtime

Nausea
persists

Lower
estrogenic
activity

No relief

Progestin-only
OC

Re-evaluate
in 3 mo.

Resolved
No side
effects

Unresolved

Consider
alternative
contraceptive
method

Ⓝ Weight
gain

Cyclic
Lower
estrogenic
activity

No relief

Progestin-only
OC

Increased
appetite
Lower
progestational
activity

Ⓞ Headaches

Exclude:
CVA

Monitor
BP

Vascular
head-
ache
Discon-
tinue
OC
Consider
alter-
native
method

Fluid
retention
Lower
estrogenic
and
progestational
activity
Follow
closely
for 1–2
cycles

Ⓟ Depression

Lower estrogenic
and/or
progestational
activity

No resolution

Discontinue
OC for 3–6
cycles and
re-evaluate

INFERTILITY

PonJola Coney, M.D.

Infertility is defined as failure of conception after 12 months of unprotected coitus. Primary infertility refers to a history of no previous conception; secondary infertility is infertility after at least one documented conception. Peak fertility rates occur up to age 29 and begin to decline thereafter. After age 35, for every 5 years the length of time for conception doubles. The incidence of conception depends on the length of exposure, coital frequency, and age. In couples considered normal and fertile, the chances of conception after 1 month of unprotected coitus are 25%; after 6 months, 70%; and after 1 year, 85%. Only an additional 5% conceive after 1–2 years without therapy. The causes of infertility are manifold and often involve both parties. In general, 40% of infertility is due to male factors, 50% to female factors, and 10% unexplained. Approximately 25% of couples have combined factors. Couples with multiple factors may require more time to achieve pregnancy. Since etiologic factors are frequently relative rather than absolute contributors to the infertility, and because therapy in general could take years and is costly, the basic evaluation along with any other indicated tests should be made very early. Despite recent advances in reproductive technology, pregnancy rates with infertility therapy are only 60%. Interview both parties together. This is very important, since the reproductive failure should be viewed as a problem of the couple. Emphasize the importance of precise timing of diagnostic testing, the complexity of the therapy, the time and expense involved, and the prognosis for pregnancy.

A. A history of pregnancy or previous infertile relationship should be obtained. Other important aspects of the history should include contraceptive use, coital frequency and techniques, practice of douching, use of lubricants, and medical and family histories, particularly DES exposure in utero. Specific history taking in women should cover age of menarche; cycle length; frequency, length, and amount of bleeding; episodes of amenorrhea and galactorrhea; previous pelvic complaints; intrauterine device (IUD) use; sexually transmitted disease; eating disorders; and chronic illnesses.

B. Perform a careful physical and pelvic examination. Pay close attention to signs of hirsutism, breast secretions, thyroid enlargement, abdominal scars, and evidence of estrogen secretion. Take cultures for *Chlamydia* and gonorrhea. Perform a Pap smear if indicated.

C. The basic or fundamental tests for infertility include semen analysis, postcoital test, basal body temperature chart (BBT), endometrial biopsy with progesterone level, hysterosalpingography, and laparoscopy.

D. Once testing is complete, review the test results with the couple. Once the diagnosis is made, develop a precise plan, review it with the couple, and initiate appropriate therapy. If the diagnosis is unclear or if specific problems are identified that require additional testing or therapy, refer the couple to an infertility center.

References

Asch RH, et al. Pregnancy after translaparosopic gamete intrafallopian transfer. Lancet 1984; 2:1035.

Buttram VC Jr, Reiter RC, eds. Surgical treatment of the infertile female. Baltimore: Williams & Wilkins, 1985.

Collins JA, et al. The postcoital test as a predictor of pregnancy among 355 infertile couples. Fertil Steril 1984; 41:703.

Lopata A. Concepts in human in vitro fertilization and embryo transfer. Fertil Steril 1983; 40:289.

Schwartz M, et al. The use of human menopausal and chorionic ganadotropin for induction of ovulation. AM J Obstet Gynecol 1980; 138:801.

Talbert LM: Clomiphene citrate induction of ovulation. Fertil Steril 1983; 39:742.

INFERTILE COUPLE

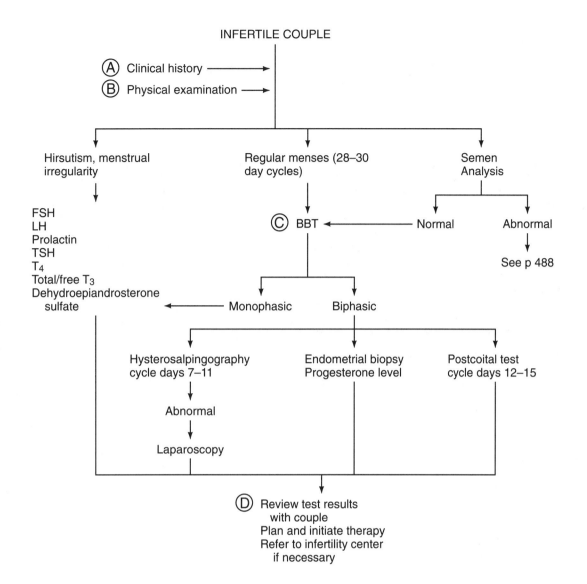

Ⓐ Clinical history

Ⓑ Physical examination

Hirsutism, menstrual
irregularity

FSH
LH
Prolactin
TSH
T₄
Total/free T₃
Dehydroepiandrosterone
  sulfate

Regular menses (28–30
day cycles)

Ⓒ BBT

Semen
Analysis

Normal   Abnormal

See p 488

Monophasic   Biphasic

Hysterosalpingography
cycle days 7–11

Endometrial biopsy
Progesterone level

Postcoital test
cycle days 12–15

Abnormal

Laparoscopy

Ⓓ Review test results
  with couple
  Plan and initiate therapy
  Refer to infertility center
    if necessary

UROLOGY

ACUTE DYSURIA OR PYURIA IN MEN

Richard F. Hoffman, M.D.

A. Dysuria is a sensation of discomfort with or after urination that often is accompanied by frequency, urgency, and nocturia. There are multiple causes, depending on the patient's age and sexual activity. Physical examination is usually unremarkable. Fever is uncommon but may be present in pyelonephritis, acute prostatitis, orchitis, or epididymitis. Inspect the genitals for evidence of urethral inflammation, discharge, and other penile lesions. Palpation may reveal swelling or tenderness of the testicles or epididymis and may elicit suprapubic or costovertebral tenderness. On rectal examination the prostate may be enlarged or tender or may have a palpable nodule.

B. A comprehensive sexual history is imperative. Sexual activity exposes a male to sexually transmitted diseases (STDs), which are not a consideration in men who are sexually inactive or in a stable, monogamous relationship. Ask patients about the number and gender of partners, whether they consort with prostitutes, and whether they use condoms.

C. Microscopic examination of the urine is most commonly performed after the specimen is centrifuged for 5 minutes at 2000 rpm. The normal upper limits of WBCs per high-power field (hpf) is 5–10. The most widely accepted normal upper limit for RBCs is 3/hpf.

D. The most worrisome cause of dysuria and hematuria is urologic cancer, especially bladder cancer. Men >40 years old, tobacco users, analgesic abusers, those with a history of pelvic irradiation or cyclophosphamide chemotherapy, and men who work with dyestuffs and rubber compounds are at increased risk for malignancy. Other considerations are bladder calculi, which usually occur in the setting of benign prostatic hypertrophy (BPH), as well as BPH itself. Cystoscopy has a sensitivity of 87% in diagnosing bladder cancer and may directly visualize stones and confirm BPH. At the Mayo Clinic, urine cytology had a sensitivity of 67% and specificity of 96% in detecting bladder cancer.

E. When pyuria is present, culture and sensitivity tests should be performed. First-void specimens and clean-catch midstream voided specimens are equally sensitive for the detection of bacteruria. In men the growth of a single or predominant organism ≥103 colony forming units (CFU)/ml indicates an infection; growth of <103 CFU/ml or multiple organisms indicates contamination. Gram-negative bacilli including *Escherichia coli, Proteus,* and *Providencia* species cause approximately 75% of infections. Gram-positive bacteria, mainly enterococci and coagulase-negative staphylococci, cause most of the remaining infection. The presence of a urinary tract infection (UTI) in men has been assumed to warrant investigation for a structural abnormality of the urinary tract. Abnormalities are frequently found but usually do not alter treatment. The need for a diagnostic work-up in men with a first UTI has not been studied. Repeated infections or those that do not respond to treatment require further investigation. Sterile pyuria may be present in nephrolithiasis or urologic neoplasms and must be excluded. First morning urine cultures for acid-fast bacilli repeated three times are positive in 90% of men with renal tuberculosis.

F. The yield of a urethral smear depends on the timing of the collection. Highest yield is obtained by examining a smear collected early in the morning before micturition. Micturition decreases the number of WBCs seen on the smear. Obtain a smear by inserting a urethral swab 1–2 cm into the distal urethra and rotating it. If no discharge is apparent, stripping of the urethra or prostatic massage may produce a discharge. The urethral swab is smeared on a slide, heat fixed, and Gram-stained. A urethral smear in a symptomatic male showing gram-negative intracellular diplococci has 98% sensitivity and 99% specificity in diagnosing gonococcal urethritis when compared with a single culture on Thayer-Martin media. Most patients with nongonococcal urethritis (NGU) have leukocytes on urethral smear (4 WBC/hpf), but 16–46% with culture-proved urethritis have <4 WBC/hpf.

G. In a recent national survey, 21% of gonococcal isolates showed resistance to penicillin, tetracycline, cefoxitin, and/or spectinomycin. All isolates were sensitive to ceftriaxone. The CDC recommends ceftriaxone, 250 mg IM, for all presumed cases of gonorrhea. Since up to 40% of patients with gonorrhea have a concomitant chlamydial infection, they should also be treated with tetracycline, 500 mg q.i.d. or doxycycline, 100 mg b.i.d. for 1 week.

H. The most frequent causes of acute NGU are *Chlamydia trachomatis* and *Ureaplasma urealyticum.* Bowie estimated that *C. trachomatis* causes 30–50% of acute cases and *U. urealyticum,* 30–40%. The role of *U. urealyticum* in urethritis is controversial, as the organism has frequently been isolated from the urethra of asymptomatic men. Some authors consider that this represents colonization. *C. trachomatis* may be grown in tissue culture. An antibody test has become available that allows direct detection of the *Chlamydia* antigen in clinical specimens. The test is based on the development of a monoclonal antibody to *C. trachomatis* antigen. Compared with culture, the test had sensitivity of 93% and specificity of 96%. *U. urealyticum* also may be grown on tissue culture. Both *C. trachomatis* and *U. urealyticum* can be treated with tetracycline, 500 mg q.i.d. or doxycycline, 100 mg b.i.d. for 7 days.

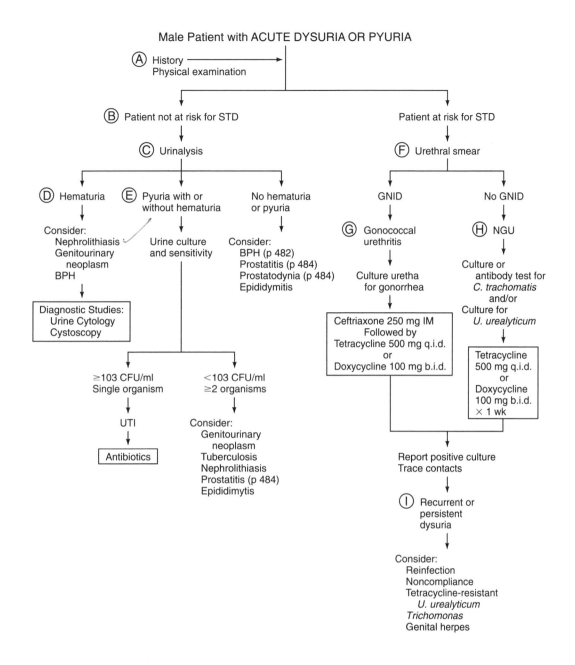

Male Patient with ACUTE DYSURIA OR PYURIA

(A) History
Physical examination

(B) Patient not at risk for STD

(C) Urinalysis

(D) Hematuria

(E) Pyuria with or without hematuria

No hematuria or pyuria

Consider:
Nephrolithiasis
Genitourinary
neoplasm
BPH

Urine culture
and sensitivity

Consider:
BPH (p 482)
Prostatitis (p 484)
Prostatodynia (p 484)
Epididymitis

Diagnostic Studies:
Urine Cytology
Cystoscopy

≥10³ CFU/ml
Single organism

<10³ CFU/ml
≥2 organisms

UTI

Consider:
Genitourinary
neoplasm
Tuberculosis
Nephrolithiasis
Prostatitis (p 484)
Epididimytis

Antibiotics

Patient at risk for STD

(F) Urethral smear

GNID

No GNID

(G) Gonococcal
urethritis

(H) NGU

Culture uretha
for gonorrhea

Culture or
antibody test for
C. trachomatis
and/or
Culture for
U. urealyticum

Ceftriaxone 250 mg IM
Followed by
Tetracycline 500 mg q.i.d.
or
Doxycycline 100 mg b.i.d.

Tetracycline
500 mg q.i.d.
or
Doxycycline
100 mg b.i.d.
× 1 wk

Report positive culture
Trace contacts

(I) Recurrent or
persistent
dysuria

Consider:
Reinfection
Noncompliance
Tetracycline-resistant
U. urealyticum
Trichomonas
Genital herpes

I. Reinfection from an untreated or new partner should be the first consideration. Noncompliance with treatment is also possible, especially in those treated with tetracycline regimens that require qid dosing and avoidance of dairy products. *U. urealyticum* resistance to tetracycline has been reported, so patients may be given a 10–21 day course of erythromycin, 500 mg q.i.d. *Trichomonas vaginalis* may cause urethritis in sexually active men. The diagnosis may be confirmed by microscopic examination of a urethral swab or by culture. Metronidazole is the drug of choice, and treatment of the sexual partner is important. Herpes simplex virus types I and II may cause urethritis, usually accompanied by external lesions on the genitalia. Herpes simplex may be isolated in tissue culture. Many other organisms may have a pathogenic role in NGU, including human papillomaviruses, *Mycoplasma hominis, Mycoplasma genitalium,* and *Neisseria meningitidis.* In at least 20–30% of cases of NGU, no organism can be identified.

References

Bowie WR. Nongonococcal urethritis. Urol Clin North Am 1984; 11:55.

Judson FN. Gonococcal urethritis: diagnosis and treatment. Arch Androl 1979; 3:329.

Lipsky BA. Urinary tract infections in men. Ann Intern Med 1989; 110:138.

Schwarcz SK. National surveillance of antimicrobial resistance in *Neisseria gonorrhoeae.* JAMA 1990; 264:1413.

Sutton JM. Evaluation of hematuria in adults. JAMA 1990; 263:2475.

Tam MR. Culture independent diagnosis of *Chlamydia trachomatis* using monoclonal antibodies. N Engl J Med 1984; 310:1146.

SCROTAL MASS

William P. Johnson, M.D.

A. Palpation of an abnormal mass within the scrotal cavity occurs frequently during a careful examination of the male external genitalia. The importance of this finding depends on the establishment of an accurate diagnosis. Often, an accurate history and physical examination are all that is required to establish a diagnosis and determine subsequent management. The presence or absence of pain must be elicited. Ask the patient how long he has been aware of the mass, change in size, previous operative procedures, and the presence or absence of dysuria. During the physical examination the size, location, and consistency of the mass are precisely documented. Examine the patient in both the supine and erect positions. Finally, the examination must include transillumination of the scrotal mass, as nearly all benign conditions transilluminate easily; the notable benign exceptions are hematocele and varicocele. A urinalysis is routinely obtained looking for evidence of bacteriuria and pyuria. When the cause of the lesion remains in doubt, scrotal ultrasonography has proved an effective means of differentiation of intrascrotal masses.

B. In patients with a history of scrotal trauma, suspect a ruptured testicle. Remember that the degree of the traumatic blow must correlate with the extent of the injury. Testicular neoplasms are more prone to rupture and should be suspected in any patient who presents with a large scrotal mass after minimal trauma.

C. A painful scrotal mass is usually due to an inflammatory process, but also consider testicular torsion or malignancy. Scrotal ultrasonography is a useful diagnostic tool in differentiating the above conditions.

D. Acute and chronic epididymitis are both extremely common clinical entities in adult males. The clinical presentation may range from an exquisitely tender scrotal mass (acute) to a low-grade process that the patient is barely aware of (chronic). In adults <40 years of age, *Chlamydia trachomatis* is often the initiating organism; in older men, gram negative bacteria are the likely cause. Follow-up examination ensures that an underlying testicular tumor is not present after the acute inflammatory process subsides.

E. Testicular neoplasms are the most common solid tumor in males 20–39 years old. These patients usually present with a mass within the substance of the testis. The masses are usually smooth or nodular, rock hard, and painless; they do not transilluminate. They often enlarge rapidly.

F. A hydrocele is the most common benign scrotal mass. It is of varying size and is located ventral, superior, and anterior to the testicle. It is nontender and transilluminates easily. It may be congenital or acquired. Because 10% of testicular tumors are associated with a hydrocele, perform aspiration if the testicle is not palpable.

G. Primary tumors arising from the epididymis are rare and usually benign, adenomatoid tumors being the most common. A spermatocele is a cystic mass containing sperm that arises as a small diverticulum from the head of the epididymis.

H. Scrotal varicoceles are common (10–15% of the normal male population). This scrotal mass represents a dilated pampiniform plexus of the spermatic cord. It is usually asymptomatic but may reach a large size, resulting in a "dragging" or heavy sensation in the scrotum.

References

Blute RD Jr. Scrotal masses. In: Greene HL, Glassock RJ, Kelley MA, eds. Introduction to clinical medicine. Philadelphia: BC Decker, 1990:289.

Spirnak JP. Adult scrotal mass. In: Resnick MI, Caldamone AA, Spirnak JP, eds. Decision making in urology. 2nd ed. Philadelphia: BC Decker, 1991:208.

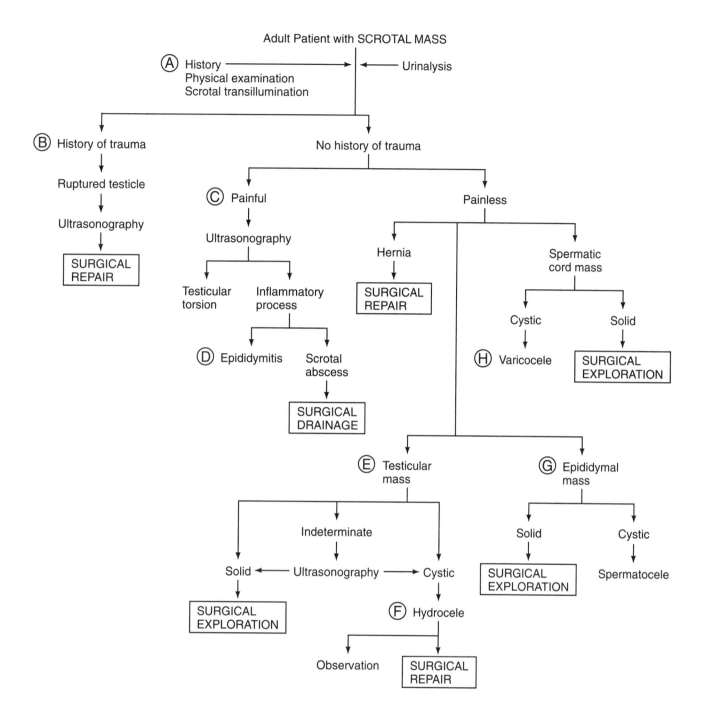

Adult Patient with SCROTAL MASS

(A) History ——————→ ←—— Urinalysis
Physical examination
Scrotal transillumination

(B) History of trauma

No history of trauma

Ruptured testicle

(C) Painful

Painless

Ultrasonography

SURGICAL
REPAIR

Ultrasonography

Hernia

Spermatic
cord mass

Testicular
torsion

Inflammatory
process

SURGICAL
REPAIR

Cystic

Solid

(D) Epididymitis

Scrotal
abscess

(H) Varicocele

SURGICAL
EXPLORATION

SURGICAL
DRAINAGE

(E) Testicular
mass

(G) Epididymal
mass

Indeterminate

Solid

Cystic

Solid ←— Ultrasonography —→ Cystic

SURGICAL
EXPLORATION

Spermatocele

SURGICAL
EXPLORATION

(F) Hydrocele

Observation

SURGICAL
REPAIR

PROSTATE NODULE OR ENLARGEMENT

Jeffrey I. Miller, M.D.
George W. Drach, M.D.

Digital rectal examination to assess the size, shape, and texture of the prostate gland should be a part of every general physical examination. The normal prostate feels smooth and rubbery on palpation. Any firmness, nodularity, or induration should be considered abnormal. Anatomically, the gland is wider at its "base," near the bladder neck. The lateral sulci and the median furrow should be well defined. Any irregularity of these landmarks should be noted. Assessment of prostatic size may be difficult: the normal average prostate triangle is about 4 cm on each side. Most patients over age 50 have some degree of benign enlargement. As enlargement occurs, the lateral sulci become deeper and the gland becomes more prominent to rectal palpation. Benign enlargement becomes clinically significant in the presence of symptoms suggesting bladder outlet obstruction. If clinically significant benign prostatic hyperplasia (BPH) or a prostate nodule is detected, initiate the appropriate evaluation before urologic consultation.

A. Detection of a smooth, symmetrically enlarged prostate should prompt a thorough inquiry into symptoms suggestive of bladder outlet obstruction. Irritative symptoms include dysuria, frequency, urgency, and nocturia. Obstructive symptoms include hesitancy, straining, decreased force and caliber of the urinary stream, a sense of incomplete emptying, and stream interruption. Patients without significant symptoms are reassured and no further work-up is indicated. Patients presenting with complete urinary retention should be catheterized and referred directly to a urologist. Obvious sources of retention (e.g., alpha-adrenergic agonists, diphenhydramine) should be removed if possible.

B. Prostate-specific antigen (PSA) is a protein found only in prostatic epithelial cells. Serum levels can be elevated in a variety of prostatic disorders, including prostatitis, BPH, and prostate adenocarcinoma. Its usefulness in screening for prostate cancer in asymptomatic men has not been determined. However, many investigators agree that a serum PSA level should be obtained in men with clinically significant symptoms suggestive of bladder outlet obstruction. Levels >10 ng/ml (Hybritech assay) suggest adenocarcinoma; however, a very large or infected benign gland may also produce elevated serum levels. Ideally, serum PSA levels should be drawn before or several weeks after prostatic manipulation (e.g., bladder catheterization) to avoid falsely elevated levels. A gentle rectal examination probably does not significantly influence serum levels.

C. A properly collected urinalysis and urine culture are crucial for detecting associated microhematuria and infection. The source of isolated microscopic hematuria may be an enlarged prostate. However, intravenous pyelography (IVP) is necessary to rule out upper tract disorders, including calculi or tumor. Even when IVP is normal, cystoscopic examination by a urologist is still required to exclude a bladder tumor or stone as the source of microhematuria. In the absence of microhematuria, IVP is generally not recommended.

D. Urinary tract infection in the older male should not simply be treated and dismissed. Residual urine may be the main contributor to infection, especially in someone with an enlarged prostate and symptoms suggestive of BPH. When there is high residual urine volume (>200–300 ml), leave a Foley catheter in place to help drain the infection. Obtain urologic consultation.

E. An elevated serum creatinine level may be the first indication of renal failure secondary to bladder outlet obstruction. Urinary symptoms may not be severe and patients often continue to void by overflow. Bilateral hydronephrosis on ultrasonography suggests bladder outlet obstruction as the source of the renal insufficiency. Residual urine volume is almost always elevated. Place a Foley catheter to decompress the bladder and upper tracts. The patient may need to be monitored for pathologic postobstructive diuresis, depending on the duration and severity of obstruction. Obtain a repeat serum creatinine level before urologic consultation.

F. The urologist rules out other causes of bladder outlet obstruction (e.g., urethral stricture, bladder tumor, neurogenic bladder) that may be contributing to the symptoms. A typical evaluation at this point might include urinary flow rate and office cystoscopy to assess the degree of apparent internal urethral obstruction. If the symptoms and physical examination suggest a neurogenic component, a urodynamic evaluation is indicated. When the patient desires treatment and his urologist is confident that the voiding symptoms are primarily related to BPH, he is offered a group of therapeutic options. These include standard transurethral resection of the prostate, transurethral prostatic incision for small prostates, open prostatic enucleation (for very large prostates), medical treatment with alpha-adrenergic blockers, or transurethral balloon dilatation of the prostate. Other options under investigation include prostatic hyperthermia or hormonal manipulation, to decrease prostatic size.

G. If a prostate nodule is palpated or there is asymmetric enlargement or induration of the gland on digital rectal examination, referral to a urologist is indicated. Obtain a serum PSA before referral; however, the result will have no bearing on the subsequent evaluation, since normal PSA and prostatic carcinoma may coexist. There is no accurate means of

ABNORMAL DIGITAL RECTAL EXAMINATION

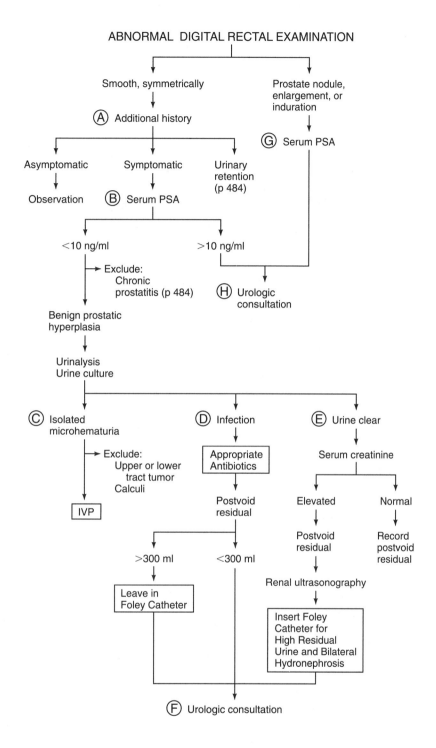

detecting prostate adenocarcinoma other than by needle biopsy.

H. All prostate nodules should be biopsied regardless of the serum PSA level or clinical symptoms. The urologist usually performs the biopsy under ultrasound guidance. A thin needle is passed transrectally or transperineally to obtain a small core of tissue for histologic analysis. Any bleeding diathesis or coagulopathy should be corrected before prostate biopsy. In addition, patients at risk for subacute bacterial endocarditis should be given prophylactic antibiotics before and after the procedure.

References

Cooner WH, Mosley BR, Rutherford CL Jr, et al. Prostate cancer detection in a clinical urological practice by ultrasonography, digital rectal examination and prostate specific antigen. J Urol 1990; 143:1146.

Oesterling JE, Bilhartz DL, Tindall DJ. Clinically useful serum markers for adenocarcinoma of the prostate. Part II—prostate specific antigen. AUA Update series, 1991; Vol 10, Lesson 18:138.

Smith DR. Physical examination of the genitourinary tract. In: Smith DR, ed. General urology. Los Altos, CA: Lange Medical Publications, 1984:40.

PROSTATITIS

Jeffrey I. Miller, M.D.
George W. Drach, M.D.

Prostatitis refers to a series of inflammatory diseases of differing causes affecting the prostate gland. It may be difficult to define a specific cause. Treatment is not always curative and recurrence is common. Patients may be assigned to one of four prostatitis syndromes: acute or chronic bacterial prostatitis, nonbacterial prostatitis, or prostatodynia. The work-up and treatment for each syndrome is quite different.

A. Acute bacterial prostatitis is a potentially serious process that can result in septicemia or abscess formation. Patients usually present with acute onset of dysuria and irritative voiding symptoms. Obstructive voiding symptoms are not uncommon. Low back pain, perineal discomfort, fever, chills, and malaise are often present. Patients with a chronic prostatitis syndrome present with low-grade irritative voiding symptoms, ill-defined pelvic or perineal discomfort, and/or pain associated with ejaculation. They are not acutely ill. The hallmark of chronic bacterial prostatitis is a history of relapsing urinary tract infection.

B. Bacteriuria is always present in acute bacterial prostatitis; enteric pathogens are usually responsible. A culture before antibiotic treatment is mandatory.

C. Gentle rectal examination confirms the diagnosis of acute bacterial prostatitis. The prostate feels enlarged and edematous and is very tender. Never perform digital massage to obtain fluid for analysis in this situation, or bacteremia and septicemia may result.

D. In acute bacterial prostatitis the barrier to drug infusion into the prostate is not as prominent as in the chronically inflamed state. Therefore, one may select any antibiotic to which the causative organism is sensitive and expect a favorable effect. Serial gentle rectal examinations, CT, or transrectal ultrasound imaging can rule out prostatic abscess (which requires surgical drainage). Suspect abscess when antibiotic treatment is unsuccessful. Urinary retention, caused by prostatic edema, may require urethral or suprapubic catheter drainage of the bladder. Hospitalization is commonly indicated. Continue antibiotic therapy for 4–6 weeks.

E. The urine culture is usually negative in chronic prostatitis. However, if present, bacteriuria should be treated first with a short course of an antibiotic that does not cross the blood-prostate barrier. Best drugs are nitrofurantoin, penicillin, or a cephalosporin. Bacterial cystitis treated in this way will not interfere with subsequent localizing studies to determine the cause of the prostatitis.

F. The prostate is usually normal to palpation in chronic prostatitis. Consider prostate carcinoma, however, if there is a nodule, induration, or asymmetry. Never attribute prostatic induration to chronic inflammation until carcinoma is ruled out by biopsy.

G. Perform digital massage to obtain expressed prostatic secretions (EPS), which should be microscopically examined under high power. In general, more than ten leukocytes/hpf and more than one or two lipid-laden macrophages suggest prostatic inflammation.

H. In the presence of prostatic inflammation, the EPS should be cultured. Isolation of bacteria from the EPS is necessary to establish a diagnosis of chronic bacterial prostatitis. This is the first screening test.

I. To be certain that the source of the bacteriuria is the prostate, obtain divided quantitative urine cultures. A first-voided specimen (VB1) identifies the urethral flora that can contaminate subsequent specimens. Obtain a midstream urine culture (VB2) to rule out coexisting bacterial cystitis. These cultures are quantitatively compared with that of the EPS. Bacteriuria is localized to the prostate when the EPS colony count is proportionately greater (by a factor of 10) than that of the VB1 and VB2.

J. In patients with chronic bacterial prostatitis, there is an intact barrier to perfusion of many antibiotics into the prostatic fluid or tissue. Effective prostatic antibiotics include trimethoprim, doxycycline, and carbenicillin. The quinolones achieve excellent therapeutic concentrations in the prostatic parenchyma and are very effective in eradicating chronic bacterial prostatitis.

K. Patients with chronic nonbacterial prostatitis have an inflammatory EPS with negative cultures. Causative agents, such as *Mycoplasma* or *Chlamydia*, cannot easily be demonstrated by present techniques. Thus, empiric treatment with long-acting doxycycline or minocycline is indicated. Trichomoniasis also should be ruled out.

L. Patients with prostatodynia have complaints of prostatic pain but there is no evidence of prostatic inflammation and no bacterial cause is found. Patients may have mild prostatic tenderness upon rectal examination and also a mild to moderate decrease in voiding flow rate. Treatment options include low-dose diazepam, 2 mg three to four times per day; this drug is used more for its smooth muscle-relaxing effect than for tranquilization. Antispasmodics such as hyoscyamine sometimes decrease the intensity of symptoms. Some patients seem to respond to alpha-adrenergic blocking agents; warn them of the side effects, including dizziness, hypotension, and loss of ejaculation.

PROSTATITIS Suspected

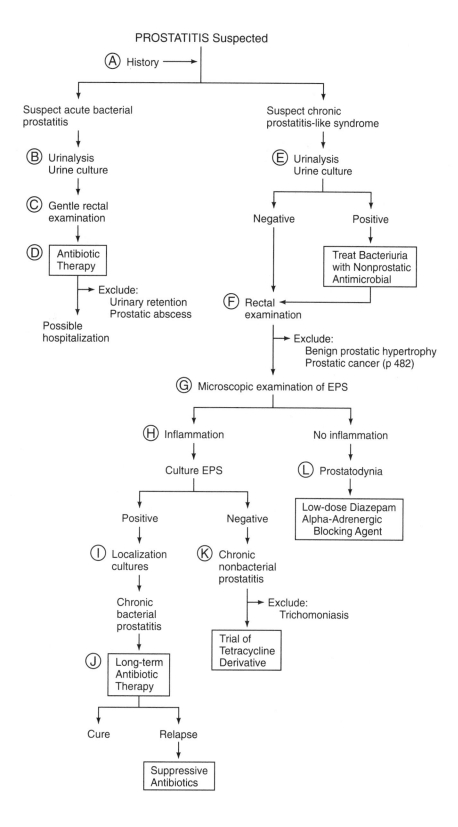

Ⓐ History

Suspect acute bacterial prostatitis

Ⓑ Urinalysis
Urine culture

Ⓒ Gentle rectal examination

Ⓓ Antibiotic Therapy

→ Exclude:
Urinary retention
Prostatic abscess

Possible hospitalization

Suspect chronic prostatitis-like syndrome

Ⓔ Urinalysis
Urine culture

Negative   Positive

Treat Bacteriuria with Nonprostatic Antimicrobial

Ⓕ Rectal examination

→ Exclude:
Benign prostatic hypertrophy
Prostatic cancer (p 482)

Ⓖ Microscopic examination of EPS

Ⓗ Inflammation   No inflammation

Culture EPS   Ⓛ Prostatodynia

Positive   Negative   Low-dose Diazepam
Alpha-Adrenergic Blocking Agent

Ⓘ Localization cultures   Ⓚ Chronic nonbacterial prostatitis

Chronic bacterial prostatitis   → Exclude:
Trichomoniasis

Ⓙ Long-term Antibiotic Therapy   Trial of Tetracycline Derivative

Cure   Relapse

Suppressive Antibiotics

References

Drach GW. Prostatitis. In: Rakel RE, ed. Conn's current therapy. Philadelphia: WB Saunders, 1987:562.

Drach GW, Mears EM Jr, Fair WR, et al. Classification of benign disease associated with prostatic pain: prostatitis or prostatodynia. J Urol 1978; 120:266.

Fowler JE Jr. Practical approach to bacteriologic investigation of chronic prostatitis. Urology 1985; 26:17.

Fowler JE Jr. Prostatitis. In: Gillenwater JY, Grayhack JT, Howards SS, Duckett JW, eds. Adult and pediatric urology. St. Louis: Mosby-Year Book, 1991:1395.

URINARY INCONTINENCE

William P. Johnson, M.D.

A. Urinary incontinence is the involuntary urethral or extraurethral loss of urine. This occurs more frequently in women (approximately 8%) than in men (approximately 3%), particularly in older women. Despite the availability of sophisticated urodynamic tests, a good urologic history and physical examination are of paramount importance in the initial evaluation and classification of the patient with urinary incontinence. The two basic stages of the normal micturition cycle are filling-storage and emptying-expulsion. The normal adult bladder capacity is about 400 ml and the average adult urinates four to eight times per day. Normally, the detrusor muscle and bladder outlet act as a coordinated unit. The following symptoms suggest specific causes: losing small amounts of urine during physical activity (stress incontinence), losing large amounts of urine without warning (neurologic), irritative voiding symptoms (inflammatory), and decreased stream (bladder outlet obstruction). Medical and surgical histories should be obtained. Any previous pelvic surgical procedures may have damaged the bladder's nerve supply and resulted in neurogenic bladder and incontinence. Medical diseases such as diabetes, multiple sclerosis, and cerebrovascular disease may also play an important etiologic role. A drug history, including both OTC and prescription medications, may be important, as a variety of medications may affect bladder or sphincter function. Physical examination of the abdomen, pelvis, and external genitalia may reveal a palpable, poorly emptying bladder; an enlarged prostate; or other abnormalities that could contribute to incontinence. The basic neurologic assessment should include evaluation of deep tendon reflexes and the presence or absence of perineal sensation, and should check for an intact bulbocavernosus reflex.

B. Urgency incontinence (detrusor instability) is the involuntary loss of urine associated with a strong desire to void. This is most commonly caused by inflammation or infection of the lower urinary tract.

C. Overflow incontinence is frequently seen in elderly males in association with previous obstructive symptoms of hesitancy, decreased urinary stream, frequency, and nocturia, thereby implicating prostatic obstruction. It may also be seen with a hypotonic overdistended bladder associated with major pelvic surgery. Drugs may be a complicating factor, including alpha-adrenergic agents, anticholinergics, calcium channel blockers, and sedatives.

D. Functional incontinence occurs when the patient is unable to reach the toilet because of difficulty ambulating or undressing, through inability to manipulate a urinal or bedpan, or because the facilities are unavailable. Prescribed medication may diminish sensory awareness and worsen this problem.

E. Reflex incontinence is classically due to suprasacral spinal cord lesions such as tumor, spondylosis, or trauma. Paraplegia or lower leg neurologic deficit may be obvious or subtle. A very active bulbocavernosus reflex or spastic lower extremities with overactive deep tendon reflexes may be suggestive.

F. With total incontinence, look for an ectopic orifice or a fistula. Total incontinence in adults is either congenital or secondary to common problems or diseases such as paraplegia, multiple sclerosis, and spina bifida. Accurate diagnosis in women may require instillation of methylene blue into the bladder to search for a fistula.

G. Stress incontinence (sphincter insufficiency) occurs when bladder neck and external sphincter incompetence produce pressures within the urethra that are lower than pressures within the bladder. Normally increased intra-abdominal pressure is transmitted equally to the bladder and urethra when the urethra is in normal position. With pelvic floor laxity, however, the proximal urethra and bladder neck herniate through the pelvic floor with increased intra-abdominal pressure. Therefore, pressure is unequally transmitted to the urethra, and incontinence occurs. Most commonly, this is secondary to urethral hypermobility from weakening of the supporting muscles and ligament structures, which occurs during childbirth. These same supporting structures may lose tissue tone and elasticity as a result of hormonal changes at menopause, psychotropic drugs, severe chronic coughing, or marked obesity. A multiparous woman may have stress incontinence secondary to an inherent weakness of the bladder neck or a short urethra. Surgery involving the urethra or prostate may cause external sphincter damage or weakness. An important clue to stress incontinence is the inability to stop the urinary stream while voiding.

References

Hopkins TB. Urinary incontinence. In: Greene HL, Glassock RJ, Kelly MA, eds. Introduction to clinical medicine. Philadelphia: BC Decker, 1990:289.

Spirnak JP. Urinary incontinence in adults. In: Resnick MI, Caldamone AA, Spirnak JP, eds. Decision making in urology. 2nd ed. Philadelphia: BC Decker, 1991:26.

Patient with URINARY INCONTINENCE

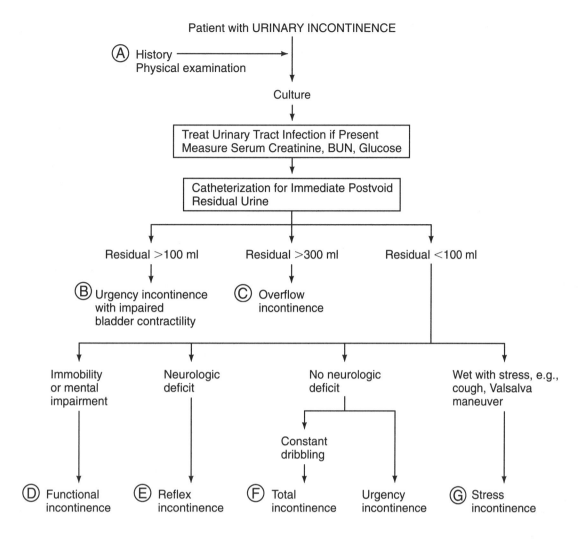

MALE INFERTILITY

PonJola Coney, M.D.

Approximately 15% of couples of reproductive age in the United States experience difficulty achieving pregnancy after 12 months of unprotected coitus. Of these, 25% have abnormalities affecting both parties. A male factor is responsible in 40% of cases of infertility. Traditionally, the female seeks evaluation from the gynecologist first for infertility. Always perform an initial evaluation of semen during the basic infertility evaluation. If marginal to abnormal semen parameters are found, urologic evaluation of the male is in order. Evaluation and treatment of the male should be systematic and thorough and conducted with that of the female. There are five categories of male infertility: pretesticular, testicular, post-testicular, infectious, and immunologic. The goal of evaluation is to distinguish the probably fertile male from the infertile male.

A. Semen specimens should be collected by masturbation and examined within 1 hour of collection. The specimen should not be exposed to extremes of temperature during transportation. Measurement of sperm numbers, motility, and morphology and interpretation of semen characteristics are the components of an initial semen analysis. There are current opinions of what constitutes a normal semen analysis, but not of what constitutes "fertile" or "infertile" when parameters fall outside the established normal range. Marginal male infertility may be compensated by optimal female fertility. It is emphasized that both parties must be evaluated and treated simultaneously if indicated.

B. Testicular causes are usually the result of a direct insult to the testes and spermatogenesis (toxins, trauma, genetic, radiation, chemotherapy) are generally untreatable and often present with azoospermia. Post-testicular causes (obstruction, retrograde ejaculation, systemic disease, cryptorchism) are generally untreatable, with some exceptions. The important distinction is the presence or absence of spermatozoa.

C. The infectious, immunologic, and pretesticular (endocrinopathies) causes are generally treatable with proper diagnosis and appropriate therapy.

D. Treatment for male infertility, if possible, is often long term.

References

Greenberg SH, et al. Experience with 425 subfertile male patients. J Urol 1978; 119:507.

Ng SC, et al. Micromanipulation: its relevance to human IVF. Fertil Steril 1990; 53:203.

Santiago BO. Andrological consultation in human spermatozoa. In: Acosta AA, et al, eds. Assisted reproduction. Baltimore: Williams & Wilkins, 1990:24.

Santoro N, et al. Hypogonadotropic disorders in men and women: diagnosis and therapy with pulsatile gonadotropin-releasing hormone (GnRH). Endocr Rev 1986; 7:11.

World Health Organization. WHO Laboratory Manual for the examination of human semen and semen–cervical mucus interaction. Cambridge, England: Cambridge University Press, 1987.

Yovich JL, et al. The management of oligospermic infertility by IVF. Ann NY Acad Sci 1985; 442:276.

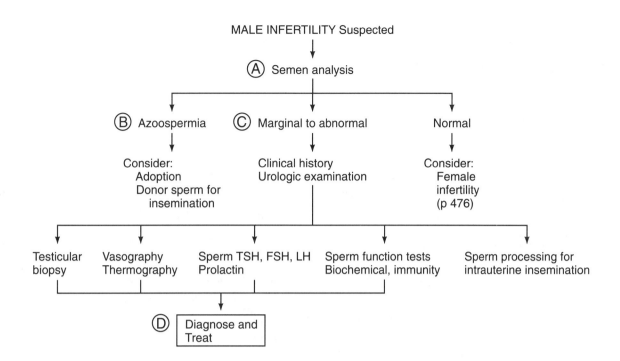

MALE INFERTILITY Suspected

Ⓐ Semen analysis

Ⓑ Azoospermia | Ⓒ Marginal to abnormal | Normal

Consider:
Adoption
Donor sperm for
insemination

Clinical history
Urologic examination

Consider:
Female
infertility
(p 476)

Testicular
biopsy

Vasography
Thermography

Sperm TSH, FSH, LH
Prolactin

Sperm function tests
Biochemical, immunity

Sperm processing for
intrauterine insemination

Ⓓ Diagnose and
Treat

BEHAVIORAL MEDICINE
ALCOHOLISM

Michael E. Scott, M.D.
Myra M. Kerstitch, M.D.

Patients with an alcohol problem rarely present with a chief complaint of problem drinking. More commonly they exhibit various complications of alcohol abuse. Some are psychological in nature (fatigue, anxiety, depression, insomnia); others are somatic (palpitations, weakness, gastric upset, headaches). Emergency room physicians commonly encounter intoxicated patients brought in by police because of assaultive behavior, public intoxication, or drunk driving. Alcoholism is the primary diagnosis in 25% of suicides. The physician must maintain a *high index of suspicion* to avoid missing this common diagnosis. Consider alcohol-related problems in nearly every patient.

A. History is the key to a diagnosis of alcohol or drug abuse or dependence; however, patients often distort the history and minimize the problem. Denial is a strong defense in all alcohol and drug abusers. It is often necessary to interview family members to obtain accurate information. Review patients' alcohol and drug use history in detail. Look for problems in social (divorce, job loss, family arguments), legal (DUI), and medical (gastritis, peptic ulcer, hepatitis) areas of the patient's life. It is important to identify negative consequences that suggest loss of control and support a diagnosis of dependence. Compulsive use and preoccupation with drinking complete the criteria for dependence or addiction. The mnemonic CPR (compulsivity, preoccupation, relapse) is useful for recalling the essential features of dependence. Also review the family history, since alcoholism shows strong family trends. Physiologic dependence is often present but not required for the diagnosis of alcohol dependence.

B. Physical examination should be detailed and thorough. Patients with cirrhosis, ascites, edema, rhinophyma, peripheral neuropathy, and jaundice characterize end-stage alcoholism. These patients have usually been drinking uncontrollably for >10 years. Physical complications of alcohol are late findings and may not be evident early in the disease.

C. Laboratory screening can be informative. Look for elevations in aspartate aminotransferase (AST) (serum glutamic-oxaloacetic transaminase [SGOT]), alanine aminotransferase (ALT) (serum glutamic-pyruvic transaminase [SGPT]), and gamma glutamyltransferase (GGT). Typically the AST is greater than the ALT. The GGT is the most sensitive indicator of alcohol-induced liver damage. The CBC frequently shows elevated MCV and MCH with prolonged regular use of alcohol. Hypercholesterolemia and hyperlipidemia are often present. Blood alcohol level >300 mg/dl in an alert patient indicates significant tolerance.

D. Using the data thus far collected, the physician can usually make a diagnosis of alcohol abuse, dependence, or polysubstance dependence. The DSM III-R lists the criteria used; two are listed for abuse. Diagnosis requires only one of these. Dependence requires at least three of the nine criteria listed. Polysubstance abuse/dependence is becoming much more common. It is important to note that physiologic tolerance to alcohol (or other drugs) is no longer required for a diagnosis of alcohol abuse or dependence, although it is usually present with alcohol.

E. Dual diagnosis refers to alcohol abuse or dependence *plus* another major psychiatric diagnosis such as depression, bipolar disorder, schizophrenia, or anxiety disorder. These patients can be extremely difficult to diagnose and treat. Psychiatric consultation is suggested. Successful treatment of alcohol problems requires identification and treatment of all other comorbid psychiatric problems.

F. Individualize treatment to the particular needs of the patient. Merely telling the patient to quit drinking is futile and potentially dangerous. Consultation with an experienced psychiatrist or addictionist is strongly recommended. Referral to AA or other support group is an excellent place to begin but may not be enough for patients with advanced disease or comorbid psychiatric disorders.

References

Addiction medicine (special issue). Smith DE (special editor). West J Med 1990; 152:502.

American Psychiatric Association. Diagnostic and statistical manual of mental disorders. 3rd ed, revised. Washington, DC: American Psychiatric Association. Elmsford, NY: Pergamon Press, 1987.

Knott DH. Alcohol problems. Pergamon Press, 1986.

Hays JT, Spickard WA Jr. Alcoholism: early diagnosis and intervention. J Gen Intern Med 1987; 2:420.

Milhorn JT Jr. The diagnosis of alcoholism. Am Fam Physician 1988; 37:175.

Reid, WH, Wise MG. DSM-III-R Training Guide. 3rd ed. New York: Brunner/Mazel, 1989.

Patient with DRINKING PROBLEM

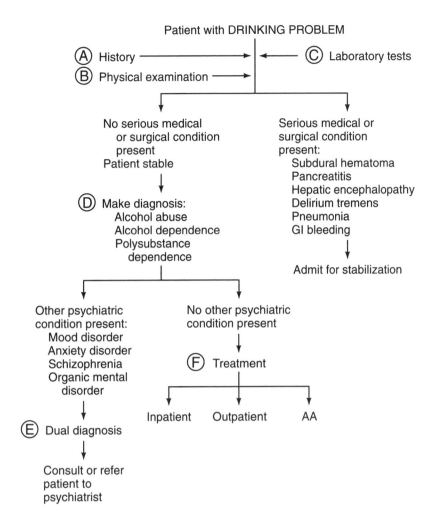

Ⓐ History

Ⓑ Physical examination

Ⓒ Laboratory tests

No serious medical or surgical condition present
Patient stable

Serious medical or surgical condition present:
Subdural hematoma
Pancreatitis
Hepatic encephalopathy
Delirium tremens
Pneumonia
GI bleeding

Admit for stabilization

Ⓓ Make diagnosis:
Alcohol abuse
Alcohol dependence
Polysubstance dependence

Other psychiatric condition present:
Mood disorder
Anxiety disorder
Schizophrenia
Organic mental disorder

No other psychiatric condition present

Ⓕ Treatment

Inpatient   Outpatient   AA

Ⓔ Dual diagnosis

Consult or refer patient to psychiatrist

ANXIETY

Eric M. Reiman, M.D.

A. Everyday stressors such as illness, injury, and loss can produce anxiety in patients and their families. Compassion, patience, and understanding can reduce feelings of helplessness and social isolation and increase patients' confidence and self-esteem. A benzodiazepine may be prescribed if patients understand that it is a temporary measure and if they have no history of a psychoactive substance use disorder.

B. Organic factors can produce symptoms of anxiety: e.g., patients frequently experience anxiety during the initial stages of dementia (these patients may respond to sedative-hypnotics with increased anxiety and memory impairment). Diagnose and treat the underlying problem. However, the presence of a nonpsychiatric medical disorder does not always exclude the possibility of a concurrent anxiety disorder.

C. Anxiety is a feature of almost all psychiatric disorders: e.g., it is a common symptom of major depression. Diagnose and treat the underlying problem.

D. Panic disorder is characterized by frequent panic attacks, sudden episodes of severe apprehension or fear associated with at least four of the following symptoms: shortness of breath; choking or smothering sensations; palpitations or tachycardia; chest discomfort; dizziness, trembling, or shaking; numbness or tingling; hot flashes or chills; sweating; nausea or abdominal distress; feelings of unreality; a fear of dying; and a fear of going crazy or losing control. Look for abrupt onset (maximal intensity within 10 minutes of onset) and short duration (typically, 2–30 minutes). Many patients see cardiologists or emergency room doctors seeking a medical explanation of the problem. Indeed, they account for >30% of patients with atypical or nonanginal chest pain. Several medications can block anxiety attacks, including antidepressants such as imipramine (start low, go slow, warn the patient of an exacerbation in symptoms early in treatment), monoamine oxidase (MAO) inhibitors such as phenelzine (provide a list of dietary and medication restrictions), and high-potency benzodiazepines such as alprazolam (use standing doses to prevent attacks, warn patients about withdrawal symptoms and the related need for slow discontinuation, and avoid in patients with a history of a psychoactive substance use disorder). Recent evidence suggests that cognitive-behavioral therapy can prevent anxiety attacks in patients with panic disorder. This standardized, short-term treatment should be administered by a well-trained professional; it is designed to help patients identify and revise their habit of responding to normally innocuous physical sensations as dangerous. Once the panic attacks are addressed, patients who have panic disorder with agoraphobia are encouraged to confront and learn to overcome their fears through repeated, frequent, intense exposure.

E. Phobias, irrational fears that are recognized by the individual as excessive, are extremely common. Agoraphobia is an irrational fear of situations from which it may be difficult or embarrassing to escape. Always consider the possibility of panic attacks in patients with this disorder. A social phobia is an irrational fear of activities that may lead to embarrassment; the most common social phobia is a fear of public speaking. A simple phobia is an irrational fear of particular objects or situations (e.g., animals, closed places, heights). Exposure therapy encourages patients to gradually confront and learn to overcome the feared object, activity, or situation; frequency, duration, and intensity of exposures are directly related to outcome. Prescribe a benzodiazepine if patients understand that it is a temporary measure and if there is no history of a psychoactive substance use disorder. Social phobias may benefit from P.R.N. dose of a beta-blocker or benzodiazepines or standing doses of a MAO inhibitor as an adjunct to exposure.

F. Obsessions are recurrent, intrusive, unwanted ideas that insistently enter the mind; they are distressing and typically recognized as senseless by the individual. Compulsions are repetitive, ritualistic behaviors typically performed to neutralize an obsession and reduce distress; most of these individuals recognize that their behaviors are unreasonable and excessive. The Yale-Brown Obsessive Compulsive Scale Symptom Checklist may help identify additional problems in these patients. Many patients benefit from a trial of a serotonin-reuptake inhibitor (clomipramine or fluoxetine), behavioral therapy (e.g., a structured, short-term protocol that involves repeated exposure to the obsession-eliciting situation together with a mandate to suppress anxiety-reducing compulsions), or a combination of the two. Some patients benefit from participation in a support group. Occasionally, consider stereotactic surgery, such as bilateral anterior cingulotomy, in patients with extremely disabling symptoms that are unresponsive to the arsenal of more conventional treatments.

G. Consider post-traumatic stress disorder (PTSD) in individuals who have been exposed to stressors outside the range of normal human experience (e.g., rape, accidental or natural disasters, military combat). Symptoms include recurrent, intrusive thoughts of the traumatic event; increased arousal (e.g., insomnia, hypervigilance, startle, irritability, anger); and restrictions in range of affect and interpersonal relationships. Consider individual or group psychotherapy to increase self-esteem, decrease social isolation, and support coping resources; antidepressants or MAO inhibitors to reduce symptoms of anxiety; and referral

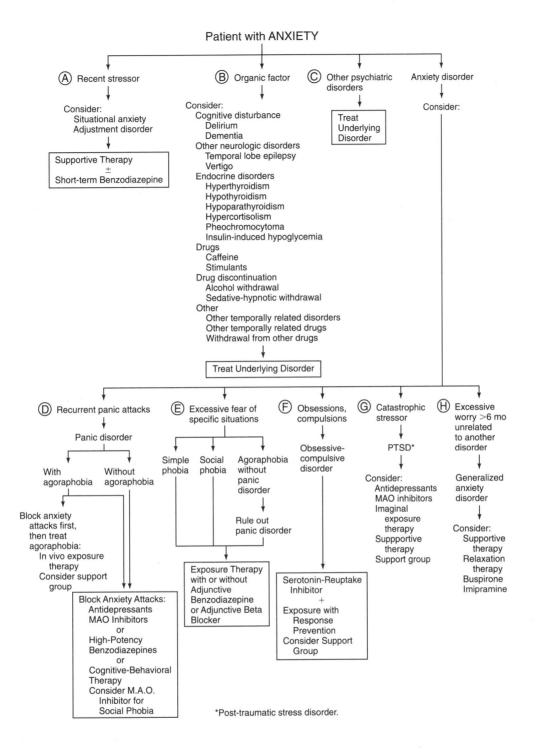

Patient with ANXIETY

A Recent stressor

Consider:
Situational anxiety
Adjustment disorder

Supportive Therapy
±
Short-term Benzodiazepine

B Organic factor

Consider:
Cognitive disturbance
Delirium
Dementia
Other neurologic disorders
Temporal lobe epilepsy
Vertigo
Endocrine disorders
Hyperthyroidism
Hypothyroidism
Hypoparathyroidism
Hypercortisolism
Pheochromocytoma
Insulin-induced hypoglycemia
Drugs
Caffeine
Stimulants
Drug discontinuation
Alcohol withdrawal
Sedative-hypnotic withdrawal
Other
Other temporally related disorders
Other temporally related drugs
Withdrawal from other drugs

Treat Underlying Disorder

C Other psychiatric disorders

Treat
Underlying
Disorder

Anxiety disorder

Consider:

D Recurrent panic attacks

Panic disorder

With agoraphobia   Without agoraphobia

Block anxiety attacks first, then treat agoraphobia:
In vivo exposure therapy
Consider support group

Block Anxiety Attacks:
Antidepressants
MAO Inhibitors
or
High-Potency Benzodiazepines
or
Cognitive-Behavioral Therapy
Consider M.A.O. Inhibitor for Social Phobia

E Excessive fear of specific situations

Simple phobia   Social phobia   Agoraphobia without panic disorder

Rule out panic disorder

Exposure Therapy with or without Adjunctive Benzodiazepine or Adjunctive Beta Blocker

F Obsessions, compulsions

Obsessive-compulsive disorder

Serotonin-Reuptake Inhibitor
+
Exposure with Response Prevention
Consider Support Group

G Catastrophic stressor

PTSD*

Consider:
Antidepressants
MAO inhibitors
Imaginal exposure therapy
Supportive therapy
Support group

H Excessive worry >6 mo unrelated to another disorder

Generalized anxiety disorder

Consider:
Supportive therapy
Relaxation therapy
Buspirone
Imipramine

*Post-traumatic stress disorder.

for participation in a structured program of behavioral therapy, one that involves frequent imagined exposures to the stressor.

H. Generalized anxiety disorder is a diagnosis of exclusion. Consider the other disorders in the algorithm (e.g., panic disorder, major depression) first. Consider nonpharmacologic therapy or buspirone first; consider an antidepressant such as imipramine second; use benzodiazepines sparingly, especially in patients with cognitive impairment or a psychoactive substance use disorder; and discontinue medications that fail to work.

References

American Psychiatric Association. Diagnostic and statistical manual of mental disorders. 3rd ed, revised. Washington, DC: American Psychiatric Association, 1987.

Arana GW, Hyman SE. Handbook of psychiatric drug therapy. 2nd ed. Boston: Little, Brown, 1991.

Barlow DH. Anxiety and its disorders: the nature and treatment of anxiety and panic. New York: Guilford Press, 1988.

DEPRESSION

Iris R. Bell, M.D., Ph.D.

Mood disorders, especially dysphoria, occur in 5% of the general population, with women and persons aged 25–44 years most at risk. The full syndrome of major depression carries significant morbidity and mortality in terms of suicide risk and poorer outcome of concomitant medical disorders. Many patients with depression present first to the primary care physician with somatic concerns and seek a medical diagnosis or treatment for anxiety or "nerves," while the proper diagnosis and treatment are often overlooked.

A. Depression is a clinical syndrome without a specific laboratory test to confirm the diagnosis; comprehensive clinical assessments provide the main data.

B. Criteria for diagnosis of major depression include at least five of nine symptoms present daily or almost daily during the same 2-week period and indicative of a change from previous functioning. Symptoms are (1) depressed mood, (2) markedly reduced interest or pleasure in activities, (3) significant weight loss or gain or decrease or increase in appetite, (4) insomnia or hypersomnia, (5) psychomotor agitation or retardation, (6) fatigue or low energy, (7) feelings of worthlessness or inordinate guilt, (8) difficulty concentrating or indecisiveness, and (9) recurrent thoughts of death or suicide or a suicide attempt. Broad differential diagnosis must include organic mood disorder, depressed, and a major depression.

C. A screening battery of laboratory tests helps rule out specific organic causes. In combination with the history and physical examination, findings may suggest more specific laboratory studies (see D). Specialized tests sensitive but not specific to major depression include the dexamethasone suppression test, the thyrotropin releasing hormone stimulation test, and polysomnography.

D. Differential diagnosis for organic causes includes substance abuse and prescription drugs such as antihypertensives, hormones, analgesics, anticancer drugs, antiparkinsonian drugs, antianxiety and hypnotic drugs, GI drugs; endocrine and metabolic disorders (especially thyroid and adrenal); nutritional deficiencies (vitamins B_1, niacin, folate, B_{12}); and heavy metal toxicity (e.g., lead). Depression in alcoholics may resolve with abstinence. Depressive symptoms follow stroke in up to 60% of cases within 2 years. Treatment of underlying medical problems may lead to resolution of depression; if not, standard antidepressant treatment strategies are often effective.

E. Initial antidepressant regimens usually involve secondary amine tricyclics (nortriptyline, desipramine) to minimize side effects and maximize compliance, in combination with psychotherapy. If tricyclics fail or are contraindicated, second-generation antidepressants (fluoxetine, bupropion, trazodone) or monoamine oxidase inhibitors (MAOIs) (phenelzine, tranylcypromine) are alternatives. Choose medication to target symptoms (e.g., agitated versus retarded) and address side effect profile. Watch for drug interactions with MAOIs and fluoxetine; MAOIs require a tyramine- free diet. Stimulants may mobilize apathetic, medically ill patients, but their long-term efficacy for major depression is uncertain.

F. Up to 50% of unipolar depressed patients with partial or no response to an antidepressant alone may respond more fully to the addition of lithium. More controversial augmentation strategies include thyroid supplementation, combination fluoxetine with tricyclic, combination MAOI with tricyclic; the last two approaches involve a significant risk of drug interactions.

G. Growing evidence suggests that bright light therapy may suffice in some cases of winter depression; more standard somatic therapies are also effective.

H. Recent studies have shown the need for a combination of antidepressant and antipsychotic drugs rather than single-agent therapy to treat psychotic depression.

I. Bipolar patients may switch into manic episodes during treatment with antidepressant medications alone. This may necessitate concomitant coverage with lithium or another mood-stabilizing agent.

J. Electroconvulsive therapy is the most effective treatment for major depression, especially the subtype with psychotic features. It is the treatment of choice for acute suicidality, severe cachexia and dehydration secondary to poor intake, many medically complex major depressions, and antidepressant medication failures.

K. A chronic course of at least 2 years and a less severe depressive picture suggests a dysthymic disorder, which can co-occur with major depression. Dysphoria or fluctuating mood instability are characteristic of a range of chronic personality disorders that vary in their responsiveness to psychotherapeutic interventions.

L. An identifiable stressor, maladaptive symptoms lasting <6 months, and a generally less severe depressive picture suggest an adjustment disorder with depressed mood, which usually resolves with time and supportive psychotherapy.

Patient with DYSPHORIC MOOD

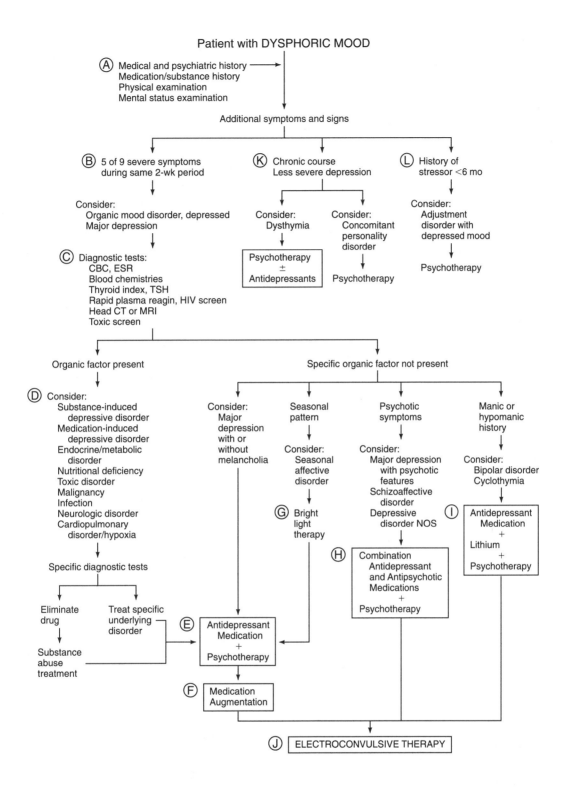

References

Baldessarini R. Current status of antidepressants: clinical pharmacology and therapy. J Clin Psychiatry 1989; 50:117.

Hirschfeld RMA, Goodwin FK. Mood disorders. In: Talbott JA, Hales RE, Yudofsky SC, eds. Textbook of psychiatry. Washington, DC: American Psychiatric Press, 1988: 403–441.

Keller MB. Diagnostic issues and clinical course of unipolar illness. In: Frances AJ, Hales RE, eds. Review of psychiatry. Vol 7. Washington, DC: American Psychiatric Press, 1988:188–212.

Nierenberg AA, Amsterdam JD. Treatment-resistant depression: definition and treatment approaches. J Clin Psychiatry 1990; 51 (6, Suppl):39.

Wise MG, Taylor SE. Anxiety and mood disorders in medically ill patients. J Clin Psychiatry 1990; 51 (1, Suppl):27.

EMOTIONAL DISORDERS WITH SOMATIC EXPRESSION

John Misiaszek, M.D.

Patients with emotionally based somatic complaints are largely unaware of their emotional conflicts. Often labeled as "crocks," they receive poor and fragmented treatment, although their tendency to express their emotional conflicts through somatizing behavior does not immunize them against bona fide physical illness. Furthermore, many physical disorders such as thyroid disease, multiple sclerosis, and temporal lobe epilepsy may initially or primarily present as an emotional disorder, causing delays in diagnosis and treatment. The physical, emotional, and iatrogenic morbidity of patients who somaticize their psychic distress can be largely reduced by having a physician provide consistency, support, and reassurance while minimizing invasive procedures and redundant evaluations. These patients are emotionally impaired; rejection only serves to heighten their impairment.

A. The medical history should include a review for similar, previously undiagnosed disorders in the patient and family members. Often the somaticizing coping behavior has been modeled or reinforced earlier in life. Early traumatic emotional development may result in more severe somatoform expression such as a factitious disorder. Personal or family history may also suggest a proclivity for one of the major psychiatric disorders.

B. Patients with acute or chronic psychoses may have bizarre somatic complaints (e.g., an alien force has turned their intestines inside out). Their overall thought disturbance is readily manifest in their report. It is sometimes difficult to differentiate between the complaint as a delusion or a symbolic and personalized interpretation of a genuine physical discomfort. Patients with psychotic depression or monodelusional disorders (e.g., delusions of parasitosis) may have more focused or fixed somatic concerns that may or may not diminish when treated with high-potency antipsychotics such as haloperidol or pimozide.

C. Although delirious or demented patients may misperceive or fabricate somatic symptoms, their primary psychiatric problem is differentiated from "functional psychosis" by the presence of periodic or persistent confusion and disorientation. Antipsychotic medication may decrease the somatic delusions and behavioral difficulties, but treatment of the underlying disorder may be curative.

D. Depression may be masked by a complaint of headache or generalized fatigue. Vegetative signs of depression may be variably present, along with diminished self-esteem and a depressive affect; these often precede or coincide with somatic sensations. A primary depression must be distinguished from a secondary (or reactive) depression that is a result, not the cause, of a somatic problem.

E. Patients with a generalized anxiety disorder present with a variety of somatic symptoms: tachycardia, motor tension, autonomic hyperactivity. Patients with panic attacks may fear cardiac or pulmonary disorders. A primary anxiety disorder needs to be differentiated from a secondary apprehension about a physical symptom.

F. A hypochondriacal reaction is distinguished from classical hypochondriasis in that it follows a recent stressful event, is short-lived, and responds to reassurance. Examples include an individual who is concerned about minor chest discomfort after a cardiac-related death of a close friend, a medical student who has a phobia about the "disease of the day," and a luncheon crowd's hysteria in response to the erroneous report of a food-poisoning victim in their midst.

G. Conversion disorder is likely if there is loss or alteration in physical function after a stressful event. The resultant psychic conflict is not readily apparent to the individual or evaluator. The diagnosis also requires that the physical problem cannot be explained by a known physical disorder. "La belle indifference" has been widely overstated as a characteristic symptom and is of little diagnostic value. Use caution when assigning this diagnosis. Studies have shown that 13–30% of patients so diagnosed later develop physical problems that could have explained their original physical complaint.

H. Conscious deceit is subdivided into malingering when secondary gain is apparent, and factitious disorder when reasons for the deceit are not understood by the patient or the physician. A military draft inductee who feigns a disorder to avoid conscription is malingering, whereas patients with factitious disorders (e.g., Munchausen's syndrome) have complex, convoluted reasons for faking somatic disorders, are angry and emotionally traumatized, have unsettled lives, and displace hostility onto others. They are difficult patients to treat either medically or psychiatrically; confrontation in the absence of a comprehensive medical psychiatric treatment plan rarely works and risks escalating maladaptive behavior.

I. Hypochondriasis is the misinterpretation of physical signs or sensations as serious disease. Patients are typically fearful, do not respond readily to support and reassurance, return for further evaluation and treatment, or seek other physicians. These patients have been described as hostile, masochistic, and demanding individuals who deny their needs for dependence, or (less commonly) individuals who are clinging, passive, and overtly dependent in their relationship with their doctor. Related terms are somatization disorder, in which patients develop multiple "review of systems" complaints as an early life-coping mech-

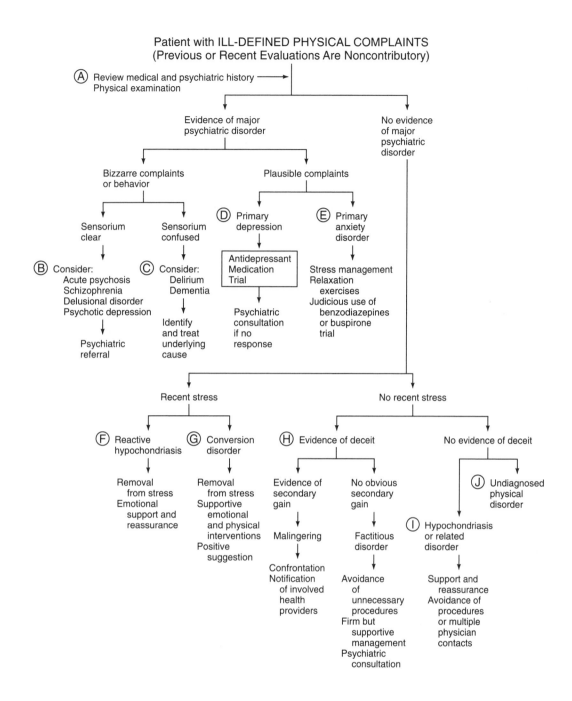

Patient with ILL-DEFINED PHYSICAL COMPLAINTS
(Previous or Recent Evaluations Are Noncontributory)

Ⓐ Review medical and psychiatric history →
Physical examination

Evidence of major psychiatric disorder

No evidence of major psychiatric disorder

Bizzarre complaints or behavior

Plausible complaints

Sensorium clear

Sensorium confused

Ⓓ Primary depression

Ⓔ Primary anxiety disorder

Ⓑ Consider:
Acute psychosis
Schizophrenia
Delusional disorder
Psychotic depression

↓

Psychiatric referral

Ⓒ Consider:
Delirium
Dementia

↓

Identify and treat underlying cause

Antidepressant Medication Trial

↓

Psychiatric consultation if no response

Stress management
Relaxation exercises
Judicious use of benzodiazepines or buspirone trial

Recent stress

No recent stress

Ⓕ Reactive hypochondriasis

Ⓖ Conversion disorder

Ⓗ Evidence of deceit

No evidence of deceit

Removal from stress
Emotional support and reassurance

Removal from stress
Supportive emotional and physical interventions
Positive suggestion

Evidence of secondary gain

No obvious secondary gain

Ⓙ Undiagnosed physical disorder

↓

Malingering

↓

Confrontation
Notification of involved health providers

Factitious disorder

↓

Avoidance of unnecessary procedures
Firm but supportive management
Psychiatric consultation

Ⓘ Hypochondriasis or related disorder

↓

Support and reassurance
Avoidance of procedures or multiple physician contacts

anism, and somatoform pain disorder, when pain is the specific hypochondriacal concern.

J. The absence of a physical finding or inability to establish a physical diagnosis by itself is insufficient for a diagnosis of a major psychiatric or somatoform disorder. These diagnoses can be made only when the associated psychiatric characteristics are present and when the dysfunction and somatic problems are a consequence of such characteristics. Since life stress or misfortune is found in most medical patients and nonpatients alike, take care not to magnify such occurrences when there is no obvious connection to the physical impairment.

References

Cassem NH. Functional somatic symptoms and somatoform disorders. In: Hackett TP, Cassem NH, eds. Massachusetts General Hospital handbook of general hospital psychiatry. 2nd ed. Littleton, MA: PSG Publishing, 1987.

Ekkehard D. Somatization disorder. Psychiatr Ann 1988; 18:330.

Ford CV. The somatizing disorders: illness as a way of life. New York: Elsevier Biomedical, 1983.

GRIEF

Gail L. Schwartz, M.D.

A. Normal grief responses are variable. The process of grieving may be seen as occurring in three stages: initial shock or numbing, acute mourning, and a period of resolution or recovery. A lack of perceived social support is one predictor of difficulty in recovery. Those seen as grieving most intensely early in the bereavement may have a poorer outcome after 1 year than those with a relative absence of mourning. There is little evidence to support the efficacy of treatment for people experiencing uncomplicated bereavement.

B. Neurovegetative symptoms of depression are common in bereavement. Sleep disturbance may last for up to 1 year. Appetite usually returns within 4 months after the loss. However, motor retardation, ruminative guilt, and a feeling of worthlessness are not typical symptoms of bereavement and suggest the need for psychiatric evaluation and treatment.

C. Persistent symptoms of anxiety and depression warrant a more detailed psychiatric evaluation. Clinically depressed patients are most often treated with a combination of antidepressant medication and psychotherapy.

D. Over 40% of bereaved spouses have at least one type of anxiety disorder during the first year of bereavement. A history of anxiety disorder is a strong predictor of its presenting during bereavement. Anxiety symptoms include somatic distress, obsessions and compulsions, phobias, and panic attacks.

E. Antidepressants are useful in the treatment of most anxiety disorders and may be preferred to benzodiazepines because of the lack of dependence potential.

F. A history of an addictive disorder is a strong predictor of substance abuse during grieving. Because there is a significant risk of morbidity and mortality with substance abuse, it is imperative that a careful history be taken and that bothersome symptoms of anxiety and sleeplessness be treated nonpharmacologically or with medications that have minimal addiction potential.

G. In normal grief the intensity of the emotional pain gradually decreases; significant resolution occurs by 1 year. Theories of attachment behavior have been used to explain the difficulties that complicate the grieving process for some people (Table 1).

H. It is suggested that expressive psychotherapy is most appropriate for conflicted grief syndromes, cognitive treatment may be particularly useful for dependent grief syndrome, and treatments developed specifically for persons suffering from post-traumatic stress disorder may be most useful for those who have had a sudden, unexpected loss.

TABLE 1 Pathologic Grief Syndromes

Dependent	A stable sense of self is dependent on presence of the lost person
Unexpected loss	A post-traumatic stress syndrome with hyperreactivity, intrusive memories, and nightmares alternating with affect constriction and numbing
Conflicted	Ambivalence toward the lost person is unacceptable, and the grieving person turns the negative feelings on himself or herself

References

Clayton PJ. Bereavement and depression. J Clin Psychiatry 1990; 51 (Suppl):34.

Middleton W. Bereavement. Psychiatr Clin North Am 1987; 10:329.

Rynearson EK. Psychotherapy of pathologic grief. Psychiatr Clin North Am 1987; 10:487.

Zisook S. Anxiety and bereavement. Psychiatr Med 1990; 8:83.

Patient Has Experienced SIGNIFICANT LOSS

History

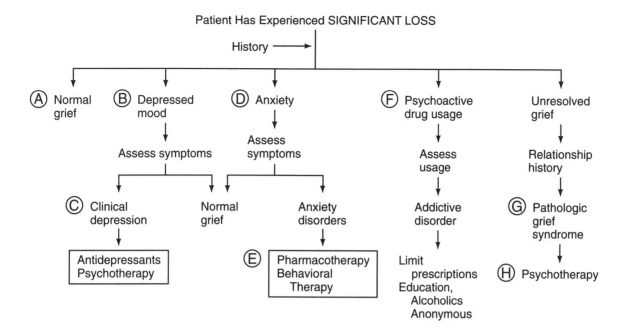

PSYCHOSIS

Alan J. Gelenberg, M.D.

A psychotic episode is typified by deranged thinking, speech, and behavior, often manifesting as hallucinations (false sensory impressions: visual, auditory, olfactory, gustatory, tactile), delusions (false fixed beliefs), difficulty distinguishing reality from fantasy, disorganized thinking, and strange and inappropriate behavior.

A. Confronted with an acutely psychotic patient, the physician's first task is to ensure the safety of the patient and others against injury or possible death. A calm, low-stimulus environment with nonthreatening behavior by staff is essential. Force should not be threatened unless overwhelming force is available. The patient should not be left alone and an examining physician should be accompanied by at least one other person. Some patients may need to be restrained. Patients should be questioned about any thoughts of suicide or injuring others, which must be taken extremely seriously.

B. A medical history is essential in the evaluation of a psychotic patient. Given the patient's mental status, the most valuable information will probably come from others who know him or her. Inquire about the time course of the emerging bizarre behavior and possible relation to any medical conditions, recent-onset physical symptoms, exposure to infectious or toxic agents, medication use, drug abuse, or recent surgery or trauma.

C. Possible medical causes of acute psychotic behavior should be considered and ruled out immediately. Despite the difficulties, perform as complete a physical examination as possible, including pupils and, to the extent possible, fundi. Examine carefully the patient's entire body for evidence of trauma, substance abuse, or disease.

D. Address such readily treatable (and potentially hazardous) conditions as hypoglycemia by such means as immediate drawing of blood followed by IV injection of a concentrated dextrose solution.

E. If the history (usually from others), a careful physical examination, and indicated laboratory tests fail to reveal any organic causes of psychosis, consider a psychiatric differential diagnosis.

F. Schizophrenia is a lifelong chronic condition marked by acute psychotic episodes interspersed with periods of less disturbed but still abnormal behavior. Between episodes, schizophrenics often show poor motivation and social awkwardness. Acute schizophrenic episodes are typically treated with antipsychotic agents, which usually are maintained at lower doses to mitigate the likelihood and severity of future episodes. Use benzodiazepine sedation as needed as an adjunct to antipsychotic drugs during acute episodes.

G. Mania often presents as an acute psychosis. A history typically reveals past episodes of mania or major depression. A mental status examination shows the patient to be highly excited, emotionally labile, overtalkative, pressured in speech, hypersexual, and with grandiose ideas. Acute treatment consists of antipsychotic drugs as needed, often with adjunctive lithium. Lithium is the mainstay therapy for most bipolar (manic-depressive) patients. Electroconvulsive therapy (ECT) is usually effective for patients who fail to benefit or cannot tolerate these medications. Use benzodiazepines adjunctively to control an acute episode.

H. Psychotic depression may become manifest either as a recurrent mood disorder itself or as an episode in the course of a bipolar illness. Delusions and hallucinations commonly manifest such depressive themes as guilt and punishment. Effective treatments include ECT and combined antipsychotic and antidepressant drugs. Guard against suicide, an omnipresent hazard in these patients.

I. Delusional (paranoid) disorder is a chronic condition characterized by a fixed and focused delusional system in the midst of otherwise intact thinking. It is often refractory to biologic and psychologic treatments.

J. Demented patients often manifest psychotic behaviors that can complicate long-term management. Rule out acute medical conditions and, if possible, handle disruptive behaviors through behavioral and environmental means. If this is not possible, low doses of antipsychotic drugs may assist management.

References

American Psychiatric Association. Treatment of psychiatric disorders: a task force of the American Psychiatric Association. Washington, DC: American Psychiatric Association, 1989:1485, 1655, 1725.

Gelenberg AJ. Psychosis. In: Gelenberg AJ, Bassuk EL, Schoonover SC, eds. The practitioner's guide to psychoactive drugs. 3rd ed. New York: Plenum, 1991:125.

Kaplan HI, Sadock BJ, eds. Comprehensive textbook of psychiatry. Vol. 1. 5th ed. Baltimore: Williams & Wilkins, 1989:699, 830, 859.

PSYCHOTIC PATIENT

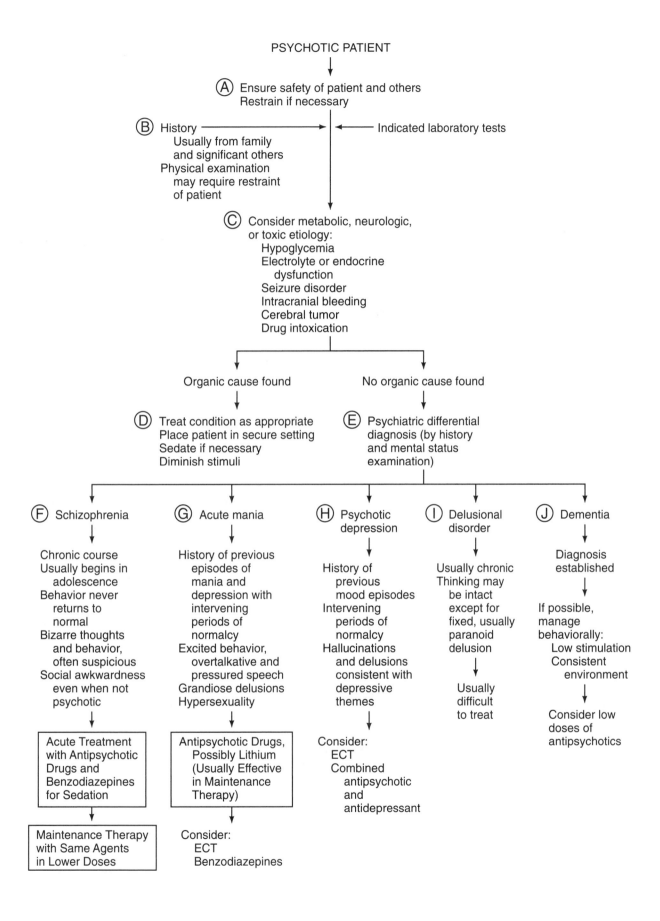

(A) Ensure safety of patient and others
Restrain if necessary

(B) History ——————
Usually from family
and significant others
Physical examination
may require restraint
of patient

Indicated laboratory tests

(C) Consider metabolic, neurologic,
or toxic etiology:
Hypoglycemia
Electrolyte or endocrine
dysfunction
Seizure disorder
Intracranial bleeding
Cerebral tumor
Drug intoxication

Organic cause found

No organic cause found

(D) Treat condition as appropriate
Place patient in secure setting
Sedate if necessary
Diminish stimuli

(E) Psychiatric differential
diagnosis (by history
and mental status
examination)

(F) Schizophrenia

Chronic course
Usually begins in
adolescence
Behavior never
returns to
normal
Bizarre thoughts
and behavior,
often suspicious
Social awkwardness
even when not
psychotic

Acute Treatment
with Antipsychotic
Drugs and
Benzodiazepines
for Sedation

Maintenance Therapy
with Same Agents
in Lower Doses

(G) Acute mania

History of previous
episodes of
mania and
depression with
intervening
periods of
normalcy
Excited behavior,
overtalkative and
pressured speech
Grandiose delusions
Hypersexuality

Antipsychotic Drugs,
Possibly Lithium
(Usually Effective
in Maintenance
Therapy)

Consider:
ECT
Benzodiazepines

(H) Psychotic
depression

History of
previous
mood episodes
Intervening
periods of
normalcy
Hallucinations
and delusions
consistent with
depressive
themes

Consider:
ECT
Combined
antipsychotic
and
antidepressant

(I) Delusional
disorder

Usually chronic
Thinking may
be intact
except for
fixed, usually
paranoid
delusion

Usually
difficult
to treat

(J) Dementia

Diagnosis
established

If possible,
manage
behaviorally:
Low stimulation
Consistent
environment

Consider low
doses of
antipsychotics

SMOKING CESSATION

Harry L. Greene, M.D.
Lawrence A. Garcia, M.D.

The Surgeon General has determined that the leading preventable cause of death and disability in the United States is cigarette smoking. About 30% of adult Americans (32% of men and 27% of women) smoke regularly. Although 75% of all adults visit a physician at least once a year, the smoker will visit more often due to increased illness. The first step in smoking cessation is to identify the smoker by simply asking: "Do you smoke?" Although a few may be evasive about their smoking, most admit it, and surveys show that 80% say they would like to quit.

A. Congratulate patients who are nonsmokers. Counsel preteenagers and teenagers about peer pressure, targeted advertising, and the fallacy of smoking as a way to be more grown-up. Encourage those who have quit to maintain their cessation.

B. Inform smokers of the adverse health consequences of smoking and the benefits of stopping, emphasize the damage or disease already present, motivate them to consider quitting, and give firm and unequivocal advice to quit. Judith Ockene of the University of Massachusetts recommends using guided questions such as "Are you aware of the effects of smoking on your health?" Make the patient aware of any physical findings that are present and related to smoking, in an effort to personalize the effects of smoking. Mention the benefits of quitting now, including lower risk of cancer, sudden death, or myocardial infarction (MI); and longer active life (at any age). Many smokers are fatalistic and unaware of the reversibility of smoking-related disease and risk. Make a statement such as: "As your physician, I must advise you that smoking is bad for your health."

C. One can sense whether a patient is contemplating quitting by asking questions such as: "How do you feel about being a smoker? What reasons do you have to quit? Were you able to stop smoking in the past? How did you do it that time? What caused you to start again? If you had that chance again what would you do differently?" The purpose of these questions is to allow insight, build confidence, problem solve, and begin a plan for a new successful cessation attempt. A critical series of questions are next posed: "Have you thought about stopping? Do you think you can stop now? How will you do it?"

D. At this point, some patients do not show adequate motivation or are unwilling to discuss or plan a cessation attempt. These people often lack the confidence that they can be successful and are unwilling to risk their self-esteem if they fail. Some investigators believe that these patients should sign a waiver stating they have been informed of the risks and for the moment are choosing to smoke against the physician's advice. They can be given a brochure to read and the subject can be broached again on subsequent visits. Watch for a possible critical incident (e.g., acute illness; MI in patient, friend, or relative; cancer; pregnancy; death of a valued person) as a time when contemplation can be changed to action.

E. Ambivalent patients are often unwilling to choose a quit date or sign a contract to quit but may be willing to do other things. A smoking diary can help document when, where, what they were doing, with whom, and the value of the cigarette from 1 (crucial) to 5 (not very important). The diary helps build awareness. It can be accompanied by tapering (i.e., eliminating the not very important cigarettes). Other techniques include switching to cigarettes with lower tar and nicotine content and smoking fewer each day. These measures are mainly directed at building confidence for a successful cessation attempt. Until patients are ready to change it is better not to court failure.

F. For patients ready to quit, a quit date should be set and a contract signed. These can be preprinted or simply written in the chart. The contract can serve as an additional reminder if it is on duplicate paper with a chart copy and another one is placed in a prominent place selected by the patient (e.g., refrigerator, mirror). Some patients may keep a smoking diary for a few days to increase awareness of when, where, and why they smoke. Once the quit date is chosen, develop an action plan in conjunction with the patient to determine who will be the support people at home and at work and how weight gain will be handled (increased exercise, low-calorie diet). As the lungs return to normal, patients often begin to cough; it is worth emphasizing this in a positive light (i.e., cleansing of the lungs). Tell patients to use a cough suppressant only as a last resort to help them sleep.

(Continued on page 504)

Patient for SMOKING PREVENTION OR CESSATION

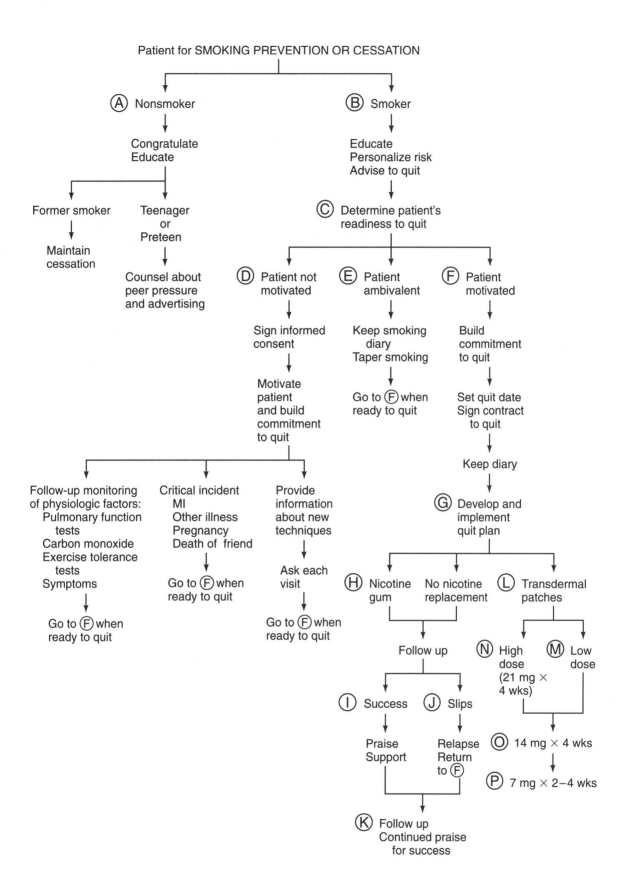

(A) Nonsmoker

Congratulate
Educate

Former smoker

Maintain
cessation

Teenager
or
Preteen

Counsel about
peer pressure
and advertising

(B) Smoker

Educate
Personalize risk
Advise to quit

(C) Determine patient's
readiness to quit

(D) Patient not
motivated

Sign informed
consent

Motivate
patient
and build
commitment
to quit

Follow-up monitoring
of physiologic factors:
  Pulmonary function
  tests
  Carbon monoxide
  Exercise tolerance
  tests
  Symptoms

Go to (F) when
ready to quit

Critical incident
  MI
  Other illness
  Pregnancy
  Death of friend

Go to (F) when
ready to quit

Provide
information
about new
techniques

Ask each
visit

Go to (F) when
ready to quit

(E) Patient
ambivalent

Keep smoking
diary
Taper smoking

Go to (F) when
ready to quit

(F) Patient
motivated

Build
commitment
to quit

Set quit date
Sign contract
to quit

Keep diary

(G) Develop and
implement
quit plan

(H) Nicotine
gum

No nicotine
replacement

(L) Transdermal
patches

Follow up

(I) Success

Praise
Support

(J) Slips

Relapse
Return
to (F)

(N) High
dose
(21 mg ×
4 wks)

(M) Low
dose

(O) 14 mg × 4 wks

(P) 7 mg × 2–4 wks

(K) Follow up
Continued praise
for success

G. The decision to use nicotine replacement therapy is made based on whether the patient is heavily addicted to nicotine. This can be ascertained by the response to two questions: "Do you smoke within 30 min of arising in the morning?" and "Do you smoke more than 25 cigarettes/day?" These patients may do better with nicotine replacement therapy. The choice of whether to use nicotine policricex gum or transdermal patches is a matter of choice by the physician and patient. Some patients cannot chew gum because of dental work or TMJ problems or have tried the gum before and lack confidence in it. For these patients transdermal patches may be indicated. Others may be smoking a small number of cigarettes each day or may prefer not to use nicotine replacement; for these patients a trial of cessation without replacement therapy may be appropriate.

H. For heavily addicted patients, offer nicotine (Nicorette) gum. This can be done on a timed schedule and gradually tapered after the psychologic aspects of addiction have abated. Many people who are unsuccessful in stopping do not use enough Nicorette gum or may use it incorrectly. For all patients beginning cessation, maintain close follow-up or contact over the first several days or weeks. This can be accomplished by a call from a staff member or by having patients call in with a report of how they are doing. The purpose of this is to identify slips (brief relapses) early and plan how to manage them and start the cessation attempt again. One slip is not a failure, and most patients who are successful have had to deal with three or four relapses.

I. For successful patients, praise and support should be part of the maintenance plan.

J. For those who relapse, starting again at F makes sense, or they can be referred to a more specialized program. Two forms of Nicorette are available, 2 or 4 mg. Depending on patients' overall pack-year history and smoking pattern, an initial 2-mg dose helps taper craving for the nicotine in the cigarettes. David Sachs of Stanford suggests that a rule of four's be followed with an eventual taper (i.e., 1 pack per day [ppd], 12 pieces Nicorette/day; 1.5 ppd, 16 pieces/day; 2 ppd, 20 pieces/day). He also suggests a chew, stop, and park regimen for the user (i.e., chew slowly until a tingle is felt, stop chewing and park the medication between cheek and gum, restart chewing when the tingle is gone, and stop when the tingle returns).

K. All future physician visits should include follow-up questions on cessation with reinforcement and praise for continued success.

L. For those individuals who are addicted and for whom the transdermal nicotine patches are appropriate, the first dose is determined by amount of smoking and patient size.

M. Those weighing less than 105 lbs or smoking less than 20 cigarettes per day or who have frequent angina attacks should be considered for a 14 mg starting dose. Also those who do not tolerate the 21 mg patch due to excess nicotine symptoms may do better on the lower dose. The 14 mg dose is continued for at least 1 month.

N. Most smokers who are heavily addicted (with the exceptions noted in M) should begin on the 21 mg transdermal patch. This is continued for 1 month. Patients frequently comment on vivid, altered, or increased dreaming on the 21 mg patch. Most will get erythema beneath the patch. Patches should be moved to a new location each day. The manufacturer's instructions should be carefully followed. The *patient must not smoke and use patches,* since this can lead to nicotine toxicity, increased angina, or myocardial infarction. A small percent of patients develop severe skin reactions (1–3%) at the patch site. These patients should be managed using gum.

O. After 1 month these patients should be given a 14 mg patch and this continued for 4–6 weeks depending on how well the habit and psychologic components of smoking are doing.

P. Finally a 7 mg patch should be used for 2–4 weeks and then discontinued. Continue close follow-up and support as outlined under I and K. The patient who relapses while using patches should stop using them and pick a new quitting date and start again at F.

References

Albright CL, Farquhar JW. Principles of behavioral change. In: Greene HL, Glassock RJ, Kelly MA, eds. Introduction to clinical medicine. Philadelphia: BC Decker, 1991:596.

Bronson DC, et al. Smoking cessation counseling during periodic health exams. Arch Intern Med 1989; 149:1653.

Cummings SR, et al. Training physicians in counseling about smoking cessation—a randomized trial of the "quit for life" program. Ann Intern Med 1989; 110:640.

DeNelsky GY, Smoking cessation strategies that work. Cleve Clin J Med 1990; 57:416.

Huston CG, et al. How to help your patients stop smoking. Am Fam Physician 1990; 42:1017.

Ockene JK. Cigarette smoking. In: Greene HL, Glassock RJ, Kelly MA, eds. Introduction to clinical medicine. Philadelphia: BC Decker, 1991:589.

Ockene JK, Kristeller J, Goldberg R. Increasing the efficacy of physician delivered smoking interventions: a randomized clinical trial. J Gen Med 1991; 6:1.

SUICIDAL PATIENT

Rebecca Potter, M.D.

Most suicidal persons communicate their self-destructive intentions to those around them, including their physicians. As many as two thirds of those who commit suicide have seen a doctor in the weeks to months before their death. Medical students and primary care physicians should therefore, know how to evaluate the suicidal patient. Does a patient look or feel depressed and talk of "not being able to go on," giving up, and losing interest in activities? If so, a more detailed assessment of suicidal risk is in order.

A. Psychiatric disorders associated with an increased risk of suicidal ideation and attempt include depression, bipolar disorder, alcohol or drug abuse, panic attacks, and panic disorders.

B. The following psychosocial factors place people at an increased risk of committing suicide: being single, divorced, widowed, or separated; unemployment; decreased social supports; humiliating life events (e.g., the recent loss of a job or an important relationship); a chronic medical illness; or a family history of suicide. A previous suicide attempt is a predictor of future completed suicide.

C. Do not ignore or minimize references to suicide: taking risks, talk of guilt over past events, talk of "ending it all", making a will, giving away prized possessions. Ask patients directly whether they are suicidal, and if so what plan they have; assess their understanding of the lethality of the plan. Do they have the means to carry out the plan? Have there been earlier attempts? Determine patients' mood, changes in appetite and sleep, the presence of hallucinations or delusions, and quality of speech. Patients with "command" hallucinations to commit suicide are at particularly high risk. A physical examination and laboratory studies to consider contributory or concomitant physical illness are necessary.

D. If the patient has serious immediate suicidal intent, consider psychiatric consultation and voluntary or involuntary hospitalization. If the risk is not as imminent, establish and make available a therapeutic relationship. The forming of a no-suicide contract, frequent appointments, and provision of reassurance and hope are important. Allow the patient to ventilate feelings and help him or her to problem solve, communicating empathy and caring. Treat any underlying psychiatric or medical disorder.

References

Adelman SA, Peterson LG. Assessment of the suicidal patient. In: Greene HL, Glassock RJ, Kelley MA, eds. Introduction to clinical medicine. Philadelphia: BC Decker, 1991:582.

Blumenthal SJ. Suicide: a guide to risk factors, assessment, and treatment of suicidal patients. Med Clin North Am 1988; 72:937.

Roy A. Suicide. In: Kaplan HI, Sadock BJ, eds. Comprehensive textbook of psychiatry. Vol II. 5th ed. Baltimore: Williams & Wilkins, 1989.

Weissman MM, et al. Suicidal ideation and suicide attempts in panic disorder and attacks. N Engl J Med 1989; 312:1209.

SUICIDAL PATIENT

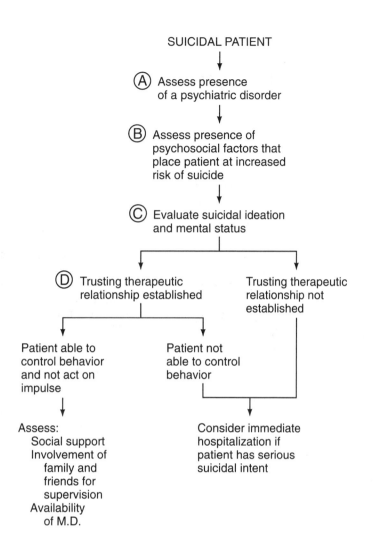

Ⓐ Assess presence
of a psychiatric disorder

Ⓑ Assess presence of
psychosocial factors that
place patient at increased
risk of suicide

Ⓒ Evaluate suicidal ideation
and mental status

Ⓓ Trusting therapeutic
relationship established

Trusting therapeutic
relationship not
established

Patient able to
control behavior
and not act on
impulse

Patient not
able to control
behavior

Assess:
Social support
Involvement of
family and
friends for
supervision
Availability
of M.D.

Consider immediate
hospitalization if
patient has serious
suicidal intent

PHARMACOLOGY

ACUTE ANTICOAGULATION

Michael D. Katz, Pharm.D.
Robert J. Lipsy, Pharm.D.

Thromboembolic disorders and medical procedures that may require anticoagulation therapy include proximal deep venous thrombosis (DVT), pulmonary embolism (PE), atrial fibrillation with embolism, acute myocardial infarction, and placement of mechanical heart valves. In situations of apparent thromboembolic disorders (as opposed to prophylaxis) that are potentially life-threatening (e.g., PE with shock), initiate heparin therapy before performing diagnostic tests.

A. Diagnostic tests vary in sensitivity and specificity. In patients with PE, a high degree of clinical suspicion may necessitate therapy even when the ventilation-perfusion scan is negative.

B. Contraindications to heparin are relative: the risks must be weighed against the potential benefits. In most cases, patients with previous hypersensitivity or heparin-induced thrombocytopenia, active bleeding, intracranial hemorrhage, GI bleeding, hemophilia, thrombocytopenia, severe hypertension, or recent surgery of the brain, spinal cord, or eye should not receive heparin therapy. In PE patients in whom there are contraindications to heparin therapy, consider placement of an inferior vena cava (IVC) filter.

C. In patients with massive PE or those with hemodynamic compromise, consider thrombolytic therapy with streptokinase or urokinase. However, clinical trials have shown no clear advantage of thrombolytic therapy over heparin in patients with venous thromboembolism.

D. Heparin dosages must be based on body weight and the disease being treated. Patients with PE are relatively hypercoagulable and have more rapid heparin clearance. Therefore, they should receive the higher initial bolus and infusion dose. Partial thromboplastin time (PTT) should be checked no sooner than 6 hours after a heparin bolus; PTT checked sooner may be falsely elevated.

(Continued on page 510)

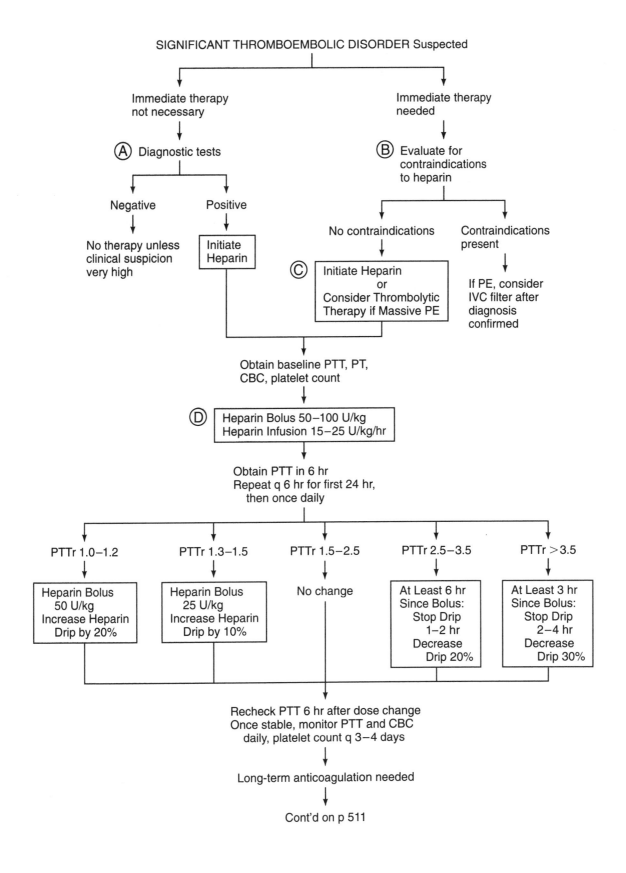

SIGNIFICANT THROMBOEMBOLIC DISORDER Suspected

Immediate therapy not necessary

Immediate therapy needed

Ⓐ Diagnostic tests

Ⓑ Evaluate for contraindications to heparin

Negative

Positive

No contraindications

Contraindications present

No therapy unless clinical suspicion very high

Initiate Heparin

Ⓒ Initiate Heparin or Consider Thrombolytic Therapy if Massive PE

If PE, consider IVC filter after diagnosis confirmed

Obtain baseline PTT, PT, CBC, platelet count

Ⓓ Heparin Bolus 50–100 U/kg
Heparin Infusion 15–25 U/kg/hr

Obtain PTT in 6 hr
Repeat q 6 hr for first 24 hr,
then once daily

PTTr 1.0–1.2

PTTr 1.3–1.5

PTTr 1.5–2.5

PTTr 2.5–3.5

PTTr >3.5

Heparin Bolus
50 U/kg
Increase Heparin
Drip by 20%

Heparin Bolus
25 U/kg
Increase Heparin
Drip by 10%

No change

At Least 6 hr
Since Bolus:
Stop Drip
1–2 hr
Decrease
Drip 20%

At Least 3 hr
Since Bolus:
Stop Drip
2–4 hr
Decrease
Drip 30%

Recheck PTT 6 hr after dose change
Once stable, monitor PTT and CBC
daily, platelet count q 3–4 days

Long-term anticoagulation needed

Cont'd on p 511

E. If long-term anticoagulation is indicated, initiate warfarin as soon as the heparin dose and PTT are stable and therapeutic. The initial dose should be the expected maintenance dose. Early warfarin therapy allows earlier patient discharge. In elderly patients or those who have liver dysfunction or are receiving drugs that inhibit the metabolism of warfarin, the initial dose should be reduced. Administration of larger initial warfarin doses has no pharmacologic rationale and makes subsequent monitoring more difficult. Because the pharmacologic effects of warfarin depend on decreased synthesis of vitamin K–dependent factors and the catabolism of those factors already formed, the effects of a given warfarin dose are not seen for 3–4 days.

F. Continue heparin for at least 4 days after initiation even if the prothrombin time (PT) is in the therapeutic range earlier. Patients are not truly anticoagulated on warfarin until depletion of factors IX and X occurs; early increases of PT are related to depletion of factor VII.

G. Education of the patient and family or caretaker is mandatory with warfarin therapy. Patients must understand the reason for taking the medication, the importance of not changing the brand, possible drug and diet interactions, laboratory monitoring, potential adverse effects, and post-discharge follow-up. If possible, refer patients to an Anticoagulation Clinic for long-term maintenance.

References

Carter BL. Therapy of acute thromboembolism with heparin and warfarin. Clin Pharm 1991; 10:503.

Harrington R, Ansell J. Risk-benefit assessment of anticoagulant therapy. Drug Safety 1991; 6:54.

Hyers TM, Hull RD, Weg JG. Antithrombotic therapy for venous thromboembolic disease. Chest 1989; 95 (Suppl): 37S.

Kelley MA, Carson JL, Palevsky HI, Schwartz JS. Diagnosing pulmonary embolism: new facts and strategies. Ann Intern Med 1991; 114:300.

Mohr DN, Ryu JH, Litin SC, Rosenow EC. Recent advances in the management of venous thromboembolism. Mayo Clin Proc 1988; 63:281.

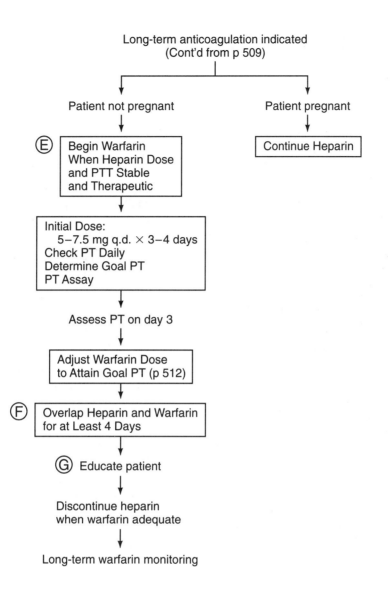

Long-term anticoagulation indicated
(Cont'd from p 509)

Patient not pregnant

(E) Begin Warfarin
When Heparin Dose
and PTT Stable
and Therapeutic

Initial Dose:
  5−7.5 mg q.d. × 3−4 days
Check PT Daily
Determine Goal PT
PT Assay

Assess PT on day 3

Adjust Warfarin Dose
to Attain Goal PT (p 512)

(F) Overlap Heparin and Warfarin
for at Least 4 Days

(G) Educate patient

Discontinue heparin
when warfarin adequate

Long-term warfarin monitoring

Patient pregnant

Continue Heparin

LONG-TERM ANTICOAGULATION

Michael D. Katz, Pharm.D.

A. Contraindications to long-term anticoagulant therapy include those listed under acute anticoagulation (p 508), as well as patients who are severely debilitated and malnourished, those who fall or undergo significant trauma, alcoholics, and those who are unlikely to understand or comply with therapy. As always, the risk-benefit ratio must be considered.

B. Patients with recurrent thromboembolism on warfarin therapy should first be evaluated for compliance and adequacy of anticoagulation. If low-intensity anticoagulation was used, consider high-intensity therapy with a prothrombin time ratio, measured control (PTr), of 1.5–2.0. Alternatively, consider twice daily subcutaneous heparin therapy. In patients with frequent recurrences of thromboembolism, consider the presence of malignancy or other hypercoagulable state.

C. Most thromboembolic disorders require low-intensity warfarin therapy. In most settings, the therapeutic PTr is 1.3–1.5. However, determination of a therapeutic range is complicated by the differing sensitivities of the various PT assays available. The sensitivity of a given assay is determined by the international sensitivity index (ISI). The published low-intensity PT range is based on an ISI of 2.4; the clinician therefore must know the ISI of the assay being used. In an attempt to standardize for different assays, the international normalized ratio (INR) may be calculated. For low-intensity therapy, the therapeutic INR is 2.0–3.0; for high-intensity therapy, the desired INR is 3.0–4.5. The INR may be calculated using the following formula:

$$INR = \frac{PT \text{ (observed)}}{PT \text{ (control)}}$$

D. Tailor outpatient monitoring of warfarin therapy to the patient. Frequent monitoring is needed as therapy is titrated; less frequent visits are adequate as the patient becomes stable. The use of flow sheets facilitates monitoring of doses and PTr. At each visit, review patient education information.

E. If the PTr is not in the therapeutic range, evaluate the patient for noncompliance or interacting drugs. If these factors are identified and corrected, continue the previous warfarin dose. In previously stable patients with minor deviations of the PT, the dose should be maintained and the PT rechecked in 1 week. If a dosage change is necessary, it should be relatively small; alteration of the weekly dose by 15–20% is adequate in most cases. When the PT is extremely high, warfarin should be held and therapy with vitamin K or fresh frozen plasma considered if the patient is bleeding. With any dosage change, recheck the PT in 3 days if a major change is made or in 1–2 weeks with minor dose adjustments.

F. The duration of anticoagulant therapy is determined by the underlying disease and risk of recurrent thromboembolism. For patients with a first deep venous thrombosis (DVT) or pulmonary embolism (PE), 3–6 months of therapy is adequate. However, in patients with recurrent DVT or PE, atrial fibrillation with embolism or mechanical valves will require long-term therapy.

G. Bleeding complications may occur in the presence of excessive or therapeutic anticoagulation. In any case, if there is a significant bleeding episode, re-evaluate the need for anticoagulation. If the PT is excessive and anticoagulation is still needed, adjust the dose. If the PT is therapeutic, discontinue warfarin and consider alternative therapy. With episodes of GI bleeding or hematuria and a therapeutic PT, consider a diagnostic work-up for a GI or urinary tract lesion.

References

Carter BL. Therapy of acute thromboembolism with heparin and warfarin. Clin Pharm 1991; 10:503.

Hirsh J, Poller L, Deykin D, et al. Optimal therapeutic range for oral anticoagulants. Chest 1989; 95 (Suppl):5S.

Levine MN, Raskob G, Hirsh J. Hemorrhagic complications of long-term anticoagulation. Chest 1989; 95 (Suppl):26S.

Stults BM, Dere WH, Caine TH. Long-term anticoagulation: indications and management. West J Med 1989; 151:414.

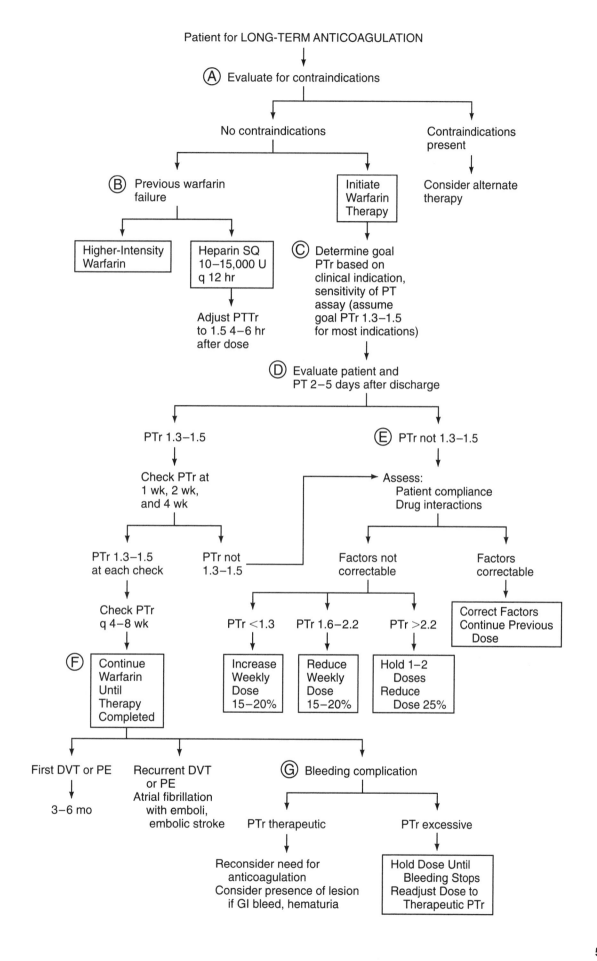

Patient for LONG-TERM ANTICOAGULATION

Ⓐ Evaluate for contraindications

No contraindications

Contraindications present

Consider alternate therapy

Ⓑ Previous warfarin failure

Initiate Warfarin Therapy

Higher-Intensity Warfarin

Heparin SQ 10–15,000 U q 12 hr

Adjust PTTr to 1.5 4–6 hr after dose

Ⓒ Determine goal PTr based on clinical indication, sensitivity of PT assay (assume goal PTr 1.3–1.5 for most indications)

Ⓓ Evaluate patient and PT 2–5 days after discharge

PTr 1.3–1.5

Ⓔ PTr not 1.3–1.5

Check PTr at 1 wk, 2 wk, and 4 wk

Assess:
Patient compliance
Drug interactions

PTr 1.3–1.5 at each check

PTr not 1.3–1.5

Factors not correctable

Factors correctable

Check PTr q 4–8 wk

PTr <1.3

PTr 1.6–2.2

PTr >2.2

Correct Factors Continue Previous Dose

Ⓕ Continue Warfarin Until Therapy Completed

Increase Weekly Dose 15–20%

Reduce Weekly Dose 15–20%

Hold 1–2 Doses Reduce Dose 25%

First DVT or PE

Recurrent DVT or PE
Atrial fibrillation with emboli, embolic stroke

Ⓖ Bleeding complication

3–6 mo

PTr therapeutic

PTr excessive

Reconsider need for anticoagulation
Consider presence of lesion if GI bleed, hematuria

Hold Dose Until Bleeding Stops Readjust Dose to Therapeutic PTr

513

ANAPHYLAXIS

Michael D. Katz, Pharm.D.

The common signs and symptoms of anaphylaxis include an aura, rhinitis, cough, pruritus, urticaria, laryngeal edema, generalized edema, decreased sensorium, shock, bronchospasm, GI cramps, and vomiting. Rarely, patients may develop heart failure, pulmonary edema, and disseminated intravascular coagulation. Other conditions such as vasovagal reactions, hyperventilation, globus hystericus, and hereditary angioedema may mimic aspects of anaphylaxis and should be ruled out before aggressive therapy is initiated.

A. Anaphylaxis can be caused by a variety of agents such as drugs (beta-lactam antibiotics, sulfonamides, anesthetics, chymopapain, protamine, dextran, radiocontrast media), foreign proteins such as animal sera, desensitization sera and blood products, foods, bees from the Hymenoptera order, and latex. In any patient with anaphylaxis, obtain a complete exposure history, including any previous reactions.

B. Local reactions usually consist of redness, swelling, and pain at the site of injection. Systemic signs and symptoms may develop rapidly. Measures to slow absorption of the antigen from the injection site, such as application of ice or use of a venous- (not arterial) occluding tourniquet, may be useful in the field until the patient reaches medical attention.

C. Base the initial management of anaphylaxis on support of vital signs. Place all patients in the Trendelenburg position and give supplemental oxygen. In patients with cardiac or respiratory arrest or serious arrhythmias, initiate basic and advanced cardiac life support measures.

D. Epinephrine is the mainstay of therapy for anaphylaxis; no other drug has proved as effective. Epinephrine reverses the effects of the mediators of anaphylaxis and may reduce the further release of these mediators. In most adults, give 0.3 ml of 1:1000 solution by subcutaneous (SQ) injection (in children, the dose is 0.01 ml/kg). However, if the patient is in shock, epinephrine should be given through a central vein or instilled into the endotracheal tube. If the desired response is not achieved and no adverse effects occur, repeat epinephrine in 10 minutes. Monitor elderly patients, especially those with underlying cardiac disease, very closely.

(Continued on page 516)

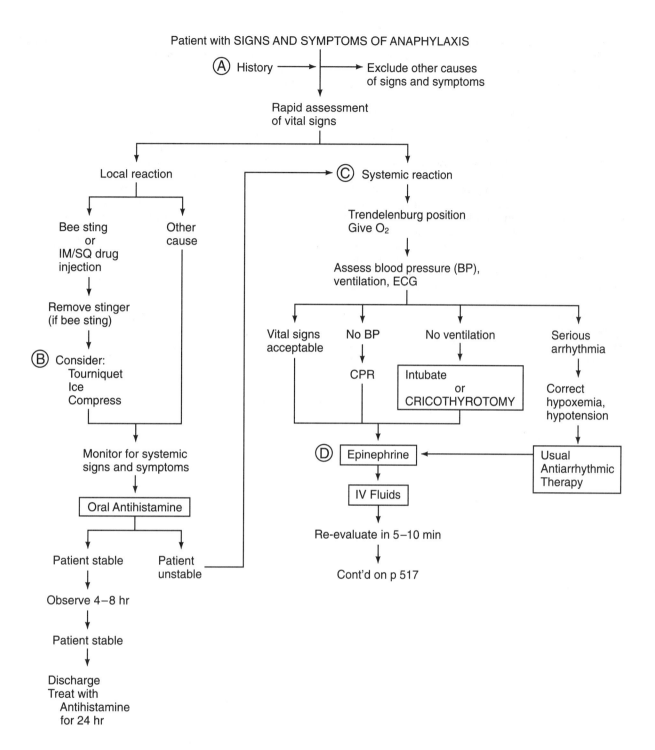

Patient with SIGNS AND SYMPTOMS OF ANAPHYLAXIS

(A) History → Exclude other causes of signs and symptoms

Rapid assessment of vital signs

Local reaction

Bee sting or IM/SQ drug injection

Other cause

Remove stinger (if bee sting)

(B) Consider:
Tourniquet
Ice
Compress

Monitor for systemic signs and symptoms

Oral Antihistamine

Patient stable

Patient unstable

Observe 4–8 hr

Patient stable

Discharge
Treat with
Antihistamine
for 24 hr

(C) **Systemic reaction**

Trendelenburg position
Give O₂

Assess blood pressure (BP), ventilation, ECG

Vital signs acceptable

No BP

CPR

No ventilation

Intubate or CRICOTHYROTOMY

Serious arrhythmia

Correct hypoxemia, hypotension

Usual Antiarrhythmic Therapy

(D) Epinephrine

IV Fluids

Re-evaluate in 5–10 min

Cont'd on p 517

E. In patients with severe bronchospasm, epinephrine and inhaled β_2 agonists (albuterol, metaproterenol) are the most effective treatment. There is no evidence that IV theophylline is effective in the treatment of acute, severe bronchospasm, and it may increase the risk of cardiac arrhythmias. However, in a patient with refractory bronchospasm, a loading dose of theophylline (5 mg/kg aminophylline) may be administered.

F. Corticosteroids and antihistamines, although commonly used to treat anaphylaxis, have not been shown to relieve symptoms or improve outcome. Theoretically, corticosteroids may help prevent further mast cell degranulation and prolonged symptoms. The onset of action of corticosteroids is at least 4–6 hours; therefore, use them only as secondary therapy. An initial IV dose of 50–100 mg methylprednisolone may be followed in 6 hours with oral prednisone. Since the major signs and symptoms of anaphylaxis are not histamine mediated, there is little rationale for administration of antihistamines such as diphenhydramine. These agents may be useful in relieving pruritus. While there are cases of refractory anaphylaxis responding to the H_2 blocker cimetidine, there is no evidence to support routine use of this agent.

G. Instruct all patients with anaphylaxis in ways to avoid future exposure to the inciting agent. The cause of the episode, if known, should be clearly documented in the patient's medical record, especially in drug-induced anaphylaxis.

H. In some instances, specific preventive therapy may be indicated. Consider patients with bee sting allergy who cannot easily avoid future exposures for desensitization. In patients with frequently recurrent idiopathic anaphylaxis, prophylactic therapy with corticosteroids and antihistamines has proved effective. Autoinjectors containing epinephrine may also be used by the patient at risk for another serious reaction.

References

Corren J, Schocket AL. Anaphylaxis, a preventable emergency. Postgrad Med 1990; 87:167.

Fisher M. Anaphylaxis Dis Man. 1987; 33:433.

Wong S, Yarnold PR, Yango C, et al. Outcome of prophylactic therapy for idiopathic anaphylaxis. Ann Intern Med 1991; 114:133.

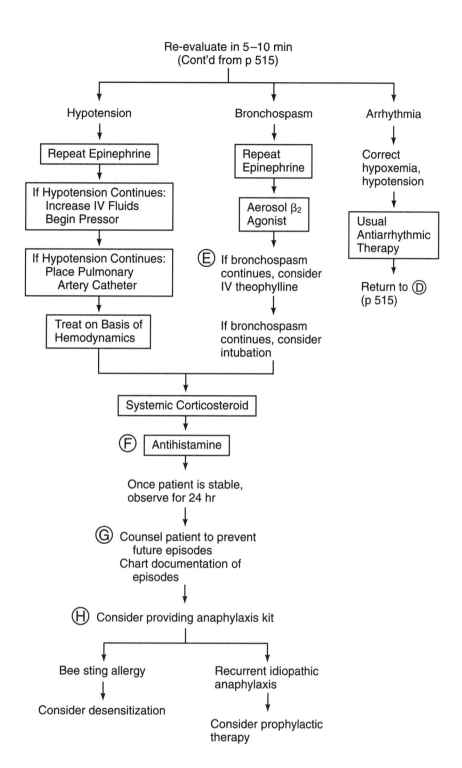

Re-evaluate in 5–10 min
(Cont'd from p 515)

Hypotension

Repeat Epinephrine

If Hypotension Continues:
Increase IV Fluids
Begin Pressor

If Hypotension Continues:
Place Pulmonary
Artery Catheter

Treat on Basis of
Hemodynamics

Bronchospasm

Repeat
Epinephrine

Aerosol β₂
Agonist

Ⓔ If bronchospasm
continues, consider
IV theophylline

If bronchospasm
continues, consider
intubation

Arrhythmia

Correct
hypoxemia,
hypotension

Usual
Antiarrhythmic
Therapy

Return to Ⓓ
(p 515)

Systemic Corticosteroid

Ⓕ Antihistamine

Once patient is stable,
observe for 24 hr

Ⓖ Counsel patient to prevent
future episodes
Chart documentation of
episodes

Ⓗ Consider providing anaphylaxis kit

Bee sting allergy

Consider desensitization

Recurrent idiopathic
anaphylaxis

Consider prophylactic
therapy

ADVERSE DRUG REACTIONS

Robert J. Lipsy, Pharm.D.

An adverse drug reaction (ADR) is any response to a drug that is noxious and unintended and that occurs at doses used in humans for prophylaxis, diagnosis, or treatment, excluding failure to accomplish its intended purpose. Drugs frequently contribute to the occurrence of iatrogenic diseases, which in turn may generate as many as one in every 40 physician consultations. The incidence of ADRs has been estimated at 1–28% on the basis of various surveys, and ADRs are responsible for 2.9–6.2% of all hospital admissions. In the Boston Collaborative Surveillance Program, 5–10% of reactions were rated as having major severity, and fatal ADRs were calculated at 0.31%. FDA records show an increased risk for the elderly, with patients >60 accounting for nearly half of ADR-associated deaths. Accurate assessment of a possible adverse effect has an important impact both on the morbidity of the reaction and on the appropriate treatment of the original condition requiring drug therapy.

A. Establishing a temporal association is often the most difficult part of the evaluation. Most ADRs manifest within the first day or two of treatment, and nearly all by the second week of therapy. The temporal relationship is drug, patient, and reaction specific. To establish a clear-cut temporal relationship, compare the time of onset of the reaction with that expected based on previous reported reactions or the known or proposed pathophysiologic mechanism. If the reaction has not been seen with the suspected drug, compare similar agents or drugs within the same class. Take into account patient specificity: e.g., type I hypersensitivity reactions may be immediate in nature in a previously exposed patient, or delayed 5–10 days in a naive patient.

B. If possible, the suspected drug should be discontinued or held or the dose reduced, depending on the type of reaction. Cross reactivity with drugs of similar structure or agents in the same class may occur; these should be avoided.

C. Like the onset of a reaction, resolution varies according to the specific nature of the reaction and the patient. Be aware that some adverse reactions, such as ototoxicity from aminoglycosides or nephrotoxicity from amphotericin B, may resolve only after long periods or may have permanent sequelae.

D. Rechallenge should not be undertaken unless the benefits outweigh the risks and should not be used merely to confirm the association between the ADR and the suspected drug. Be aware that there may be a different manifestation of the adverse reaction upon rechallenge, particularly in cases of allergic reactions. These changes may be in the temporal relationship or in the severity of the reaction.

E. Various clinical conditions can affect one or multiple organ systems, causing signs and symptoms resembling a wide spectrum of adverse drug effects. When a temporal relationship or resolution of the ADR is unclear or when discontinuation of a drug or rechallenge does not occur, the association between a suspected adverse effect and the drug can be made less clear by these conditions. If the suspected reaction has been previously reported with the drug, a stronger association may be implied. Less common adverse drug reactions of newly marketed drugs (<3 years) may not be known, as these drugs are often tested in fewer than 2000 patients before FDA approval. Contacting the manufacturer or the FDA may be the only way to determine whether an adverse reaction has been previously reported.

References

Jick H. Adverse drug reactions: the magnitude of the problem. J Allergy Clin Immunol 1984; 74:555.

McQueen K. ADR monitoring: rationale, impact and cost issues. Cal J Hosp Pharm 1990; 2:5.

Middleton RK. Hospital-based adverse drug reaction reporting and evaluation. Cal J Hosp Pharm 1990; 2:7.

Miller RR. Drug surveillance utilizing epidemiologic methods. A report from the Boston Collaborative Drug Surveillance Program. Am J Hosp Pharm 1973; 30:584.

Patterson R. Early recognition of allergic reactions to new drugs. J Allergy Clin Immunol 1984; 74:641.

Patient with POSSIBLE ADVERSE DRUG REACTION

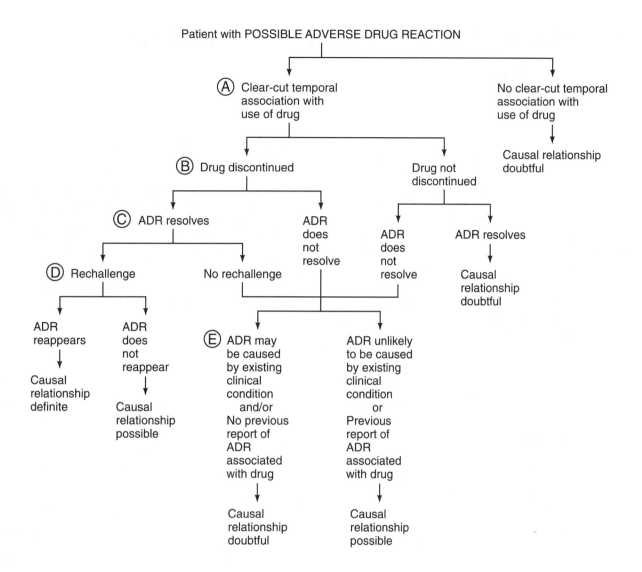

(A) Clear-cut temporal association with use of drug

No clear-cut temporal association with use of drug

Causal relationship doubtful

(B) Drug discontinued

Drug not discontinued

(C) ADR resolves

ADR does not resolve

ADR does not resolve

ADR resolves

Causal relationship doubtful

(D) Rechallenge

No rechallenge

ADR reappears

ADR does not reappear

Causal relationship definite

Causal relationship possible

(E) ADR may be caused by existing clinical condition and/or No previous report of ADR associated with drug

ADR unlikely to be caused by existing clinical condition or Previous report of ADR associated with drug

Causal relationship doubtful

Causal relationship possible

NONSURGICAL ANTIMICROBIAL PROPHYLAXIS

Brian L. Erstad, Pharm.D.
Collin Freeman, Pharm.D.

A. Patients undergoing surgery who require bacterial endocarditis prophylaxis include those with prosthetic valves, previous bacterial endocarditis, congenital cardiac malformations, acquired valvular dysfunction, hypertrophic cardiomyopathy, and mitral valve prolapse with valvular regurgitation.

B. Dental procedures in which prophylaxis is indicated include those known to cause gingival or mucosal bleeding, including cleaning. Surgical procedures in which prophylaxis may be required include tonsillectomy and adenoidectomy, bronchoscopy performed with a rigid bronchoscope, sclerotherapy performed for esophageal varices, surgical procedures involving mucosa of the respiratory or intestinal tracts, gallbladder surgery, cystoscopy, urethral dilatation, urethral catheterization or urinary tract surgery in a patient with a urinary tract infection, prostate surgery, vaginal hysterectomy, vaginal delivery with an infection of the birth canal, and incision and drainage of infected tissue.

C. Prophylaxis against *Pneumocystis carinii* pneumonia (PCP) is given to HIV-positive patients who have a history of PCP, a CD4 cell count <200, or a CD4 cell count that is <20% of the total lymphocyte count. Consult the most recent Centers for Disease Control (CDC) guidelines.

D. Traveler's diarrhea is likely in persons traveling to countries where hygiene is poor. Most diarrhea is self-limiting. It is best to avoid foods that are not fully cooked and unboiled water (even ice) in underdeveloped countries. If medications are used, they should be continued for the duration of the trip and 2 days to 2 weeks after leaving the underdeveloped country.

E. Influenza prophylaxis is given in the fall and winter months to high-risk contacts, patients with chronic illness, the elderly, and immunocompromised patients.

F. Consult the most recent CDC guidelines for malaria prophylaxis.

G. Indications for patients requiring tuberculosis prophylaxis include a close contact to a person with known active tuberculosis of <2 months previously. A second indication would be in a patient with a recent skin test (<2 years) that has now converted to positive, being 10 mm induration or greater. Finally, a skin test that has been positive for an unknown length of time in a patient who also is immunocompromised or shows positive lesions on chest films indicates prophylaxis.

References

ASHP Commission on Therapeutics. ASHP therapeutic guidelines on nonsurgical antimicrobial prophylaxis. Clin Pharm 1990; 9:423.

Centers for Disease Control. Guidelines for prophylaxis against *Pneumocystis carinii* pneumonia for persons infected with human immunodeficiency virus. MMWR 1989; 262 (Suppl 5):335.

Dajani AS, Bisno AL, Chung KJ, et al. Prevention of bacterial endocarditis: recommendations by the American Heart Association. JAMA 1990; 264:2919.

Douglas RG. Prophylaxis and treatment of influenza. N Engl J Med 1990; 322:443.

Drugs for parasitic infections. Med Lett Drugs Ther 1990; 32:23.

Drugs for tuberculosis. Med Lett Drugs Ther 1988; 30:43.

Hughes WT, Bodey GP, Feld R, et al. Guidelines for the use of antimicrobial agents in neutropenic patients with unexplained fever. J Infect Dis 1990; 161:381.

Suavez J, Salamon FR. Management and prevention of bacterial diarrhea. Clin Pharm 1988; 7:746.

Wilhelm MP, Edson RS. Antimicrobial agents in urinary tract infections. Mayo Clin Proc 1987; 62:1025.

NONSURGICAL ANTIMICROBIAL PROPHYLAXIS

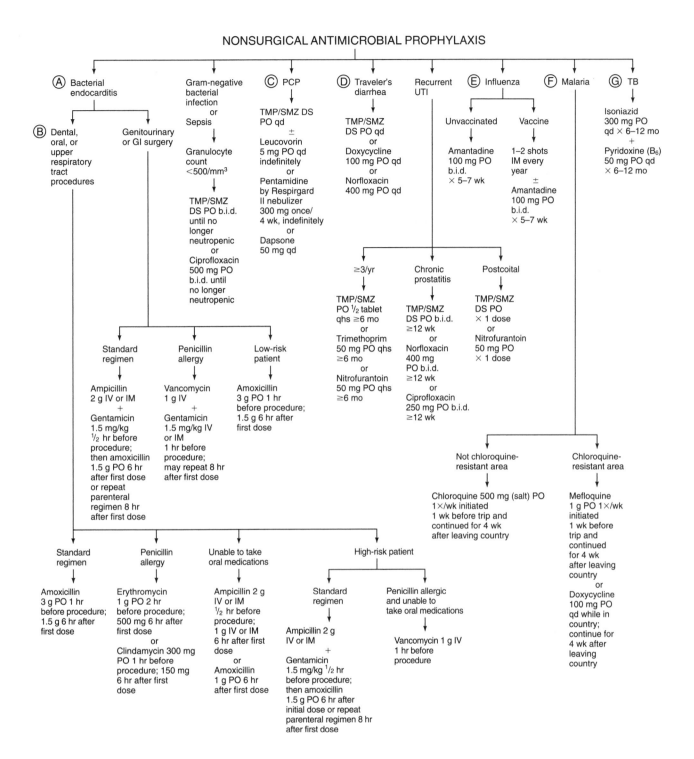

Ⓐ Bacterial endocarditis

Ⓑ Dental, oral, or upper respiratory tract procedures

Genitourinary or GI surgery

Gram-negative bacterial infection or Sepsis

Granulocyte count <500/mm³

TMP/SMZ DS PO b.i.d. until no longer neutropenic or Ciprofloxacin 500 mg PO b.i.d. until no longer neutropenic

Ⓒ PCP

TMP/SMZ DS PO qd ± Leucovorin 5 mg PO qd indefinitely or Pentamidine by Respirgard II nebulizer 300 mg once/ 4 wk, indefinitely or Dapsone 50 mg qd

Ⓓ Traveler's diarrhea

TMP/SMZ DS PO qd or Doxycycline 100 mg PO qd or Norfloxacin 400 mg PO qd

Recurrent UTI

≥3/yr

TMP/SMZ PO ½ tablet qhs ≥6 mo or Trimethoprim 50 mg PO qhs ≥6 mo or Nitrofurantoin 50 mg PO qhs ≥6 mo

Chronic prostatitis

TMP/SMZ DS PO b.i.d. ≥12 wk or Norfloxacin 400 mg PO b.i.d. ≥12 wk or Ciprofloxacin 250 mg PO b.i.d. ≥12 wk

Postcoital

TMP/SMZ DS PO × 1 dose or Nitrofurantoin 50 mg PO × 1 dose

Ⓔ Influenza

Unvaccinated

Amantadine 100 mg PO b.i.d. × 5–7 wk

Vaccine

1–2 shots IM every year ± Amantadine 100 mg PO b.i.d. × 5–7 wk

Ⓕ Malaria

Not chloroquine-resistant area

Chloroquine 500 mg (salt) PO 1×/wk initiated 1 wk before trip and continued for 4 wk after leaving country

Chloroquine-resistant area

Mefloquine 1 g PO 1×/wk initiated 1 wk before trip and continued for 4 wk after leaving country or Doxycycline 100 mg PO qd while in country; continue for 4 wk after leaving country

Ⓖ TB

Isoniazid 300 mg PO qd × 6–12 mo + Pyridoxine (B₆) 50 mg PO qd × 6–12 mo

Standard regimen

Ampicillin 2 g IV or IM + Gentamicin 1.5 mg/kg ½ hr before procedure; then amoxicillin 1.5 g PO 6 hr after first dose or repeat parenteral regimen 8 hr after first dose

Penicillin allergy

Vancomycin 1 g IV + Gentamicin 1.5 mg/kg IV or IM 1 hr before procedure; may repeat 8 hr after first dose

Low-risk patient

Amoxicillin 3 g PO 1 hr before procedure; 1.5 g 6 hr after first dose

Standard regimen

Amoxicillin 3 g PO 1 hr before procedure; 1.5 g 6 hr after first dose

Penicillin allergy

Erythromycin 1 g PO 2 hr before procedure; 500 mg 6 hr after first dose or Clindamycin 300 mg PO 1 hr before procedure; 150 mg 6 hr after first dose

Unable to take oral medications

Ampicillin 2 g IV or IM ½ hr before procedure; 1 g IV or IM 6 hr after first dose or Amoxicillin 1 g PO 6 hr after first dose

High-risk patient

Standard regimen

Ampicillin 2 g IV or IM + Gentamicin 1.5 mg/kg ½ hr before procedure; then amoxicillin 1.5 g PO 6 hr after initial dose or repeat parenteral regimen 8 hr after first dose

Penicillin allergic and unable to take oral medications

Vancomycin 1 g IV 1 hr before procedure

ANTIMICROBIAL PROPHYLAXIS IN SURGICAL PATIENTS

Brian L. Erstad, Pharm.D.

A. A classification system for expected postoperative wound infection rates related to surgical procedures was developed by the National Academy of Sciences–National Research Council in the 1960s. This system categorized surgery as clean (Cl), clean-contaminated (CC), unknown contamination (UC), contaminated (CO), or dirty (D), depending on associated infection rates; rates of infection are generally less than 2% for clean and approximately 40% for dirty procedures. However, infection rates for the same operation may vary at different institutions; physician- and institution-specific rates should be recorded and used in the consideration of prophylaxis. Treatment, not prophylaxis, is needed for contaminated or dirty surgical procedures, as well as complicated trauma (e.g., colon injury with delayed surgery).

B. Do not base the decision to use antimicrobial prophylaxis solely on postoperative wound infection rates. Total hip replacement is classified as a clean operative procedure according to criteria developed by the National Academy of Sciences–National Research Council, but a postoperative infection of the prosthesis may be catastrophic. Hence, a clinically significant decrease in the incidence of an unacceptable complication may be sufficient justification for prophylaxis. Such justification is often used for the prophylaxis of bacterial endocarditis.

C. Cefazolin is the standard with which other antimicrobials should be compared for most surgical procedures. Cefazolin is inexpensive, has a moderately long half-life, has a spectrum against most predominant pathogens, and has demonstrated activity in clinical trials. Vancomycin, 1 g IV, may be used in hospitals where methicillin-resistant *Staphylococcus* is a problem.

D. Cefoxitin (or oral agents in the case of colorectal operations) is used when anaerobes, in particular *Bacteroides fragilis,* are expected pathogens. Other agents such as cefotetan have been substituted for cefoxitin, although in vivo supporting data are limited. Give IV antimicrobials within 30 minutes of the first incision to ensure adequate concentrations. Additional doses of the antimicrobial may be needed during extended procedures, depending on its pharmacokinetic properties: e.g., a second dose of cefazolin should be given 4 hours and cefoxitin 2 hours from the start of an operation. With the possible exceptions of coronary bypass and arthroplastic procedures, there is little benefit from antibiotic administration beyond 24 hours after surgery. Some studies have shown efficacy when single preoperative doses were administered. Recommended dosages are listed in Table 1.

TABLE 1 Drug Dosages for Surgical Antimicrobial Prophylaxis

Cefazolin	1 g IV q8h
Cefoxitin	1 g IV q6h
Vancomycin	1 g IV q12h
Clindamycin	300 mg IV q8h
Gentamicin	1.7 mg/kg IV q8h
Penicillin	1 million units IV q4h
Erythromycin	1 g PO × 3 doses*
Neomycin	1 g PO × 3 doses*

*Give at 1 PM, 2 PM, and 11 PM the day before surgery.

References

Antimicrobial prophylaxis in surgery. Med Lett Drugs Ther 1989; 31:105.

Burnakis TG. Surgical antimicrobial prophylaxis: principles and guidelines. Pharmacotherapy 1984; 4:248.

Cruse PJE, Foord R. A five-year prospective study of 23,649 surgical wounds. Arch Surg 1973; 107:206.

Kaiser AB. Antimicrobial prophylaxis in surgery. N Engl J Med 1986; 315:1129.

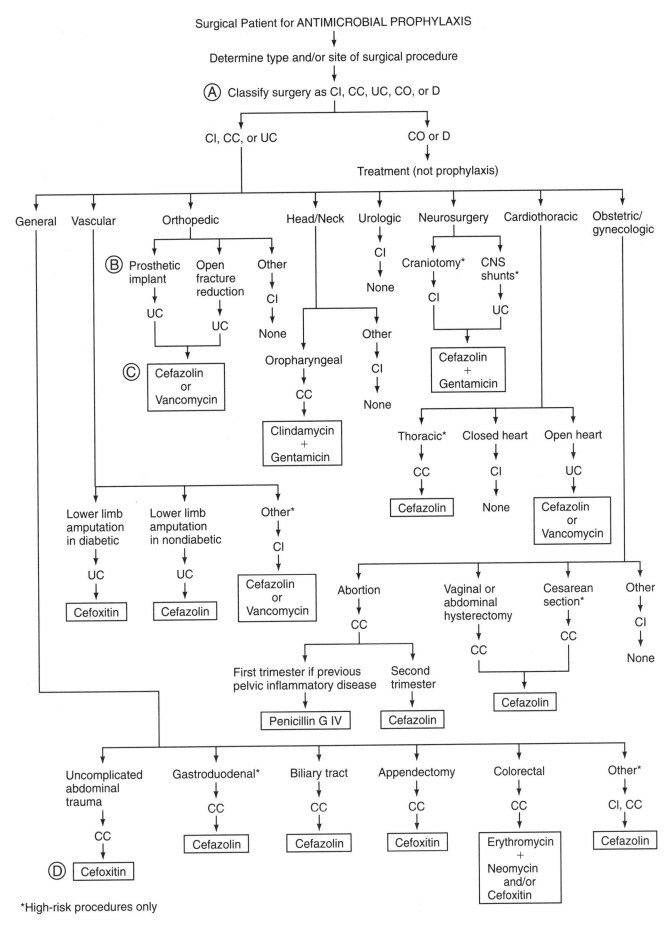

Surgical Patient for ANTIMICROBIAL PROPHYLAXIS

Determine type and/or site of surgical procedure

(A) Classify surgery as CI, CC, UC, CO, or D

CI, CC, or UC

CO or D

Treatment (not prophylaxis)

General   Vascular   Orthopedic   Head/Neck   Urologic   Neurosurgery   Cardiothoracic   Obstetric/gynecologic

(B) Prosthetic implant   Open fracture reduction   Other

UC

UC

(C) Cefazolin or Vancomycin

CI

None

Oropharyngeal

CC

Clindamycin + Gentamicin

CI

None

Other

CI

None

Craniotomy*   CNS shunts*

CI

UC

Cefazolin + Gentamicin

Thoracic*   Closed heart   Open heart

CC

CI

UC

Cefazolin

None

Cefazolin or Vancomycin

Lower limb amputation in diabetic   Lower limb amputation in nondiabetic   Other*

UC

UC

CI

Cefoxitin

Cefazolin

Cefazolin or Vancomycin

Abortion   Vaginal or abdominal hysterectomy   Cesarean section*   Other

CC

CC

CC

CI

First trimester if previous pelvic inflammatory disease   Second trimester

Cefazolin

None

Penicillin G IV

Cefazolin

Uncomplicated abdominal trauma   Gastroduodenal*   Biliary tract   Appendectomy   Colorectal   Other*

CC

CC

CC

CC

CC

CI, CC

(D) Cefoxitin

Cefazolin

Cefazolin

Cefoxitin

Erythromycin + Neomycin and/or Cefoxitin

Cefazolin

*High-risk procedures only

523

CHOOSING APPROPRIATE ANTIMICROBIAL THERAPY

Michael D. Katz, Pharm.D.

The choice of appropriate antimicrobial therapy should be based on several factors, including pathogens being treated, the antimicrobial spectrum, and a variety of patient-specific factors. Antibiotic choices should be based on a sound rationale.

A. Empiric therapy is based on a presumptive diagnosis of infection or clinical syndrome. Especially in the hospital setting, empiric therapy is broad in spectrum, designed to cover the most likely pathogens in the specific patient. Before initiating empiric therapy, obtain appropriate specimens for culture and sensitivity. Empiric therapy is indicated when the infection is potentially rapidly life threatening (sepsis, pneumonia) or causes significant morbidity (urinary tract infection, otitis media).

B. The most likely pathogens at a site of infection may be based on normal flora at that site, tropism of certain pathogens for various tissues or organs, and patient-specific factors such as previous antimicrobial therapy, nosocomial versus community-acquired infection, and patient immune status. Not every possible pathogen requires coverage: just those that are most likely.

C. Patient-specific factors include history of previous adverse reactions to antimicrobials, patient age, pregnancy or lactation, concomitant drugs, excretory organ function, immune status, and site of infection. For very ill patients, IV administration is preferable to ensure adequate drug concentrations at the site of infection.

D. Combination therapy is indicated when broad-spectrum coverage is desired (sepsis), in polymicrobial infections (intraperitoneal abscesses), to prevent the emergence of resistance (tuberculosis), or to provide antimicrobial synergy (streptococcal endocarditis, beta-lactam/aminoglycoside for *Pseudomonas aeruginosa* infections, amphotericin/5- flucytosine for cryptococcal meningitis).

E. The cost of drug therapy is based not only on the drug cost but on the cost of administration, supplies, and monitoring. If all else is equal, choose the least expensive regimen. However, therapeutic efficacy is of primary importance.

F. Definitive therapy occurs when a microbiologic as well as a clinical diagnosis is confirmed. Definitive therapy is narrow in spectrum and generally requires only one drug. If the patient was previously receiving empiric therapy, determine the need for continued treatment.

G. Sensitivity data is useful in determining definitive data, but there are certain pitfalls. If the reported sensitivities do not fit usual patterns for that organism, the reliability of the information is suspect. If minimal inhibitory concentrations (MICs) are present, in general, any drug in the sensitive MIC range will be effective.

H. Even with positive cultures, broad-spectrum therapy may be indicated. Base the choice of antimicrobial regimen on clinical judgment as well as laboratory data.

I. A variety of drug-specific factors must be considered. Certain agents do not penetrate well into certain tissues (aminoglycosides in CNS infections). If a relatively new antimicrobial is considered, there should be clinical trials documenting efficacy compared with the conventional regimen for that infection. Consider drug toxicity; reserve more toxic drugs (aminoglycosides, amphotericin B) for higher-risk patients.

J. If the patient is not very ill and has adequate GI tract function, give oral antimicrobials as soon as possible. However, in some cases, long-term or home IV antimicrobial therapy is indicated if oral agents are not available for the specific infection.

References

Guglielmo BJ, Brooks GF. Antimicrobial therapy: cost-benefit considerations. Drugs 1989; 38:473.

Kim JH, Gallis HA. Observations on spiraling empiricism: its causes, allure, and perils with particular reference to antibiotic therapy. Am J Med 1989; 87:201.

Moellering RC. Principles of anti-infective therapy. In: Mandell GL, Douglas RG, Bennet JE. Principles and practice of infectious diseases. 3rd ed. New York: Churchill Livingstone, 1990:206.

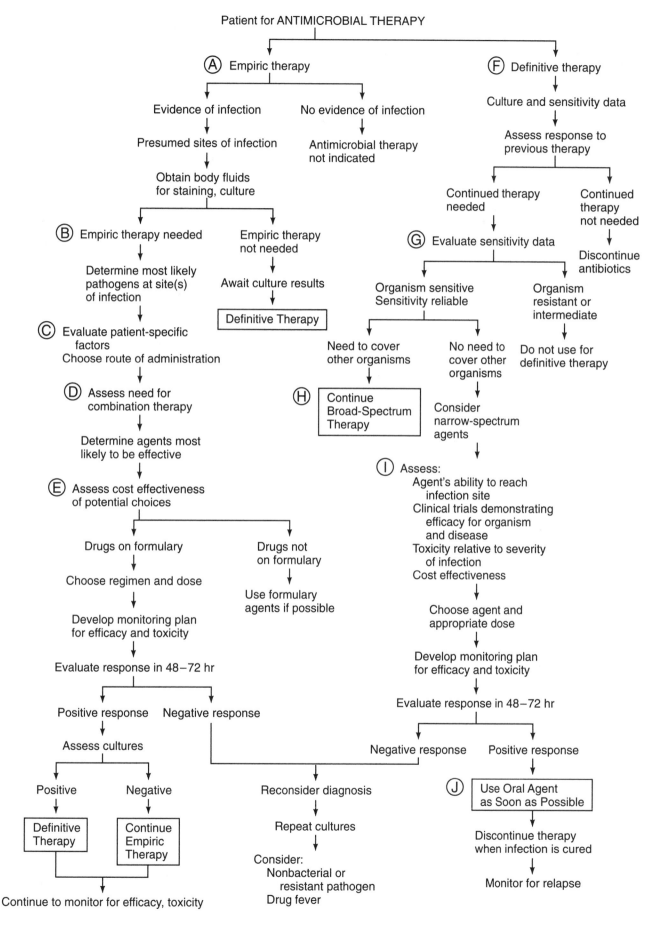

Patient for ANTIMICROBIAL THERAPY

(A) Empiric therapy

Evidence of infection → Presumed sites of infection → Obtain body fluids for staining, culture

No evidence of infection → Antimicrobial therapy not indicated

(B) Empiric therapy needed → Determine most likely pathogens at site(s) of infection

(C) Evaluate patient-specific factors
Choose route of administration

(D) Assess need for combination therapy → Determine agents most likely to be effective

(E) Assess cost effectiveness of potential choices

Empiric therapy not needed → Await culture results → Definitive Therapy

Drugs on formulary → Choose regimen and dose → Develop monitoring plan for efficacy and toxicity → Evaluate response in 48–72 hr

Drugs not on formulary → Use formulary agents if possible

Positive response → Assess cultures
Positive → Definitive Therapy
Negative → Continue Empiric Therapy
Continue to monitor for efficacy, toxicity

Negative response → Reconsider diagnosis → Repeat cultures → Consider:
Nonbacterial or resistant pathogen
Drug fever

(F) Definitive therapy → Culture and sensitivity data → Assess response to previous therapy

Continued therapy needed → (G) Evaluate sensitivity data

Continued therapy not needed → Discontinue antibiotics

Organism sensitive
Sensitivity reliable

Organism resistant or intermediate → Do not use for definitive therapy

Need to cover other organisms → (H) Continue Broad-Spectrum Therapy

No need to cover other organisms → Consider narrow-spectrum agents

(I) Assess:
Agent's ability to reach infection site
Clinical trials demonstrating efficacy for organism and disease
Toxicity relative to severity of infection
Cost effectiveness

Choose agent and appropriate dose → Develop monitoring plan for efficacy and toxicity → Evaluate response in 48–72 hr

Negative response

Positive response → (J) Use Oral Agent as Soon as Possible → Discontinue therapy when infection is cured → Monitor for relapse

525

HISTORY OF HYPERSENSITIVITY TO BETA-LACTAM ANTIBIOTICS

Michael D. Katz, Pharm.D.

A. Beta-lactam antibiotics (penicillins, cephalosporins, monobactams, carbapenems) are widely prescribed agents for a variety of infections. Many patients relate a history of an "allergy" to one of these agents. Decide whether this history of a previous reaction requires a change in therapy. It is important to obtain a detailed history of the type of reaction (immediate hypersensitivity, skin rash), the specific drug involved, and when the reaction occurred.

B. Immediate hypersensitivity reactions, especially anaphylaxis, are the most severe immunologically mediated reactions. The overall incidence of anaphylaxis due to penicillin is 0.01%, with a fatality rate of 9%. Urticarial reactions occur in 4.5% of patients with no history of previous hypersensitivity. The cross allergenicity among beta-lactam agents (i.e., risk of reaction from cephalosporin with previous penicillin allergy) is not known. Widely quoted figures of 5–10% are not based on scientific studies of modern beta-lactam agents. The risks are probably drug- and patient-specific. Aztreonam, a monobactam, does not appear to cross react and can be used safely in patients with immediate reactions to other beta-lactam agents. The risk of cross reactivity with imipenem is not known. Most immediate reactions are IgE mediated, with antibodies directed against a drug metabolite rather than the parent drug.

C. Because effective alternative agents are usually available, the need for skin testing and desensitization is now greatly diminished. Skin testing only identifies patients with immediate (IgE-mediated) hypersensitivity. Skin testing should never be done simply to document the presence of drug allergy. Testing must be done with parent drug and metabolites and is associated with a risk of anaphylaxis. Skin testing is associated with false-positive and false-negative results. Desensitization must be carried out cautiously, with epinephrine and resuscitation equipment at hand.

D. Maculopapular rashes are the most common hypersensitivity reactions. The immunologic nature of these reactions is not clear. Skin rashes associated with ampicillin therapy, often seen with concomitant Epstein-Barr virus and cytomegalovirus infection and allopurinol therapy, are not usually immunologic in nature. A previous maculopapular reaction does not increase the risk of immediate reactions with subsequent exposure. Patients may be at higher risk of recurrent skin rash with rechallenge, although the actual risk is not known. If a maculopapular rash occurs, management depends on the severity of symptoms such as pruritus and the availability of effective alternatives. The rash often resolves even if therapy with the inciting agent continues.

E. Document all information on the history of previous reactions and response to subsequent drug therapy in the medical record. Nonhypersensitivity reactions should not be called "allergies," and patients should be warned of the risk of subsequent reactions and drug classes to avoid.

References

Anderson JA. Cross-sensitivity to cephalosporins in patients allergic to penicillin. Pediatr Infect Dis J 1986; 5:557.

Idsoe O, Guthe T, Willcox R, De Weck AL. Nature and extent of penicillin side-reactions, with particular reference to fatalities from anaphylactic shock. Bull World Health Organ 1968; 38:159.

Saxon A. Immediate hypersensitivity reactions to beta-lactam antibiotics. Ann Intern Med 1987; 107:204.

Smith JW, Johnson JE, Cluff LE. Studies on the epidemiology of adverse drug reactions. II. An evaluation of penicillin allergy. N Engl J Med 1966; 274:998.

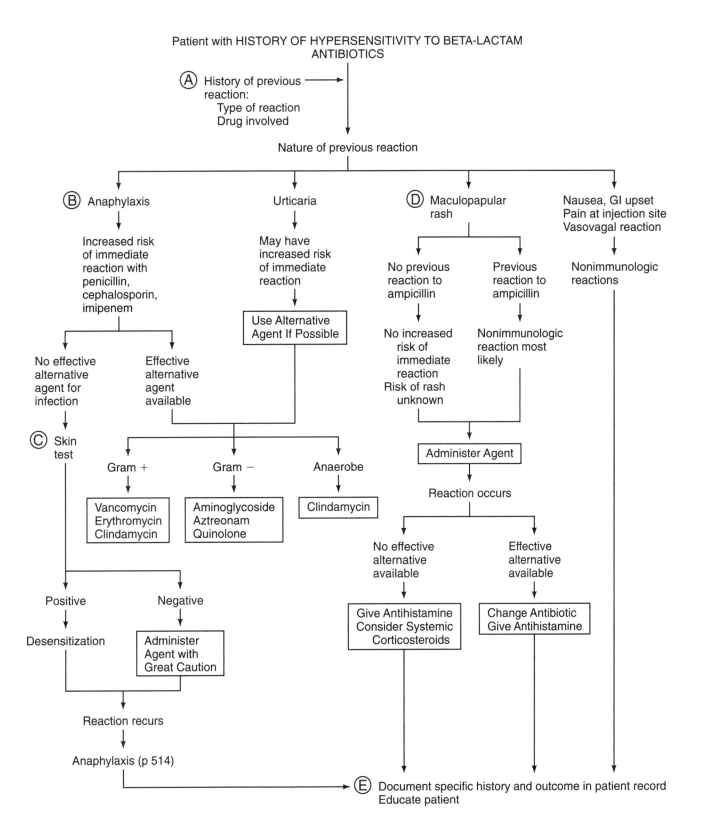

Patient with HISTORY OF HYPERSENSITIVITY TO BETA-LACTAM ANTIBIOTICS

(A) History of previous reaction:
Type of reaction
Drug involved

Nature of previous reaction

(B) Anaphylaxis

Increased risk of immediate reaction with penicillin, cephalosporin, imipenem

No effective alternative agent for infection

Effective alternative agent available

(C) Skin test

Gram +

Vancomycin
Erythromycin
Clindamycin

Gram −

Aminoglycoside
Aztreonam
Quinolone

Anaerobe

Clindamycin

Positive

Desensitization

Negative

Administer Agent with Great Caution

Reaction recurs

Anaphylaxis (p 514)

Urticaria

May have increased risk of immediate reaction

Use Alternative Agent If Possible

(D) Maculopapular rash

No previous reaction to ampicillin

No increased risk of immediate reaction
Risk of rash unknown

Previous reaction to ampicillin

Nonimmunologic reaction most likely

Administer Agent

Reaction occurs

No effective alternative available

Give Antihistamine Consider Systemic Corticosteroids

Effective alternative available

Change Antibiotic Give Antihistamine

Nausea, GI upset
Pain at injection site
Vasovagal reaction

Nonimmunologic reactions

(E) Document specific history and outcome in patient record
Educate patient

USE AND MONITORING OF AMINOGLYCOSIDE ANTIBIOTICS

Brian L. Erstad, Pharm.D.

Gentamicin (G), tobramycin (T), netilmicin (N), and amikacin (A) are members of a class of antiinfectives known as the aminoglycosides. They are injectable antimicrobials primarily used for their excellent activity against gram-negative aerobic bacteria, with a few important exceptions (e.g., *Xanthomonas maltophilia*). The agents tend to have similar spectrums, although tobramycin may be particularly useful for *Pseudomonas aeruginosa* in institutions with gentamicin-resistant strains. The aminoglycosides are particularly useful for their additive or synergistic actions with other antimicrobials in serious infections. They are commonly used in combination with penicillins for synergism when treating enterococcal infections. Many infectious disease experts also recommend the addition of an aminoglycoside to beta-lactam therapy for serious infections due to organisms such as *P. aeruginosa*.

A. Although the loading dose of an aminoglycoside can be readily calculated on the basis of body weight, the subsequent maintenance doses need to be calculated with consideration of the patient's renal function. Equations and computer programs have been developed for dosing the aminoglycosides, but less complicated nomograms have been developed that can be used until blood levels have been obtained. The nomogram of Sarubbi and Hull is widely used (see reference). Further documentation of the efficacy and lowered toxicity of extended interval dosing schedules (e.g., every 24 hours), may allow for more optimal use of the aminoglycosides.

B. One interaction between aminoglycosides and penicillins deserves special mention. Aminoglycoside concentrations may be lowered in vivo and in vitro by concomitant administration of penicillins. Therefore, the schedules of these antimicrobials should be spread as far apart as possible to avoid this potential interaction.

C. Remember to monitor the patient and not just the serum aminoglycoside levels. Potential nephro- and ototoxicity concerns have led to the availability of aminoglycoside assays at many hospitals. When used appropriately, these assays can be valuable monitoring tools. However, the levels should not become a substitute for an appropriate clinical evaluation. Aminoglycoside levels may be in the therapeutic range, but the patient may not be clinically improving, which may require a change or re-evaluation of the current therapy. Aminoglycoside levels may not be needed for expected therapy <5 days in patients with stable renal function and fluid balance. For patients in whom aminoglycoside levels are needed, diligent attention to the collection and analysis of the levels is crucial. Aminoglycoside doses may be skipped or given at unexpected times. Blood may be drawn from a line containing the aminoglycoside or not drawn at all.

The draw may not be at the proper time. Assuming the level is ordered and drawn correctly, the specimen may not be properly stored before analysis.

D. The definitions of the pharmacokinetic terms "peak" and "trough" have not been standardized in the medical literature. In this chapter a peak level refers to the blood concentration of an aminoglycoside drawn 30 minutes after a 30-minute infusion. The trough level refers to the concentration 30 minutes before a dose of the aminoglycoside.

E. The introduction of antimicrobials with enhanced gram-negative activity has allowed the clinician more choices for treating such infections. Fears of aminoglycoside toxicity have limited the use of this class of compounds in many institutions. However, with proper selection and monitoring of patients, the incidence of major toxicity is acceptable. It is thought that the nephrotoxicity associated with aminoglycosides is primarily related to prolonged high trough concentrations; there is little evidence that isolated high peak levels of the aminoglycosides increase the risk of nephrotoxicity. Other factors associated with aminoglycoside toxicity include liver disease, shock, and congestive heart failure, as well as the age and sex of the patient (higher in the elderly and females). Fortunately, when nephrotoxicity does occur, it usually presents as a reversible, nonoliguric renal failure. Ototoxicity related to the aminoglycosides is usually seen in patients with renal failure who receive the agents for prolonged periods.

F. The optimal duration of aminoglycoside therapy has not been well studied. In general, extended courses (e.g., weeks) are necessary for more severe infections such as osteomyelitis caused by gram-negative bacteria. Uncomplicated wound or urinary tract infections often resolve after 3–5 days of the aminoglycosides. Take into account the site, severity, and clinical response in deciding when to discontinue therapy.

References

Gilbert DN. Once-daily aminoglycoside therapy. Antimicrob Agents Chemother 1991; 35:399.

Henderson JL, Polk RE, Kline BJ. In vitro interaction of gentamicin, tobramycin, and netilmicin by carbenicillin, azlocillin, or mezlocillin. Am J Hosp Pharm 1981; 38:1167.

Sarubbi FA, Hull JH. Amikacin serum concentrations: prediction of levels and dosage guidelines. Ann Intern Med 1978; 89:612.

Yee GC, Evans WE. Reappraisal of guidelines for pharmacokinetic monitoring of aminoglycosides. Pharmacotherapy 1981; 1:55.

USE OF AMINOGLYCOSIDE ANTIBIOTIC INDICATED

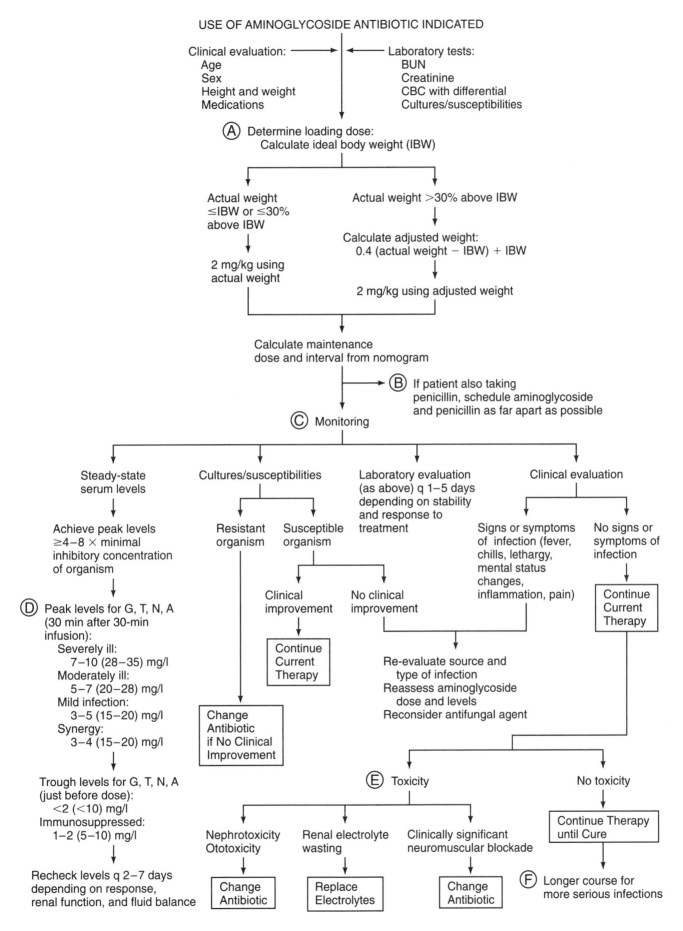

USE AND EVALUATION OF SERUM DRUG LEVELS

Collin Freeman, Pharm.D.
Brian L. Erstad, Pharm.D.

A. Certain medications have a pharmacokinetic characteristic known as a narrow therapeutic index (NTI). This means there is a narrow range, or window, between a serum level at which a drug will have a minimal therapeutic effect and a minimal toxic effect. Some examples of these medications include, but are not limited to, theophylline, phenytoin, carbamazepine, digoxin, procainamide, quinidine, and aminoglycoside antibiotics (see p 528 for specific evaluation and dosing of aminoglycoside antibiotics). These drugs generally have a relationship between the effect of the drug and the patient's serum drug level (SDL). Not all drugs with an assay for obtaining an SDL have this relationship (e.g., benzodiazepines). Other drugs may be monitored by SDLs only under certain circumstances (e.g., aspirin in Kawasaki's syndrome).

B. Therapeutic drug monitoring (TDM) involves patients receiving drugs with an NTI and requires obtaining SDLs at appropriate times to maximize efficacy and minimize toxicity of that particular drug therapy. The use of pharmacokinetics is often helpful to develop a personal drug-dosing regimen based on SDLs. A patient's specific parameters (weight, height, age, sex, renal and hepatic laboratory values) should be obtained, since these factors can all affect an SDL and the response to drug therapy.

C. Most therapeutic ranges of NTI drugs are based on a trough level, which is usually defined as an SDL obtained 30 minutes or less before the next scheduled dose of the drug. Reference ranges for SDLs in the literature are usually based on trough levels. It is therefore difficult to judge what an SDL means clinically when it is drawn too early. Drawing an SDL too early may also cause an erroneously high level to be reported (e.g., digoxin). This can occur if the blood is drawn during the distribution phase of the drug (the period in which the drug in the plasma is equilibrating with the tissues and other fluids into which it will distribute). An SDL is more useful when the patient's blood is drawn after it has achieved steady state (SS). Steady state is that condition in which the rate of the drug administered is equal to the rate of its elimination. Drawing blood and determining an SDL before the drug has reached SS usually results in a lower level being reported than will occur at SS. Four to five half-lives is the time frame considered necessary before a drug achieves SS. Therefore, to calculate when a drug will reach SS, the clinician must first obtain the appropriate half-life of the drug for the particular patient.

D. It is important that the patient's response to the medication be considered rather than the reported SDL.

E. Changing a drug dosage regimen on the basis of an SDL should be carefully considered. All benefits and risks of a dosage change need to be taken into account (e.g., when a theophylline level has been reported correctly as 19.0 [normal 10–20] μg/ml but the patient has not experienced clinical benefit). It is probably more prudent to try an additional therapy or discontinue the theophylline and try another kind of bronchodilating therapy rather than attempt to obtain an SDL of 20 μg/ml.

References

Melamed AJ, Dnistrian A, Muller RJ, et al. A table for therapeutic drug monitoring. Hosp Pharm 1988; 23:743.

Taylor WJ, Caviness MHD, eds. A textbook for the clinical application of therapeutic drug monitoring. Irving, TX: Abbott Laboratories, Diagnostic Division, 1986.

Winter ME. Basic clinical pharmacokinetics. 2nd ed. Vancouver, WA: Applied Therapeutics, 1988.

EVALUATION OF SERUM DRUG LEVEL Requested

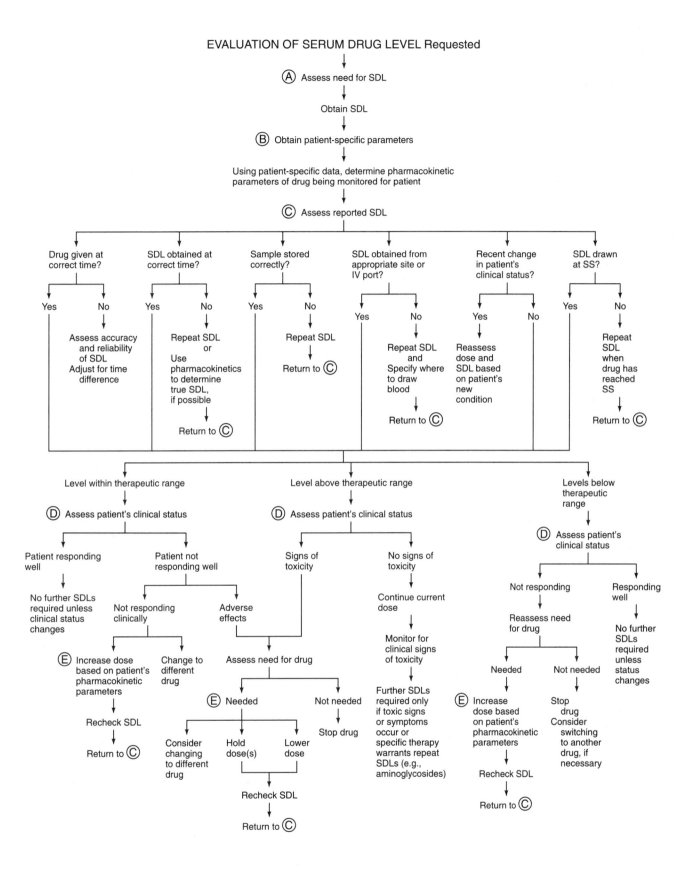

EVALUATION OF A DRUG STUDY

Gary H. Smith, Pharm.D.

A. The title, abstract, and introduction of a clinical drug trial should give the reader a concise, objective summary of the study. The title should not be misleading or overstated. The abstract should identify the study purpose, research design, and methodology and make a brief review of the results and conclusions. It also should not be overstated or contain biased language. The introduction should be brief and lay the framework for the purpose of the study, including reference to other published literature. The author(s) should have good credentials (e.g., faculty members of a college of medicine or pharmacy).

B. A good study design is the single most important step of the drug study without which the results will be of questionable value. Drug studies ideally should be prospective, double-blind, randomized, comparative, and controlled. The design should allow for a comparison between two drugs of similar action or at the least between a drug and a placebo. Retrospective studies do not show a cause-and-effect relationship and are usually reserved for epidemiologic data collection for assessing an association between a drug and an effect. Prospective studies that are not blinded or controlled are often referred to as having an open-label design and are usually fraught with bias.

C. It is important that the study is representative of the population in which the drug will ultimately be used. Thus, a randomized selection from a larger population is important to ensure a representative sample. Also, the sample size should be large enough to show a difference between comparative groups if a difference exists. This is referred to as power. Generally, 50 subjects in each arm of the study are required for most comparative drug studies. A power test ideally should be performed in advance to determine the sample size and should be stated in the paper. Inclusion and exclusion criteria should be clearly stated and consistent with the objectives of the study.

D. Treatment allocation should be random. Standard therapeutic doses should be used for each active treatment group as well as the control group if a drug is used. The dosage form should be the same as is commercially available if possible, to eliminate any difference that may occur as a result of a specialized dosage form. Treatment should last long enough to show an effect of the drug if one exists (e.g., at least 1 month with tricyclic antidepressants). Compliance should be monitored if a drug is given outside a controlled environment (e.g., ambulatory setting).

E. A description of the evaluation procedures should be complete. Evaluation instruments should be described and should be appropriate for measuring the desired end points. The instruments should also be sensitive and specific enough to provide meaningful results. A plan for statistical analysis of the data should be described. Many drug studies published in the medical literature fail to subject data to appropriate statistical analysis, thus rendering the study invalid.

F. The results section should organize the raw data so as to make it easily understood by the reader. The data should be complete enough to allow the reader to subject it to an independent analysis. Tables and figures should contain the data in an easily understood format. Dropouts should be accounted for and included in the final analysis. All adverse drug reactions (ADRs) should be noted and presented in a tabular form with a brief explanation of any unusual reactions. The results of the statistical analysis should be presented here.

G. The discussion/conclusion section should provide a commentary on the results of the study. A comparison of the results with previously published studies of a similar nature should be made, and any differences discussed. Any deviation from the original objectives should be explained here. The conclusion should be based on the results, and any exaggeration of the results should be questioned by the reader. The discussion and conclusion should be stated objectively and free from any bias.

References

Chalmers TC, Smith H, Blackburn B, et al. A method for assessing the quality of a randomized control trial. Controlled Clin Trials 1981; 2:31.

Cuddy PG, Elenbaas RM, Elenbaas JK. Evaluating the medical literature, part 1: abstract, introduction, methods. Ann Emerg Med 1983; 12:549.

Elenbaas JK, Cuddy PG, Elenbaas RM. Evaluating the medical literature, part 3: results and discussion. Ann Emerg Med 1983; 12:679.

Elenbaas RM, Elenbaas JK, Cuddy PG. Evaluating the medical literature, part 2: statistical analysis. Ann Emerg Med 1983; 12:610.

Miller BS, Smith GH. Self-paced learning module in drug literature evaluation. Kalamazoo, MI: Upjohn, 1991.

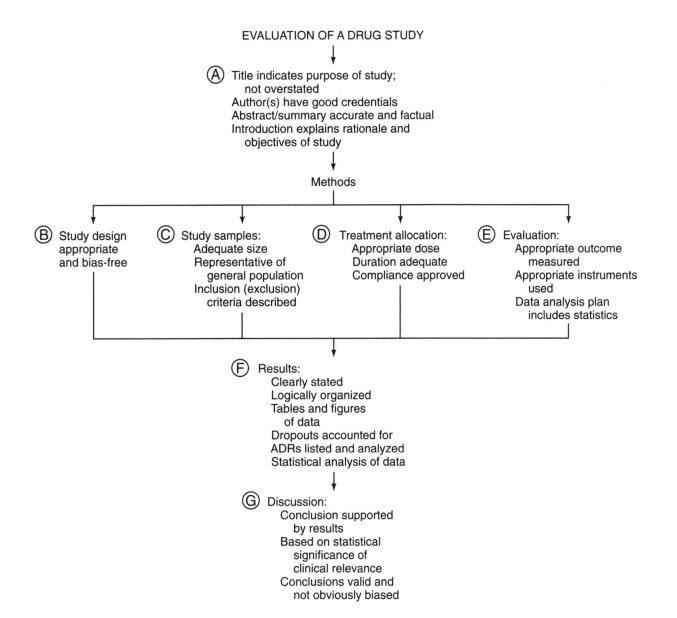

EVALUATION OF A DRUG STUDY

(A) Title indicates purpose of study;
    not overstated
    Author(s) have good credentials
    Abstract/summary accurate and factual
    Introduction explains rationale and
        objectives of study

Methods

(B) Study design
    appropriate
    and bias-free

(C) Study samples:
    Adequate size
    Representative of
        general population
    Inclusion (exclusion)
        criteria described

(D) Treatment allocation:
    Appropriate dose
    Duration adequate
    Compliance approved

(E) Evaluation:
    Appropriate outcome
        measured
    Appropriate instruments
        used
    Data analysis plan
        includes statistics

(F) Results:
    Clearly stated
    Logically organized
    Tables and figures
        of data
    Dropouts accounted for
    ADRs listed and analyzed
    Statistical analysis of data

(G) Discussion:
    Conclusion supported
        by results
    Based on statistical
        significance of
        clinical relevance
    Conclusions valid and
        not obviously biased

EVALUATION OF A DRUG FOR CLINICAL USE OR INCLUSION IN A FORMULARY

Terra A. Robles, Pharm.D.

The systematic evaluation of drugs is the foundation for guiding clinicians in the selection of safe and effective agents for therapy. As new drugs become available, more effective agents should replace those that are less effective on the basis of well-designed therapeutic trials. FDA approval covers a drug's safety and efficacy for its labeled indications. However, the FDA does not address whether a drug is safer or more effective than other agents for a given indication. Systems for maximizing rational drug use are necessary in organized health care settings owing to the multiplicity of drugs, the complexities of their use, and the necessity of cost-effective practices. Pharmacy and Therapeutics Committees (P&T) were developed to assist as advisory and educational bodies to medical staffs on issues regarding the therapeutic use of drugs. The Joint Commission on Accreditation of Healthcare Organizations (JCAHO) requires hospitals to have a functioning P&T Committee and drug formulary. The formulary is a list of pharmaceuticals that, in the judgment of the P&T Committee and the medical staff, permits high-quality yet cost-effective therapy. The P&T Committee continuously evaluates agents for comparative efficacy and safety, and develops and enforces policies that prevent the use of agents likely to lead to suboptimal, hazardous, or unnecessarily costly health outcomes. All clinicians who prescribe drugs should use the same techniques developed by P&T Committees to evaluate new drugs. This process involves the evaluation of drug studies (p 532).

A. A drug or drug class is selected for evaluation based on at least one of the following: (1) a new drug entity; (2) a drug with a newly approved or changed drug use; (3) a drug has a new approved dosage form, a new method of administration, or a new combination of active ingredients; (4) there has been a significant change in the drug's profile: pharmacology, pharmacokinetics, drug interactions, adverse effects, safety profile, or cost; (5) inappropriate prescribing, drug cost, or drug monitoring requires the development of specific guidelines or criteria of use; (6) local practice standards warrant evaluation of a drug for an unlabeled use; (7) a drug has decreased utility; (8) the use or cost of the drug is greater than expected; (9) the prescriber has requested consideration for the drug's addition to the formulary.

B. Appropriate medical literature must be available documenting the safety and the efficacy of the drug to be evaluated. Pharmaceutical manufacturer-provided information should not be the sole source for such data. Nonbiased, blinded, randomized, controlled studies offer credibility.

C. Decide whether an entire drug review or only portions of a review are required. It is important to include all areas that will provide the evaluator with the information necessary for a comprehensive review.

D. When a summary of information is presented to the P&T Committee, it should be organized in a format that can easily be critiqued and assimilated, including all the areas decided upon in C.

E. The FDA classifies drugs as 1AA (a "high priority" new entity drug with important therapeutic advances, for AIDS drugs); IA (new drug entity with major therapeutic gain; generally, no other similar drugs are currently on the market); IB (new drug entity with modest therapeutic gain; there may be similar drugs on the market, but the new entity may have a property that differs, such as a different mechanism of action); or IC (new drug entity with little or no therapeutic gain).

F. Determine whether the differences between the new agent and other similar agents are clinically significant. For example, the agent evaluated may be hepatically cleared while the formulary agent is renally cleared. Will lowering the dose of the formulary agent achieve the same outcome as using the new agent in patient with decreased renal function? Consider any information that may affect outcomes (e.g., drug interaction potential for highly protein-bound agents or drugs that undergo cytochrome P-450 metabolism).

G. Summary of well-designed clinical trials that evaluate therapeutic outcomes. Is in vitro data only available or is there meaningful clinical information? The lack of meaningful clinical data is an especially important consideration with new antimicrobial agents.

H. An older drug may have much documentation on its adverse reactions while a new agent in the same class may not. Keep in mind the potential, as yet unreported adverse effect that a new agent may have.

I. Consider a drug's potential to reduce overall cost (e.g., decreased length of stay). This should be determined for all therapeutically similar agents as compared with the new drug being reviewed. Consider if the additional cost of an agent associated with marginal benefit justifies its use.

J. Follow-up is necessary, especially for drugs that require monitoring or surveillance programs. Delete from the formulary, if possible, drugs the new agent is replacing.

REQUEST FOR FORMULARY ADDITION OR DRUG REVIEW

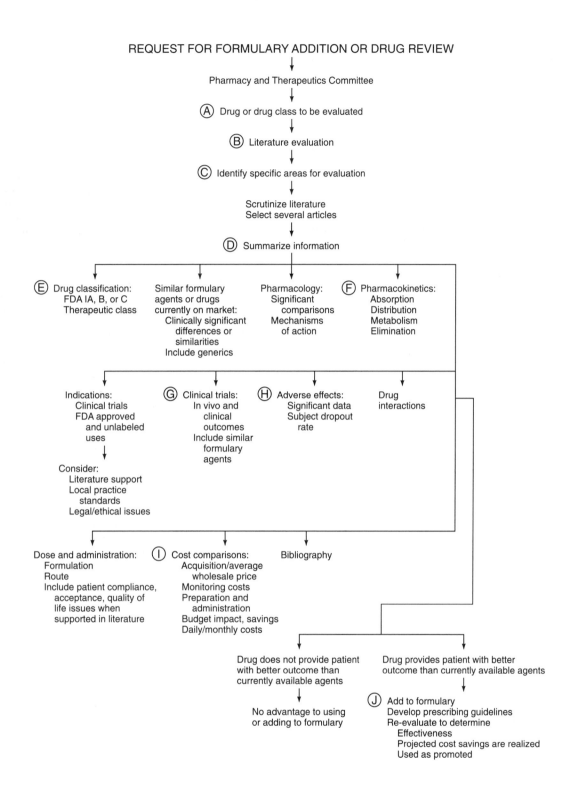

Pharmacy and Therapeutics Committee

Ⓐ Drug or drug class to be evaluated

Ⓑ Literature evaluation

Ⓒ Identify specific areas for evaluation

Scrutinize literature
Select several articles

Ⓓ Summarize information

Ⓔ Drug classification:
FDA IA, B, or C
Therapeutic class

Similar formulary
agents or drugs
currently on market:
Clinically significant
differences or
similarities
Include generics

Pharmacology:
Significant
comparisons
Mechanisms
of action

Ⓕ Pharmacokinetics:
Absorption
Distribution
Metabolism
Elimination

Indications:
Clinical trials
FDA approved
and unlabeled
uses

Ⓖ Clinical trials:
In vivo and
clinical
outcomes
Include similar
formulary
agents

Ⓗ Adverse effects:
Significant data
Subject dropout
rate

Drug
interactions

Consider:
Literature support
Local practice
standards
Legal/ethical issues

Dose and administration:
Formulation
Route
Include patient compliance,
acceptance, quality of
life issues when
supported in literature

Ⓘ Cost comparisons:
Acquisition/average
wholesale price
Monitoring costs
Preparation and
administration
Budget impact, savings
Daily/monthly costs

Bibliography

Drug does not provide patient
with better outcome than
currently available agents

Drug provides patient with better
outcome than currently available agents

No advantage to using
or adding to formulary

Ⓙ Add to formulary
Develop prescribing guidelines
Re-evaluate to determine
Effectiveness
Projected cost savings are realized
Used as promoted

References

American Society of Hospital Pharmacists. ASHP statement on the pharmacy and therapeutics committee. Am J Hosp Pharm 1986; 43:2481.

American Society of Hospital Pharmacists. ASHP statement of the formulary system. Am J Hosp Pharm 1983; 40:1384.

Liang FZ, Greenberg RB, Hogan GF. Legal issues associated with formulary product-selection when there are two or more recognized drug therapies. Am J Hosp Pharm 1988; 45:2372.

Pilkington MA, Dolinsky D. Selecting alternate drug therapies. Med Care 1991; 29:152.

Sesin GP. Therapeutic decision-making: a model for formulary evaluation. Drug Intell Clin Pharm 1986; 20:581.

Schumacher GE. Multiattribute evaluation in formulary decision making as applied to calcium-channel blockers. Am J Hosp Pharm 1991; 48:301.

INPATIENT PARENTERAL NUTRITION

Michael D. Katz, Pharm.D.

The use of total parenteral nutrition (TPN) has become standard practice in the past 10 years. However, the provision of TPN is complex and is associated with a variety of potentially severe complications. Patient management by a multidisciplinary nutritional support team has been shown to reduce TPN-associated complications. If such a team does not exist, a clinician skilled in the provision of TPN should be consulted to guide the management of these patients.

A. The choice between parenteral and enteral support is based primarily on the functional status of the GI tract. A variety of factors and underlying conditions may temporarily preclude the use of the GI tract for nutrition. Common conditions include GI surgery, ileus, GI obstruction, enterocutaneous fistulas, severe trauma, sepsis, severe pancreatitis, and severe diarrhea. Parenteral nutrition should not be considered primary treatment of any disease (other than malnutrition) but a method to support the patient while the underlying conditions are being managed. Enteral feeding should be provided, even if total enteral support is not possible. Recent studies indicate that TPN is associated with villous atrophy and translocation of intestinal bacteria, resulting in an increased risk of infection.

B. Consider ethical issues when evaluating patients for TPN. Patients who are terminally ill and not receiving specific therapy for the underlying disease and have a short life expectancy will not benefit from TPN. The risks of catheter placement and metabolic and infectious complications associated with TPN must be weighed against the potential benefits.

C. Not all patients with GI tract dysfunction require TPN. Most patients tolerate up to 5 days of starvation without significant morbidity. The decision to initiate TPN must be based on the expected duration of GI tract dysfunction, degree of baseline malnutrition, and level of metabolic stress. Patients with severe malnutrition or severe metabolic stress (e.g., trauma, burns) may benefit from earlier nutritional intervention.

D. Peripheral parenteral nutrition (PPN) is indicated for unstressed patients who are expected to need support for at most 10 days. The provision of nutrition via a peripheral vein is limited by the osmolality of the solution and tolerance of the veins for these solutions, as well as the ability of the patient to receive large volumes of fluid. Most unstressed adults receive adequate calories and protein with 2000–2500 ml of a peripheral formula if a large proportion of calories are provided as fat emulsion. The concentration of irritating electrolytes such as K and Ca should be limited, and the total osmolality of the solution should be no greater than 900 mOsm/kg.

E. Ideally, a new or unused single-lumen subclavian catheter should be used for TPN. Internal jugular catheters, while easier to place, may be associated with a higher risk of catheter sepsis. Multilumen catheters may be used if a lumen has been reserved for TPN. Previously used catheters are associated with a higher incidence of catheter sepsis. Catheters used for TPN should not be used for other solutions (e.g., drugs, blood products) or hemodynamic monitoring.

(Continued on page 538)

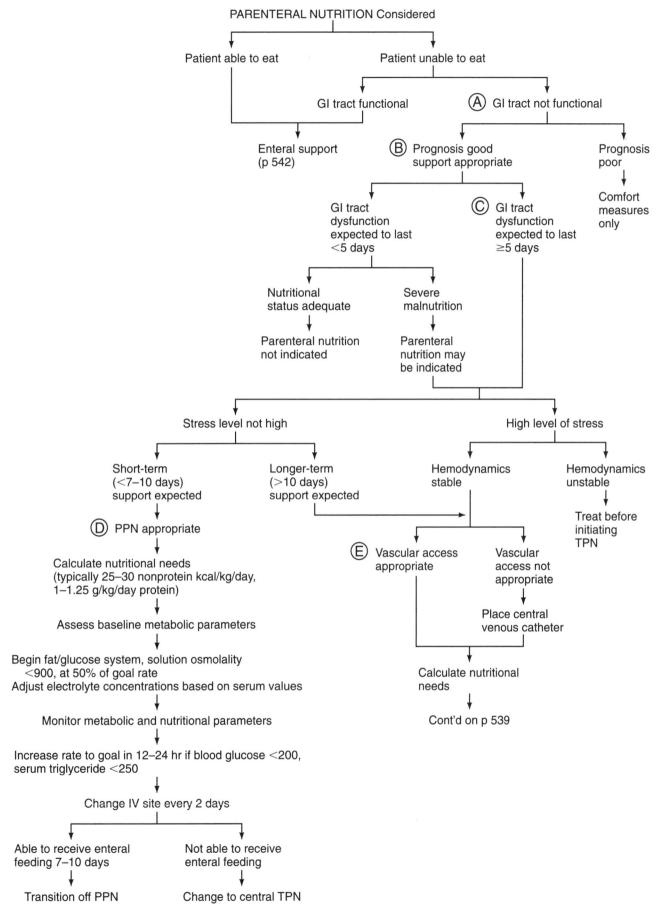

PARENTERAL NUTRITION Considered

Patient able to eat   Patient unable to eat

GI tract functional   Ⓐ GI tract not functional

Enteral support
(p 542)

Ⓑ Prognosis good
support appropriate

Prognosis
poor

Comfort
measures
only

GI tract
dysfunction
expected to last
<5 days

Ⓒ GI tract
dysfunction
expected to last
≥5 days

Nutritional
status adequate

Severe
malnutrition

Parenteral nutrition
not indicated

Parenteral
nutrition may
be indicated

Stress level not high

High level of stress

Short-term
(<7–10 days)
support expected

Longer-term
(>10 days)
support expected

Hemodynamics
stable

Hemodynamics
unstable

Ⓓ PPN appropriate

Treat before
initiating
TPN

Calculate nutritional needs
(typically 25–30 nonprotein kcal/kg/day,
1–1.25 g/kg/day protein)

Ⓔ Vascular access
appropriate

Vascular
access not
appropriate

Assess baseline metabolic parameters

Place central
venous catheter

Begin fat/glucose system, solution osmolality
<900, at 50% of goal rate
Adjust electrolyte concentrations based on serum values

Calculate nutritional
needs

Monitor metabolic and nutritional parameters

Cont'd on p 539

Increase rate to goal in 12–24 hr if blood glucose <200,
serum triglyceride <250

Change IV site every 2 days

Able to receive enteral
feeding 7–10 days

Not able to receive
enteral feeding

Transition off PPN

Change to central TPN

F. The nonprotein calorie and protein requirements are determined by lean body weight (or actual weight if the patient is below ideal), level of metabolic stress, and organ function. High-level metabolic stress as seen in trauma (especially head trauma), sepsis, acute renal failure, ARDS, and burns primarily increases protein needs. Metabolic stress is suggested by the underlying problem, presence of hyperglycemia, elevated serum lactate levels, and severe protein catabolism. Patients with renal and liver failure do not tolerate protein well, but those receiving dialysis tolerate somewhat more protein. The nutritional response to the initial formula must be assessed frequently, especially as the patient's clinical status changes. Provision of excessive calories, whether glucose or fat, will not speed the patient's nutritional repletion and may result in significant morbidity. Overfeeding may result in respiratory failure or difficulty in weaning from mechanical ventilation, liver dysfunction, and sepsis.

G. The caloric source provided depends on the patient's glucose and fat tolerance. There is increasing evidence that providing calories as a mixture of glucose and fat is associated with fewer metabolic complications than glucose alone. If glucose alone is used, fat emulsion should be given twice weekly to prevent essential fatty acid deficiency. A pharmacist skilled in the provision of TPN should be consulted to assist in determining the appropriate solution for a patient.

H. TPN solutions contain a variety of components in addition to macronutrients. Many institutions have standard formulas that are suitable for many patients. Most TPN solutions should contain Na, Cl, K, PO_4, Mg, Ca, and acetate as well as multivitamins, vitamin K, and trace elements. Heparin may be added to reduce catheter clotting, and certain patients (e.g., alcoholics) may require folic acid and thiamine supplementation. The literature and/or consultants should be used to determine appropriate concentrations of these components. Most drugs are not chemically or physically compatible with TPN solutions.

I. Patients on TPN must receive metabolic and nutritional monitoring. During the initiation and titration of TPN, assess serum electrolytes, serum triglyceride (if receiving fat emulsion for calories), and renal function daily. Check fingerstick glucose levels every 6 hours until the patient's TPN rate and blood glucose are stable. Check serum Ca, Mg, PO_4, CBC, and liver enzymes periodically. A short half-life protein (transferrin or prealbumin) should be checked once or twice weekly to assess the adequacy of nutritional support. In general, the laboratory monitoring of patients receiving TPN must be individualized on the basis of patient stability and development of complications.

(Continued on page 540)

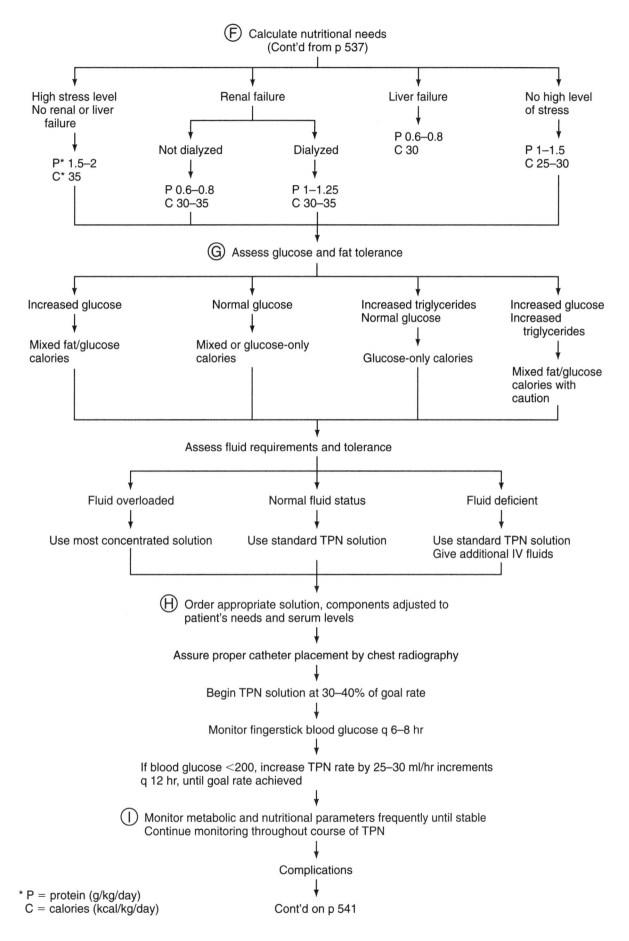

F Calculate nutritional needs
(Cont'd from p 537)

High stress level
No renal or liver
failure

P* 1.5–2
C* 35

Renal failure

Not dialyzed

P 0.6–0.8
C 30–35

Dialyzed

P 1–1.25
C 30–35

Liver failure

P 0.6–0.8
C 30

No high level
of stress

P 1–1.5
C 25–30

G Assess glucose and fat tolerance

Increased glucose

Mixed fat/glucose
calories

Normal glucose

Mixed or glucose-only
calories

Increased triglycerides
Normal glucose

Glucose-only calories

Increased glucose
Increased
triglycerides

Mixed fat/glucose
calories with
caution

Assess fluid requirements and tolerance

Fluid overloaded

Use most concentrated solution

Normal fluid status

Use standard TPN solution

Fluid deficient

Use standard TPN solution
Give additional IV fluids

H Order appropriate solution, components adjusted to
patient's needs and serum levels

Assure proper catheter placement by chest radiography

Begin TPN solution at 30–40% of goal rate

Monitor fingerstick blood glucose q 6–8 hr

If blood glucose <200, increase TPN rate by 25–30 ml/hr increments
q 12 hr, until goal rate achieved

I Monitor metabolic and nutritional parameters frequently until stable
Continue monitoring throughout course of TPN

Complications

* P = protein (g/kg/day)
  C = calories (kcal/kg/day)

Cont'd on p 541

J. A variety of complications can occur with TPN. Most are predictable and severe problems can be avoided by compulsive clinical and biochemical monitoring. Hyperglycemia is the most common complication, more severe in patients receiving glucose as the sole caloric source, and in patients with severe stress or diabetes mellitus. With frequent monitoring of blood glucose, severe hyperglycemia with hyperosmolar coma should no longer occur. Blood glucose levels below 200 mg/dl are acceptable. The management of hyperglycemia associated with TPN depends on the severity. Severe hyperglycemia reflects the inability to utilize glucose; therefore, these patients should receive less glucose and more fat for calories. Insulin used for mild to moderate hyperglycemia may be initiated as a sliding scale to titrate the dose, with insulin added to the TPN solution subsequently. In patients with rapidly fluctuating blood glucose, a continuous insulin infusion may allow more rapid titration and reduce wastage of expensive TPN solutions.

K. As the patient's GI tract dysfunction resolves, the patient should receive enteral feeding. The TPN should not be suddenly stopped but slowly weaned as the patient is able to tolerate increasing amounts of food or tube feeding. In patients with chronic GI dysfunction that is not expected to resolve, long-term TPN may be considered.

References

American Society for Parenteral and Enteral Nutrition standards for nutrition support. Nutr Clin Pract 1988; 3:28.

Driscoll DF, Blackburn GL. Total parenteral nutrition 1990. A review of its current status in hospitalised patients, and the need for patient-specific feeding. Drugs 1990; 40:346.

Nehme A. Nutritional support of the hospitalized patient: the team concept. JAMA 1980; 243:1906.

Rombeau JL, Caldwell MD. Parenteral feeding. Philadelphia: WB Saunders, 1984.

Sitzmann JV, Pitt HA. American Gastroenterological Society statements on guidelines for total parenteral nutrition. Dig Dis Sci 1989; 34:489.

Vo NM, Waycaster M, Acuff RV, Lefemine AA. Effects of postoperative carbohydrate overfeeding. Am Surg 1987; 58:632.

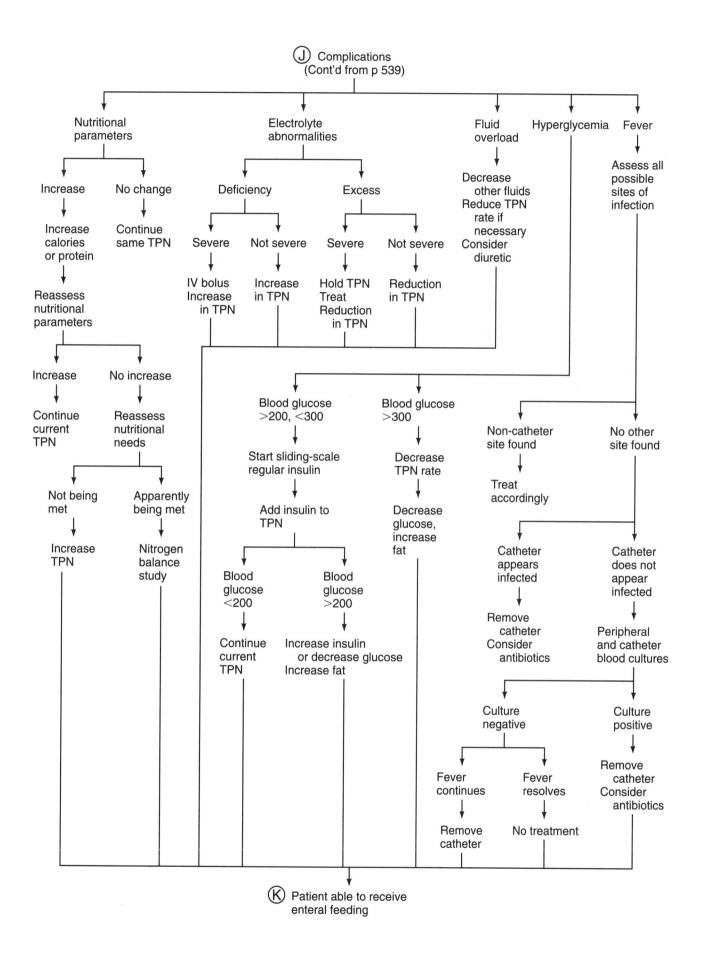

J Complications
(Cont'd from p 539)

Nutritional parameters

Increase → Increase calories or protein → Reassess nutritional parameters

Increase → Continue current TPN

No increase → Reassess nutritional needs

Not being met → Increase TPN

Apparently being met → Nitrogen balance study

No change → Continue same TPN

Electrolyte abnormalities

Deficiency

Severe → IV bolus Increase in TPN

Not severe → Increase in TPN

Excess

Severe → Hold TPN Treat Reduction in TPN

Not severe → Reduction in TPN

Blood glucose >200, <300 → Start sliding-scale regular insulin → Add insulin to TPN

Blood glucose <200 → Continue current TPN

Blood glucose >200 → Increase insulin or decrease glucose Increase fat

Blood glucose >300 → Decrease TPN rate → Decrease glucose, increase fat

Fluid overload → Decrease other fluids Reduce TPN rate if necessary Consider diuretic

Hyperglycemia

Fever → Assess all possible sites of infection

Non-catheter site found → Treat accordingly → Catheter appears infected → Remove catheter Consider antibiotics

No other site found → Catheter does not appear infected → Peripheral and catheter blood cultures

Culture negative

Fever continues → Remove catheter

Fever resolves → No treatment

Culture positive → Remove catheter Consider antibiotics

K Patient able to receive enteral feeding

541

INPATIENT ENTERAL NUTRITION

Michael D. Katz, Pharm.D
Cynthia Thomson, M.S., R.D.

A. When considering the initiation of nutritional therapy, determine the need for immediate intervention and what type of intervention is appropriate. Patients' nutritional needs for calories and protein as well as micronutrients (vitamins, minerals) must be assessed. Calorie and protein requirements will be based on body mass, level of metabolic stress, and organ function. Patients' baseline degree of malnutrition, as evidenced by history of weight loss, and biochemical parameters, often determines the need for immediate intervention. Patients who are not expected to be able to eat within 5–7 days should be considered for support, especially if there is metabolic stress or baseline malnutrition.

B. Consider ethical issues when evaluating patients for enteral feeding. Patients who are terminally ill, are not receiving therapy for the underlying disease, and have a short life expectancy are not likely to benefit from nutritional support. The discomfort of tube placement and potential adverse effects of support must be weighed against the potential benefits.

C. If the GI tract is functional, enteral nutritional support is appropriate. In these patients, an effort should be made to provide enteral support, with total parenteral nutrition (TPN) reserved for those who do not tolerate enteral feedings or have nonfunctioning GI tracts (see p 536).

D. Patients with alterations in digestive (pancreatic insufficiency, lactase deficiency) or absorptive (villous atrophy, malabsorption syndromes, mucosal damage) capacity usually do not tolerate intact proteins and complex carbohydrates. In these patients, partially digested formulas containing hydrolyzed proteins and simple sugars may be better tolerated. A variety of protein hydrolyzed formulas exist, including elemental formulas that are enteral formulations of TPN.

E. A large and increasing array of tube feeding (TF) formulas are available. A dietitian skilled in the provision of tube feeding should be consulted in order to choose the best formula for a given patient. A variety of specific brands exist within each category of TF. The institution should develop a formulary and stock one brand from each category.

F. Renal or liver failure alters nutritional needs as well as protein, carbohydrate, and electrolyte tolerance. In some instances, specialized formulas, while expensive, may be appropriate to avoid providing excessive protein and electrolytes such as potassium.

(Continued on page 544)

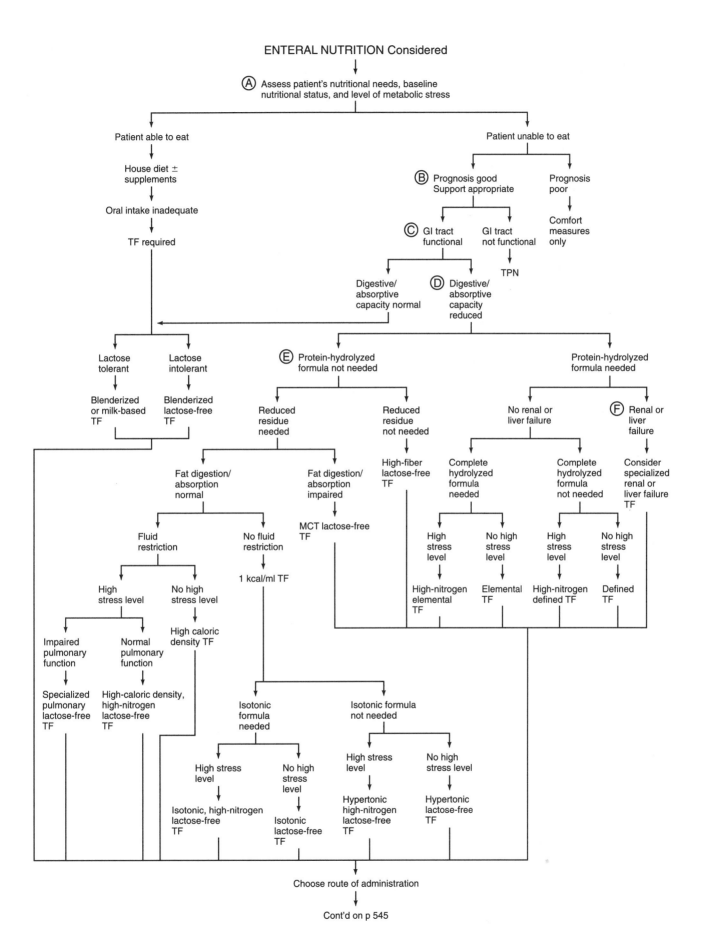

ENTERAL NUTRITION Considered

Ⓐ Assess patient's nutritional needs, baseline nutritional status, and level of metabolic stress

Patient able to eat

House diet ± supplements

Oral intake inadequate

TF required

Patient unable to eat

Ⓑ Prognosis good Support appropriate

Prognosis poor

Comfort measures only

Ⓒ GI tract functional

GI tract not functional

TPN

Digestive/ absorptive capacity normal

Ⓓ Digestive/ absorptive capacity reduced

Lactose tolerant

Lactose intolerant

Ⓔ Protein-hydrolyzed formula not needed

Protein-hydrolyzed formula needed

Blenderized or milk-based TF

Blenderized lactose-free TF

Reduced residue needed

Reduced residue not needed

No renal or liver failure

Ⓕ Renal or liver failure

Fat digestion/ absorption normal

Fat digestion/ absorption impaired

High-fiber lactose-free TF

Complete hydrolyzed formula needed

Complete hydrolyzed formula not needed

Consider specialized renal or liver failure TF

Fluid restriction

No fluid restriction

MCT lactose-free TF

High stress level

No high stress level

High stress level

No high stress level

High stress level

No high stress level

High caloric density TF

1 kcal/ml TF

High-nitrogen elemental TF

Elemental TF

High-nitrogen defined TF

Defined TF

Impaired pulmonary function

Normal pulmonary function

Specialized pulmonary lactose-free TF

High-caloric density, high-nitrogen lactose-free TF

Isotonic formula needed

Isotonic formula not needed

High stress level

No high stress level

High stress level

No high stress level

Isotonic, high-nitrogen lactose-free TF

Isotonic lactose-free TF

Hypertonic high-nitrogen lactose-free TF

Hypertonic lactose-free TF

Choose route of administration

Cont'd on p 545

543

G. The type of tube placed depends on several factors. In patients requiring short-term TF, the relative risk of aspiration should be assessed. A nasoenteric tube is possibly safer in patients at risk for aspiration (e.g., stroke, coma). The passage of a tube through the pylorus may be hastened by administration of metoclopramide for 24 hours. In patients with oral, nasal, or esophageal obstruction or damage, who cannot have a nasogastric or enteric tube placed, parenteral support may be most appropriate for short-term therapy. Patients requiring long-term support, for whatever reason, should have a gastrostomy (percutaneous endoscopic gastrostomy [PEG]) or jejunostomy placed for their comfort.

H. Assess laboratory tests before initiating TF to determine nutritional and metabolic status. Metabolic parameters should include electrolytes; BUN and creatinine; blood glucose; serum Ca, Mg, and PO_4; liver enzymes; CBC; and serum triglyceride. Nutritional parameters should include serum albumin, hemoglobin, hematocrit, serum iron, and a short half-life protein such as transferrin or prealbumin (transthyretin). The frequency of subsequent monitoring depends on the stability of the patient and tolerance of TF.

I. Assess the patient's ability to tolerate TF. Abdominal cramping, distention, and nausea are common complaints and are often due to too rapid infusion or rate titration. Large residuals of TF formula in the stomach signify poor gastric emptying and may be due to intrinsic motility problems or the effects of fat. With large gastric residuals, the risk of aspiration may be increased.

J. Diarrhea is another common complaint; it often is not due to TF but to a drug or infection. Hyperosmolar oral agents (KCl, Mg salts, PO_4 salts) should be diluted to become isotonic. In patients receiving long-term antibiotics, *Clostridium difficile* may be the cause of the diarrhea. If no other cause for the diarrhea is identified, the TF rate should be decreased or, if a hypertonic TF is used, it should be diluted or changed to an isotonic formula. If the diarrhea persists, consider a more elemental formula. Avoid pharmacologic treatment of diarrhea with narcotics. However, if an antimotility agent is desired, loperamide is the preferred agent.

References

Chen M, Hares DW, Curtas MS. A decision tree for selecting an appropriate enteral formula. Nutrition 1987; 3:257.

Edes TE, Walk BE, Austin JL. Diarrhea in tube-fed patients: feeding formula not necessarily the cause. Am J Med 1990; 88:91.

Rombeau JL, Caldwell MD. Clinical nutrition: enteral and tube feeding. 2nd ed. Philadelphia: WB Saunders, 1990.

Talbot JM (ed). Guidelines for the scientific review of enteral food products for special medical purposes. Federation of American Societies for Experimental Biology, FDA Contract No. 223-88-2124, Task order no. 6, Dec. 1990.

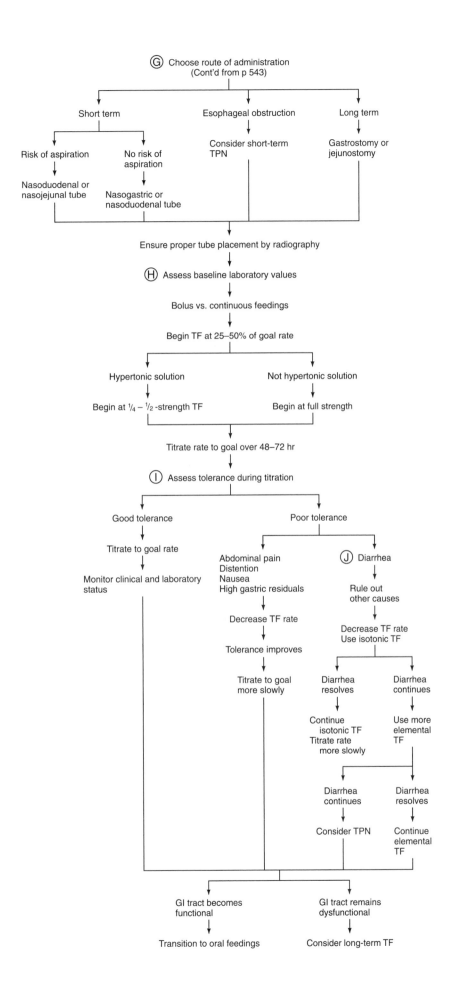

INDEX

A

Abdomen
    acute, 458–459
    scanning of, 159
Abetalipoproteinemia, 334
ABO compatible granulocytes, 202
Abscess
    epidural, 396
    lung, 364, 434, 436
    prostatic, 484
Abuse
    alcohol, 490–491
    substance, 312–315
ABVD; see Adriamycin, bleomycin, vinblastine, dacarbazine
Acetaminophen, 302, 303
Achalasia, 140
ACHES, mnemonic, 472
Acid phosphatase, 218
Acidosis, metabolic, 287
Acids ingestion, 438
Acquired immunodeficiency syndrome, 378–379, 450
Acromioclavicular separation, 394
Acyclovir, 452
Addiction, alcohol, 490
Adenocarcinoma
    of prostate, 482–483
    of uterus, 454
Adenoma
    pituitary gland, 122, 124–125, 462
    thyroid-stimulating hormone–secreting, 110
Adenopathy, mediastinal, 206, 370–371
ADR; see Drugs, adverse reactions to
Adrenal glands
    congenital hyperplasia of, 128
    mass in, 120–121
    suppression of, 38
Adrenergic blocking agents
    incontinence and, 486
    in prostatodynia, 484
    Raynaud's phenomenon and, 410
Adrenocorticotropic hormone, 122
Adriamycin, bleomycin, vinblastine, dacarbazine, 206
Ageusia, 349
Agoraphobia, 492
Airway
    foreign body in, 434–437
    obstructive disease of, 366
Akathisia, 336
Albumin
    ascites and, 152
    in edema, 14
Albuterol, 516
Alcohol
    in behavior changes, 342, 346
    in gait disturbances, 326
    in hypomagnesemia, 290, 291
    memory loss from, 312–315
    muscle weakness and, 416
    in neuropathies, 334
    seizures and, 318–319
    suicidal patient and, 506
Alcoholism, 490–491
Aldosterone-secreting tumors, 120
Aldosteronism, 58
Alkali burns, 438
Alkaline phosphatase, 426–427
Alkalosis, metabolic, 287
Alkylating agents

    in leukopenia, 188
    in polycythemia, 184–185
Allergy
    granulomatosis in, 92
    in rhinitis, 28
    transfusions and, 204
    urticaria and, 88
    in vaginal discharge, 450
Allopurinol, 414
Alpha-adrenergic blocking agents
    incontinence and, 486
    in prostatodynia, 484
Alpha-fetoprotein, 218
Alpha-interferon, 208
Alpha-methyldopa, 424
Alprazolam, 492
ALT; see Aminotransferases
Alzheimer's disease, 312, 344–347
Amantadine, 330, 344
Amaurosis fugax, 304, 306–307
Amenorrhea, 126–127
Amikacin, 528
Amiloride, 289
Aminoglycosides
    neutropenia and, 220
    use and monitoring of, 528–529
Aminotransferases, 176
Amiodarone, 334
Amnesia, 312–315
Amobarbital, 312
Amoxicillin, 452
Amoxicillin and clavulanate, 460
Amphotericin, 202, 220
Ampicillin, 452, 460
Amylase
    ascites and, 152
    elevated serum, 180–181
Amyloidosis, 210
ANA test; see Antinuclear antibody test
Analgesics in headache, 302, 303
Anaphylaxis, 514–517, 526
Anemia, 182–183
Anesthesia
    anaphylaxis and, 514
    in status epilepticus, 320
Angina, 48–51
Angioplasty, percutaneous coronary, 48
Angiotensin-converting enzyme inhibitors, 288–289
Angrelide, 185
Anorexia, 4, 138–139
Anosmia, 348–349
Antibiotics
    anaphylaxis and, 514
    in chemotherapy-induced neutropenia, 220
    hypersensitivity to, 526–527
    serum drug levels of, 530
    in urinary tract infection, 460
    use and monitoring of, 528–529
Antibodies
    antinuclear, 424–425
    antithyroglobulin, 108
    in scleroderma, 406
    in Sjögren's syndrome, 408
    thyroid antimicrosomal, 108
Anticentromere antibody, 406
Anticholinergics
    in behavior changes, 342
    in incontinence, 486
    in memory loss, 312

Anticholinergics—*cont'd*
  in Parkinson's disease, 330
Anticoagulants, 36
  in deep venous thrombosis, 193
  oral, 193
  in stroke, 308–309, 310–311
  in transient ischemic attacks, 304
Anticoagulation, 508–513
Anticonvulsants, 424
Antidepressants
  in confusional states, 344
  depression and, 494
  grief and, 498
  in migraine, 302, 303
  panic disorder and, 492
  in sleep disturbances, 351
Antiepileptics, 318, 319, 320
Antihistamines, 410, 516
Antimetabolites, 184–185, 188
Antimicrobial prophylaxis
  in chemotherapy-induced neutropenia, 220
  choice of, 524–525
  nonsurgical, 520–521
Antimicrobial therapy, 220, 440
Antinuclear antibody, 406, 408
Antinuclear antibody test, 424–425
Antispasmodics, 172, 484
Antithrombin III, 192
Antithyroid agents, 424
Anus
  disorders of, 166
  manometry and, 174
Anxiety, 492–493
  confusional states and, 342
  dizziness in, 316–317
  fatigue and, 2
  grief and, 498
  somatic disorders and, 496
Aortic coarctation, 59
Apheresis, 198
Apnea
  in brain death, 356–357
  in near-drowning, 446–449
  sleep, 72
Appetite loss, 138
Apraxia, 326
Arrest, cardiac, 76–77
Arrhythmias
  in hypokalemia, 286
  myocardial infarction and, 80
  palpitations and, 62
Arsenic, 334, 346
Arterial ulcer, 86
Arteriography
  of abdominal vessels, 159
  bronchial, 358–359
  in pulseless extremity, 432
Arteriovenous malformations, 374
Arteritis
  giant cell, 416–417
  temporal, 300–301, 306
Arthritis
  foot pain in, 404
  gout and, 414–415
  knee and, 402
  monoarticular, 384–385
  polyarticular, 386–387
  rheumatoid, 386, 400
  seronegative, 388–389
Arthro-ophthalmopathy, 418
Arthropathy, inflammatory, 398
Asbestos, 382–383
Ascites, 152–153, 490
Aspiration

  of foreign body, 360
  of joint, 384
  pulmonary nodules and, 372, 374
  of thyroid gland, 114
Aspirin
  in headache, 302, 303
  in myocardial infarction, 80
  in transient ischemic attacks, 304
AST; *see* Aminotransferases
Asterixis, 328
Asthma, 362
Ataxia, 326
Atelectasis, 434, 436
Athetosis, 336
Atrial fibrillation, 62
Atrioventricular block, 42–43
Atrium, 66
Atrophy
  peripheral muscular, 334
  villous, 536
Atropine, 77
Audiography, 32
Austin Flint murmur, 54
Autoantibodies, 194
Autoimmune disorders, 362
Autologous transfusion, 200
AVMs; *see* Arteriovenous malformations
Axillary lymph node, 214, 216

B

B-cell neoplasm, 210
Babinski sign, 326
Back pain, 396–397
Bacteria
  in arthritis, 384
  diarrhea and, 164
  in prostatitis, 484–485
  transfusions and, 204
Bacteriuria, 484
Bacteroides fragilis, 522
Ballismus, 336
Balloon thrombectomy, 433
Barium enema
  constipation and, 166
  in flatulence, 172
  guaiac-positive stools and, 170
Barrett's esophagus, 142
Battery ingestion, 434, 438–439
BCM; *see* Birth control method
Behavior changes, 342–347
Belching, 146–147
Bell's palsy, 332
Benzodiazepines
  anxiety and, 492
  grief and, 498
  in sleep disturbances, 351
Benzyl penicillin, 440
Bereavement, 498–499
Beta blockers
  asthma from, 362
  in headache, 302, 303
  in hyperkalemia, 288–289
  in myocardial infarction, 80
  Raynaud's phenomenon and, 410
Beta-human chorionic gonadotropin, 218
  abdominal pain and, 458
  in carcinoma of unknown primary site, 218
  in gynecomastia, 131
Beta-lactam antibiotics, 220, 526–527
Bethesda classification system, 464
Bicarbonate of sodium, 288, 289
Biceps inflammation, 390

Bile duct obstruction, 150, 154
Biliary tract disease, 426
Biopsy
    of breast, 212
    in carcinoma, 218
    cervical, 452
    endometrial, 454
    of liver, 176
    in lung disease, 376
    lymph node, 206, 210, 214
    muscle, 428
    prostate, 483
    temporal artery, 416
Bipolar disease, 494, 506
Birth control method, 468–471
Bites, 440–441
Bladder
    calculi of, 478
    neurogenic, 486
    tumor of, 482
Bleeding
    as complication of long-term anticoagulation, 512
    disorders of, 194–197
    gastrointestinal, 156–159
    rectal, 160–161
    vaginal, 454–457
Bleomycin, 206, 218
Blepharitis, 26
Blood
    autologous transfusion of, 200–201
    coagulation of, 194–197
    in diarrhea, 164
    expectoration of, 358–359
    glucose in, 100–103
    in joint diffusions, 384
Blood gases
    in brain death, 356–357
    in polycythemia, 184
Blood pressure
    gastrointestinal bleeding and, 158
    oral contraceptives and, 474
Bone marrow transplantation, 208
Botulinum toxin, 336, 337
Bouchard's nodes, 386
Bowel
    flatulence and, 172
    inflammatory disease of, 162, 388
    irritable, 164
Bradycardia, 42–43, 62–63
Brain death, 356–357
Brain in organic brain syndrome, 342–343
Breakthrough bleeding, 472–475
Breast
    cancer of, 216–217, 218, 462
    discharge from, 462–463
    mass in, 212–213
Bretylium, 77
Bromocriptine
    in confusional states, 344
    in mastodynia, 466
    in Parkinson's disease, 330
Bronchial artery embolization, 358–359
Bronchiectasis, 364
Bronchitis, 364
Bronchodilators, 362
Bronchoscopy, 360, 364
    in AIDS, 378
    in diffuse interstitial lung disease, 376
    in pulmonary nodules, 372, 374
    in wheezing, 362
Bronchus
    foreign body in, 434
    tumor in, 364
Brudzinski's sign, 354

Bulimia, 4, 138
Bundle branch block, 46
Bupropion, 494
Burping, 146–147
Bursa, 402
Bursitis, 390, 398
Busulfan, 208
Bypass graft, coronary artery, 48, 50

C

Café au lait spots, 84
Caffeine, 302, 303, 410
Calcinosis, 406
Calcium
    in hyperkalemia, 288, 289
    hypocalcemia and, 104
    in hypophosphatemia, 292
Calcium channel blockers, 302, 303, 486
Calcium pyrophosphate deposition disease, 384, 386
Calculus, bladder, 478
Calorie requirements, 540
Cancer
    abdominal pain and, 458
    of breast, 216–217
    fever in, 220
Candida, 450
Captopril, 289
Carbamazepine, 530
Carbidopa, 330
Carbohydrate tolerance, 102
Carbon monoxide, 342
Carboxyhemoglobin, 184
Carcinoma, 464
    of adrenal gland, 120
    of breast, 212–213, 462
    colorectal, 160, 166, 170
    metastatic, 374
    prostate, 484
    of thyroid, 114
    of unknown primary site, 218–219
Cardiac dyspnea, 78–79
Cardiac risk index, 34
Cardiac tamponade, 60
Cardiology, 42–83
Cardiomegaly, 14, 66–67
Cardiopulmonary resuscitation, 446–449
Carotid artery, 304–306
Carpal tunnel syndrome, 400
Cathartics, 438
Catheter
    for balloon thrombectomy, 433
    cardiac, 74
    sepsis and, 536
    Swan-Ganz, 60
Cauda equina syndrome, 396
Caustics ingestion and exposure, 438–439
Cefazolin, 522
Cefoperazone, 220
Cefoxitin, 478, 522
Ceftriaxone, 452, 478
Cephalosporins, 484
    in bite wounds, 440
    in cervicitis, 452
    in chemotherapy-induced neutropenia, 220
    hypersensitivity to, 526
    in urinary tract infection, 460
Cerebral artery in stroke, 308–309
Cerebrospinal fluid in status epilepticus, 320
Cerebrovascular accident, 474
Cerebrum, depression of, 356–357
Cervical cap, 470
Cervical cytopathology, 464–465
Cervical intraepithelial neoplasia, 464

Cervical spine, 392
Cervicitis, 452–453
CFI; see Clenched fist injury
Charcot-MariTooth disease, 334
Chemicals
    injury from, 438–439
    sweating and, 20
Chemotherapy, 218
    in breast cancer, 216–217
    in breast mass, 212
    in Hodgkin's disease, 206
    multiple myeloma and, 210
    in myelogenous leukemia, 208
    neutropenia induced by, 220
    in plasmacytoma, 210
    Raynaud's phenomenon and, 410
    in testicular cancer, 218
    Waldenström's macroglobulinemia and, 211
Chest radiography
    in AIDS, 378
    in cough, 364
Chlamydia
    in cervicitis, 452
    in dysuria or pyuria, 478–479
    gonorrhea and, 478
    in prostatitis, 484
    scrotal mass and, 480
    in vaginal bleeding in pregnancy, 456
    vaginal discharge and, 450
Chlorambucil, 211
Chloroquine, 322
Cholangiography, 150
Cholangiopancreatography, 150
Cholecystitis, 458
Cholecystography, 146, 154
Cholesterol, 96
Chronic obstructive pulmonary disease, 34
Churg-Strauss syndrome, 92
Chvostek's sign, 104
Chymopapain, 514
Cigarette smoking, 502–505
CIN; see Cervical intraepithelial neoplasia
Cingulotomy, 492
Ciprofloxacin, 460
Cirrhosis, 490
Cisplatin, 218
    in hypomagnesemia, 290–291
    in neuropathies, 334
Clavicle pain, 394
Clavulanate; see Amoxicillin and clavulanate
Clenched fist injury, 440
Clindamycin, 522
Clofibrate, 322
Clomipramine, 492
Clonazepam, 351
Clostridium, 544
Clotrimazole, 450
Clotting in disseminated intravascular coagulation, 190
Clotting time, 194–197
Coagulation abnormalities, 194–197
Coarctation of aorta, 59
Coccidioidomycosis, 374
Coccygodynia, 168
Cognitive-behavioral therapy, 492
Colchicine, 322, 414
Colic, biliary, 154–155
Collagen vascular disease, 298, 376
Colloids, sulfur, 159
Colon
    polyp of, 170
    transit times of, 166
Colonoscopy, 164
    guaiac-positive stools in, 170
    rectal bleeding and, 160

Colony stimulating factors, 186
Colorectal carcinoma
    constipation and, 166
    guaiac-positive stools in, 170
    rectal bleeding and, 160
Coma, 354–355
Compulsions, 492
Computerized tomography
    in carcinoma of unknown primary site, 218
    in gastrointestinal bleeding, 156, 158
    in headache, 300–301
    in lymphadenopathy, 214
    status epilepticus and, 320
    in stroke, 308–309
    in transient ischemic attacks, 304–305
Condoms, 470
Confusion, 342–343
Conjunctivitis, 22–25
Consciousness, 342
Constipation, 166–167
Continuous positive alveolar pressure, 448
Contraception, 468–471
Contraceptives
    oral, 472–475
    in premenstrual syndrome, 466
    Raynaud's phenomenon and, 410
    vaginal bleeding and, 454
Contractures, 340
Conversion disorder, 496
Cor pulmonale, 72–73
Coronary angioplasty, 48
Coronary artery bypass grafting, 48, 50
Coronary artery disease
    heart failure and, 68
    hyperlipidemia and, 96
    hypotension and, 60
    palpitations and, 62–63
Corticosteroids
    in anaphylaxis, 516
    in leukocytosis, 186
    muscle weakness and, 416
    in myopathies, 428
    osteopenia and, 412
    in transfusion therapy, 202
Cortisol, 122
Costochondritis, 134
Cosyntropin stimulation test, 100
Cough, 364–365
CPAP; see Continuous positive alveolar pressure
CPPD; see Calcium pyrophosphate deposition disease
Cramps, 340–341
Creatine kinase, 428–429
Creatinine, 414, 482
Crepitus, 422
CREST syndrome, 406
Crithidia, 424
Cryptorchism, 488
Culture of stool, 162
Cushing's disease, 124
Cushing's syndrome, 122–123
    adrenal mass and, 120
    hypertension and, 59
Cyclosporine, 298
Cyst, ovarian, 458
Cystitis, 460
Cytology in pleural effusion, 368
Cytomegalovirus, 298–299

D

Dacarbazine, 206
Danazol, 466
Dapsone, 334
Death, brain, 356–357

Decongestants, 410
Defecography, 167, 174
Defibrillation, 76
Degeneration of joint, 400, 422
Degenerative disease, 312
Dehydroepiandrosterone sulfate, 128
Déjérine-Sottas disease, 334
Delirium, 342–343
Deltoid muscle bursitis, 390
Delusions, 500
Dementia, 344–347, 500
    memory loss and, 312
    somatic disorders and, 496
Dependence, alcohol, 490
Depo-Provera, 468
Depressants, 494
Depression, 494–495
    bereavement and, 498
    cerebral, 356–357
    confusional states and, 342
    fatigue and, 2
    in memory loss, 312
    oral contraceptives and, 474
    somatic disorders and, 496
    suicidal patient and, 506
Dermatitis, 90
Dermatofibroma, 84
Dermatology, 84–95
Dermographism, 88
DES; see Diethylstilbestrol
Desbuquois' syndrome, 418
Desipramine, 494
Detrusor muscle, 486
Dexamethasone, 124, 322
Dexamethasone suppression test, 122, 494
Dextran, 514
Dextrose
    in hypothermia, 444
    in status epilepticus, 320–321
DHEA-S; see Dehydroepiandrosterone sulfate
Diabetes mellitus, 38, 102–103
    gestational, 102
    vaginal yeast infection and, 450
Dialysis, 37, 288, 289, 294–295
Diaphram as contraceptive device, 470
Diarrhea
    acute, 162–163
    chronic, 164–165
    enteral nutrition and, 544
    traveler's, 520
Diastolic murmur, 54–55
Diazepam
    nipple discharge and, 462
    in prostatodynia, 484
    in status epilepticus, 320
DIC; see Disseminated intravascular coagulation
Dichloralphenazone, 302, 303
Dicyclomine, 172
Diet
    in hyperkalemia, 288–289
    in hypokalemia, 286
    very low calorie, 10
Diethylstilbestrol, 470
Digitalis, 288, 289
Digoxin, 530
Dihydroergotamine, 302, 303
Diphenhydramine, 516
Dipyridamole-thallium testing, 48
Disc disease, 392
Disc herniation, 396
Discharge
    nipple, 462–463
    vaginal, 450–451
Disdiadochokinesia, 328

Disease
    Alzheimer's, 312, 344–347
    Cushing's, 124
    Erdheim's, 418
    Graves', 110
    Hodgkin's, 206–207
    Meniere's, 316–317
    Osgood-Schlatter, 402
    Paget's, 396, 426
    Parkinson's, 330–331
    Pick's, 344–347
    Refsum's, 334
    Reiter's, 388
    von Willebrand's, 196
Dislocation, glenohumeral, 394
Disseminated intravascular coagulation, 190–191
Disulfiram, 334
Diuretics
    in hyperkalemia, 288–289
    hypokalemia and, 286
    in hypomagnesemia, 290, 291
    in leukopenia, 188
    weakness and, 322
Diverticulitis, 458
Dizziness, 316–317
Donor for kidney transplantation, 296
Dopamine, 336
Doxorubicin, 322
Doxycycline
    in cervicitis, 452
    in dysuria or pyuria, 478
    in prostatitis, 484
Drowning, 446–449
Drugs
    abdominal pain and, 134
    adverse reactions to, 518–519
    in behavior changes, 342, 346
    in confusional states, 344
    depression and, 494
    diarrhea and, 164
    fatigue and, 2
    formulary of, 534–534
    in gastrointestinal bleeding, 156
    gynecomastia and, 130
    hirsutism and, 128
    hypercalcemia and, 106
    in hyperkinesia, 336
    in leukopenia, 188
    in lupus syndrome, 424
    in neuropathies, 334
    obesity and, 10
    seizures and, 318–319
    serum levels of, 530–531
    in sleep disturbances, 351
    study of, 532–533
    suicidal patient and, 506
    sweating and, 20
    in taste disturbances, 348–349
    transplantation and, 298
    in urticaria, 88
    weakness and, 322
Dry eye, 26
Dual diagnosis, 490
Duroziez' sign, 54
Dysesthesia, 332
Dysgeusia, 349
Dyspepsia, 134–135, 148–149
Dysphagia, 140–141
Dysphoria, 494
Dysplasia, 418
Dyspnea
    cardiac, 78–79
    pulmonary, 366–367
Dysthymic disorder, 494

Dystonia, 336
Dystrophy, muscular, 322
Dysuria, 460, 478–479

E

Ear, dizziness and, 316–317
Eating disorders, 4–5
Echocardiography, 74
Ectasia, 418
Ectopic pregnancy, 458
Ectopic urethral orifice, 486
Ectopy, ventricular, 62
Edema, 14–17
   in alcoholic, 490
   laryngeal, 360
   pulmonary, 70–71
EE; see Ethinyl estradiol
Effusion
   joint, 384
   pleural, 368–369
      asbestos and, 382
      dyspnea in, 366
EGD; see Esophagogastroduodenoscopy
Ehlers-Danlos syndrome, 418–421
Ejaculation
   premature, 12
   retrograde, 488
Ejection murmur, 52
Eldepryl; see Selegiline
Elderly
   anorexia in, 138
   gastrointestinal bleeding in, 156
   transfusions and, 204
Electrocoagulation, 158
Electroconvulsive therapy, 494, 500
Electroencephalography, 318, 319
Electromechanical dissociation, 76
Electromyography, 332, 392
Electrophoresis, 210–211
Electrophysiology, 332
Embolism
   foot pain in, 404
   pulmonary, 192–193, 508
   in pulseless extremity, 432
   in stroke, 310–311
Embolization of bronchial artery, 358–359
Emergency, 432–449
Emetine, 322
EMG; see Electromyography
Emotional disorders, 496–497
Encephalitis, 312
Encephalopathy
   toxic-metabolic, 342–343, 354
   Wernicke's, 312
End-stage renal disease; see Renal failure
Endocarditis, bacterial, 520
Endocervical scraping, 464
Endocervicitis, gonococcal, 452
Endocrine system
   disorders of, 96–131
      hyperglycemia in, 102
      in hyperhidrosis, 20
      multiple neoplasia in, 120
      obesity and, 10
   surgical risks and, 38
Endometrium, 454
Endoscopic retrograde cholangiopancreatography, 154
Endoscopy
   in belching, 146
   in biliary colic, 154
   in heartburn, 142
   in noncardial chest pain, 144
Endotoxin, 186

Enema, barium; see Barium enema
Enteral nutrition, 542–545
Enterobacteriaceae, 460
Enterococcus
   in pyuria, 478
   in urinary tract infection, 460
Enzymes
   asymptomatic increased, 176–177
   deficiencies of, 340
Eosinophils, 406
Ependymoma, 168
Epicondylitis, 390
Epididymis, 480
Epididymitis, 478, 480
Epilepsy, 312, 318–319
Epinephrine
   in anaphylaxis, 514–516
   cardiac arrest and, 76
   in laryngospasm, 360
   in leukocytosis, 186
   in snake bites, 442
Episcleritis, 22
ERCP; see Endoscopic retrograde cholangiopancreatography
Erdheim's disease, 418
Ergotamine, 302, 303, 410
Eructation, 146–147
Erythema in acute red eye, 24
Erythromycin, 479, 522
Erythropoietin, 184
Escherichia coli, 460, 478
Esophagitis, 364
Esophagogastroduodenoscopy, 140
Esophagus
   disorders of, 140, 144, 406
   foreign body in, 434–437
Estrogen
   amenorrhea and, 125
   in breast cancer, 212
   nipple discharge and, 462
   oral contraceptives and, 472–475
Estrogen receptor negative tumor, 216
Ethics
   enteral nutrition and, 542
   parenteral nutrition and, 536
Ethinyl estradiol, 472
Ethynodiol diacetate, 472
Etoposide, 218
Eustachian tube, 30
Exercise, muscle cramps in, 340
Exercise test
   symptom-limited, 82
   treadmill, 48
Exposure therapy, 492
Exposure to caustics, 438–439
Expressive psychotherapy, 498
Extrapyramidal syndromes, 344
Extremity, pulseless, 432–433
Exudate in pleural effusion, 368
Eye burns, 22

F

Factitious disorder, 496
Factors, blood, 194–197
Farr assay, 424
Fasciitis, eosinophilic, 406
Fatigue, 2–3
Fecal incontinence, 174–175
Femur fracture, 398
Fertility awareness methods, 470
Fetoproteins, 218
Fetus, 456
Fever, 220–221
   sweating in, 20

transfusions and, 204
Fibrillation
  atrial, 62
  ventricular, 76
Fibrin, 190, 194
Fibrinogen, 191, 194–197, 432
Fine needle aspiration biopsy
  in breast mass, 212
  in carcinoma, 218
  in lymphadenopathy, 214
Finkelstein's test, 400
Fistula, 486
Flatulence, 172–173
Fluids, intravenous, 158
Fluoroquinolone, 460
Fluoxetine, 492, 494
Follicle-stimulating hormone, 125
Foot pain, 404–405
Foreign body
  aspiration of, 360
  ingestion of, 434–437
Formulary, drug, 534–535
Formulas in enteral nutrition, 542
Fracture
  femoral, 398
  neck pain in, 392
  pelvic, 398
  of temporal bone, 32
  vertebral compression, 396
Freckles, 84
Free thyroxine index, 108
Fungal infection
  in chemotherapy-induced neutropenia, 220
  foot pain and, 404
  transplantation and, 298–299

G

Gait disturbances, 326–327
Galactorrhea, 462–463
Gallstones, 146, 154
Gammopathy, monoclonal, 210–211
Gardnerella vaginalis, 450
Gas, intestinal, 172
Gastric emptying study, 136
Gastric surgery, 10
Gastritis, 408
Gastroenterology, 132–181
Gastroesophageal reflux disease, 142, 144
Gastrointestinal system
  bleeding from, 156–159
  disorders of, 138
  flatulence and, 172
Gastrostomy, 544
Gemfibrosil, 322
Generalized anxiety disorder, 493
Genital herpes, 452
Genital tract cancer, 454
Gentamicin, 522, 528
  in chemotherapy-induced neutropenia, 220
  in urinary tract infection, 460
GERD; see Gastroesophageal reflux disease
Germ cell cancer, 218
Gestation, 456
Giant cell arteritis, 416–417
Glaucoma, 306
Glenohumeral dislocation, 394
Globe laceration, 22
Glucagon, 436
Glucocorticoids, 286, 288
Glucose
  blood, 100–103
  in coma, 354
  intolerance to, 102–103

in memory loss, 312
in status epilepticus, 320
Goiter, 109, 112–113, 116
Gonadotropin
  abdominal pain and, 458
  in carcinoma of unknown primary site, 218
  in gynecomastia, 131
  vaginal bleeding and, 454
Gonadotropin-releasing hormone agonists, 466
Gonadotropin-secreting tumors, 124
Gonococci in arthritis, 384
Gonorrhea, 456, 478
Gonozyme, 452
Gout, 384, 386, 414–415
Graft, coronary artery, 48, 50
Graham Steel murmur, 54
Gram-negative organisms, 478
Granulocytes, 202–203
Granuloma, 106, 374
Granulomatosis, 92
Granulomatous disease, 370
Graves' disease, 110
Grief, 498–499
Guaiac stool study, 170–171
Guanethidine, 322
Guillain-Barré syndrome, 334
Gum, nicotine, 504
Gynecology, 450–477
Gynecomastia, 130–131

H

Haemophilus influenzae, 378
Hager's criteria for salpingitis, 452
Hallucinations, 500, 506
Hand pain, 400–401
Hashimoto's thyroiditis, 109, 116
Head
  injury to
    anosmia and, 348–349
    coma and, 354
    memory loss and, 312
  lymphadenopathy and, 214
  neck cancer and, 218
Headache, 300–303
Hearing loss, 32–33
Heart, 66–67
  block of, 42–43, 46
  disease of
    chest pain in, 144
    creatine kinase and, 428
    prevention of, 82
    valvular, 68
  failure of, 68–69
    diffuse interstitial lung disease and, 376
    dyspnea in, 366
  valves of, 508
Heartburn, 142–143
Heberden's nodes, 386
Heimlich maneuver, 446
Hemarthrosis, 384
Hematemesis, 156
Hematocele, 480
Hematochezia, 156
Hematologic risk, 36
Hematuria, 272
Hemiparesis, 308–309
Hemoccult test, 170
Hemochromatosis, 178
Hemodialysis, 294–295
Hemoglobin
  in polycythemia, 184
  in transfusion therapy, 200

Hemolysis
  in anemia, 182
  in transfusion reaction, 204
Hemolytic anemia, 190
Hemophilia, 196
Hemoptysis, 358–359
Hemorrhage
  abdominal, 132
  in normal sclera, 22
  stigmata of recent, 158
  subarachnoid, 354
  transfusions in, 200
Henoch-Schönlein purpura, 92
Heparin
  in coagulation abnormalities, 194, 508
  in deep venous thrombosis, 193
  in disseminated intravascular coagulation, 190
  in myocardial infarction, 80
  pulseless extremity and, 432
  in stroke, 308, 311
  in transient ischemic attacks, 304
Hepatitis, 204
Hereditary disorders
  of hearing, 32
  weakness and, 322
Herniation of disc, 396
Heroin, 322
Herpes simplex
  in cervicitis, 452
  in urethritis, 479
  vaginal discharge and, 450
Hilum, 370
Hip pain, 398–399
Hirsutism, 128–129
Histamine receptor agonist, 148
Histamine receptor antagonist, 142
Histamine receptor blocker, 442
Histoplasmosis, 374
Hodgkin's disease, 206–207
Homan sign, 192
Homocystinuria, 418
Hormones
  in breast cancer, 212, 216
  in pituitary tumors, 124
  postcoital, 470
  in thyroid disease, 109
Human chorionic gonadotropin, 454, 458
Hybritech assay, 482
Hydralazine, 334
Hydrocele, 480
Hydrocephalus, 310–311
Hydrofluoric acid, 438
Hydroxychloroquine, 322
Hydroxyurea, 184–185, 208
Hyoscyamine, 484
Hyperaldosteronism, 290
Hyperamylasemia, 180
Hypercalcemia, 106–107
Hyperglycemia, 102–103, 540
Hyperhidrosis, 20
Hyperkalemia, 288–289
Hyperkinesia, 336–339
Hyperlipidemia, 96–99
Hypermobility of joints, 418–421
Hypernatremia, 284–285
Hyperparathyroidism, 104, 106
Hyperpigmentation, 84
Hyperprolactinemia, 125–126
Hypersensitivity vasculitis, 92
Hypersomnia, 351
Hypersplenism, 182
Hypertension, 56–59
  heart failure and, 68
  portal, 152
  pulmonary, 72

Hyperthyroidism, 38, 110–111, 116
Hypertrophic cardiomyopathy, 52
Hyperuricemia, 414–415
Hyperventilation, 316–317
Hypoalbuminemia, 104
Hypocalcemia, 104–105
Hypochondriasis, 496–497
Hypoglycemia, 100–101, 318–319, 500
Hypokalemia, 286–287
Hypomagnesemia, 104, 290–291
Hyponatremia, 282–283
Hypoparathyroidism, 104
Hypophosphatemia, 292–293
Hypotension, 60–61
Hypothermia, 444–449
Hypothyroidism, 38, 109, 112

I

Ibuprofen, 414
Ifosfamide, 218
Imipramine, 492
Immunoglobulins, elevated, 210–211
Immunologic defect, 220
Immunosuppression, 298–299, 334
Impotence, 12
Incontinence
  fecal, 174–175
  urinary, 486–487
Infarction, myocardial, 80–81
Infection
  abdominal pain and, 458
  diarrhea and, 164
  fungal, 220, 404
  headache and, 300–301
  in leukopenia, 188
  neutropenia and, 220
  in peripheral neuropathy, 334
  postoperative wound, 522
  in stroke, 310–311
  sweating and, 20
  from transfusions, 204
  in transplant patient, 298–299
  upper respiratory, 364
  urinary tract, 460–461, 478, 482, 484
  viral, 376
Infertility, 476–477, 488–489
Infiltrates in lungs, 378–379
Inflammation
  arthropathy and, 398
  of bowel, 388
  foot pain and, 404
  of knee, 402
  low back pain in, 396
  in polyarthritis, 386
  in prostatitis, 484–485
Influenza, 520
Ingestion
  of caustics, 438–439
  of foreign body, 434–437
Inguinal node, 214, 218
INH; see Isoniazid
Insecticides, 342, 346
Insomnia, 350–353
Insulin
  in hyperkalemia, 288, 289
  insufficient, 102–103
  seizures and, 318–319
Insulinoma, 100
Intercourse, painful, 12
Interstitium
  asbestos and, 382
  diffuse disease of, 376–377
Intervertebral disc
  herniation of, 396

neck pain and, 392
Intestines, bacterial infections of, 164
Intrauterine devices, 468–471
Intubation, endotracheal, 362
Iodine-125 with fibrinogen, 192
Iodine in goiter, 112
IPG; see Plethysmography
Iron, 178–179
Ischemia, 304–305
  mesenteric, 134
  in stroke, 308–311
Isoenzyme tests, 428
Isometheptene, 302, 303
Isoniazid, 380, 424
IUDs; see Intrauterine devices

J

Jaundice, 150–151, 490
Jejunostomy, 544
Jod-Basedow hypothyroidism, 112
Joints
  degeneration of, 422
  hypermobility of, 418–421
Jugular venous pressure, 14–17

K

Kallmann's syndrome, 348–349
Kaposi's sarcoma, 378
Keratoconjunctivitis sicca, 408–409
Keratoses, seborrheic, 84
Kernig's sign, 354
Kidney
  failure of; see Renal failure
  hypocalcemia and, 104
  hypokalemia and, 286
  serum amylase in, 180
  transplantation of, 296–299
Kinase, creatine, 428–429
Klinefelter's syndrome, 130
Knee
  bursitis in, 390
  pain in, 402–403
Korsakoff syndrome, 312
Kyphoscoliosis, 72

L

L-thyroxine
  in goiter, 112
  in hypothyroidism, 109
  in thyroid nodule, 114
Labyrinthitis, 316–317
Laceration of globe, 22
Lactate dehydrogenase, 368
Lactation, 470
Laparoscopy, 458
Larsen's syndrome, 418
Laryngoscopy, 360, 434–437
Laryngospasm, 360
Laxatives, 286
LDH; see Lactate dehydrogenase
Lead, 346
Leg ulcer, 86–87
Lentigo, 84
LES; see Lower esophageal sphincter pressure
Leukapheresis, 202
Leukemia, 208–209
Leukocyte filters, 200
Leukocytosis, 186–187
Leukodystrophy, 334
Leukopenia, 188–189
Levodopa

in confusional states, 344
  in hyperkinesia, 336
  in Parkinson's disease, 330
Levonorgestrel, 472
Lidocaine
  cardiac arrest and, 77
  in myocardial infarction, 80
  in status epilepticus, 320
Light therapy, 494
Lipid disorders, 96–99
Lithium, 494, 500
Livedo reticularis, 94–95
Liver
  biopsy of, 176
  chronic dysfunction of, 38
  enteral nutrition and, 542
  jaundice tests and, 150
  stroke and, 310–311
Loperamide, 544
Lorazepam, 320
Lovastatin, 322
Lower esophageal sphincter pressure, 140
Lumbar puncture, 320
Lumbar spine, 398
Lumpectomy, 212
Lung
  abscess of, 364
  asbestos and, 382–383
  diffuse interstitial disease of, 376–377
  infiltrates in, 378–379
  nodules of, 372–375
Lupus anticoagulant, 194
Lupus erythematosus, systemic, 386
Lupus syndrome, drug-induced, 424
Luteinizing hormone, 125
Lymph nodes
  biopsy of, 206, 210
  in breast cancer, 216
  carcinoma of unknown primary site and, 218
  inguinal, 214
Lymphadenopathy, 214–215
Lymphoma
  non-Hodgkins, 378
  pulmonary, 374
Lymphopenia, 188

M

Macroglobulinemia, Waldenström's, 210–211
Magnesium
  hypocalcemia and, 104
  in hypomagnesemia, 290–291
  in status epilepticus, 320–321
Magnet tube, 436
Magnetic resonance imaging
  in temporomandibular pain, 422
  in transient ischemic attacks, 304–305
Malformation, arteriovenous, 374
Malignancy
  after transplantation, 298
  hypercalcemia and, 106
  mediastinal adenopathy in, 370
  in peripheral neuropathy, 334
  sweating in, 20
Malingering, 496
Mammography, 212
  in carcinoma of unknown primary site, 218
  in nipple discharge, 462
Manganese, 346
Mania, 500
Mannerisms, 336
Manometry, 148, 174
Marfan's syndrome, 418–421
Marker transit study of intestines, 166

Marrow, bone, 208
Mass
    adrenal gland, 120–121
    breast, 212–213
    lung, 382
    mediastinal, 206
    red blood cell, 184
    scrotal, 480–481
Mastectomy, 212
Mastication, 422
Mastodynia, 466
Mechlorethamine, 206
Media nerve dysfunction, 400
Mediastinal mass, 206
Mediastinoscopy, 372
Mediastinum, 370–371
Melanoma, 84
Melasma, 84
Melena, 156
Melphalan, 210
Memory loss, 312–315
Meniere's disease, 316–317
Meningitis, 354
Menkes' syndrome, 420
Menstruation, 466–467
Mercury, 346
Mesentery, 134
Mestranol, 472
Metabolism
    abdominal pain and, 134
    confusional states and, 342
    disorders of, 96–131
    in status epilepticus, 320–321
Metals, heavy
    in behavior changes, 346
    in neuropathies, 334
    as toxins, 342
Metaproterenol, 516
Metastasis, inguinal node, 218
Methotrexate, 458
Methylprednisolone, 516
Methysergide, 302, 303
Metoclopramide, 544
Metronidazole, 450, 479
Mezlocillin, 220
Miconazole, 450
Migraine, 300–303, 474
Milk in hypophosphatemia, 292
Mineralocorticoids, 286, 288, 289
Minocycline, 484
Mobitz I or II block, 42–43
Mole, 84, 456
Mongolian spot, 84
Monitoring of parenteral nutrition, 540
Monoclonal gammopathy, 210–211
Mononeuropathy, 332
Morphea, 406
Morton's neuroma, 404
Motility studies, anorectal, 166
Motor neuron, 322–325
Multidisciplinary pain center, 18
Multiple sclerosis, 316–317
Murmur, 52–54
Muscle
    creatine kinase and, 428
    of mastication, 422
    pain and soreness of, 340–341, 416–417
    weakness of, 322
Musculoskeletal disease, 428
Mycobacterium tuberculosis, 378
Mycoplasma, 479, 484
Myelitis, 322–325
Myelogenous leukemia, 208–209
Myeloma

multiple, 210
    in peripheral neuropathy, 334
Myelopathy, 322–325
Myocardial infarction, 50, 60, 80–83
Myopathy, 416–417, 428

N

Naloxone
    in coma, 354
    in hypothermia, 444
NAP; see Neutrophil alkaline phosphatase
Narcan; see Naloxone
Nasoenteric tube, 544
Nasogastric tube, 158, 448
Nausea, 136–137
Near-drowning, 446–449
Neck
    cancer of, 218
    pain in, 392–393, 394
Necrosis, avascular, 384, 398
Neisseria gonorrhoeae, 450, 452
Neisseria meningitidis, 479
Neomycin, 522
Neoplasia
    cervical, 452
    multiple endocrine, 120
Neoplasm
    b-cell, 210
    of bladder, 482
    knee pain in, 402
    testicular, 480
Nephrotoxicity, 528
Nerve root, 396
Netilmicin, 528
Neuritis, optic, 306
Neuroleptics, 344
Neurologic deficit, 304–305
Neurologic disease, 428
Neuroma, Morton's, 404
Neuron, 322
Neuronitis, vestibular, 316–317
Neuropathy
    optic, 306
    peripheral, 322–324, 332–335, 490
Neutra-Phos, 292
Neutropenia, 188–189
    fever and, 220–221
    transfusions and, 202
Neutrophil alkaline phosphatase, 208
Neutrophilia, 186–187
Nevus of Ota, 84
Nicotine
    Raynaud's phenomenon and, 410
    transdermal patches and, 504, 505
Nifedipine, 80
NIH Early Breast Cancer Concensus Development Conference, 216
Nipple discharge, 462–463
Nitrofurantoin
    in neuropathies, 334
    in prostatis, 484
    in urinary tract infection, 460
Nitroglycerin, 80
Nocardia, 298–299
Nodule
    pulmonary, 372–375
    Schmorl's, 412
Nonoxynol 9, 470
Nonsteroidal anti-inflammatory drugs
    asthma from, 362
    in gout, 414
    in hyperkalemia, 288–289
    in migraine, 302, 303
Norethindrone, 472

Norethynodrel, 472
Norfloxacin, 460
Norgestimate, 472
Norgestrel, 472
Norplant, 454, 468
Nortriptyline, 494
Nutrition
    enteral, 542–545
    parenteral, 536–541

O

Obesity, 10–11
Obsessions, 492
Obstruction
    airway, 366
    of bile duct, 154
    bladder outlet, 482, 486
    gastrointestinal, 434–437
    pulmonary, 376
Odontoid fracture, 392
Oncovin, 206
Opiates, 462
Orchitis, 478
Organic brain syndrome, 342–343
Organophosphates, 334, 346
Orgasmic dysfunction, 12
Ortho-Novum 777, 472
Osgood-Schlatter disease, 402
Osteoarthritis, 384, 386
Osteomalacia, 412, 426
Osteomyelitis, 396
Osteopenia, 412–413
Osteoporosis, 412
Ota's nevus, 84
Ovary
    cancer of, 218
    cysts of, 458
    polycystic disease of, 128
Oxygen tension, 72
Oxyhemoglobin dissociation curve, 184

P

Paget's disease, 396, 426
Pain
    abdominal, 132–135, 458–459
    acute, 18
    anorectal, 168–169
    chest, 144–145
    chronic, 18–19
    diffuse muscle, 416–417
    foot, 404–405
    hip, 398–399
    knee, 402–403
    low back, 396–397
    malignant, 18
    myofascial, 422
    neck, 392–393
    postprandial, 134
    sensitivity to, 432
    shoulder, 394–395
    soft tissue, 390–391
    temporomandibular, 422–423
    in thyroid, 116–117
    visceral, 132–133
Palpitations, 62–63
Palsy, Bell's, 332
Pancreatitis, 180, 458
Pancytopenia, 188
Panic, 492, 506
Pap smear, 464–465
Papillomavirus, 454, 464
    in cervicitis, 452

in urethritis, 479
    vaginal discharge and, 450
Paraldehyde, 320
Paralysis, 432
Paranoia, 500
Parasites, 374
Parenteral nutrition, 536–541
Paresthesia, 332, 432
Parkinson's disease, 330–331
Parosmia, 349
Paroxysmal supraventricular tachycardia, 44
Partial thromboplastin time, 190, 192, 194–197
Pasteurella multocida, 440
Patella, 402
PCWP; *see* Pulmonary capillary wedge pressure
PEEP; *see* Positive end-expiratory pressure
Pelvis
    examination of, 168
    fracture of, 398
    inflammatory disease of, 452
Penicillin
    aminoglycoside antibiotics and, 528
    anaphylaxis and, 526
    antimicrobial prophylaxis and, 522
    in bite wounds, 440
    in cervicitis, 452
    in chemotherapy-induced neutropenia, 220
    in drug-induced lupus syndrome, 424
    in gonococcal infection, 478
    hypersensitivity to, 526
    in leukopenia, 188
    neutropenia and, 220
    in prostatis, 484
Pentazocine, 322
Pentobarbital, 320
Percutaneous coronary angioplasty, 48
Perforation, gastrointestinal, 434–437
Pergolide, 330
Perioperative evaluation, 34–39
Peritonitis, 152
Phalen's sign, 400
Pharmacology, 508–545
Phenelzine, 492, 494
Phenobarbital, 320
Phenomenon, Raynaud's, 406, 408, 410–411
Phenothiazines, 188, 462
Phenytoin
    in gait disturbances, 326
    serum drug levels of, 530
    in status epilepticus, 320
Pheochromocytoma, 58, 120
Phlebotomy, 184
Phobia, 492
Phosphate
    in carcinoma of unknown primary site, 218
    hypocalcemia and, 104
    in hypophosphatemia, 292–293
Phospho-Soda, 292
Photocoagulation, 158
Pick's disease, 344–347
Pigmented lesions, 84–85
Pituitary gland adenoma, 122, 124–125, 462
Plasma
    cortisol level of, 100
    fibrin degradation in, 190
    fresh frozen, 196
Plasma erythropoietin, 184
Plasmacytoma, 210
Plasmapheresis, 196, 334
Platelets, 198–199
    in deep venous thrombosis, 192
    in disseminated intravascular coagulation, 190
    polycythemia and, 184
    transfusion of, 198–199

Plethysmography, 14–17, 192
Pleura
    effusion of, 366, 368–369
    lesions of, 382
Pneumoconioses, 376
Pneumocystis carinii, 298–299
    in AIDS, 378
    antimicrobial prophylaxis in, 520
Pneumonia
    foreign body aspiration in, 434–437
    in pleural effusion, 368
    Pneumocystis carinii, 520
    wheezing in, 362
Pneumonitis, 378
Pneumothorax, 60, 434, 436
Poisoning, snake venom, 442–443
Polycystic ovarian disease, 128
Polycythemia, 90, 184–185
Polymyalgia rheumatica, 416–417
Polymyositis, 428
Polyp, colon, 170
Polysomnography, 494
Porphyria, 334
Portal system, 152
Positive end-expiratory pressure, 448
Post-traumatic stress disorder, 492
Postnasal drip, 364
Potassium
    in hyperkalemia, 288–289
    in hypokalemia, 286–287
    in hypophosphatemia, 292
Prednisone
    in anaphylaxis, 516
    in giant cell arteritis, 416
    in Hodgkin's disease, 206
    in leukemia, 208
Pregnancy
    ectopic, 458
    molar, 456
    vaginal bleeding in, 456–457
Premature contractions, atrial, 62
Premature ejaculation, 12
Premature infant transfusion, 200
Premenstrual syndrome, 466–467
Prenif cap, 470
Pressure sensitivity, 432
Probe, transvaginal, 458
Probenecid, 414
Procainamide, 424, 530
Procaine penicillin G, 452
Procarbazine, 206
Proctalgia fugax, 168
Proctoscopy, 174
Progestasett, 468
Progesterone, 466
Progesterone antagonist, 470
Progestin, 472–475
Progestin challenge test, 126
Prolactin, 462
Prolactinoma, 124
Prophylaxis, 520–523
Prostate
    adenocarcinoma of, 482–483
    benign hypertrophy of, 478
    carcinoma of, 484
Prostate-specific antigen, 218, 482
Prostatitis, 478, 484–485
Prostatodynia, 484
Protamine
    anaphylaxis and, 514
    in coagulation abnormalities, 194
Protamine paracoagulation phenomenon test, 191
Protein electrophoresis, 210–211
Protein requirements for parenteral nutrition, 540

Proteus, 478
Prothrombin time, 510
    assays of, 512
    in coagulation abnormalities, 196
    in deep venous thrombosis, 192
    in disseminated intravascular coagulation, 190
Providencia, 478
Provocative testing in noncardial chest pain, 144
Pruritus, 90–91, 450
PSA; *see* Prostate-specific antigen
Pseudogout, 384, 386
Pseudohypoparathyroidism, 104
Pseudomonas aeruginosa, 528
Psoriasis, 386, 388
Psychosis, 500–501
    confusional states and, 342
    somatic disorder and, 496
Psychotherapy, expressive, 498
Psychotic depression, 500
PT; *see* Prothrombin time
PTCA; *see* Percutaneous coronary angioplasty
Pulmonary artery enlargement, 66
Pulmonary capillary wedge pressure, 60
Pulmonary edema, 70–71
Pulmonary embolism, 192, 508
Pulmonary hypertension, 72
Pulse, extremity, 432–433
Purpura, 92–93
Pyelography, 482
Pyelonephritis, 478
    after transplantation, 298–299
    in urinary tract infection, 460
Pylorus, 436
Pyuria, 478–479

Q

QRS complex, 44–47
Quincke's sign, 54
Quinidine, 424, 530
Quinine sulfate, 340

R

R-R interval, 46
Radial nerve dysfunction, 400
Radiation therapy
    in breast cancer, 216
    in breast mass, 212
    in Hodgkin's disease, 206
    plasmacytoma and, 210
Radioactive iodine uptake, 108
Radiography
    chest, 364, 378
    of neck, 392
    in shoulder pain, 394
    of small bowel, 172
    in temporomandibular pain, 422
Radioimmunoassay, Farr, 424
Radionuclides, 136
Radiopaque markers, 166
Random-donor unit, 198
Rash, maculopapular, 526
Raynaud's phenomenon, 406, 408, 410–411
Raynaud's syndrome, 400
RDP; *see* Random-donor unit
Rectosigmoidoscopy, 168
Rectum
    bleeding from, 160–161
    disorders of, 166
    manometry of, 174
Red blood cells, 200–201
    in anemia, 182
    in diarrhea, 162

in disseminated intravascular coagulation, 190
   polycythemia and, 184
   technetium-labeled, 159
   transfusion of, 200–201
Red eye, 22–27
Reflex incontinence, 486
Reflexes, deep tendon, 326
Reflux
   esophageal, 364
   gastroesophageal, 142, 144
Refsum's disease, 334
Regurgitation, 136
   aortic, 54
   mitral, 52, 66
   pulmonic, 54
Rehabilitation, cardiac, 82–83
Reiter's disease, 388
Reiter's syndrome, 386
Rejection of transplant, 298–299
Renal failure
   acute, 37
   enteral nutrition and, 542
   in stroke, 310–311
   transplantation and, 296–297
Renovascular disease, 58
Replacement therapy, hormone, 109, 124
Reserpine, 462
Respiratory distress syndrome, 376
Respiratory tract infection, 364
Resuscitation in near-drowning, 446–449
Rheumatism, nonarticular, 390
Rheumatoid arthritis, 386, 400
Rheumatoid factor, 408
Rheumatology, 384–429
Rhinitis, 28–29
Rhinophyma, 490
Rinne's test, 32
Rupture of tendon, 400

S

Sacrum, 168
Saline in hypomagnesemia, 290
Salpingitis, 452
Salt substitutes, 288–289
Sarcoidosis, 106
Sarcoma, Kaposi's, 378
Scanning, computerized tomography; see Computerized
   tomography
Scapula, 394
Schirmer test, 408
Schizophrenia, 500
Schmorl's nodules, 412
Sciatica, 396
Sclerodactyly, 406
Scleroderma, 406–407
Sclerosis, 158, 159, 322
Scrotum, 480–481
Sedatives
   in gait disturbances, 326
   in incontinence, 486
   in sleep disturbances, 350
Seizures, 318–321, 342
Selegiline, 330, 344
Semen specimen, 488
Sepsis, catheter, 536
Serology in lymphadenopathy, 214
Sexual dysfunction, 12–13
Sexually transmitted diseases, 464
   abnormal vaginal bleeding in, 454
   acute red eye in, 24
   cervicitis in, 452
   dysuria or pyuria and, 478
Shoulder pain, 394–395

Siderosis, 178
Sigmoidoscopy, 160
   constipation and, 166
   diarrhea and, 162
   in flatulence, 172
   in gastrointestinal bleeding, 159
   guaiac-positive stools in, 170
Sign
   Babinski, 326
   Brudzinski's, 354
   button, 84
   Chvostek's, 104
   double density, 66
   Duroziez', 54
   Homan, 192
   Kernig's, 354
   Phalen, 400
   Quincke's, 54
   Tinel, 400
   Trousseau's, 104
Sinemet, 330
Single-donor apheresis unit, 198
Sinus node disease, 42–43
Sinusitis, 28, 300–301
Sjögren's syndrome, 26, 408–409
Skin test
   beta-lactam antibiotics and, 526
   tuberculin, 380–381
Sleep
   deprivation of, 318–319
   disturbances of, 350–353
Smear
   pap, 464–465
   urethral, 478
Smell disturbances, 348–349
Smoking cessation, 502–505
Snake venom, 442–443
Sodium bicarbonate, 288, 289
Sodium phosphate, 292
Sodium polystyrene sulfonate, 288, 289
Soft tissue pain, 390–391
Solvents, 334, 346
Somatic disorders, 496–497
Sonography, 456, 458
Spectinomycin, 478
Spermatogenesis, 488
Spermicides, 470
Sphincter of Oddi, 154
Spinal cord
   anorectal pain and, 168
   lesions of, 322–325
Spine
   cervical, 392
   stenosis of, 396
Spleen
   in anemia, 182
   in polycythemia, 184
Splenomegaly, 188
Spondylitis, ankylosing, 386, 388
Spondyloarthropathy, 396
Sprain, 404
Squamous cell carcinoma, 218
Staphylococcus, 384, 460, 478
Status epilepticus, 320–321, 354
STDs; see Sexually transmitted diseases
Stenosis
   mitral, 54, 66
   spinal, 396
   tracheal, 360
   tricuspid, 54
Steroids
   in leukopenia, 188
   neutropenia and, 220
   in peripheral neuropathy, 332, 334

Steroids—cont'd
  weakness and, 322
Stickler's syndrome, 418
Stiffness of muscle, 416–417
Stimulants, 318–319
STK; see Streptokinase
Stool culture, 162, 170–171
Streptococcus pneumoniae, 378
Streptokinase, 80, 508
Stress disorder, post-traumatic, 492
Stress incontinence, 486
Stress testing, 48, 80
Stressors, 492
Stricture, urethral, 482
Stridor, 360–361
Stroke, 308–311
Substance abuse
  depression and, 494
  grief and, 498
Succinylcholine, 288, 289
Suicidal patient, 500, 506–507
Sulfonamides
  anaphylaxis and, 514
  in drug-induced lupus syndrome, 424
  in leukopenia, 188
Sulfur colloid in abdominal scanning, 159
Supraventricular arrhythmia, 62
Supraventricular tachycardia, 44, 46
Suramin, 334
Swallowing, 140–141
Swan-Ganz catheterization, 60
Sweating, 20–21
Sympathetic nervous system, 20
Syncope, 64–65, 316–317
Syndrome
  Churg-Strauss, 92
  Cushing's, 59, 120, 122–123
  Desbuquois', 418
  Ehlers-Danlos, 418–421
  Guillain-Barré, 334
  Kallmann's, 348–349
  Klinefelter's, 130
  Larsen's, 418
  Marfan's, 418–421
  Menkes', 420
  Raynaud's, 400
  Reiter's, 386
  Sjögren's, 408–409
  Stickler's, 418
  Trousseau's, 190
  Wernicke-Korsakoff, 312, 342
Synovitis, 384
Syphilis, 452

T

Tachycardia, 44–46, 62
Tamoxifen, 216
Tarsal tunnel, 404
Taste disturbances, 348–349
Technetium 99m pertechnetate, 108
Telangiectasia, 406
Temperature sensitivity, 432
Temporal artery biopsy, 416
Temporal bone fracture, 32
Temporomandibular joint pain, 422–423
Tendinitis, 390
Tendon rupture, 400
Tenosynovitis, 400
Tentorium lesion, 354
Testis
  cancer of, 218
  infertility and, 488
  mass in, 480

measurement of, 130
Testosterone, 128, 130
Tetanus, 440
Tetany, 104
Tetracycline, 452, 478–479
Thallium, 334, 346
Thallium imaging, 48
Theophylline, 516, 530
Thiamine
  in hypothermia, 444
  memory loss and, 312
  in status epilepticus, 320–321
Thoracentesis in pleural effusion, 368
Thoracotomy
  asbestos lung disease and, 383
  mediastinal adenopathy and, 371
  pleural effusion and, 369
  pulmonary nodule and, 372
Thrombectomy, 433
Thrombin time, 191
Thrombocytopenia, 188, 198
Thromboembolism, 36, 508, 512
Thrombolysis in pulseless extremity, 432
Thrombolytics, 80, 308
Thromboplastin time, partial, 194–197, 508–510
Thrombosis
  deep venous, 192–193, 508
  in pulseless extremity, 432
  in stroke, 310–311
Thyroid
  antimicrosomal antibodies and, 108
  cancer of, 114
  disease of, 38
  function tests of, 108, 118–119
  nodule of, 114–115
  painful, 116–117
  replacement therapy for, 109
Thyroid-stimulating hormone, 112, 462
Thyroid-stimulating hormone test, 108
Thyroiditis, 110, 116
Thyrotropin releasing hormone stimulation test, 494
Thyroxine
  free, 108
  in goiter, 112
  in hypothyroidism, 109
  in thyroid nodule, 114
TIAs; see Transient ischemic attacks
Ticlopidine hydrochloride, 304
Tics, 336
Tinel's sign, 400
Tinnitus, 30–31
Tissue plasminogen activator, 80
Tobramycin, 528
Toenail, ingrown, 404
Torulopsis, 450
Total parenteral nutrition, 536–541
Touch sensitivity, 432
Toxins, 334, 344
TPN; see Total parenteral nutrition
Tranquilizers
  in gait disturbances, 326
  in headache, 302, 303
Transaminases, 176–177
Transdermal patch, nicotine, 504, 505
Transfusion therapy, 198–205
Transient global amnesia, 312
Transient ischemic attacks, 304–305
Transplantation
  bone marrow, 208
  fever after, 298–299
  patient selection for, 296–297
Transvaginal probe, 458
Tranylcypromine, 494
Trauma to head, 348–349, 354

Trazodone, 494
Treadmill test, 48
Tremor, 328–330
Tri-Levelen, 472
Tri-Norinyl, 472
Triamterene, 289
Trichomonas vaginalis, 450, 479
Trichomoniasis, 484
Tricyclic antidepressants, 462, 494
Triglycerides, 96–99
Triiodothyronine, 108
Trimethoprim and sulfamethoxazole, 460
Triphasil, 472
Trochanter, 390, 398
Trousseau's sign, 104
Trousseau's syndrome, 190
TSH; *see* Thyroid stimulating hormone
Tubal ligation, 468
Tube feeding, 542
Tuberculin skin test, 380–381
Tuberculosis
    AIDS and, 378
    antimicrobial prophylaxis and, 520
    pulmonary nodules in, 374
    skin test for, 380–381
Tumor
    anosmia and, 348–349
    endobronchial, 364
    estrogen receptor negative, 216
    markers for, 218
    of pituitary gland, 122, 124–125

U

Ulcer
    cervical, 452
    corneal, 22
    leg, 86–87
Ulnar nerve dysfunction, 400
Ultrasonography
    abdominal pain and, 458
    in biliary colic, 154
    in deep venous thrombosis, 192
    in transient ischemic attacks, 304
    visual loss and, 306
Uncinate fits, 348
Ureaplasma, 478–479
Urethral smear, 478
Urethral stricture, 482
Urethritis, 478
Uric acid, 208, 414
Urinary tract infection
    after transplantation, 298–299
    in men, 478
    prostate enlargement and, 482
    prostatitis in, 484
    in women, 460–461
Urine
    human chorionic gonadotropin and, 454
    hypokalemia and, 286
    incontinence of, 486–487
Urokinase, 432, 508
Urology, 478–489
Urticaria, 88–89
Uterine adenocarcinoma, 454

V

Vaccine in leukocytosis, 186
Vagina
    abnormal bleeding from, 454–457
    discharge from, 450–451

Vaginitis, 450–451
Valsalva maneuver, 52
Vancomycin, 220, 522
Varicocele, 480
Vascular disease, 376
Vasculitis
    in keratoconjunctivitis, 408
    in peripheral neuropathy, 334
    septic, 92
    wheezing in, 362
Vasectomy, 468
Venom, 186, 442–443
Venous insufficiency, 86
Venous thrombosis, 192–193
Ventricle, right
    in cor pulmonale, 72
    enlargement of, 66, 72
    failure of, 74–75
Ventricular fibrillation, 76
Vertebral neck pain, 392
Vertigo, 316–317
Vestibular disorders, 316–317
Vinblastine, 206
Vincristine, 208, 334
Virilization, 120, 128
Virus
    in anosmia, 348–349
    in diffuse interstitial lung disease, 376
Vision loss, 306–307
Vitamin B$_6$, 466
Vitamin D, 104, 412
Vitamins
    in neuropathies, 334
    in status epilepticus, 320
Vomiting, 136–137
von Willebrand's disease, 196
Vulvovaginitis, 450–451

W

Waldenström's macroglobulinemia, 210–211
Warfarin, 432, 510, 512
Weakness, 2, 322–325
Weber's test, 32
Weight loss, 6–9
Wernicke-Korsakoff syndrome, 312, 342, 346
Wheezing, 362–363
White blood cells
    in chronic myelogenous leukemia, 208
    in diarrhea, 162
    in leukocytosis, 186
    in leukopenia, 188
    polycythemia and, 184
Whole blood in transfusion, 198
Wolff-Chaikoff effect, 112
Wounds, bite, 440–441
Wrist pain, 400–401

X

Xanthomonas, 528
Xenography, 192
Xerosis, 90
Xerostomia, 408

Y

Yeast infection, 450

Z

Zidovudine, 322